# SURGERY OF THE THYROID AND PARATHYROID GLANDS

# SURGERY OF THE THYROID AND PARATHYROID GLANDS

THIRD EDITION

**BLAKE CADY, M.D.**

*Chief of Surgical Oncology*
*New England Deaconess Hospital*
*Associate Professor of Surgery*
*Harvard Medical School*
*Boston, Massachusetts*

**RICARDO L. ROSSI, M.D.**

*Chairman*
*Department of General Surgery*
*Lahey Clinic Medical Center*
*Burlington, Massachusetts*
*Assistant Clinical Professor of Surgery*
*Harvard Medical School*
*Boston, Massachusetts*

**1991**

W.B. SAUNDERS COMPANY

*Harcourt Brace Jovanovich, Inc.*

Philadelphia ▪ London ▪ Toronto ▪ Montreal ▪ Sydney ▪ Tokyo

**W. B. SAUNDERS COMPANY**
Harcourt Brace Jovanovich, Inc.

The Curtis Center
Independence Square West
Philadelphia, PA 19106

**Library of Congress Cataloging-in-Publication Data**

Surgery of the thyroid and parathyroid glands.—3rd ed. / [edited by] Blake Cady, Ricardo L. Rossi.

p. cm.

ISBN 0-7216-3462-1

1. Thyroid gland—Surgery. 2. Parathyroid glands—Surgery. I. Cady, Blake. II. Rossi, Ricardo L.

[DNLM: 1. Parathyroid Glands—surgery. 2. Thyroid Glands—surgery. WK 280 S961]

RD599.5.T46S93 1991
617.5′39—dc20

DNLM/DLC
for Library of Congress 90-8766
CIP

*Editor:* Edward H. Wickland, Jr.

*Designer:* Joan Sinclair

*Production Manager:* Frank Polizzano

*Illustration Coordinator:* Matt Andrews

*Indexer:* Helene Taylor

SURGERY OF THE THYROID AND PARATHYROID GLANDS ISBN 0-7216-3462-1



Printed in the United States of America.

Last digit is the print number: 9 8 7 6 5 4 3 2 1

*To Cornelius E. Sedgwick, M.D., master surgeon*
*Our mentor and friend*

# CONTRIBUTORS

**CHARLES F. ANDREWS, M.D.**

Active Staff, Department of Radiation Oncology, The Allentown Hospital-Lehigh Valley Hospital Center, Allentown, Pennsylvania

*External Beam Radiotherapy in Carcinoma of Thyroid Gland*

**JOSEPH N. ATTIE, M.D.**

Clinical Associate Professor of Surgery, Albert Einstein School of Medicine; Clinical Associate Professor of Surgery, New York University School of Medicine; Director, Head and Neck Surgery, Long Island Jewish Medical Center, New Hyde Park, and North Shore University Hospital, Manhasset, New York

*Commentary: Surgical Complications and Their Management*

**MELVIN A. BLOCK, M.D., Ph.D.**

Clinical Professor of Surgery, University of California San Diego School of Medicine; Department of Surgery, Scripps Clinic Medical Group, Inc.; Active Staff, Green Hospital of Scripps Clinic, La Jolla, California

*Familial Hyperparathyroidism and Hyperparathyroidism Associated with Multiple Endocrine Neoplasia Syndromes*

**BLAKE CADY, M.D.**

Associate Professor of Surgery, Harvard Medical School; Chief of Surgical Oncology and Member, Surgical Staff, New England Deaconess Hospital, Boston, Massachusetts

*History of Thyroid and Parathyroid Surgery; Embryology and Development Abnormalities; Surgical Anatomy; Commentary: Use of Needle Biopsy Data in Diagnosis and Management of Thyroid Nodules; Differentiated Carcinoma of Thyroid Gland; Commentary: Medullary Thyroid Carcinoma; Undifferentiated Carcinoma and Lymphoma of Thyroid Gland; Surgery of Thyroid Gland; Surgery of Parathyroid Glands; Surgical Complications and Their Management*

**ORLO H. CLARK, M.D.**

Professor of Surgery, University of California San Francisco School of Medicine; Staff Surgeon, Veterans Administration Medical Center, and Consulting Surgeon, Letterman General Hospital, San Francisco, California

*Commentary: Surgery of Thyroid Gland*

**EUGENE P. CLERKIN, M.D.**

Chairman, Department of Medicine, Section of Endocrinology, Lahey Clinic Medical Center, Burlington; Assistant Clinical Professor, Harvard Medical School, Boston, Massachusetts

*Hyperparathyroidism*

**STEVEN DE JONG, M.D.**

Assistant Professor of Surgery, Loyola University Stritch School of Medicine, Maywood; Staff Physician, Loyola University

Medical Center, and Hines Veterans Administration Hospital, Hines, Illinois

*Commentary: Surgery of Parathyroid Glands*

**JOHN M. DUGAN, M.D.**

Staff Pathologist, Department of Anatomic Pathology, Lahey Clinic Medical Center, Burlington, Massachusetts

*Cytopathology of Fine Needle Aspiration of Thyroid Gland*

**RANDALL D. GAZ, M.D.**

Assistant Professor of Surgery, Harvard Medical School; Assistant Surgeon, Endocrine Surgical Unit, Department of Surgery, Massachusetts General Hospital, Boston, Massachusetts

*Recurrent or Persistent Hyperparathyroidism: Surgical Approach*

**JOEL I. HAMBURGER, M.D.**

Southfield, Michigan

*Use of Needle Biopsy Data in Diagnosis and Management of Thyroid Nodules*

**STUART W. HAMBURGER, M.D.**

Clinical Professor of Surgery, University of Michigan Medical School, Ann Arbor; Chairman, Department of Surgery, Sinai Hospital of Detroit, Detroit, Michigan

*Use of Needle Biopsy Data in Diagnosis and Management of Thyroid Nodules*

**MARY BETH HODGE, M.D.**

Section of Endocrinology, Lahey Clinic Medical Center, Burlington, Massachusetts

*Thyroid Physiology and Function Tests; Role of Thyroid-Stimulating Hormone Suppression and Radioactive Iodine in Differentiated Carcinoma of Thyroid Gland; Thyroid and Parathyroid Disease During Pregnancy*

**BARBARA K. KINDER, M.D.**

Associate Professor of Surgery, Yale University School of Medicine; Attending Surgeon, Yale New Haven Hospital, Chief of Surgery, West Haven Veterans Administration Hospital, New Haven, Connecticut

*Commentary: Carcinoma of Parathyroid Glands*

**CARL R. LARSEN, M.D.**

Head, Section of Cross-Sectional Imaging, Department of Diagnostic Radiology, Lahey Clinic Medical Center, Burlington; Assistant Clinical Professor of Radiology, Boston University School of Medicine; Lecturer in Radiology, Harvard Medical School, Boston, Massachusetts

*Cross-Sectional Imaging of Thyroid Gland; Cross-Sectional Imaging of Parathyroid Glands*

**ANN M. LAWRENCE, M.D., Ph.D.**

Professor of Medicine and Biochemistry, Loyola University Stritch School of Medicine; Maywood; Associate Chief of Staff for Education, Hines Veterans Administration Hospital, Hines; Attending Physician, Loyola University Medical Center, Maywood, Illinois

*Commentary: Surgery of Parathyroid Glands*

**EDWARD PALOYAN, M.D.**

Professor of Surgery, Loyola University Stritch School of Medicine, Maywood; Associate Chief of Staff of Research, Hines Veterans Administration Hospital, Hines; Chief, Endocrine Surgery, Loyola University Medical Center, Maywood, Illinois

*Commentary: Surgery of Parathyroid Glands*

**RICARDO L. ROSSI, M.D.**

Chairman, Department of General Surgery, Lahey Clinic Medical Center, Burlington; Assistant Clinical Professor of Surgery, Harvard Medical School, Boston, Massachusetts

*Surgical Anatomy; Nontoxic Multinodular Goiter and Mediastinal Goiter; Differentiated Carcinoma of Thyroid Gland; Commentary: Medullary Thyroid Carcinoma; Undifferentiated Carcinoma and Lymphoma of Thyroid Gland; Surgery of Thyroid Gland; Commentary: Surgical Treatment of Intrathoracic Goiter; Surgery of Parathyroid Glands; Carcinoma of Parathyroid Glands; Surgical Complications and Their Management*

**FERDINAND A. SALZMAN, M.D., F.A.C.R.**

Emeritus Staff, Department of Radiotherapy, Lahey Clinic Medical Center, Burlington; Research Affiliate, Laboratory for Electromagnetic and Electronic Systems, Massachusetts Institute of Technology, Cambridge; Consultant Emeritus, Children's Hospital, Boston, Massachusetts

*External Beam Radiotherapy in Carcinoma of Thyroid Gland*

**LAURA E. SANDERS, M.D.**

Staff General Surgeon, Lahey Clinic Medical Center, Burlington, Massachusetts

*Embryology and Developmental Abnormalities; Nontoxic Multinodular Goiter and Mediastinal*

*Goiter; Surgical Complications and Their Management*

**DAVID M. SHAHIAN, M.D.**

Chairman, Department of Thoracic and Cardiovascular Surgery, Lahey Clinic Medical Center, Burlington; Assistant Clinical Professor of Surgery, Harvard Medical School, Boston, Massachusetts

*Surgical Treatment of Intrathoracic Goiter*

**MARK L. SILVERMAN, M.D.**

Chairman, Department of Anatomic Pathology, Lahey Clinic Medical Center, Burlington; Assistant Clinical Professor of Pathology, Harvard Medical School, Boston, Massachusetts

*Pathology of Thyroid and Parathyroid Glands*

**ALLAN E. SIPERSTEIN, M.D.**

Assistant Professor of Surgery, University of California, San Francisco School of Medicine; San Francisco, California

*Commentary: Surgery of Thyroid Gland*

**DAVID I. SOYBEL, M.D.**

Chief Resident in Surgery, Barnes Hospital/ Washington University School of Medicine, St. Louis, Missouri

*Medullary Thyroid Carcinoma*

**KENNETH R. STOKES, M.D.**

Instructor in Radiology, Harvard Medical School; Director of Angiography and Interventional Procedures, Department of Radiology, New England Deaconess Hospital, Consultant, Department of Radiology, Dana Farber Cancer Institute, Boston, Massachusetts

*Invasive Radiologic Evaluation of Hyperparathyroidism*

**CHIU-AN WANG, M.D.**

Lecturer, Harvard Medical School; Attending Physician, Massachusetts General Hospital, Boston, Massachusetts

*Commentary: Undifferentiated Carcinoma and Lymphoma of Thyroid Gland*

**SAMUEL A. WELLS, Jr., M.D.**

Bixby Professor and Chairman, Department of Surgery, Washington University School of Medicine; Surgeon-in-Chief, Barnes Hospital (St. Louis), and St. Louis Children's Hospital, St. Louis, Missouri

*Medullary Thyroid Carcinoma*

**PETER F. WINTER, M.D.**

Head, Section of Nuclear Medicine, Department of Diagnostic Radiology, Lahey Clinic Medical Center, Burlington; Associate Clinical Professor of Radiology, Boston University School of Medicine, Boston, Massachusetts

*Imaging of Thyroid Gland with Radionuclides; Imaging of Parathyroid Glands with Radionuclides*

**JOHN H. WOLFF, M.D.**

Staff Physician, Section of Medical Oncology, Lahey Clinic Medical Center, Burlington; Clinical Instructor in Medicine, Harvard Medical School, Boston, Massachusetts

*Chemotherapy for Carcinoma of Thyroid Gland*

**MARVIN S. WOOL, M.D., M.P.H.**

Senior Staff Physician, Lahey Clinic Medical Center, Medical Director, Lahey Clinic Health Maintenance Organization, Burlington; Clinical Instructor of Medicine, Harvard Medical School, Boston, Massachusetts

*Evaluation of Thyroid Nodules; Hyperthyroidism; Thyroiditis*

# PREFACE

This new edition of *Surgery of the Thyroid and Parathyroid Glands* has been written by a group of authors from the Lahey Clinic and invited authorities from across the country in areas of their acknowledged expertise.

The book is focused on practical management schemes in diseases of these two interesting endocrine organs, and we hope it provides a pragmatic guide to the conduct of diagnostic work-up and therapy as well as background information on anatomy, embryology, and epidemiology.

The editors thank all the authors for their exceptional contributions, which are extraordinarily comprehensive and thorough and present the state of the art in their fields at the present time.

We particularly want to thank Polly Zorolow, supervisor of the Editorial Department at the Lahey Clinic, for her personal involvement and responsibility for this edition. We thank Cornelius Sedgwick, with whom the previous edition of the book was written, for his wisdom and guidance in our developing an interest in this area and his role as our mentor at the Lahey Clinic. Dr. Sedgwick was a true disciple of Dr. Lahey's approach to diseases of the thyroid and carried on the basic Lahey Clinic pragmatic approach to thyroid surgery through the years.

The opportunity to study a large volume of cases handled in a relatively uniform fashion by a small group of physicians who developed close working relationships through the years is a unique experience and one that is both gratifying and productive in terms of developing a practical approach to the management of patients. Much is new and interesting in the management of patients with diseases of these organs, and we hope we have been able to provide a contemporary guide for surgeons and physicians who wish to become expert in this area.

BLAKE CADY, M.D.

RICARDO L. ROSSI, M.D.

# CONTENTS

# 1

# HISTORY OF THYROID AND PARATHYROID SURGERY

*Blake Cady, M.D.*

The history of surgery of the thyroid and parathyroid glands offers interesting contrasts. In the former, clinical surgeons, operating on huge goiters that produced symptoms resulting from anatomic derangements, stimulated physiologists to seek laboratory answers to complications of thyroid removal and thereby brought about a precise understanding of thyroid function. In parathyroid disease, such anatomic derangement is absent, and physiologists first had to develop accurate understanding of the hormonal function of the gland and of the bony and renal complications of the disease. Only then did clinical surgeons cautiously attack these small glands in attempts to relieve the physiologic diseases.

Although goiter has been recognized as a disease since earliest recorded history, consistent methods of surgery of the thyroid gland, with few exceptions, date back only 100 years. Before that time, only a few intrepid, or foolhardy, men attempted removal of goiters for relief of dyspnea or dysphagia. Halsted stated that the first well-documented operation was performed in 1595, but apparently successful excision of a goiter had been carried out as early as A.D. 1000 by Albucasis, and several reports cited operations performed throughout the 16th century.

In 1872, after becoming professor at Bern, Switzerland, Kocher performed his first thyroidectomy, emulating his predecessor Lücke's apparently successful operations. Billroth at this time had abandoned thyroid operations because of the great mortality from sepsis and hemorrhage. In 1876 Bruberger was able to document only 124 cases of operative removal of goiter. Kocher, through his safe, meticulous surgery, served as the model for Halsted, who was then studying in Europe. In his first two years at Bern, Kocher performed 13 thyroidectomies and in 1883 reported his first 100 cases of which 30 were total excision of the gland. In all of these latter patients "cachexia strumipriva" developed; this was later recognized as the surgical counterpart of myxedema first described by Curling in 1850 but named by Ord in 1877. Thereafter, Kocher avoided total thyroidectomy if at all possible and in 1895 reported 900 cases of thyroidectomy with an operative mortality rate of just over 1 per cent in instances of goiter not caused by hyperthyroidism or carcinoma. In this report only one instance of operative myxedema occurred in what was to be the only total excision performed. Furthermore, only one patient had permanent tetany. In 1898 Kocher reported 600 additional thyroidectomies with only a single operative death in a patient with euthyroid benign disease and that was caused by anesthesia. By 1901 Kocher had performed 2000 thyroid operations, including those for hyperthyroidism and cancer, with an overall operative mortality of 4.5 per cent.

During this era, thyroid and parathyroid physiologic research was developing rapidly and was spurred on by clinical surgeons. In 1884 Shiff reported 60 dogs in which death followed total thyroidectomy unless the animals had been provided with a previous graft of thyroid tissue, thus confirming that this fatal complication was caused by the loss of thyroid tissue. Von Eiselsberg in 1890 had noted tetany in humans after operations for goiter and for the first time distinguished it from "cachexia strumipriva." Bley in 1891 and von Eiselsberg in 1892 produced tetany in animals by excision of the parathyroid glands alone.

Stimulated by the relief of experimental myxedema with transplanted thyroid tissue, Murray in 1891 and Horowitz in 1892 began the clinical use of thyroid extracts for the treatment of myxedema. In 1906, Payr transplanted maternal thyroid tissue to the spleen of a myxedematous daughter for whom relief was achieved.

Halsted in 1906 relieved clinical tetany after thyroid operations with dietary supplements of parathyroid glands from cattle. Leischner in 1907 and Halsted in 1908 confirmed that tetany produced experimentally in animals could be relieved by injections of parathyroid extracts or transplantation of parathyroid glands. Working with Halsted at Johns Hopkins, MacCollum and Voegtlin in 1908 demonstrated that calcium salts relieved tetany also and thus linked the parathyroid glands with calcium metabolism.

The Nobel prize in medicine was awarded to Theodor Kocher in 1909 for his outstanding contributions to the understanding of thyroid disease through both clinical surgery and research.

Leadership in the surgery and research of thyroid and parathyroid disease shifted largely to the United States in the 20th century, begining with the elegant studies and careful operative techniques of Halsted and his colleagues. In 1912 Mayo reported on 278 patients with exophthalmic goiter operated on without a death. Crile, Lahey, and the Mayos founded their private clinics largely on the basis of performing safe thyroid surgery on large numbers of patients. This surgery was immeasurably aided by the utilization of iodine solutions to relieve hyperthyroidism temporarily before operation, as first reported by Plummer in 1923. Previously, Marine and Lenhardt had virtually eliminated endemic goiter through the use of iodized salt in a group of schoolgirls in Akron, Ohio, in the years 1917 to 1920. The chemical description of thyroxine, isolated by Kendall in 1904, was reported by Harrington in 1926 and by Harrington and Barger in 1927.

Halsted wrote the most complete early history of thyroid disease and thyroid surgery in "The Operative Story of Goiter" published in 1920. An excellent review of thyroid surgery was given by Becker as the presidential address to the Southern Surgical Society, and recently a delightful historical overview was presented by Beahrs as the presidential address to the American Society of Endocrine Surgery.

Von Recklinghausen in 1891 described a bone disease marked by cystic lesions. The relationship between this bone disease and parathyroid enlargement was first suggested by Askanazy in 1904, but the parathyroid abnormality was believed by Erdheim (1907) to be secondary to bone disease. Removal of parathyroid tumors for relief of von Recklinghausen's disease of bone was suggested in 1915 by Schlagenhaufer but was not actually carried out until 1925 by Mandl in Vienna. Mandl's patient had previously been treated for more than a year with parathyroid extracts and implantation of homologous parathyroid glands following the then current but mistaken belief that the bone disease was caused by parathyroid insufficiency. The enlarged glands were presumed to be related to hormonal insufficiency, much as goiter and myxedema were related. Only in desperation was the "illogical" removal of the enlarged gland undertaken. The operation was relatively simple, and a single adenoma was found promptly. In the United States, the relation between bone disease and enlarged hyperactive parathyroid glands was so soundly based on physiologic understanding that the first patient at the Massachusetts General Hospital underwent exploration seven times before the adenoma was discovered within the mediastinum.

In 1925 Collip first isolated parathormone. Barr and Bulger reported the first successful American case of excision of parathyroid adenoma for bone disease in 1930, and Albright and his colleagues reported successful treatment of renal calculi without bone disease by excision of a parathyroid adenoma in 1932. Varieties of parathyroid gland hyperplasia were reported by Castleman and Mallory in 1935 and by Cope and associates in 1958. The complexity and difficulty of the development of parathyroid surgery has been documented by Cope (1966). Tertiary hyperparathyroidism was carefully defined by Davies and coworkers in 1968.

Treatment of hyperthyroidism with propylthiouracil was described by Astwood and MacKenzie in 1943, and by 1946 radioiodine was introduced for diagnostic and therapeutic use by Chapman. The link between childhood radiation of the thyroid gland occurring inadvertently during treatment of acne, lymphoid hyperplasia, and thymic enlargement and later thyroid carcinoma was first reported by Duffy and associates in 1950 and has been well documented many times since. This work has been instrumental in addressing the cause of thyroid cancer.

A distinctive variety of thyroid carcinoma, medullary carcinoma, was reported by Horn in 1951 and was substantiated and clarified by Hazard and associates in 1959. In 1962 Copp and coworkers reported the discovery of a new hormone, calcitonin. Melvin and Tashjian (1968) linked the carcinoma of parafollicular C cells—medullary carcinoma—with excessive production of calcitonin and prompted the use of this tumor marker in clinical practice.

Interest in medullary carcinoma has paralleled the recognition of the multiple endocrine adenopathies and the variety of hormonal products elaborated, such as gastrointestinal-stimulating peptides, which may produce diarrhea in patients with medullary carcinoma. The unifying aspects of the concept of APUD (Amino Precursor-Uptake and Decarboxylation) cells were first described by Pearse in 1968. The historical background of medullary carcinoma is given in Chapter 15 of this book.

The introduction of automatic screening of serum for hypercalcemia, beginning in the 1970s, led to enormous increases in parathyroid surgery. Comparing the few years before 1970 with the late 1970s, the number of parathyroidectomies performed increased by fourfold to sixfold in most institutions. Recently, the volume of parathyroid surgery has declined appreciably as if a large stable pool of relatively asymptomatic patients with chronically mildly elevated levels of calcium from mild hyperparathyroidism has gradually been depleted by surgical therapy. With the advent of screening programs, the paradoxical increase in the median age of patients suggests that patients with hyperparathyroidism and parathyroid adenoma have a bimodal age distribution with older patients displaying milder, more prolonged, less commonly recognized disease because of fewer and less specific symptoms. Population studies indicate a high incidence of disease in elderly women particularly. The greatest challenge in hyperparathyroid disease in the near future is to define its biologic behavior and to explain the fluctuating, irregular, and difficult to predict variations in hormone secretion, symptoms, variations in presentation, and clinical progress of patients with hypercalcemia.

In thyroid disease, the greatest challenge in the future is to comprehend the biology of thyroid carcinoma, because without a clear appreciation of the biology of the disease, logical surgical therapy cannot be designed. This fact can be appreciated currently in the conflict regarding the extent of thyroid surgery between some physicians who advocate total thyroidectomy and others who emphasize conservative removal of the thyroid gland. Thyroid needle biopsy has greatly altered the diagnostic and therapeutic approach to thyroid nodules. The prospect of utilizing flow cytometry for DNA histography on needle aspiration cytology promises still further advances in diagnostic sophistication by predicating biologic behavior for therapy.

Surgical interest in parathyroid and thyroid glands remains high, and the historical aspects of therapy of these glandular disorders are still unfolding. However, the essence of surgical therapy can profitably be repeated from a speech made by Cushing in 1913: "The accurate and detailed methods, in the use of which Kocher and Halsted were for so long the notable examples, have spread into all clinics—at least into those clinics where you or I would wish to entrust ourselves for an operation. Observers no longer expect to be thrilled in an operating room; the spectacular public performances of the past, no longer condoned, are replaced by the quiet, rather tedious procedures which few beyond the operator, his assistants, and the immediate bystanders can profitably see. The patient on the table, like the passenger in a car, runs greater risks if he has a loquacious driver, or one who takes close corners, exceeds the speed limit, or rides to applause."

Careful surgery is based on comprehensive historical, physiologic, and anatomic antecedents, which we must all comprehend to provide the finest clinical care of patients.

## SUGGESTED READING

Albright, F., Baird, P. C., Cope, O., et al.: Studies on physiology of parathyroid glands: Renal complications of hyperparathyroidism. Am. J. Med. Sci., *187*:49–65, 1934.

Beahrs, O. H.: Presidential address: Lest we forget. Surgery, *102*:893–897, 1987.

Becker, W. F.: Presidential address: Pioneers in thyroid surgery. Ann. Surg., *185*:493–503, 1977.

Castleman, B., and Mallory, T. B.: Pathology of parathyroid glands in hyperparathyroidism: Study of 25 cases. Am. J. Pathol., *11*:1–72, 1935.

Churchill, E. D., and Cope, O.: Parathyroid tumors associated with hyperparathyroidism: 11 cases treated by operation. Surg. Gynecol. Obstet., *58*:255–271, 1934.

Collip, J. B.: Extraction of a parathyroid hormone which will prevent or control parathyroid tetany and which regulates level of blood calcium. J. Biol. Chem., *63*:395–438, 1925.

Cope, O.: The study of hyperparathyroidism at the Massachusetts General Hospital. N. Engl. J. Med., *274*:1174–1182, 1966.

Cope, O., Keynes, W. M., Roth, S. I., et al.: Primary chief-cell hyperplasia of the parathyroid glands: A new entity in the surgery of hyperparathyroidism. Ann. Surg., *148*:375–388, 1958.

Copp, D. H., Cameron, E. C., Cheney, B. A., et al.: Evidence for calcitonin—a new hormone from the parathyroid that lowers blood calcium. Endocrinology, *70*:638–649, 1962.

Cushing, H.: Address in surgery on realignments in greater medicine: Their effect upon surgery and the influence of surgery upon them. Delivered before the Seventeenth International Congress of Medicine. Br. Med. J., *2*:290–297, 1913.

Davies, D. R., Dent, C. E., and Watson, L.: Tertiary hyperparathyroidism. Br. Med. J., *2*:395–399, 1968.

DeGroot, L. J. (ed.): Radiation-Associated Thyroid Carcinoma. New York, Grune & Stratton, Inc., 1977.

Duffy, B. J., Jr., and Fitzgerald, P. J.: Thyroid cancer in childhood and adolescence: Report on 28 cases. J. Clin. Endocrinol., *10*:1296–1308, 1950.

Garrison, F. H.: An Introduction to the History of Medicine. 4th ed. Philadelphia, W. B. Saunders Co., 1929.

Halsted, W. S.: The operative story of goiter: The author's operation. Johns Hopkins Hosp. Rep., *19*:71–257, 1920.

Hazard, J. B., Hawk, W. A., and Crile, G., Jr.: Medullary (solid) carcinoma of the thyroid: A clinicopathologic entity. J. Clin. Endocrinol., *19*:152–161, 1959.

Horn, R. C., Jr.: Carcinoma of the thyroid: Description of distinctive morphological variant and report of 7 cases. Cancer, *4*:697–707, 1951.

Horowitz, A., and Degenshein, G. A.: Milestones in Modern Surgery. New York, Paul B. Hoeber, Inc., 1958.

Melvin, K. E., and Tashjian, A. H., Jr.: The syndrome of excessive thyrocalcitonin produced by medullary carcinoma of the thyroid. Proc. Natl. Acad. Sci., *59*:1216–1222, 1968.

Pearse, A. G.: Common cytochemical and ultrastructural characteristics of cells producing polypeptide hormones (the APUD series) and their relevance to thyroid and ultimobranchial C cells and calcitonin. Proc. Roy. Soc. (Biol.), *170*:71–80, 1968.

# 2

# EMBRYOLOGY AND DEVELOPMENTAL ABNORMALITIES

*Laura E. Sanders, M.D., and Blake Cady, M.D.*

## THYROID EMBRYOLOGY

The surgeon dealing with thyroid, parathyroid, and parafollicular abnormalities must be familiar with their embryologic antecedents, for only through this knowledge can variations in glandular location, shape, or number and rationale for surgical maneuvers be appreciated. The thyroid takes its origin from epithelial cells in the midline of the floor of the pharyngeal anlage (Fig. 2–1). When thickening develops, a process of evagination takes place in a variety of forms. Following the path of the heart and great vessels, the thyroid anlage descends along the path of the thyroglossal duct (Fig. 2–2). This duct arises at the foramen cecum at the base of the tongue, the remnant of its pharyngeal origin, and wraps around anterior to the hyoid bone as that structure rotates forward.[1] It divides into two lobes before it comes to rest anterior to the trachea at about the seventh week, acquiring the shape of a shield. The distal end of the duct may become the pyramidal lobe (Fig. 2–3). Normally, the epithelium of the thyroglossal duct degenerates, atrophies, and disappears.

Anatomic abnormalities of the thyroid can nearly always be attributed to variations in the descent of the gland. Along the path of the descent, the two surgically important anomalies that can occur during development are persistence of a thyroglossal duct or cyst and persistence of thyroid tissue (Fig. 2–4).

## THYROGLOSSAL CYSTS AND FISTULAS

After enlarged lymph nodes, thyroglossal cysts are the most commonly found midline masses. They occur in both sexes in an even distribution. Although they can present in patients of any age, they are usually first noted in infancy or childhood.[7] Usually in the midline, they are more often found to the left than to the right. Although they can be found anywhere from the base of the tongue to the suprasternal notch, they are often (75

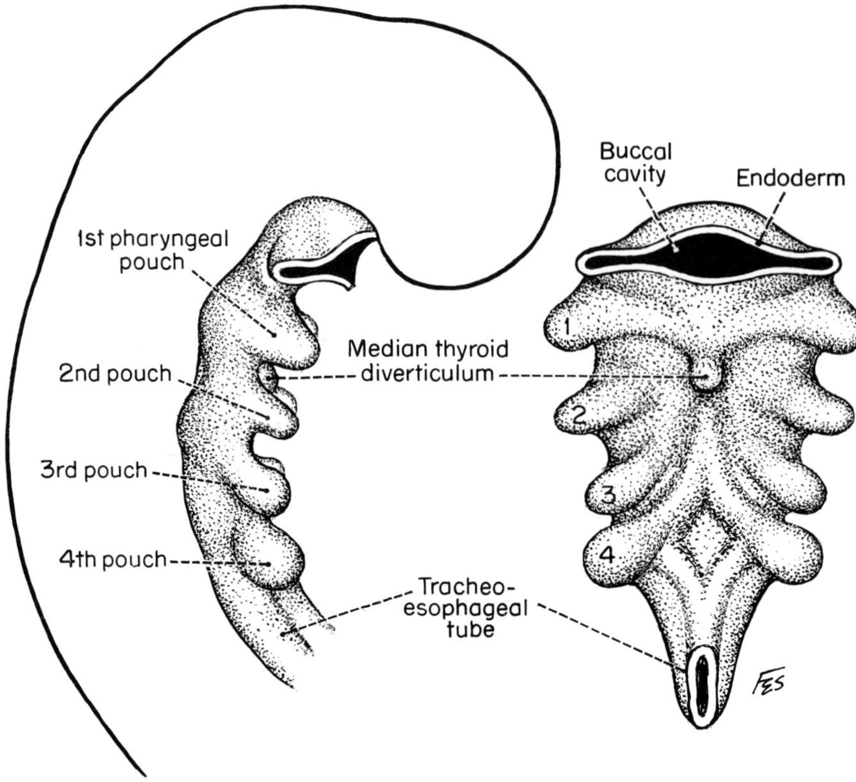


**FIGURE 2–1.** Early embryologic development of pharyngeal anlage.

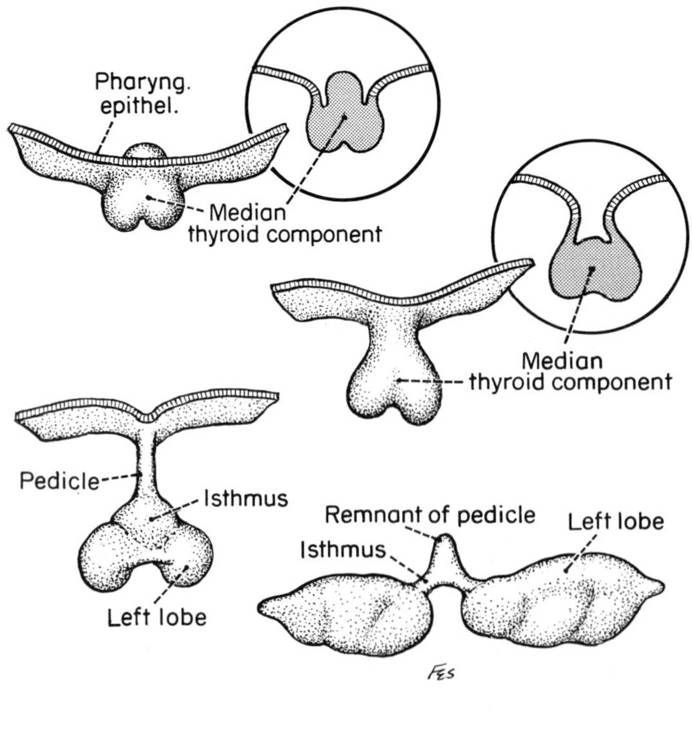


**FIGURE 2–2.** Schematic representation of early thyroid gland development from midline floor of pharyngeal anlage with later downward growth and division into lobes connected by an isthmus. (After Gray and Skandalakis.)

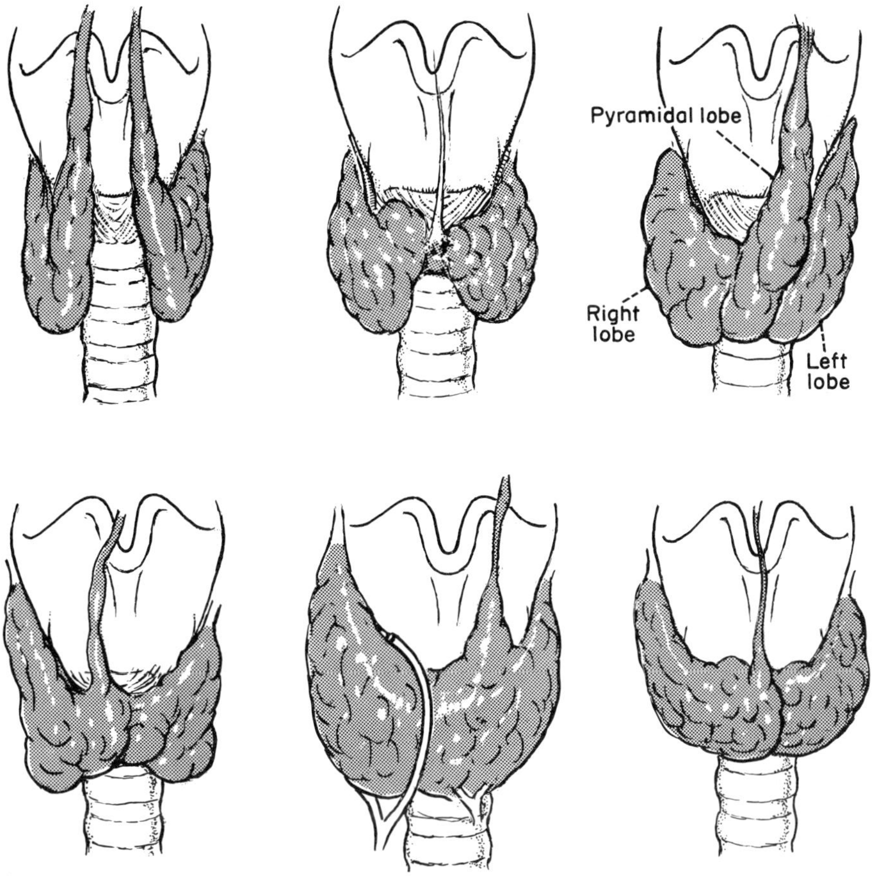


**FIGURE 2–3.** Variations of normal adult thyroid anatomy resulting from the embryologic descent and division of the thyroid gland. (After Gray and Skandalakis.)

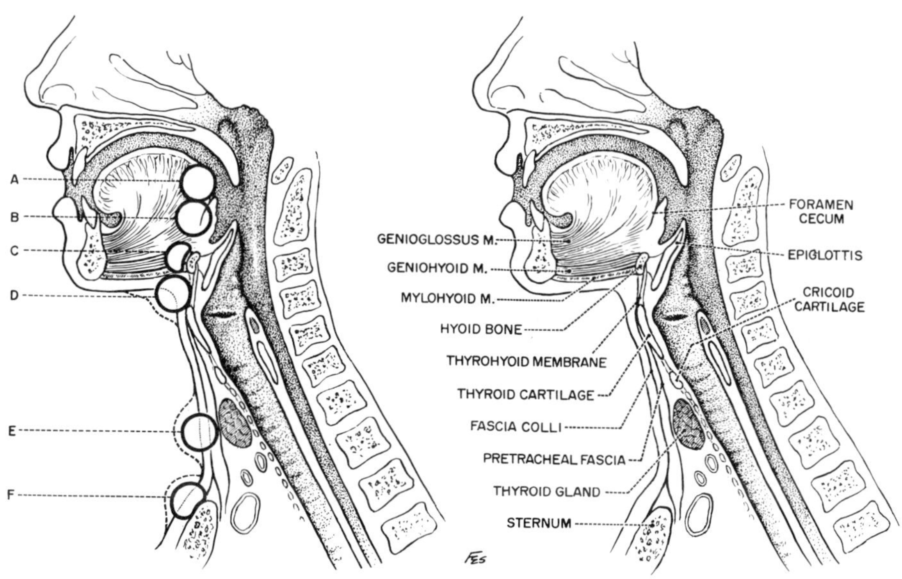


**FIGURE 2–4.** Location of thyroglossal cysts. *A*, In front of foramen cecum; *B*, at foramen cecum; *C*, suprahyoid; *D*, infrahyoid; *E*, area of thyroid gland; and *F*, suprasternal. (After Ward and Hendrick.)

per cent) found in the neck below the hyoid bone.[1] In this location, a thyroglossal cyst can be mistaken for a thyroid adenoma in the pyramidal lobe. An adenoma will elevate during swallowing, whereas the thyroglossal cyst elevates with protrusion of the tongue.

Symptoms vary with location. In an intralingual or suprahyoid location, cysts can cause choking, dysphagia, or dysphonia.[1] When this duct is patent up to the foramen cecum, a cyst may drain pus or fluid into the mouth. Thyroglossal cysts are prone to infection, and this is the main reason why patients seek medical attention. When infected, cysts can be drained, but this will result in recurrence of the cyst or in a fistula.

Because thyroid tissue is usually present in the wall of the duct, cysts have the potential for malignant transformation. Thyroglossal duct carcinoma is a rare lesion presenting usually as a midline neck mass in the middle-aged patient. Although 85 per cent of cysts contain papillary adenocarcinoma, all of the usual types of thyroid carcinoma have been reported except for medullary carcinoma, which has a parafollicular cell origin.[8] Surgical treatment is the same as for any thyroglossal cyst, with neck dissection reserved for a patient with clinically positive nodes. The patient with a thyroglossal duct papillary carcinoma has an excellent prognosis after the carcinoma has been resected.

The treatment of a patient with a benign or malignant cyst is surgical excision, which must include the entire path of the duct. As Sistrunk[10] noted in 1920, it is necessary to remove a core of tissue including the central portion of the hyoid bone up to the foramen cecum. Before the hyoid bone was removed, recurrence rates of up to 50 per cent were reported.[7] The defect in the hyoid bone need not be closed, but if the core extends to the lingual epithelium, that defect can be closed from below with a pursestring suture.

## ECTOPIC THYROID

Ectopic thyroid rests can be found anywhere along the path of descent of the gland. The most common ectopic thyroid is the pyramidal lobe and occurs so frequently (50 per cent)[5] that it can hardly qualify as an abnormality. In thyroidectomy for Graves' disease, the pyramidal lobe should not be overlooked because it can be the cause of recurrent hyperthyroidism.

Lingual thyroid glands, at the base of the tongue, account for 90 per cent of other ectopic thyroid tissue (Fig. 2–5). They can present as an asymptomatic incidental finding or, when enlarged, with hyperthyroidism, dysphagia, dysphonia, dyspnea, pain, or rarely bleeding.[5] In 70 per cent of patients, the lingual thyroid is the patient's only functioning thyroid tissue.[2, 6] In addition to being found in the normal course of the duct, ectopic thyroid tissue has rarely been seen in

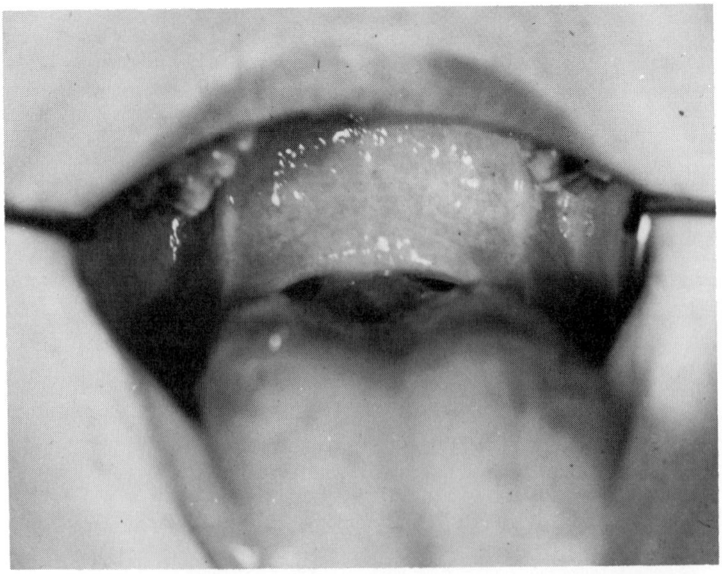

**FIGURE 2–5.** Intralingual goiter can be seen at the base of the tongue.

the suprasternal location and rarely within the larynx or trachea.[3] Mediastinal thyroid tissue has occasionally been reported to arise from displacement of thyroid remnants into the mediastinum by the heart as it migrates downward.[10] This is usually an acquired rather than a congenital lesion and is caused by the action of gravity on an enlarged goitrous gland.

Ultrasonography can distinguish between cystic and solid midline neck masses, and computed tomography can define thyroid tissue as a high density mass because of its iodine content.[7] The iodine-131 or technetium 99m scan is still the most useful study, however, both to identify a lingual or midline neck mass as thyroid tissue and to confirm that it is the patient's only functioning thyroid tissue (Fig. 2–6).

The treatment of a patient with an ectopic

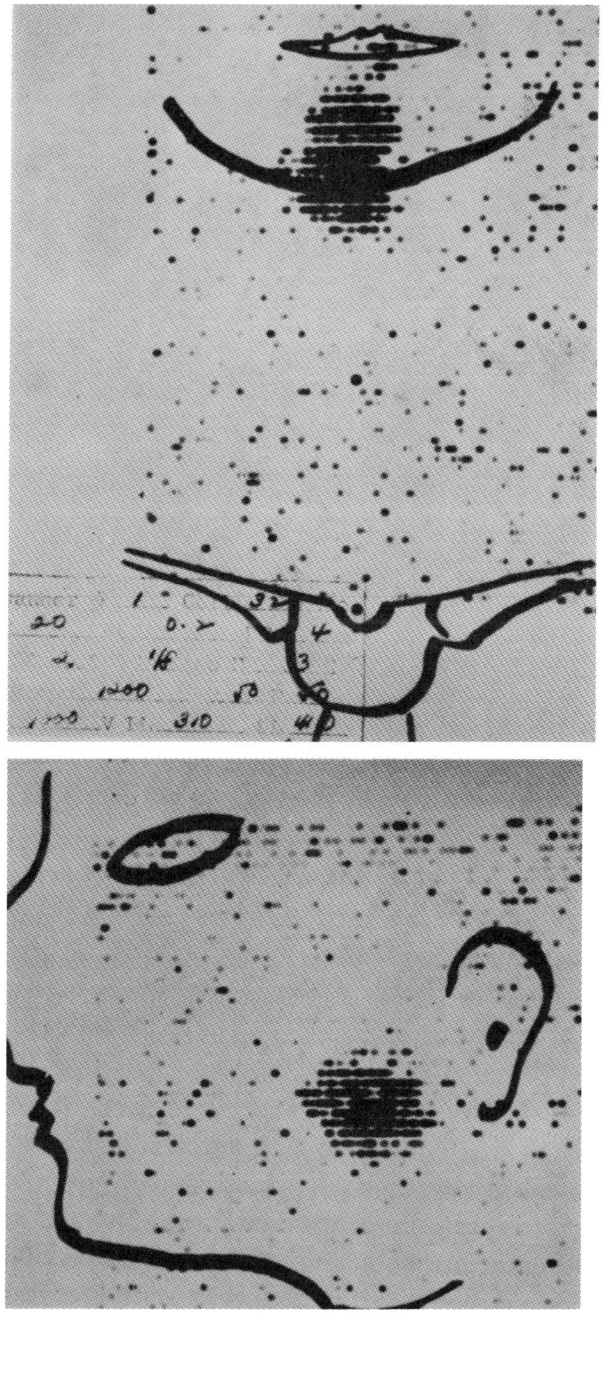

**FIGURE 2–6.** Thyroid scan of a 4-year-old girl showing lingual location of the thyroid with no other evidence of thyroid tissue. *Top*, front view; *bottom*, side view. (From Rogers, W.M.: Normal and anomalous development. *In* Werner, S.C., and Ingbar, S.H. (eds.): The Thyroid: A Functional and Clinical Text. 3rd ed. New York, Harper & Row, 1971.)

thyroid depends on the presence of symptoms and on concerns about malignancy. Ectopic thyroid tissue appears to have the same malignant potential as normal thyroid tissue and should be subject to the same evaluation by needle aspiration or biopsy. When the thyroid mass is causing acute symptoms, when carcinoma cannot be excluded, or when the patient has cosmetic objections to the neck mass, surgery and replacement thyroid therapy are recommended.[5] When the mass is asymptomatic and carcinoma is not a concern, no treatment is needed other than thyroid replacement for suppression. Excellent reviews[4, 9] may be found in the literature.

## PARATHYROID EMBRYOLOGY

The parathyroid bodies arise as endodermal cell proliferations at the lateral tips of the third and fourth pharyngeal pouches (Figs. 2–1 and 2–7). The third pouch gives rise not only to parathyroid glands but also to the thymus, which will migrate to the mediastinum. The fourth pouch and its eventual parathyroid tissue become less closely associated with the migrating thymus and more closely associated with the laterally developing thyroid lobes. Although the fourth pouch in its ventral portion seems also to produce some thymus tissue, this does not migrate or persist in the adult, although such thymic remnants are sometimes found in infants. The ultimobranchial bodies in many animals are clearly noted to arise from the fifth pouch, but in humans the fourth and fifth pouches cannot be distinguished, and the ultimobranchial body appears to arise from the fourth pouch (Fig. 2–7). These ultimobranchial bodies, which are the origin of the parafollicular C cells, are considered to be analogues of parathyroid tissue, and the fact that parafollicular cells also help govern calcium metabolism seems to bear out this embryologic point. In humans, the ultimobranchial bodies are noted as ventral portions of the fourth pouch and are incorporated into the laterally developing thyroid tissue, although in primitive vertebrates they frequently remain as separate and discrete structures.

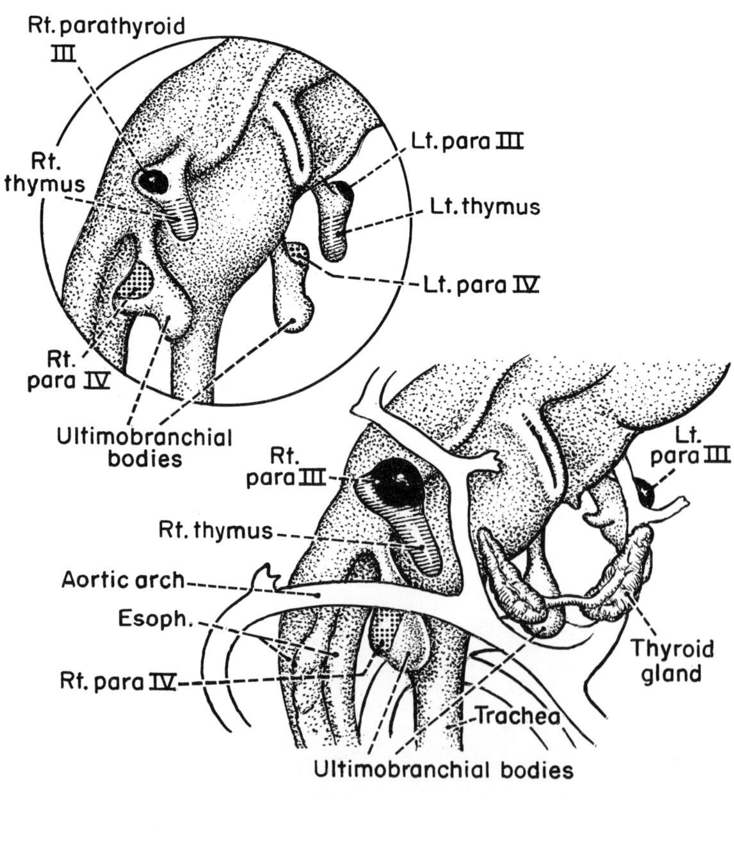


**FIGURE 2–7.** Origin of parathyroid glands at lateral tips of the third and fourth pharyngeal pouches. Note the thymus origin on the medial tips of the third pouch and the ultimobranchial body origins on the medial tips of the fourth pouch. (After Gray and Skandalakis.)

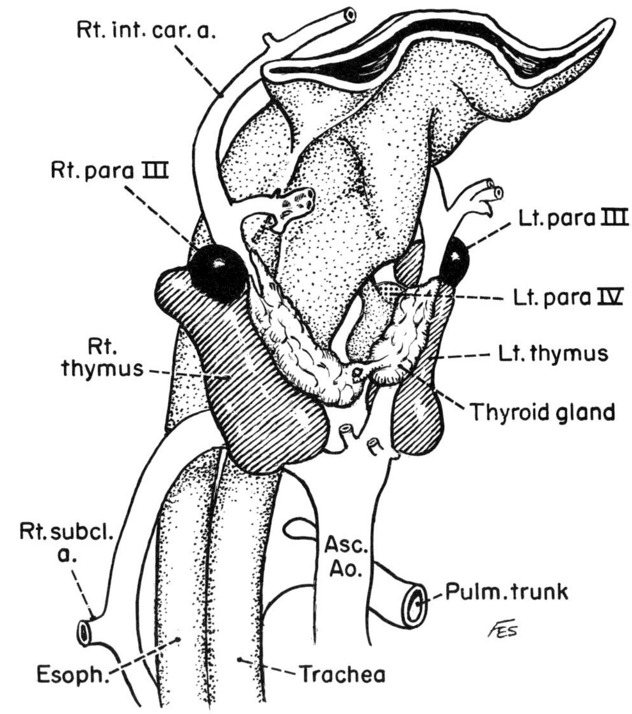


**FIGURE 2–8.** Further embryologic development stage illustrating the downward thrust of the third pouch components and the close approximation of the fourth pouch and the thyroid lobes. (After Gray and Skandalakis.)

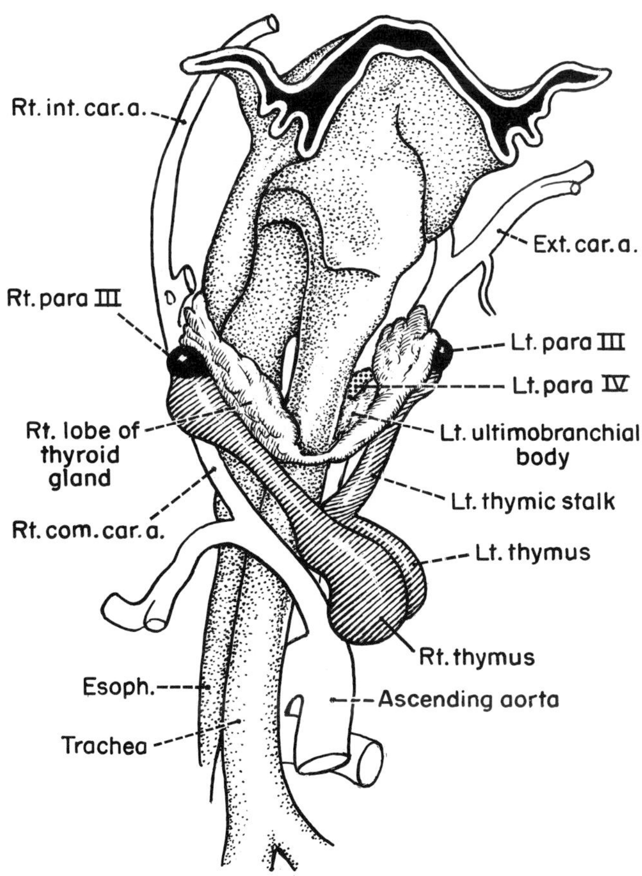


**FIGURE 2–9.** The lower thymic tissue has now migrated into the upper chest, and a rough approximation of the eventual adult location of thyroid, parafollicular, and parathyroid tissues is noted. (After Gray and Skandalakis.)

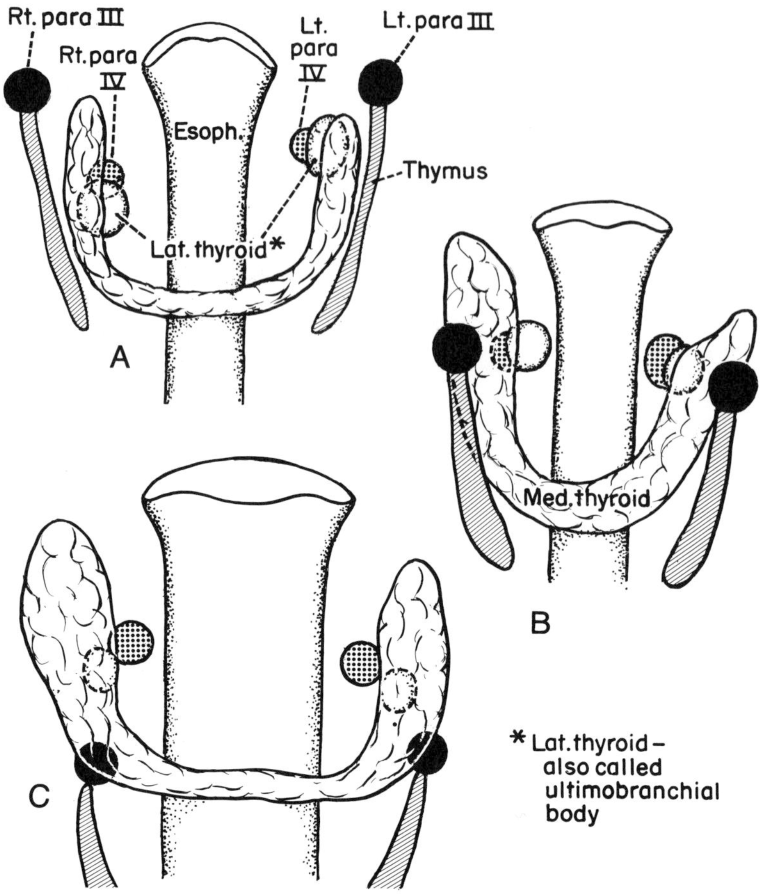


**FIGURE 2–10.** *A* and *B*, A schematic view of the shifts in location of thyroid, parafollicular, and parathyroid tissues is shown. *C*, Approximates the adult location. (After Gray and Skandalakis.)

Figures 2–8 and 2–9 graphically depict the development and early migration of the thymus and parathyroid in three dimensions and illustrate the potential for the wide variation in location of the inferior parathyroid. Figure 2–10 *A* and *B* shows in schematic form the later embryologic positioning of the thymus, parathyroids, and ultimobranchial bodies (or lateral thyroid). Finally, Figure 2–10*C* demonstrates the eventual adult location of the superior parathyroids derived from the fourth pouch and the inferior parathyroids derived from the third pouch.

## REFERENCES


1. Allard, R. H. B.: The thyroglossal cyst. Head Neck Surg., *5*:134–146, 1982.
2. Buckman, L. T.: Lingual thyroid. Laryngoscope, *46*:765–784, 878–897, and 935–955, 1936.
3. Donegan, J. O., and Wood, M. D.: Intratracheal thyroid—familial occurrence. Laryngoscope, *95*:6–8, 1985.
4. Fish, J., and Moore, R. M.: Ectopic thyroid tissue and ectopic thyroid carcinoma: A review of the literature and report of a case. Ann. Surg., *157*:212–222, 1963.
5. Haddad, A., Frenkiel, S., Costom, B., et al.: Management of the undescended thyroid. J. Otolaryngol., *15*:373–376, 1986.
6. Montgomery, M. L.: Lingual thyroid: A comprehensive review. West. J. Surg., *43*:661–669, 1935.
7. Noyek, A. M., and Friedberg, J.: Thyroglossal duct and ectopic thyroid disorders. Otolaryngol. Clin. North Am., *14*:187–201, 1981.
8. Nussbaum, M., Buchwald, R. P., Ribner, A., et al.: Anaplastic carcinoma arising from median ectopic thyroid (thyroglossal duct remnant). Cancer, *48*:2724–2728, 1981.
9. Shepard, G. H., and Rosenfeld, L.: Carcinoma of thyroglossal duct remnants: Review of the literature and addition of two cases. Am. J. Surg., *116*:125–129, 1968.
10. Sistrunk, W. E.: Surgical treatment of cysts of thyroglossal tract. Ann. Surg., *71*:121–123, 1920.


## SUGGESTED READING


Cady, B.: Management of tracheal obstruction from thyroid diseases. World J. Surg., *6*:696–701, 1982.

Gray, S. W., and Skandalakis, J. E.: Embryology for Surgeons. Philadelphia, W. B. Saunders Co., 1972.

# 3

# SURGICAL ANATOMY

*Ricardo L. Rossi, M.D., and Blake Cady, M.D.*

Surgeons attempting operations on the thyroid gland must be well informed on the anatomy of the neck, including the thyroid gland, its blood supply and its nerve supply, as well as its adjacent structures—the trachea, the larynx, the esophagus, and the parathyroid glands. The macroscopic and microscopic description of the thyroid gland is supplied elsewhere (Chapter 4). This chapter deals with the surgical anatomy of the thyroid as it applies to surgical procedures discussed elsewhere in this book. It is presented in a topographic manner, describing the anatomy as it is encountered in thyroidectomy.

## THE SKIN

The skin of the neck may reveal several transverse folds that may be of value in deciding the site of an incision. Of the folds just above the sternum and clavicle, one may be ideal for a low collar incision.

## THE MUSCLES

The *platysma* is a thin, sheetlike muscle immediately beneath the skin in the subcutaneous area, spreading fanlike from below the clavicle laterally to the mandibles above, leaving a space in the midline (Fig. 3–1). When the skin flaps are turned up to expose the underlying muscles, the skin, subcutaneous fat, and platysma should be dissected as a single layer. By this means, unnecessary bleeding will be avoided because the fascial plane between the platysma and the fascia covering the prethyroid muscles is avascular.

The muscles that must be dealt with during thyroid surgery are the two lateral *sternocleidomastoid* muscles, forming the lateral boundaries, and the *sternohyoid* and *sternothyroid* muscles, forming the superficial and anterior boundaries (Fig. 3–2). Both the sternohyoid, lying more anterior, and the sternothyroid, just beneath and covering the thyroid capsule, arise from the sternum. The sternohyoid attaches above to the hyoid, and the sternothyroid attaches to the thyroid cartilage. The fascia of the anterior medial border of the sternocleidomastoid fuses with the fascia of the lateral border of the sternohyoid. This is divided vertically during exposure of the thyroid to permit retraction of the sternocleidomastoid laterally and the sternohyoid medially. The nerve supply to the sternohyoid and sternothyroid is the ansa hypoglossi. This nerve descends along the lateral border of the sternohyoid and enters the muscles low in the neck. When the sterno-

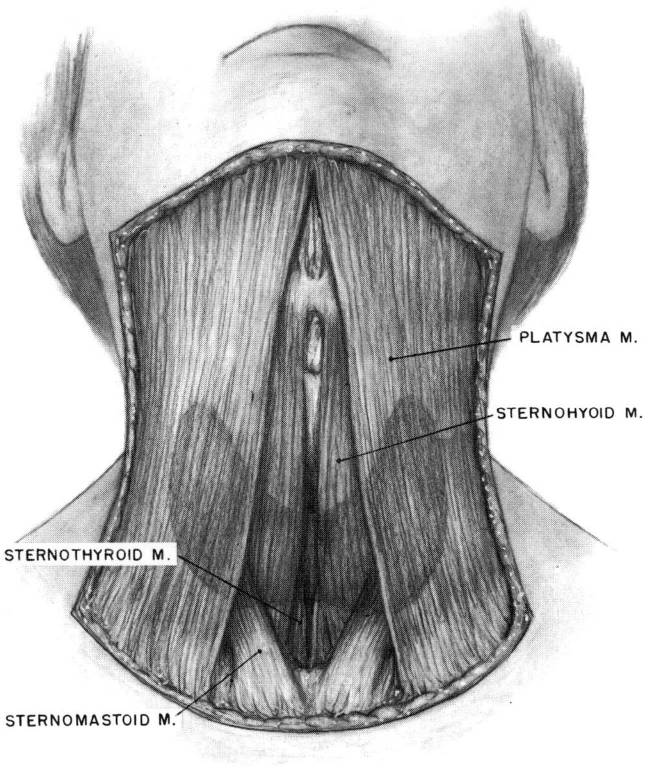


**FIGURE 3–1.** Fanlike spread of platysma from mandibles to clavicles. The sternohyoid and sternothyroid muscles are seen in the midline. The platysma fibers are best visualized for excision at lateral margins.

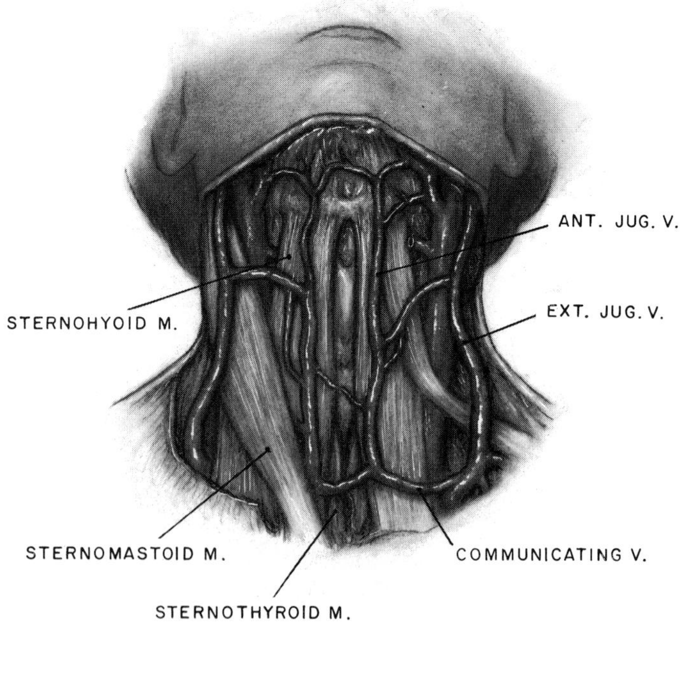


**FIGURE 3–2.** *Right side*, The muscles. *Lateral,* The sternocleidomastoid muscle passes upward from the sternoclavicular joint to the mastoid process. *Medial,* The sternohyoid passes from the sternum to the hyoid. The sternothyroid, posterior to the sternohyoid, is visualized low in the neck close to its attachment to the sternum. *Left side*, The superficial veins. The sternocleidomastoid muscle has been removed. Note communicating veins between the external and anterior jugular veins.

hyoid and sternothyroid are to be divided transversely, they must be transected high to preserve the motor function of this muscle.

## THE BLOOD VESSELS

The principal blood vessels to and from the thyroid gland are external to the capsule. The superior and inferior thyroid arteries constitute the main arterial supply. Occasionally, a branch from the aorta or innominate artery, the lowest thyroid artery (arteria thyroidea ima), and the inferior thyroid veins (vena thyreoidea ima) enter from below. The veins, in general, drain areas supplied by the corresponding arteries.

### *The Veins*

The *superficial jugular veins* lie beneath the platysma (Fig. 3–2). They are easily visualized and should present no problem for the thyroid surgeon. The external jugular veins are lateral and cross over the belly of the sternocleidomastoid muscle. The anterior jugular veins immediately overlie the sternohyoid muscles. A plexus of communicating veins may be present between the external and anterior jugular veins. In large goiters, the superficial veins may be of considerable size. Care should be exercised in turning up the skin flaps with the platysma so that the veins are not cut. If the fascia between the sternocleidomastoid and the sternohyoid muscles is divided carefully, the communicating veins may be ligated and divided. The external jugular vein may be retracted laterally along with the sternocleidomastoid muscle. The anterior jugular vein is suture ligated and divided when the sternohyoid and sternothyroid muscles are transected.

The *deep thyroid veins* leave the gland in relationship to the thyroid arteries mainly at the superior and inferior poles and the lateral aspect of the gland (Fig. 3–3). They are less constant than the arteries in number, posi-

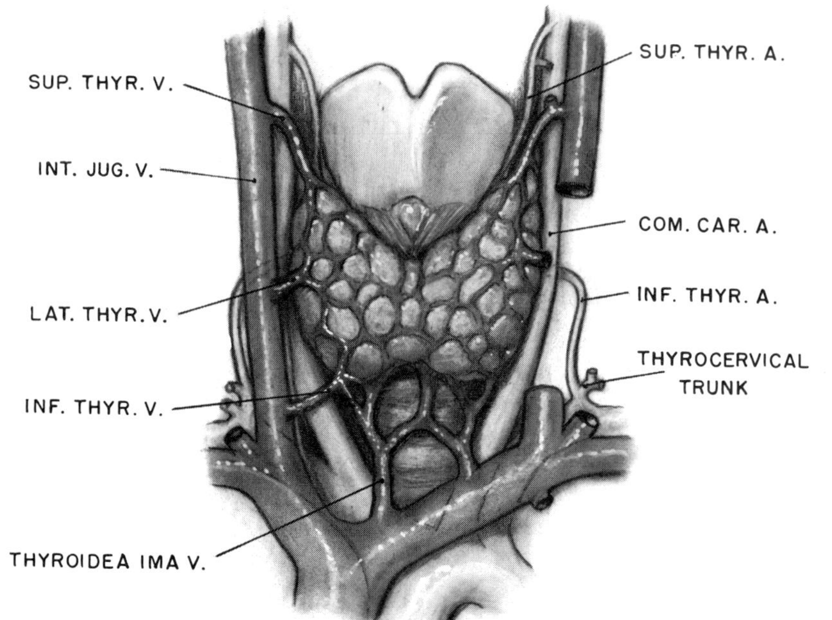


**FIGURE 3–3.** *Right*, The deep veins drain into the internal jugular veins. The superior thyroid vein is lateral to the superior thyroid arteries. The lateral or medial thyroid veins may vary in number from one to four. The inferior thyroid veins may form a plexus emptying into the internal jugular vein or present as the thyroidea ima vein emptying into the innominate vein. *Left*, The arteries. The superior thyroid artery, a branch of the external carotid artery, gives off a branch to the pyramidal lobe and isthmus. The inferior thyroid artery arises from the thyrocervical trunk, passes upward posterior to the carotid sheath, and loops downward into the midsection of the gland.

tion, and size. The deep veins may be a serious threat during thyroid surgery because they are numerous and may be torn easily with ensuing hemorrhage. This is particularly true in patients with a large substernal goiter. In such patients, the clavicle may act as a tourniquet and produce great dilatation and increased pressure in the veins. When uncontrolled hemorrhage occurs, the lower pole and the substernal extension of the goiter must be mobilized quickly out of the mediastinum. Release of the tourniquet effect of the clavicle will permit the veins to collapse, and the bleeding will be brought under control.

The *superior thyroid vein* leaves the gland at the superior pole just anterior and lateral to the superior thyroid artery. It empties into the cricothyroid tributary of the internal jugular vein. It should be ligated separately from the superior thyroid artery during thyroidectomy.

The *lateral* or *middle* veins vary in number. They pass directly from the lateral border of the lobes and enter into the internal jugular vein. During thyroidectomy, they must be divided to permit access to the lateral compartment. In pathologically enlarged glands, the jugular vein and the middle thyroid veins may be pushed close to the capsule of the thyroid. In such instances, they may be mistaken for veins in the thyroid capsule, and the fascial plane between the thyroid and the jugular vein may be difficult to find. The middle veins may override the capsule and must be identified and divided before an attempt is made to enucleate the gland.

The *inferior thyroid vein* leaves the lower pole in one or more trunks, frequently forming a plexus of veins. The inferior thyroid vein is not adjacent to the inferior thyroid artery, which is in the region of the middle third of the gland. The inferior thyroid artery is more closely associated with the middle or lateral thyroid veins. The inferior thyroid vein empties into the internal jugular vein and at times directly into the innominate vein. Occasionally, a vein (v. thyreoidea ima) drains the isthmus, passing downward on the trachea to enter the left innominate vein. The inferior thyroid veins may be closely interwoven with the recurrent nerve as it ascends. This area is vulnerable to injury to the recurrent laryngeal nerve.

## The Arteries

The *superior thyroid artery* arises as the first branch from the external carotid artery at about the level of the bifurcation of the common carotid artery (Fig. 3–3). It runs downward and medially on the surface of the inferior constrictor muscles, entering the upper pole of the thyroid on its anteromedial surface. In its downward course, it is just inferior and lateral to the superior laryngeal nerve. The superior laryngeal nerve usually turns medial from the superior thyroid artery about 1 cm above the pole, but it can be intertwined in its branches. Care must be exercised in ligating the superior thyroid artery close to its entrance to the gland to avoid injury to the superior laryngeal nerve. In many pathologically enlarged thyroid glands, a lingula of thyroid tissue is found above and lateral to the point of entry of the superior thyroid artery and the superior laryngeal nerve. This lingula represents the upper pole, and the artery may be ligated too high with possible damage to the superior laryngeal nerve. Occasionally, a branch of the superior thyroid artery to the pyramidal lobe and isthmus may arise high, and bleeding may occur from the upper pole after ligation of the superior thyroid artery simply because the artery was ligated below the origin of this branch to the pyramidal lobe.

The *inferior thyroid arteries* arise from the thyrocervical trunks shortly after their origin from the subclavian arteries. They ascend upward behind the jugular veins and carotid arteries to a level well above the inferior pole of the thyroid. They make a loop downward and medially and enter the gland at its midportion, not at the inferior pole as is stated frequently in the literature. The surgeon's first glimpse of the inferior thyroid artery usually comes when the thyroid gland is retracted medially and the jugular vein is retracted laterally. It appears from beneath the carotid artery opposite the midsection of the thyroid. Before entering the thyroid, the inferior thyroid artery may divide into one or more branches and be intimately associated with one or more branches of the recurrent laryngeal nerve (see description of nerve). One branch of the inferior thyroid artery supplies the inferior parathyroid gland, and a small branch frequently supplies the superior gland also.

The *lower thyroid artery* may be present, although this is unusual in our experience. It arises from the aorta or innominate artery and passes directly upward in front of the trachea to enter the lower border of the isthmus. It is usually ligated with the inferior thyroid veins.

## THE LYMPHATIC SYSTEM

Knowledge of the lymphatic drainage of the thyroid gland is obtained from anatomic dissection, injection techniques, and radiologic contrast study (lymphangiography).[6, 13] One important characteristic of the lymphatic drainage system of the thyroid is that it is extensive and may flow in a variety of directions: vertically as far as the mediastinum or upper neck and horizontally as far as the lateral neck or the retropharyngeal area and even to the opposite side.

Regional nodes of the thyroid gland are the paraglandular nodes; pretracheal nodes; paratracheal nodes; recurrent laryngeal nerve chain; anterosuperior mediastinal nodes; upper jugular, middle jugular, and lower jugular group both anterior and lateral to the subclavian vein; and the retropharyngeal and retroesophageal group (Fig. 3–4).

The neck is divided by the sternocleidomastoid muscle into an anterior and a posterior triangle. The inferior belly of the omohyoid muscle divides the posterior triangle into a separate muscular triangle, the caudad subclavian triangle. The lower jugular, the midjugular, and the upper jugular groups are the deep lymph nodes of the neck. All are contiguous to the internal jugular vein and the undersurface of the sternocleidomastoid muscle. The upper jugular nodes are intimately associated with the internal jugular vein and the upper end of the spinal accessory nerve as they pass deep to the posterior belly of the digastric muscle toward the jugular foramen. The subdigastric nodes in the carotid triangle are part of the jugular chain bounded by the anterior border of the ster-

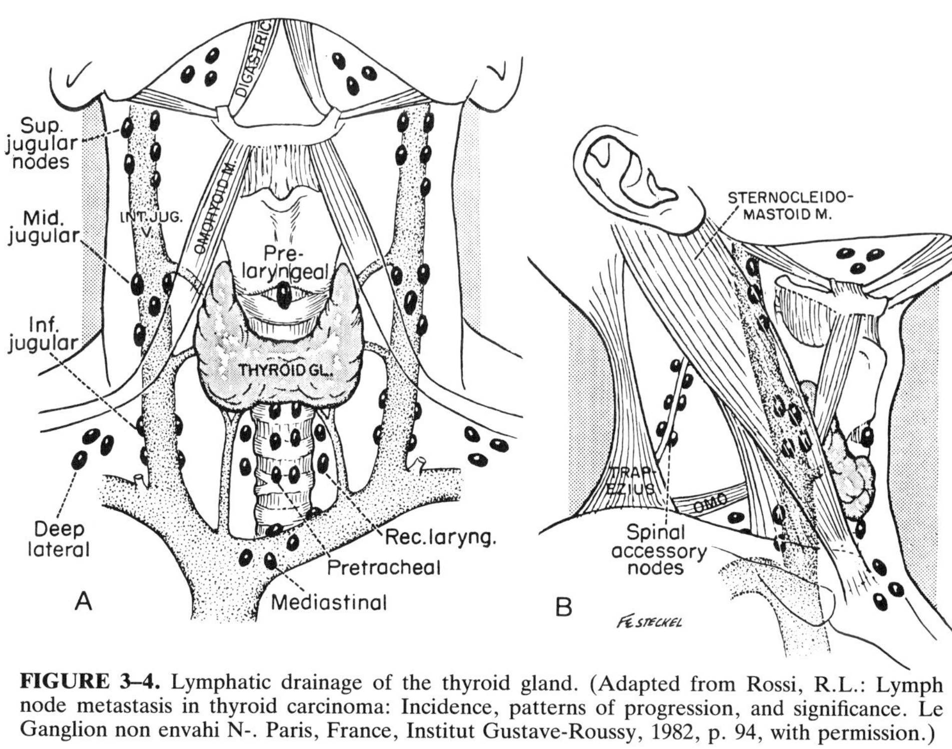


**FIGURE 3–4.** Lymphatic drainage of the thyroid gland. (Adapted from Rossi, R.L.: Lymph node metastasis in thyroid carcinoma: Incidence, patterns of progression, and significance. Le Ganglion non envahi N-. Paris, France, Institut Gustave-Roussy, 1982, p. 94, with permission.)

nocleidomastoid muscle, the superior belly of the omohyoid muscle, and the posterior belly of the digastric muscle.

Collecting lymph channels draining the intraglandular capillaries are found beneath the thyroid capsule.[13] These channels drain into the lymph vessels associated with the capsule and may cross-communicate with the isthmus and opposite lobe.

Injection studies[6, 13] have shown that lymph vessels extend upward, downward, and laterally from the thyroid gland. In general, the lymphatics accompany the veins. Those passing downward enter small lymphatic nodes on the ventral and ventrolateral surfaces of the trachea and toward nodes of the anterosuperior mediastinum just cephalad to the innominate veins. The connections with the superoanterior mediastinal nodes occur directly through lymphatics of the lower portion of the thyroid gland or lymphatics that follow the recurrent laryngeal nerves. The lymph vessels, which pass upward from the thyroid gland, connect to the prelaryngeal nodes, paraglandular nodes, deep upper cervical (superior jugular) nodes, and superficial cervical nodes. Laterally, lymphatic channels are traced to nodes situated about the carotid artery and internal jugular vein (middle and lower). Rouvière[21] described a group of lymphatics draining the posterior and superior aspect of the thyroid gland to lymphatics in the retropharyngeal area and found this to be present in one fifth of his dissections.

Metastasis to lymph nodes in the anterosuperior mediastinum may provide, in some instances, a route for spread to the contralateral neck.[5] These nodes in the retropharyngeal area and nodes in the superior mediastinum are not usually eradicated by radical neck dissection techniques. No important lymphatic communications have been identified between the anterosuperior mediastinum, the thymus, and the other mediastinal compartments.[5, 6, 14, 21] Lymph node metastases in differentiated thyroid carcinoma are estimated to occur in more than 70 per cent of patients when a systematic node dissection is performed, especially in a young patient with a papillary tumor.[3, 9, 17, 25] Noguchi et al.[17] suggested that the pattern of nodal metastasis in the early stages of thyroid cancer is directed downward and laterally toward the mediastinum and lower neck. In the later stages of disease and probably when the pretracheal and paratracheal nodes have become obstructed by tumor, metastasis follows an upward direction toward the deep upper cervical nodes (Fig. 3–5). The submaxillary nodes are infrequently involved.

## THE NERVES

The *recurrent laryngeal nerves* arise from the vagus nerves at different levels on the two sides (Fig. 3–6). The right recurrent laryngeal nerve arises where the vagus nerve crosses the first portion of the subclavian artery. The nerve hooks around the lower and posterior aspect of the subclavian artery and ascends lateral to the trachea, entering the larynx posterior to the thyroid at the cricothyroid articulation. The left recurrent laryngeal nerve leaves the vagus nerve as the vagus nerve crosses over the arch of the aorta. It hooks around the aorta and ascends again, as the right recurrent nerve does, lateral to the trachea to its terminal branches within the laryngeal muscles.

As emphasized by Fowler and Hanson,[8] the usual textbook description of the nerves ascending in the groove between the rounded surfaces of the trachea and esophagus at the lower pole of the thyroid out of harm's way was not found in their dissection of 400 recurrent nerves. They stated, and this has been our experience, that the nerves in the region of the lower pole of the thyroid gland are 1 to 2 cm lateral to the trachea. At this level, as the recurrent laryngeal nerve ascends to the middle third of the thyroid gland, it may consist of several branches closely associated with the inferior thyroid artery. It may pass posterior or superficial to the inferior thyroid artery or its branches may intertwine in innumerable variations. This is the most vulnerable area for injury to the recurrent laryngeal nerve. Rarely does the recurrent laryngeal nerve branch below the inferior thyroid artery. Therefore, it is safer to search for the nerve below the artery. Reed[18] listed 28 types of relationships of the recurrent laryngeal nerve to the inferior thyroid artery (Fig. 3–7). Investigation by Dedo[7] indicated that the recurrent laryngeal nerve has only one motor trunk innervating the laryngeal muscles (Fig. 3–8). The other extralar-

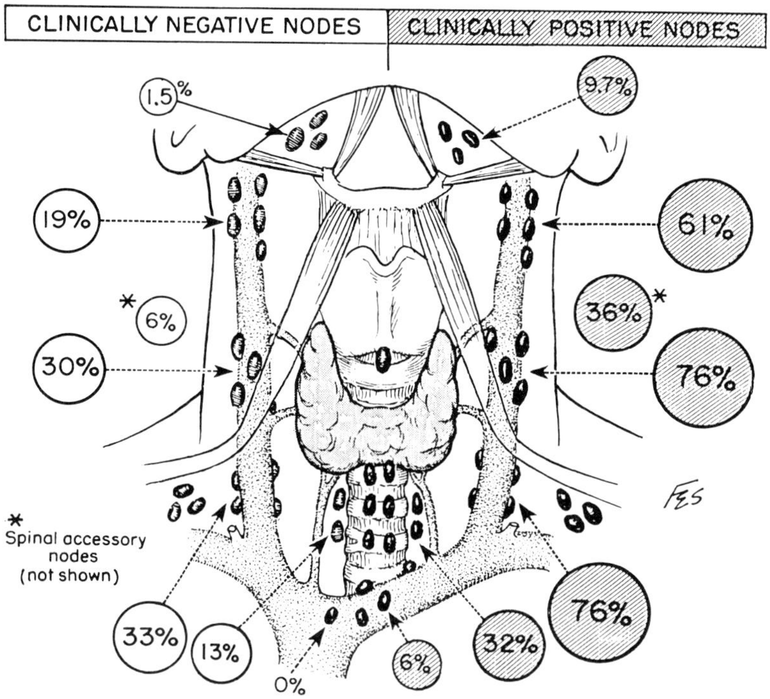


**FIGURE 3–5.** Patterns of lymph node involvement in thyroid carcinoma. In the early stages of thyroid carcinoma, involvement is directed downward and laterally toward the lower neck and mediastinum. In the later stages and when pretracheal and paratracheal nodes have become obstructed by tumor, metastasis follows an upward direction toward the upper cervical nodes. (Adapted from Frazell, E.L., Foote, F.W., Jr.: Papillary thyroid carcinoma: Pathological findings in cases with and without clinical evidence of cervical node involvement. Cancer, *8*:1164–1166, 1955.)

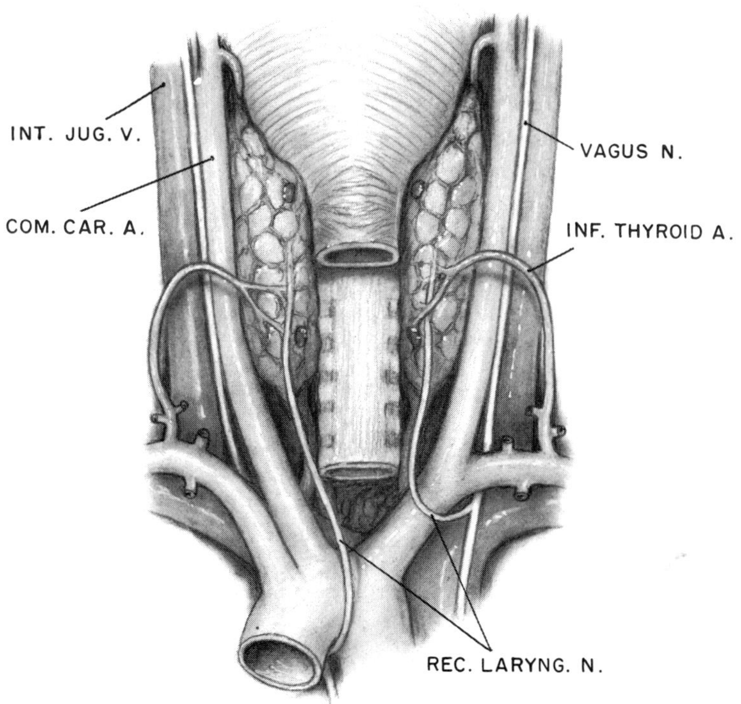


**FIGURE 3–6.** Posterior view. Recurrent laryngeal nerves and the inferior thyroid arteries. The recurrent laryngeal nerves as they ascend in the region of the lower pole of the thyroid are lateral to the tracheal groove.

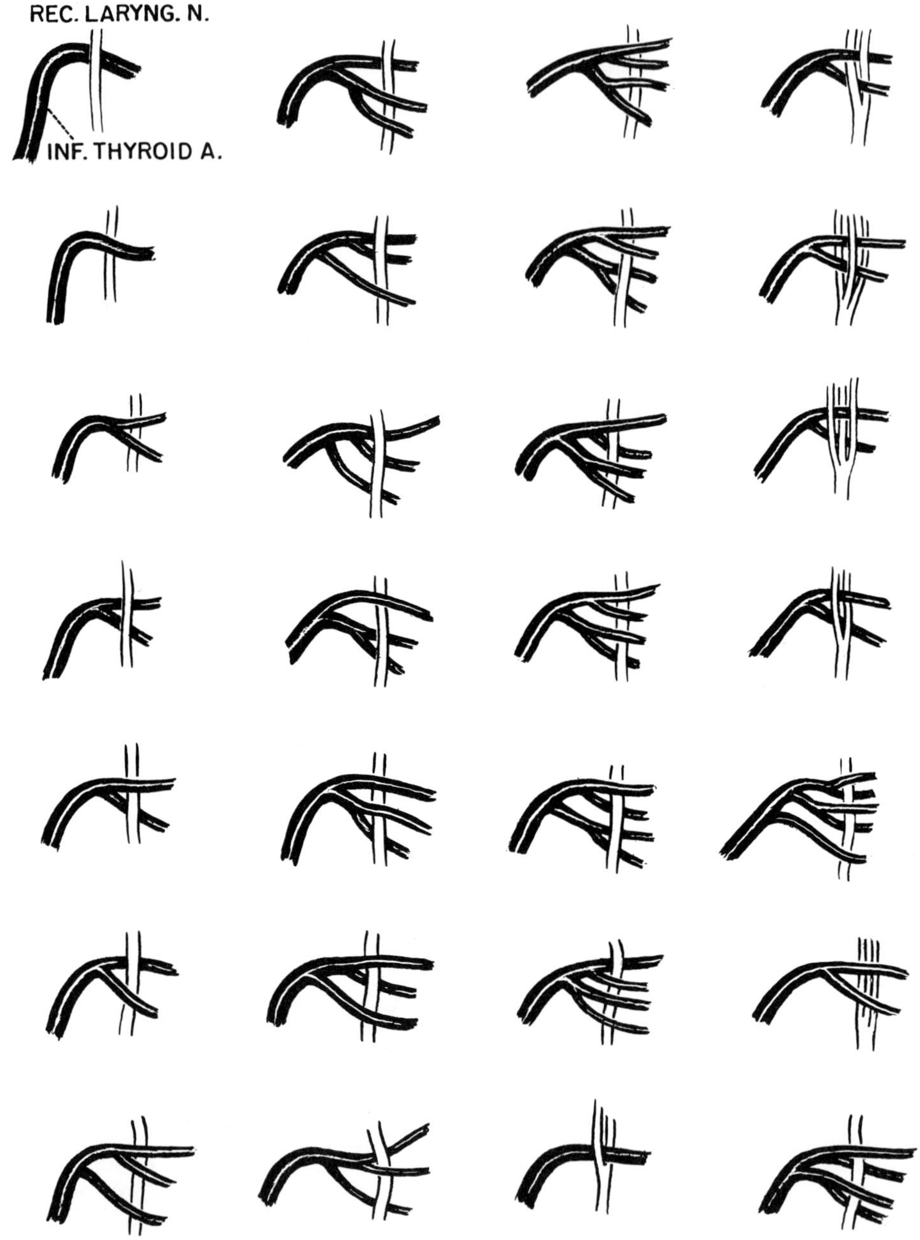


**FIGURE 3–7.** Types of relationships of the inferior laryngeal nerve to the inferior thyroid artery. (Adapted from Reed, A.F.: Relations of inferior laryngeal nerve to inferior thyroid artery. Anat. Rec., *85*:18, 1943.)

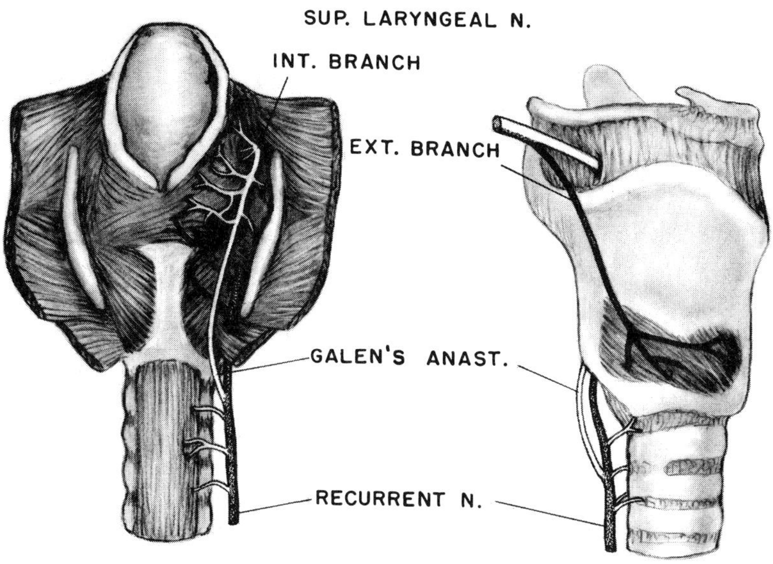


**FIGURE 3–8.** The recurrent laryngeal nerve has only one motor branch to the laryngeal muscles. The other extralaryngeal branches are sensory, one of which joins the sensory branch of the superior laryngeal nerve to form the loop of Galen. The superior laryngeal nerve divides into two branches: the internal or motor branch innervates the cricohyoid muscle, and the lateral or sensory branch forms the loop of Galen. (Adapted from Dedo, H.H.: The paralyzed larynx: An electromyographic study in dogs and humans. Laryngoscope, *80*:1467, 1970.)

yngeal branches are sensory, one of which may join the sensory branch of the superior laryngeal nerve to form the loop of Galen (Fig. 3–8).

From the practical point of view, the thyroid surgeon must consider each extralaryngeal branch of the recurrent nerve as the possible motor nerve supplying the laryngeal muscles and make every attempt to preserve them all. It continues upward and medially in close relationship with the posterior capsule of the middle third of the thyroid gland and enters the larynx between the arch of the cricoid cartilage and the inferior cornu of the thyroid cartilage. When mobilizing the posterior aspects of the gland, the surgeon must be aware of this close relationship.

The recurrent nerve, on rare occasions,

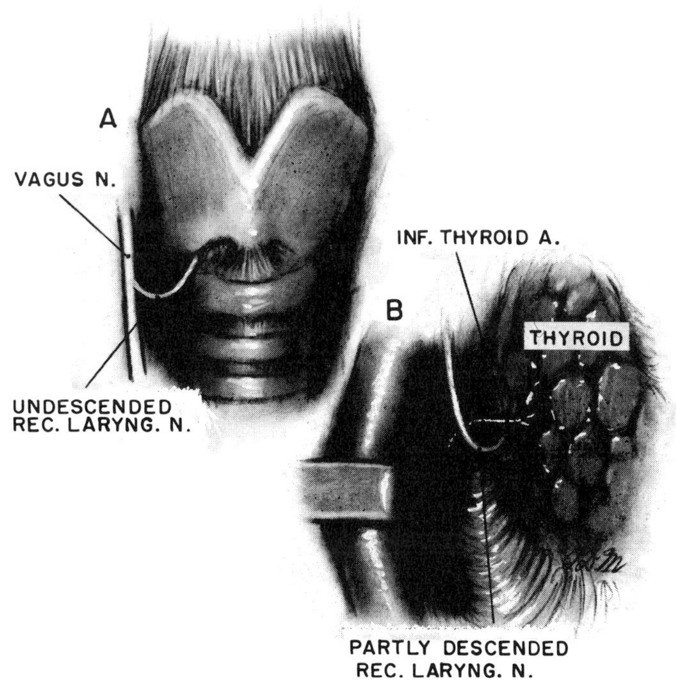


**FIGURE 3–9.** *A*, The unusual but occasional undescended inferior laryngeal nerve passing directly from vagus to beneath the horn of the thyroid cartilage (nonrecurrent laryngeal nerve). *B*, Partly descended recurrent nerve passing underneath the inferior thyroid artery but not descending into the chest.

does not recur and passes directly across from the vagus nerve either in close apposition to the superior thyroid vessels (Fig. 3–9) or in proximity to the inferior thyroid artery. For this reason, we identify the recurrent laryngeal nerve before the superior or inferior thyroid vessels are ligated.

The *superior laryngeal nerve* arises from the vagus nerve close to the base of the skull, descends medially to the carotid vessels, and, at the level of the hyoid cornu, divides into two branches. The internal branch is sensory; it penetrates the thyrohyoid membranes and may anastomose with the sensory branch of the recurrent laryngeal nerve to complete the loop of Galen (Fig. 3–8). The external branch of the superior laryngeal nerve lies on the lateral surface of the inferior pharyngeal constrictor muscle and descends to innervate the cricothyroid muscle. Both branches lie immediately adjacent to the superior thyroid artery and may be injured if the superior thyroid artery is ligated en masse or too high above its entrance into the thyroid gland.

When the recurrent nerve is injured, paralysis of the vocal cord occurs on the ipsilateral side. Controversy exists concerning an explanation for the position of the paralyzed cord and the neuromuscular mechanism involved. The laryngeal muscles (five on each side) controlling motion of the vocal cords are the abductors (the internal arytenoid and the thyroarytenoid) and the adductors (the lateral and the posterior cricoarytenoids) and are innervated by the recurrent laryngeal nerve. The cricothyroid muscle, which determines range of voice (the tensors of the vocal cord), is innervated by the internal branch of the superior laryngeal nerve. Early investigators, particularly Rosenbach[20] (1880) and Semon[23] (1881), postulated that the abductor fibers of the recurrent nerve are more susceptible to pressure than the adductor fibers—the Semon-Rosenbach law. Wagner[26] (1890) and Grossmann[12] (1897) stated that paralysis of the vocal cord in the paramedian position was the result of injury to the recurrent laryngeal nerve and that paralysis of the cord in the intermediate position was the result of injury to the recurrent laryngeal nerve and the superior laryngeal nerve—the Wagner-Grossmann theory. Another popular theory was based on the extralaryngeal branchings of the recurrent nerves.[2, 4, 15, 16, 22, 29] This hypothesis assumed that the extralaryngeal branches went to abductors or adductors. Division of the adductor branch would place the cords in an abducted position, and injury to the abductor fibers would place the cord in an adductor position.

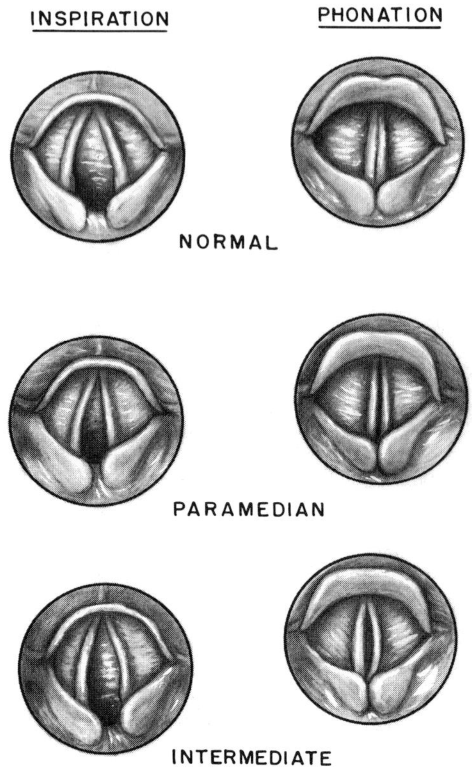


**FIGURE 3–10.** Human vocal cord shape and position during inspiration and phonation caused by specific laryngeal nerve paralyses. *Normal,* recording position of electrodes in intrinsic muscles; *paramedian,* right recurrent nerve paralysis; *intermediate,* right recurrent and superior laryngeal nerve paralysis. Note the medial prominence of vocal process seen best during inspiration. (Adapted from Dedo, H.H.: The paralyzed larynx: An electromyographic study in dogs and humans. Laryngoscope, *80*:1470, 1970.)

Dedo,[7] in an excellent paper, reviewed the many theories on the innervation of the larynx and the mechanism of laryngeal paralysis. He also studied laryngeal paralysis in dogs and human beings, correlating clinical and electromyographic findings, and concluded that the "behavior of paralyzed vocal cords is best explained by the Wagner-Grossmann theory—that complete paralysis of the recurrent nerve causes a vocal cord to be immobilized in the paramedian position, and combined paralysis of the recurrent laryngeal and superior laryngeal nerves causes a vocal cord to be paralyzed in the intermediate position" (Fig. 3–10). Furthermore, he found no evidence to support the concept of extralaryngeal branching into abductor and adductor trunks.

## THYROID GLAND

The normal thyroid gland is soft and uneven in outline and weighs about 20 g. It is spread between two lateral lobes and a connecting smaller bridge, the isthmus, a strip of thyroid tissue of variable width and thickness but much thinner than the adjacent lobes. In a thin normal person, the isthmus can be palpated overlying the trachea halfway between the cricoid cartilage and the sternal notch. It appears as a rubbery transverse ridge, perhaps 1.0 to 1.5 cm wide, when the fingers are moved up and down over the trachea. It frequently needs to be divided during tracheostomy.

The lateral lobes lie beneath the sternocleidomastoid and vertical strap muscles (see Fig. 3–1) and can be difficult to palpate even in a thin patient. The normal thyroid lobes are virtually impossible to palpate in heavyset, muscular, or short-necked individuals. Each normal lobe measures approximately 4 to 5 cm in height, 1 to 2 cm in lateral thickness, and 2 to 3 cm in anteroposterior width. The normal gland nestles in its bed (Figs. 3–3 and 3–6) surrounded closely by critical structures but largely in an anteroposterior orientation (Fig. 3–11). We so infrequently see a normal-size thyroid gland and usually only visualize abnormal glands when they are retracted vigorously anteriorly out of this bed that we forget the deep position of the posterior surface of the thyroid lobes and their predominantly anteroposterior orientation.

Frequently, a pyramidal lobe extends upward from the isthmus, usually on the left side, which represents the migratory path of the thyroid gland anlage in embryonic life. This pyramidal extension may be represented by a thin strand of tissue or a recognizable thin column of thyroid gland of 1 or 2 mm in diameter that ends a variable distance from the thyroid. This tissue must be removed in the presence of Graves' disease, goiter, or Hashimoto's thyroiditis because continued enlargement may present as an unsightly enlargement in the anterior upper neck.

## PARATHYROID GLANDS

A basic understanding of the embryologic development and normal anatomy of para-

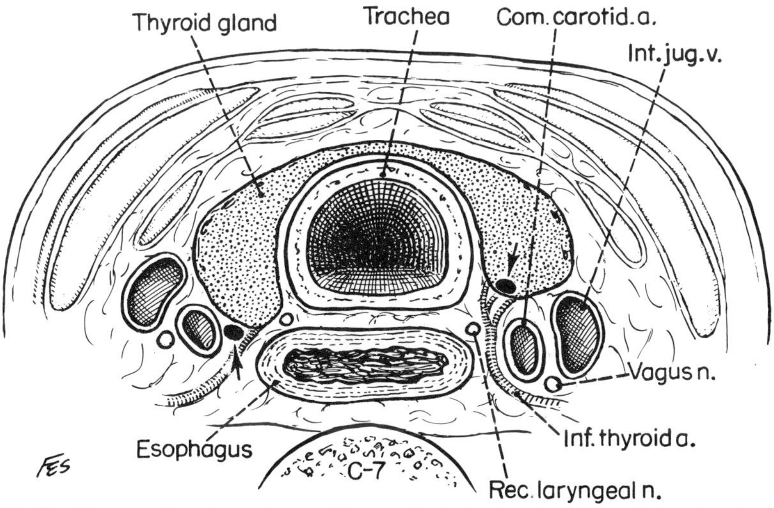


**FIGURE 3–11.** Cross-sectional anatomy of the neck at the level of the midthyroid gland. Note the posterior and medial general location of the parathyroid glands and the close approximation of the esophagus. (After Testut-Jacob.)

thyroid glands is important in performing parathyroid surgery. The surgeon must be familiar with the appearance of normal and abnormal glands to decide which gland or glands should be excised or assessed pathologically by biopsy.

The parathyroid bodies arise as a proliferation of endodermal cells at the lateral tip of the third and fourth pharyngeal pouches. The third pouch gives rise to the inferior parathyroid glands and to the thymus, which will migrate to the mediastinum. The fourth pouch gives rise to the superior parathyroid glands, is less closely associated with a migrating thymus, and is more closely associated with the lateral developing thyroid lobes.[11]

In 527 autopsies, Gilmour[10] found that about 80 per cent of the patients had four parathyroid glands, 6 per cent had five glands, and 13 per cent had three glands. The presence of as many as eight parathyroid glands has been documented, but patients with fewer than three or more than five glands are uncommon. In 160 autopsies, Wang[27] noted that three patients had five glands for an incidence of 1.9 per cent and one patient had six glands for an incidence of 0.6 per cent. He conjectured that the finding of fewer than four glands was the result of an inability to locate all glands.

In an autopsy series of 503 patients,[1] 3 per cent of patients had three glands, 84 per cent of patients had four glands, and 13 per cent of patients had a supernumerary gland. In approximately two thirds of patients, the supernumerary gland was found below the thyroid in association with a thymic liagment or the thymus on either side. In approximately one third of patients, the supernumerary gland was found in the vicinity of the thyroid between the two other glands.

The position of the glands on one side was symmetric with that on the other side in approximately 80 per cent of patients. The superior parathyroid glands were most frequently found about the intersection between the laryngeal nerve and the inferior thyroid artery. The commonest location of inferior parathyroid glands was somewhat more ventral, close to the lower thyroid pole, or in the upper thymus. In a few patients, the lower parathyroid glands were situated higher up in the neck because of failure of descent during embryologic development. Inferior parathyroid glands more than 2 cm below the lower pole of the thyroid were associated universally with thymic tissue. Only rare exceptions to this have been found, such as parathyroid glands located in the pericardium.

Parathyroid glands lying totally within the thyroid gland were not encountered by Wang[27] and were found in only 0.2 per cent of the patients reported on by Åkerström et al.[1] The anatomic locations of upper and lower parathyroid glands as dissected by Gilmour[10] are summarized in Figures 3–12 and 3–13, and the locations of the parathyroid glands as described by Wang[27] are shown in Figures 3–14 and 3–15. These findings are similar to those published by Åkerström et al.,[1] who found that the superior parathyroid glands in about 80 per cent of patients were located within a circumscribed area of 2 cm in diameter, about 1 cm above the intersection of the recurrent laryngeal nerve and the inferior thyroid artery. The glands were frequently concealed in the connective tissue fibers that bind the posterior edge of the thyroid lobe to the larynx. In 4 per cent of patients, superior parathyroid glands were located farther down and sometimes were obscured by the inferior thyroid artery, recurrent laryngeal nerve, or a protrusion of the thyroid. Superior parathyroid glands at the level of the superior pole of the thyroid gland were found in 2 per cent of patients, and location above the upper thyroid pole was found in 0.8 per cent of patients. Superior parathyroid glands were uncommonly found (1 per cent of patients) in an ectopic position, that is, more posterior in the neck in the retropharyngeal or retroesophageal space. In 61 per cent of patients, the inferior parathyroid glands were inferior, posterior, or lateral to the thyroid pole. In 17 per cent of patients, the lower glands were found anteriorly high up on the thyroid lobe closely attached to the thyroid capsule. In 26 per cent of patients, the inferior parathyroid glands were closely associated with the superior thymus. The inferior glands located in the thymus and farther down in the mediastinum were seen in only 2 per cent of patients, and only three glands (0.2 per cent of patients) were encountered below the thymus in the anterior mediastinum.

Although the studies[1, 10, 27] previously referred to were carried out in patients without

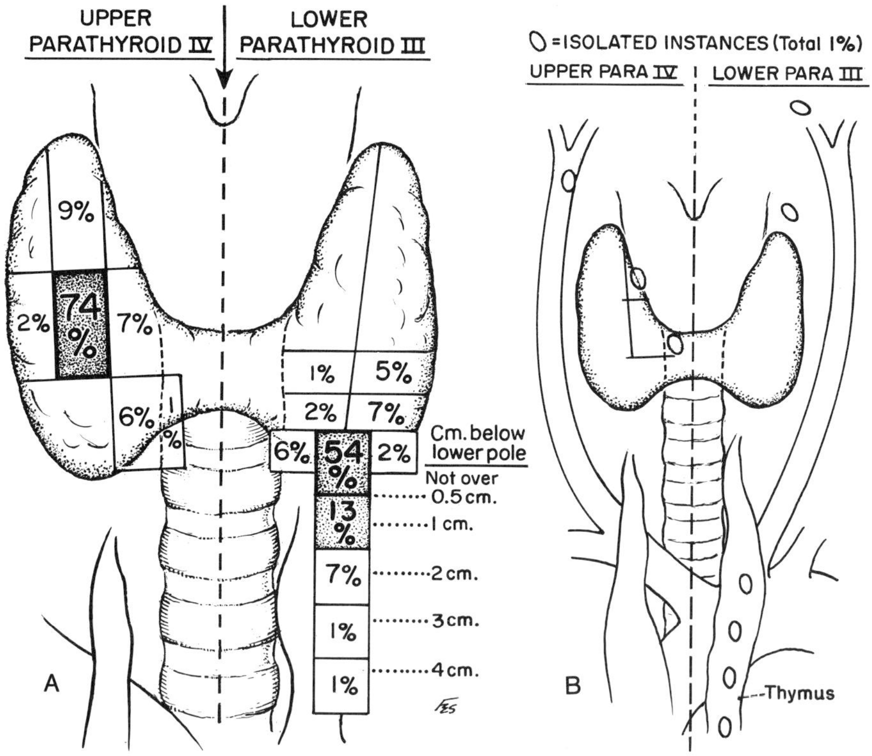


**FIGURE 3–12.** *A*, Frontal view of anatomic location of upper and lower parathyroid glands as dissected by Gilmour. *B*, Location of uncommon aberrant upper (*left*) and lower (*right*) parathyroid glands.

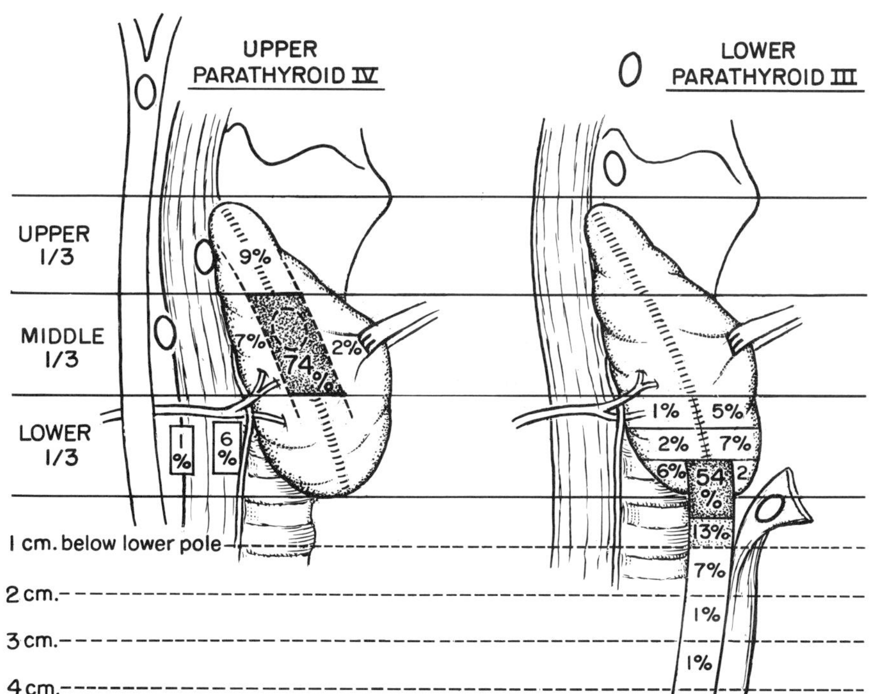


**FIGURE 3–13.** Lateral view of anatomic location of upper and lower parathyroid glands as dissected by Gilmour.

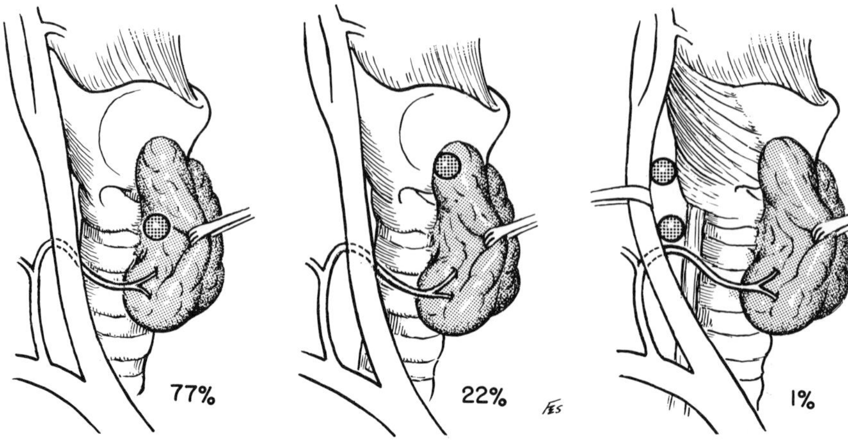


**FIGURE 3–14.** Location of upper parathyroid glands as dissected by Wang.

hyperparathyroidism, Thompson et al.[24] reported on a prospective anatomic study performed on patients with known primary hyperparathyroidism over a 4-year period. Adenoma of a single gland was found in 80 per cent of patients, hyperplasia was found in 15 per cent of patients, and two adenomas were found in 2.6 per cent of patients. In one third of patients, adenomas of the superior parathyroid glands were found in abnormal locations, that is, in retropharyngeal, retroesophageal, paraesophageal, and tracheoesophageal grooves. These neoplasms were frequently within the posterosuperior mediastinum. No superior parathyroid adenoma was intrathyroidal, although about 15 per cent were completely beneath the thyroid sheath surrounding the upper pole of the gland and were not easily identified even after the lateral aspect of the upper pole had been mobilized. Twelve per cent of adenomas of the right inferior parathyroid gland and 16 per cent of adenomas of the left inferior parathyroid gland were found in an ectopic location, such as the thymus, carotid sheath, or within the lower pole of the thyroid. Adenomas of an intrathyroidal inferior parathyroid gland were found in 2 per cent of patients. In contrast to the findings of the autopsy series of normal parathyroid glands in which only 1 per cent of the superior glands were found behind the lower pharynx or esophagus, Thompson et al.[24] found that more than one third of adenomas of superior glands were located in those abnormal positions. The incidence of adenomas of intrathymic parathyroid glands was 14 per cent and that of anterior mediastinal adenoma was only 1.8 per cent.

These studies suggest that the great majority of glands are positioned not only in a regular and symmetric fashion but also at distinct sites in relation to the thyroid. Therefore, careful exploration of the common locations with a meticulous technique is advised before direct search for unusual positions. Identification of the normal glands is important because exploration for a specific missing gland can be conducted in a logical sequence based on knowledge of the anatomy and embryology of the parathyroid glands. An awareness of the frequency of ectopic adenomas and their usual locations is helpful.

Wang[28] has also reported on 104 abnormal glands clearly localized at reexploration after a previous unsuccessful attempt to relieve hyperparathyroidism. Figures 3–16 and 3–17 demonstrate the anatomic locations of these glands. Thirty-four glands were in the posterosuperior mediastinum, and 34 were in direct association with the mediastinal thymus, of which 21 required sternotomy for extraction. The anatomic positions of these recurrent or obscure glands in hyperparathyroidism merely confirm the figures for location and incidence described previously.

In a few patients, even repeated operations will fail to reveal the tumor, thus implying that instances of extremely obscure locations occur. We[19] have reported a gland residing

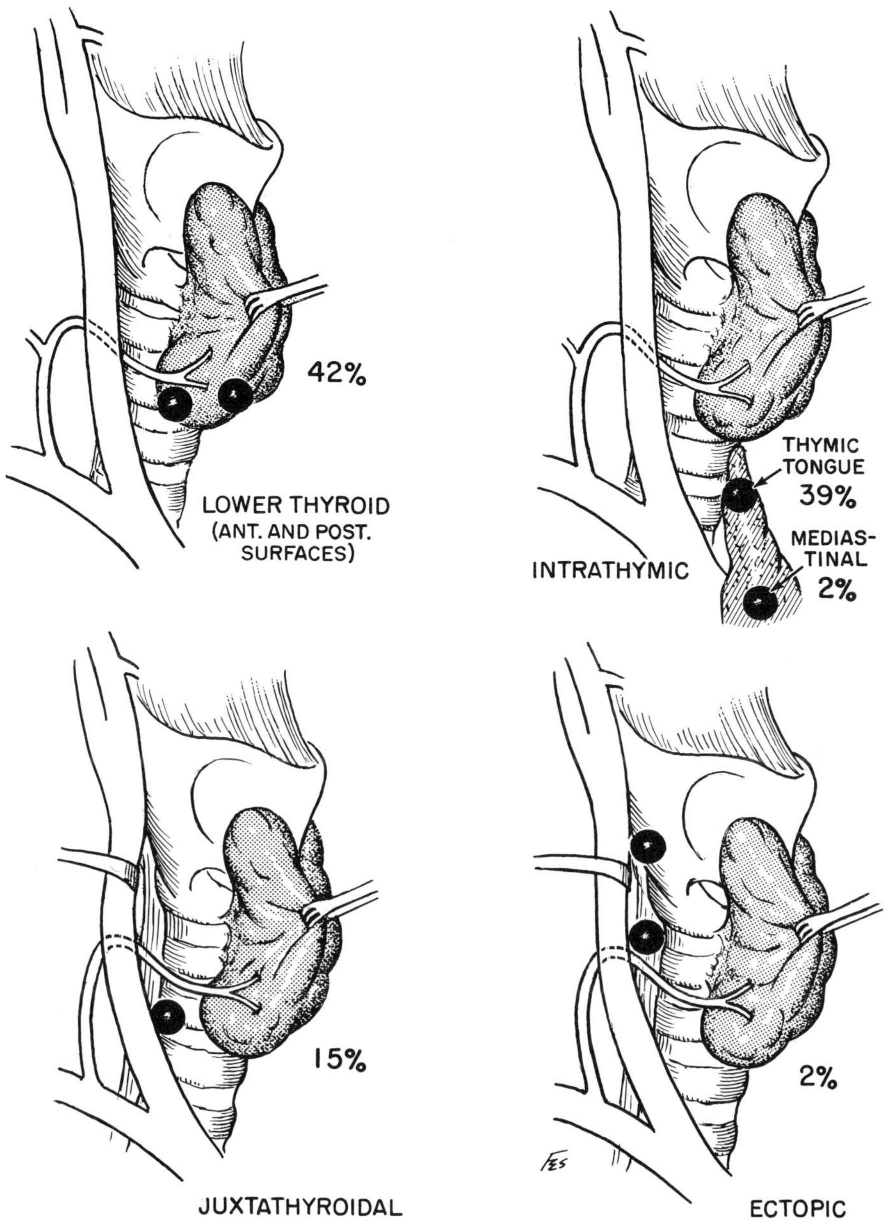


**FIGURE 3–15.** Location of lower parathyroid glands as described by Wang.

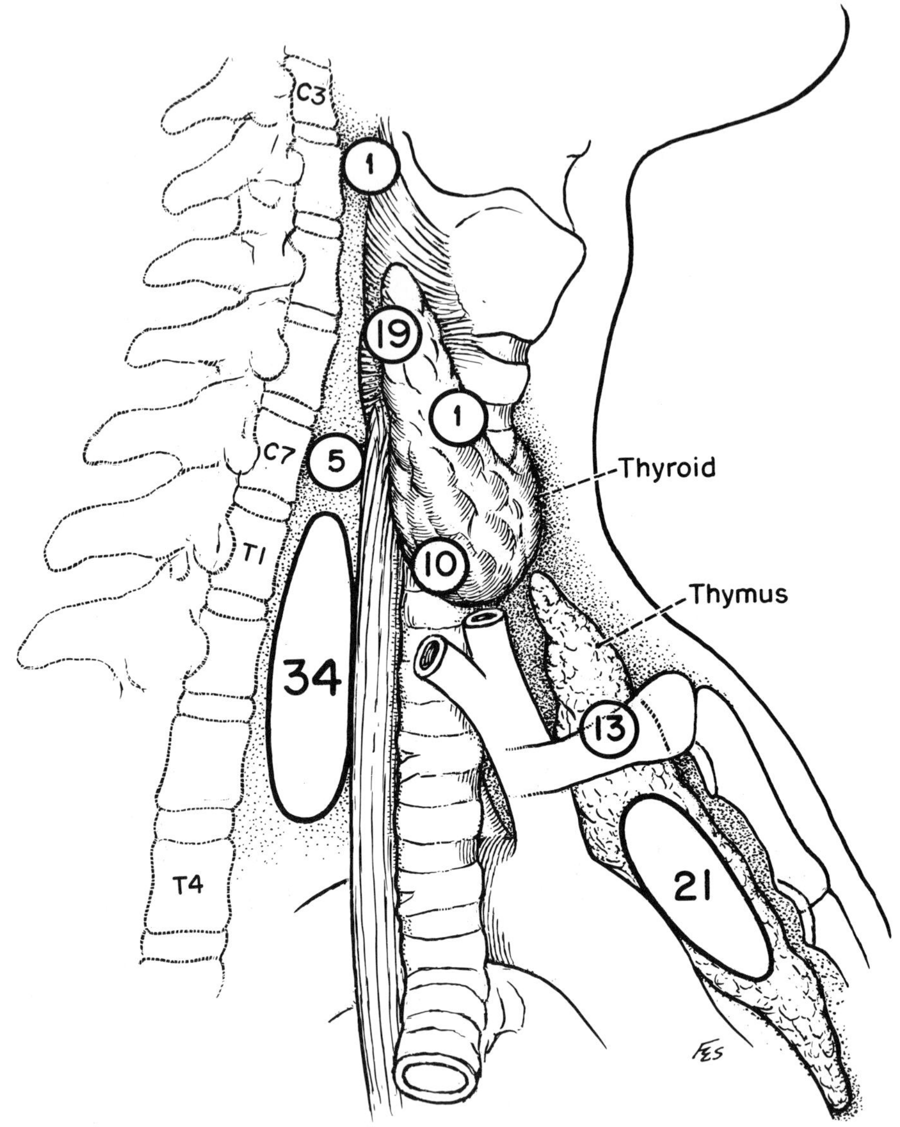


**FIGURE 3–16.** Location of parathyroid glands seen at reoperation after failure to cure hyperparathyroidism at initial surgery as described by Wang.

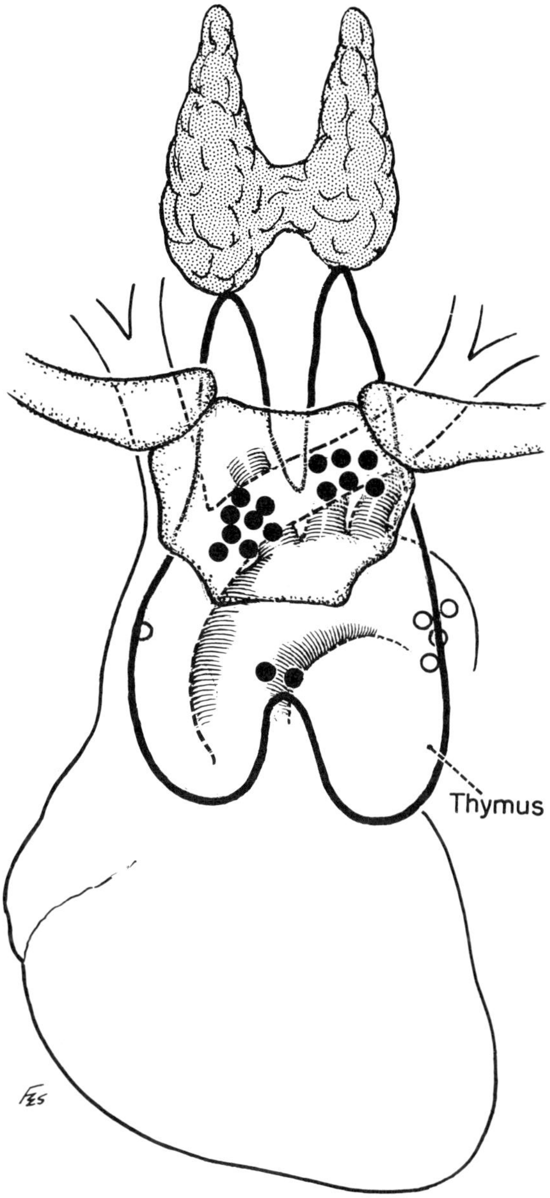


**FIGURE 3–17.** Frontal view of 21 parathyroid adenomas that required a median sternotomy for resection according to Wang. Open circles represent glands enclosed in thymus; closed circles indicate those behind thymus.

within the vagus nerve, and Wang[28] noted adenomas located at the tracheal carina, anterior to the right pulmonary artery, and behind the aortic arch. Some adenomas are so obscure that they are not found even at autopsy. Normal parathyroid glands, being far smaller, may be even more difficult to find.

Wang[28] noted that normal glands weighed, on an average, 35 to 40 mg but ranged between 10 and 78 mg. Their size was usually about 5 × 3 × 1 mm but ranged from 12 × 2 × 1 mm to 2 × 2 × 1 mm. The glands are usually yellowish tan—a color distinctive from the brighter yellow fat—although they may be surrounded by fat and thus be obscured. A reliable test at the operating table has been reported by Wang.[28] Parathyroid tissue stripped of fat always sinks in saline solution, whereas fat always floats. When the parathyroid gland is traumatized, its color, owing to hemorrhage, becomes mahogany; this color, too, is distinctive. The glands are softer than thyroid tissue or lymph nodes and may assume a wide variety of shapes. Frequently, the upper gland is beneath the thyroid capsule; less commonly, the lower gland may be subcapsular. In these situations, an incision through the posterior thyroid capsule will be required to expose the gland, which will be flat.

## REFERENCES


1. Åkerström, G., Malmaeus, J., and Bergstrom, R.: Surgical anatomy of human parathyroid glands. Surgery, *95*:14–21, 1984.
2. Armstrong, W. G., and Hinton, J. W.: Multiple divisions of recurrent laryngeal nerve: Anatomic study. Arch. Surg., *62*:532–539, 1951.
3. Attie, J. N., Khafif, R. A., and Steckler, R. M.: Elective neck dissection in papillary carcinoma of the thyroid. Am. J. Surg., *122*:464–471, 1971.
4. Berlin, D. D., and Lahey, F. H.: Dissections of recurrent and superior laryngeal nerves: Relation of recurrent to inferior thyroid artery and relation of superior to abductor paralysis. Surg. Gynecol. Obstet., *49*:102–104, 1929.
5. Block, M. A., Miller, J. M., and Horn, R. C., Jr.: Significance of mediastinal lymph node metastases in carcinoma of the thyroid. Am. J. Surg., *123*:702–705, 1972.
6. Chouke, K. S., Whitehead, R. W., and Parker, A. E.: Is there a closed lymphatic system connecting the thyroid and thymus glands? Surg. Gynecol. Obstet., *54*:865–871, 1932.
7. Dedo, H. H.: The paralyzed larynx: An electromyographic study in dogs and humans. Laryngoscope, *80*:1455–1517, 1970.
8. Fowler, C. H., and Hanson, W. A.: Surgical anatomy of thyroid gland with special reference to relations of recurrent laryngeal nerve. Surg. Gynecol. Obstet., *49*:59–65, 1929.
9. Frazell, E. L., and Foote, F. W., Jr.: Papillary thyroid carcinoma: Pathological findings in cases with and without clinical evidence of cervical node involvement. Cancer, *8*:1164–1166, 1955.
10. Gilmour, J. R.: Gross anatomy of the parathyroid glands. J. Pathol. Bacteriol., *46*:133–149, 1938.
11. Gray, S. W., and Skandalakis, J. E.: Embryology for Surgeons: Embryological Basis for Treatment of Congenital Defects. Philadelphia, W. B. Saunders Co., 1972.
12. Grossmann, M.: Experimentelle Beiträge zur Lehre von der Posticuslähmung. Arch. Laryngol. Rhinol., *6*:282–360, 1897.
13. Haagensen, C. D., Feind, C. R., Herter, F. P., Slanetz, C. A., Jr., and Weinberg, J. A.: The Lymphatics in Cancer. Philadelphia, W. B. Saunders Co., 1972.
14. Johner, C. H., and Ranniger, K.: Mediastinal lymphography. Surg. Gynecol. Obstet., *127*:1313–1316, 1968.
15. King, B. T., and Gregg, R. L.: Anatomical reason for the various behaviors of paralyzed vocal cords. Ann. Otol., *57*:925–944, 1948.
16. Morrison, L. F.: Recurrent laryngeal nerve paralysis: Revised conception based on dissection of 100 cadavers. Ann. Otol., *61*:567–592, 1952.
17. Noguchi, S., Noguchi, A., and Murakami, N.: Papillary carcinoma of the thyroid. I. Developing pattern of metastasis. Cancer, *26*:1053–1060, 1970.
18. Reed, A. F.: Relations of inferior laryngeal nerve to inferior thyroid artery. Anat. Rec., *85*:17–23, 1943.
19. Reiling, R. B., Cady, B., and Clerkin, E. P.: Aberrant parathyroid adenoma within vagus nerve. Lahey Clin. Bull., *21*:158–162, 1972.
20. Rosenbach, O.: Zur Lehre von der doppelseitigen totalen Lähmung des Nerv laryngeus inferior (recurens). Breslau Aerztl. Z., *2*:14–16, 27–30, 1880.
21. Rouvière, H.: Anatomy of the Human Lymphatic System. A compendium translated from the original "Anatomie des Lymphatiques de l'Homme" and rearranged for the use of students and practitioners by M. J. Tobias. Ann Arbor, Michigan, Edward Brothers, 1938.
22. Rustad, W. H.: Revised anatomy of recurrent laryngeal nerves: Surgical importance, based on dissection of 100 cadavers. J. Clin. Endocrinol., *14*:87–96, 1954.
23. Semon, F.: Clinical remarks on the proclivity of the abductor fibres of the recurrent laryngeal nerve to become affected sooner than the adductor fibres, or even exclusively, in cases of undoubted central or peripheral injury or disease of the roots or trunks of the pneumo-gastric, spinal accessory, or recurrent nerves. Arch. Laryngol. Rhinol., *2*:197–222, 1881.
24. Thompson, N. W., Eckhauser, F. E., and Harness, J.K.: The anatomy of primary hyperparathyroidism. Surgery, *92*:814–821, 1982.
25. Thompson, N. W., Nishiyama, R. H., and Harness, J.K.: Thyroid carcinoma: Current controversies. Curr. Probl. Surg., *15*:1–67, 1978.
26. Wagner, R.: Die Medianstellung des Stimmbandes bei Recurrenslähmung. Arch. Pathol. Anat., *120*:437–459, 1890.
27. Wang, C.-A.: The anatomic basis of parathyroid surgery. Ann. Surg., *183*:271–275, 1976.
28. Wang, C.-A.: Parathyroid re-exploration: A clinical and pathological study of 112 cases. Ann. Surg., *186*:140–145, 1977.
29. Weeks, C., and Hinton, J. W.: Extralaryngeal division of recurrent laryngeal nerve: Its significance in vocal cord paralysis. Ann. Surg., *116*:251–258, 1942.

# 4

# PATHOLOGY OF THYROID AND PARATHYROID GLANDS

*Mark L. Silverman, M.D.*

The pathologist's approach to the morphologic study of the thyroid and parathyroid glands encompasses some of the most challenging problems in diagnostic surgical pathology. In the study of thyroid disease the question is often one of determining the presence or absence of malignancy. Careful application of diagnostic criteria, experience, and considerable judgment are the pathologist's allies in this task. In the examination of parathyroid tissue, the job is different, with the emphasis on determining the cause of parathyroid gland hyperfunction.

## PATHOLOGY OF THYROID GLAND

### *Benign Lesions of Thyroid*

#### Adenomatous Goiter

The most common form of thyroid enlargement is a result of defective metabolism and does not represent a true neoplastic process. Although the term "goiter" refers to a generic enlargement of the thyroid gland, by convention it has, most commonly, come to refer only to enlargement of a metabolic nature.

A gland involved by typical goitrous change will be enlarged up to ten to 20 times the normal size and weight and will be distorted by multiple nodules often of varying size and consistency. The nodules appear grossly demarcated but are not truly encapsulated, serving to distinguish them from neoplastic adenoma (Fig. 4–1). They frequently have a mucoid or gelatinous consistency, sometimes with areas of degeneration or even calcification. The lesion may become large enough to involve the anterior mediastinum, forming the so-called *plunging goiter.* These lesions may be highly vascular and they may provide the surgeon with a difficult technical task in their extirpation.

Microscopically, the lesions are characterized by the presence of nodules, often of various sizes. The follicular epithelium in the larger more cystic areas may appear flattened

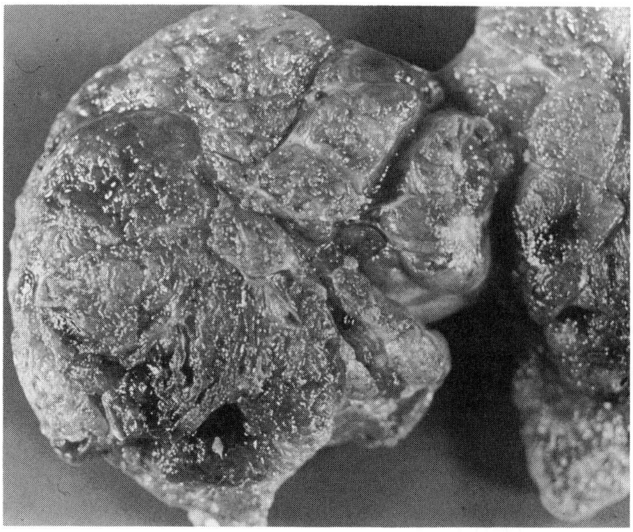

**FIGURE 4–1.** Adenomatous goiter illustrating lobulated gelatinous appearance without encapsulation.

whereas the more solid areas may show taller "hyperplastic"-appearing areas (Fig. 4–2). One cannot deduce the degree of physiologic function from a particular microscopic field in that the activity must be "summed" over the entire gland. The patient with a goitrous gland is often euthyroid, although alterations of function, e.g., mild hypothyroidism, are not uncommon. An interesting form is the so-called *toxic nodular goiter* in which one nodule is markedly hyperfunctional and produces more hormone than the entire normal gland. This situation is almost invariably benign, so a hyperfunctional scan helps to prevent some patients from undergoing unnecessary surgery.

The pathogenesis of goiter is thought to reflect cycles of thyrotropin stimulation and regression with the eventual formation of nodules due to focal failure of regression. Chronic dietary deficiency of iodine is a classic example of a goiter induced by thyroid-stimulating hormone (TSH). In that case, insufficient dietary iodine leads to ineffective hormone production with a resulting failure by the gland to "turn off" TSH. In the idiopathic variety, subtle alterations in the hypothalamic-pituitary axis may lead to the

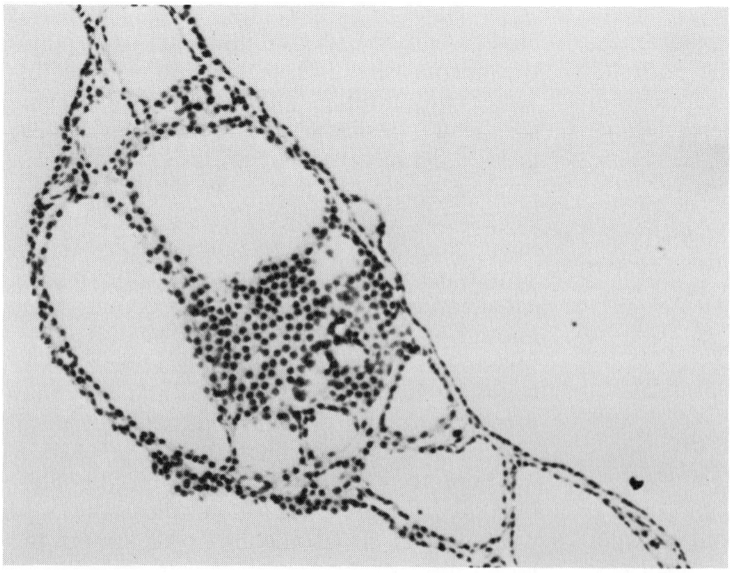

**FIGURE 4–2.** Low-power photomicrograph of typical adenomatous goiter. Note the marked variation in the size of the follicular structures as well as the flattening of the follicular epithelium (hematoxylin & eosin; 32 ×).

same phenomenon. A variant of the typical adenomatous goiter is the adenomatous nodule, which presents as a solitary dominant mass, mimicking adenoma. These come to surgical attention because they present as a nonregressing dominant mass. The adenomatous nodule is a circumscribed but unencapsulated solitary nodule. It does not fulfill the criteria for adenoma as described later. On occasion, it may be accompanied by minute nodules in the same or the opposite lobe.

## Graves' Disease (Primary Hyperplasia)

Surgery is performed for the resolution of the metabolic disorder in primary hyperplasia when the disease is refractory to medical management. The disease seldom presents a problem in terms of malignancy. In the classic untreated form, the gland is two to three times enlarged with a smooth symmetric contour similar in outline to the shape of the normal gland. Histologically, the follicles appear small with little colloid and with tall columnar epithelium. Lymphocytic infiltration of variable extent is apparent. Since most if not all glands seen surgically have been treated medically, the resected specimen will show variable regression.[3] Occasionally, an adenomatous nodule or incidental papillary carcinoma will be detected, underscoring the need for histologic examination. An examination of the capsule of the gland and its attached strap muscles may provide evidence of microscopic infiltration by follicles.[1] This should not be considered to signify malignancy. It may be found occasionally in adenomatous goiter as well.

## Thyroiditis

A variety of inflammatory conditions, which are collectively referred to as thyroiditis, may involve the thyroid gland (Fig. 4–3). In virtually all patients, these are medical entities that do not require surgical intervention. The surgical pathologist may have the occasion to see these specimens in controversial cases when the diagnosis is not readily apparent. For example, the end stage of Hashimoto's thyroiditis may produce extreme induration of the gland and with asymmetric involvement may yield the clinical findings of a mass lesion suspected of being a tumor. Riedel's thyroiditis, or chronic sclerosing thyroiditis, may closely mimic undifferentiated carcinoma by its extreme "invasiveness" and production of a stony hard mass.

Subacute thyroiditis, a probable response to a viral infection, may produce symptoms of rapid thyroid enlargement often with pain. Inflammation of the thyroid gland, sometimes with suppuration, may be caused by spread of pyogenic organisms, such as *Streptococcus* and *Staphylococcus,* from infections of the pharynx or paranasal sinuses.

Women are sometimes afflicted by chronic lymphocytic thyroiditis unassociated with the constellation of findings characteristic of

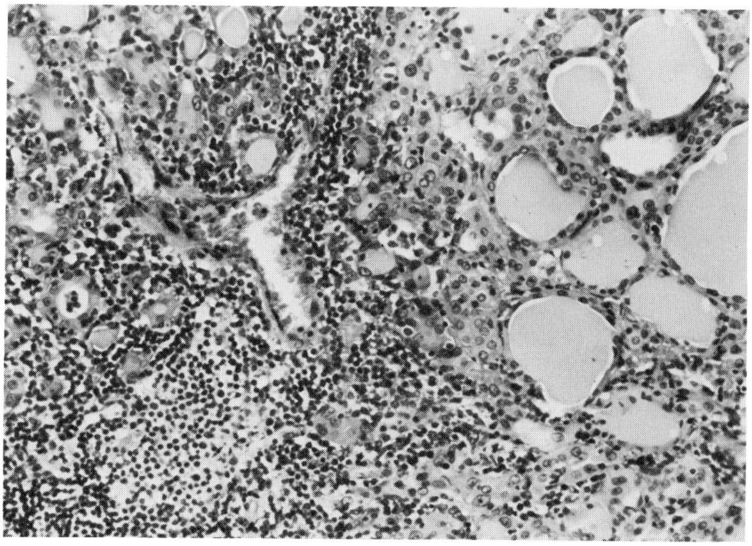

**FIGURE 4–3.** Hashimoto's thyroiditis showing typical oxyphil metaplasia (Hürthle cell change) and abundant interstitial chronic inflammation (hematoxylin & eosin; 100 ×).

Hashimoto's thyroiditis. This condition is self-limited, which underscores the need for an accurate diagnosis to obviate unnecessary surgery.

These disorders may be diagnosed without surgery by a variety of modalities, including blood values of antithyroid antibodies, nuclear imaging, and fine needle aspiration biopsy. Surgery is reserved for uncertain cases with the presence of suspected mass lesions or unusual clinical behavior.

## Lesions Related to Embryologic Development

A variety of thyroid abnormalities may be seen as a direct consequence of abnormal embryologic development. The thyroid gland develops as an outpouching of the endoderm of the foregut. It migrates caudally from a primitive opening in the tongue, the foramen cecum, leaving a tubelike pathway lined by columnar epithelium, which totally involutes normally. Its course during descent brings it in proximity to the hyoid bone.

Total failure of migration leads to a condition referred to as *lingual thyroid.* In such instances, this may constitute the only thyroid tissue, an obviously important factor in a surgical decision concerning a mass lesion of the tongue.

Thyroglossal duct cyst arises as a result of failed involution of the path of the primitive thyroid anlage. This disorder presents as a cystic mass lesion, sometimes with infection, in the midline (Fig. 4–4). This midline location helps to distinguish it from branchiogenic cysts, which are usually lateral. The midportion of the hyoid bone must be resected to extirpate the cyst totally and thus avoid recurrence.

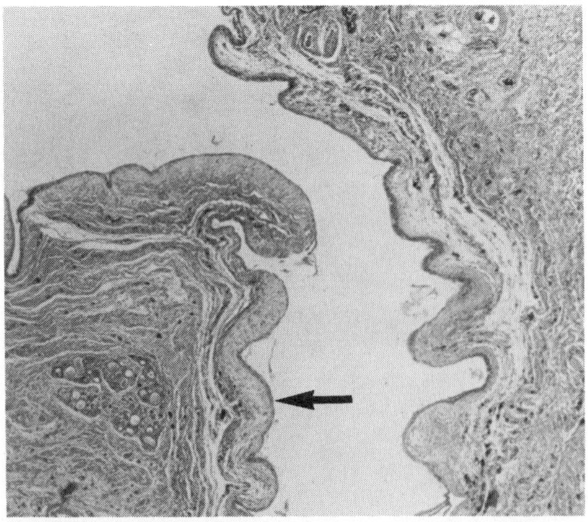

**FIGURE 4–4.** Thyroglossal duct cyst. Note columnar lining of cyst (*arrow*) with thyroid follicles embedded in wall (hematoxylin & eosin; 32 ×).

A variety of teratomatous lesions may involve thyroid tissue. An unusual one in female patients is termed *struma ovarii,* in which thyroid tissue dominates as heterotopic tissue within the ovary. It may have normal or excessive function. Its detection may require abdominal nuclear scans.

The thyroid gland during embryologic descent comes in close contact with the products of the third and fourth pharyngeal pouches, the parathyroid glands, and the thymus gland. Thus, a variety of malpositions is possible in the neck and mediastinum for each of these organs because of their close original association.

Occasionally, thyroid tissue will be found as a benign condition in cervical lymph nodes forming so-called *lateral aberrant thyroid tissue.* The thyroid follicles must have a totally normal configuration and be lacking any evidence of nuclear changes, papillary features, or psammomatous calcification to qualify as this embryologic curiosity. Understandably, the major differential diagnosis would be metastatic papillary carcinoma. Most examples of this so-called entity probably represent metastases from an occult thyroid tumor. Often, subserial section of the thyroid gland is necessary to document the presence of a primary papillary carcinoma.

Sometimes, nodules of goitrous tissue become detached from the body of the gland and give the appearance of metastatic tumor in lymph nodes, especially if there is any degree of lymphocytic infiltration. At the time of surgery this may present a problem to the unwary pathologist who may mistakenly diagnose metastatic carcinoma.

## Irradiated Thyroid

In patients who received large doses of external radiation perinatally, in childhood, or in adolescence or who have been exposed to nuclear fallout, the most common histologic change is the presence of adenomatous goiter. Thus, the thyroid nodules that are seen in such patients are often benign processes. The incidence of thyroid neoplasia is higher in these patients as well, and these tumors are primarily of the papillary low-grade type.[10] These glands may show a marked degree of nuclear hyperchromatism and atypia.

### Benign Neoplasms

The most common form of benign thyroid neoplasm is the adenoma. Its importance as an entity is largely its distinction from carcinoma. The diagnostic criteria for malignancy are discussed in the section on malignant tumors.

These lesions often present as a dominant mass, sometimes growing at an alarming rate. Rapid enlargement may, on occasion, be caused by hemorrhage. Grossly, adenomas are almost always solitary and appear well demarcated with a fairly obvious capsule. The parenchyma appears uniform without extensive evidence of necrosis. Rare instances of true multiple adenomas have been reported, although their distinction from nodular goiter is difficult.

Benign neoplasms are separated from the nodules of adenomatous goiter by the following criteria: the nodule is encapsulated, it appears different from the surrounding thyroid tissue, and it compresses the adjacent tissue.[19]

Microscopically, many patterns of growth have been identified in adenomas, including follicular, microfollicular, Hürthle cell, and embryonal patterns. However, the microscopic organization of the adenoma per se has no implication for prognosis. It is incumbent on the pathologist to examine the capsule and the blood vessels of the tumor scrupulously for signs of invasion as a way of recognizing malignant change. On rare occasions, benign-appearing follicles appear at a distant site, such as bone or brain, which is clear evidence of malignancy despite an apparently histologically benign adenoma originally. Such benign metastasizing adenomas undoubtedly represent inadequate sampling of the capsule of the original lesion.

## *Thyroid Carcinoma*

Thyroid carcinoma occupies a unique niche in the field of oncology. The incidence of these carcinomas in the general population is low, and deaths and complications are rare. Patients with some forms of differentiated carcinoma have no additional risk compared with normal individuals when these data are analyzed by actuarial methods.[5, 22]

Differentiated thyroid carcinoma is classified as either papillary or follicular. These morphologic groupings serve to distinguish the two forms of thyroid carcinoma that have different behavior patterns.

### Papillary Carcinoma

Papillary carcinoma is the most common form of differentiated carcinoma of the thyroid gland. Grossly, the carcinoma is firm yet not stony hard. It appears to merge with the surrounding tissue and does not give the impression of gross encapsulation (Fig. 4–5). In some instances of the so-called *occult sclerosing carcinoma* (Crile-Hazard tumor), it may appear as an irregular white scar in an otherwise unremarkable gland or one with the stigmata of goiter. Often these small occult tumors may be found in an area of focal calcification. Occasionally, a papillary tumor will arise in a cyst.[12] These carcinomas can be difficult to distinguish from papillary hyperplasia seen in a goiter.

Microscopically, the carcinoma, as implied in its name, is characterized by papillary

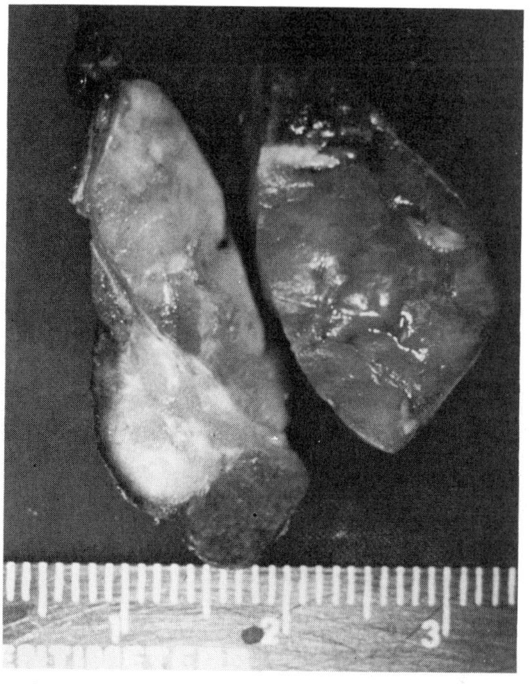


**FIGURE 4–5.** Papillary carcinoma of the thyroid. Tumor is poorly delimited from surrounding thyroid tissue.

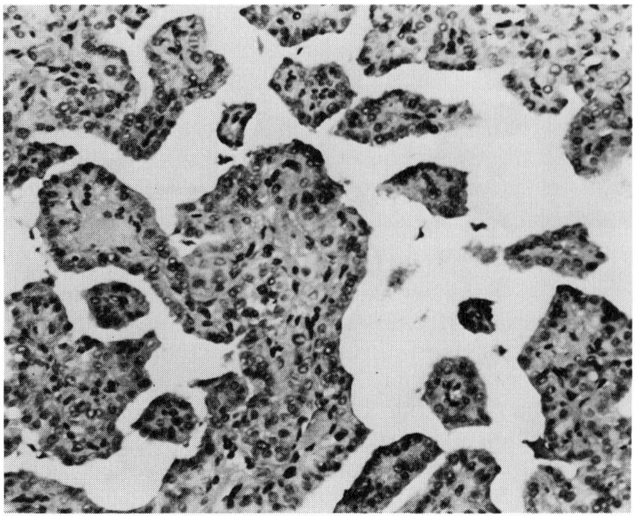

**FIGURE 4–6.** Typical papillary carcinoma illustrating well-formed stalk region. Note the lack of follicle formation and the tendency for the follicular epithelium to palisade about the periphery of the stalk (hematoxylin & eosin; 100 ×).

growth usually with a single layer of columnar cells overlying a fibrous stalk (Fig. 4–6). The stalks are most often devoid of vascularity and follicle formation, making them distinct from the papillary hyperplasia that may be seen with goiter. Laminated calcifications called psammoma bodies are found in the stalk region in a large proportion of tumors (Fig. 4–7). Psammoma bodies are highly characteristic of papillary carcinomas in general and may be seen in primary ovarian or even some lung carcinomas of the papillary type. Their presence in neck structures, such as cervical lymph nodes, should raise a strong suspicion of malignancy on the part of the pathologist. Their absence, however, should not be interpreted as a benign process.

The structure of the nucleus of the epithelial cell is helpful in the diagnosis of papillary carcinoma. The prototypical nucleus is "optically clear" without obvious chromatin structure or condensation and has been likened to the eyes of the cartoon character Little Orphan Annie (Fig. 4–8).[13] Although highly characteristic, this nuclear change should not be used to diagnose malignancy in the absence of other features. Sometimes the nucleus will appear dense, and, in these instances, nuclear grooving should be evaluated as a potentially helpful criterion.[7]

Important aspects of papillary carcinoma are its propensity for multifocal involvement and intraglandular metastasis. Careful examination of patients who have had total or subtotal thyroidectomy reveals multifocality in a high percentage.[19]

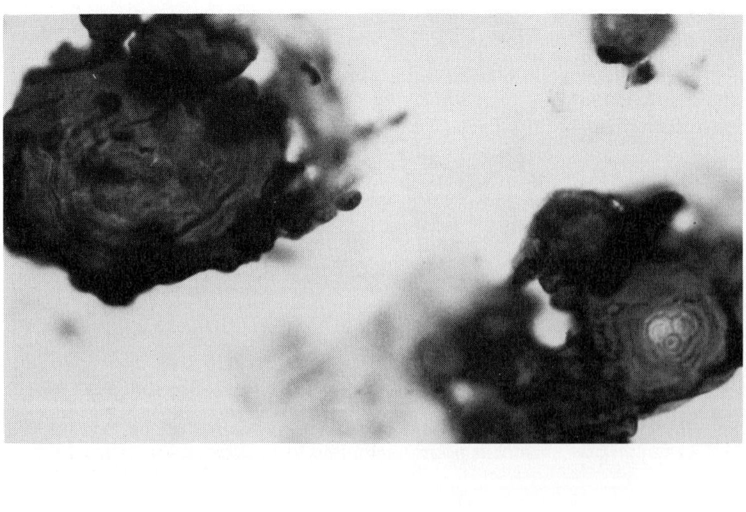

**FIGURE 4–7.** Classic psammoma bodies illustrating their concentricity. These are virtually diagnostic of papillary carcinoma when found in thyroid or cervical lymph node tissue (hematoxylin & eosin; 400 ×).

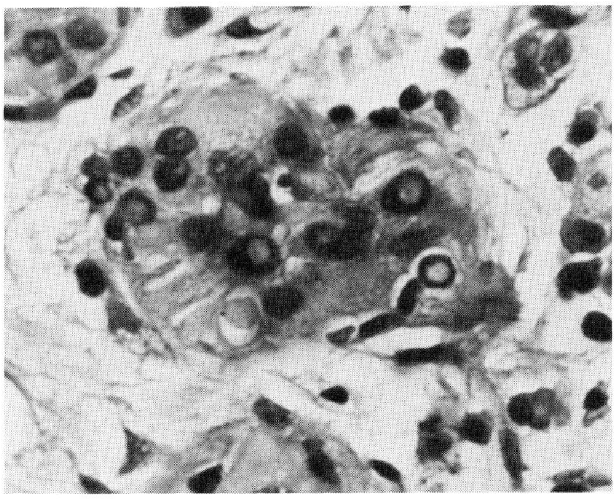

**FIGURE 4–8.** Papillary carcinoma illustrating the characteristic nuclear clearing referred to as Little Orphan Annie nuclei. In the appropriate histologic context, this finding is virtually diagnostic of papillary carcinoma. It can be seen focally in some non-neoplastic situations, but in these cases the other aspects rarely resemble carcinoma (hematoxylin & eosin; 400 ×).

Although tumors may be of papillary or follicular pattern, usually mixed papillary and follicular tumors are seen. The papillary extent may vary in these tumors. In terms of survival, prognosis, and biologic behavior, these carcinomas are identical to pure papillary carcinoma in contradistinction to pure follicular carcinoma. Some authors[19] conclude that mixed tumors are more likely to respond to radioactive iodine than the pure papillary type.

A special category is tumors classified as the follicular variant of papillary carcinoma. They appear entirely follicular and yet have the nuclear morphology of the papillary tumor (Fig. 4–9). Their prognosis is that of papillary carcinoma.[8]

Occasionally, carcinoma arises in association with thyroglossal duct cyst or its remnants.[16] These are often papillary in nature, although follicular tumors and mixed patterns have been described. The occurrence of other types would be distinctly unusual.

Microscopic papillary carcinoma may be found in a surprisingly high number of glands at autopsy. The importance of this phenomenon relates to what the surgeon should do when one of these minute occult carcinomas is discovered in a gland operated on for some other reason, such as adenomatous nodule. One should avoid overreacting to the presence of a solitary microscopic focus of papillary carcinoma in a gland operated on for another reason.[22] In particular, one should avoid reoperation in this situation.

Papillary thyroid carcinoma spreads predominantly by lymphatic and to some extent hematogenous routes. Thus, the cervical lymph nodes are the first site of extraglandular spread. The carcinoma may remain localized in lymph nodes for decades without progressive growth. Indeed, lymph node metastasis may not be an adverse prognostic factor if other circumstances are favorable, such as age and sex.[5] The carcinoma may also metastasize to the lungs, where it often creates a diffuse pattern rather than mass lesions. Pleural metastases and effusion are also seen as well as other blood-borne sites.

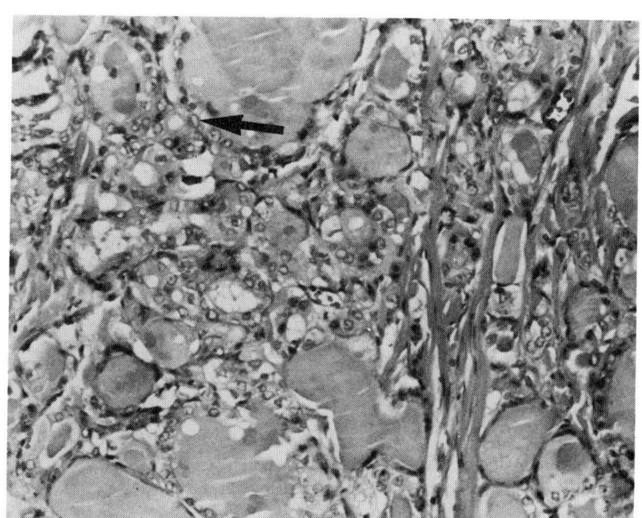

**FIGURE 4–9.** Follicular variant of papillary carcinoma. Although this tumor forms only follicles without the presence of papillary structures, it is diagnosable by the characteristic nuclear clearing (*arrow*). Its prognosis and biologic behavior are similar to ordinary papillary carcinoma (hematoxylin & eosin; 100 ×).

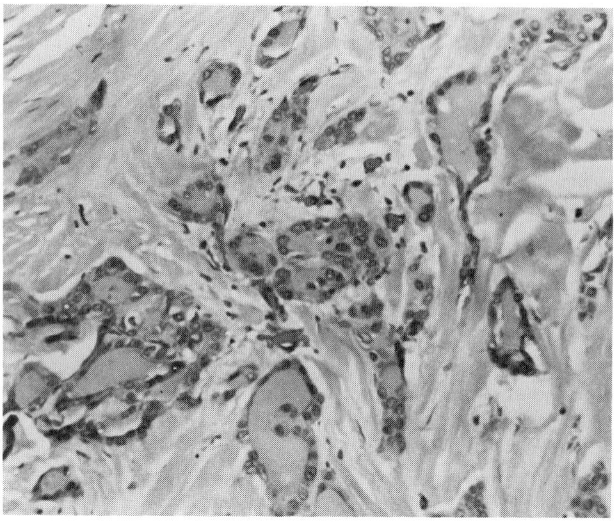

**FIGURE 4–10.** Follicular carcinoma illustrating invasive component. Tumor freely infiltrates fibrous tissue fulfilling the most important criterion for malignancy, which is invasion (hematoxylin & eosin; 100 ×).

## Follicular Carcinoma

Follicular carcinoma presents as a well-circumscribed mass often in fairly sharp contrast to the surrounding gland. Usually, it is encapsulated or appears so on gross inspection. The texture is somewhat softer than that of a papillary carcinoma. The lesion most often presents as a solitary mass and is unusual as an incidental finding in a goitrous gland.

Evaluation of follicular carcinoma is different from that of papillary carcinoma. Determination of malignancy is based on the relationship of the lesion to the surrounding gland and not on the histologic pattern of the cells (Fig. 4–10).

The most important factor in establishing the diagnosis of follicular carcinoma is invasion. As most of these lesions are at least partially encapsulated, the capsule is the first place to examine for invasion. In many patients, areas of capsular invasion may be small and difficult to find.[20] This may be particularly vexatious to the pathologist performing frozen section evaluation of these nodules. Indeed, the pathologist and the surgeon alike must anticipate that at least 5 per cent of the encapsulated lesions called benign by frozen section at surgery will eventually prove malignant when examined with multiple permanent sections of the capsule.

Areas of capsular invasion disclose neoplastic follicular epithelium in fibrous exaggerations of the capsule, often with a "buttonhole" type of pattern or with follicular structures bulging into the neighboring non-neoplastic tissue.

Another important criterion of carcinoma is the presence of vascular invasion.[19] Thyroid carcinoma and, in particular, follicular carcinoma show a propensity to invade small venous channels in the capsule. Meissner[20] strongly advocates this as the most important criterion for the diagnosis of cancer, and virtually all lesions with this finding will prove to be malignant. The problem is that various authors disagree as to the basis for identification of this phenomenon. Kahn and Perzin[14] accept subendothelial protrusions as evidence of invasion whereas Meissner[20] demands the presence of intraluminal tumor thrombus with adherence to the vessel wall.

Much of the preceding discussion has emphasized the criteria for diagnosing malignant follicular thyroid tumors. There is also great value in segregating this group into two categories for the sake of more accurate prognostication. The distinction has been drawn between tumors that are malignant by reason of frank invasion of the capsule or of contiguous structures and those that are malignant by reason of angioinvasion. This angioinvasive group consists of neoplasms that closely resemble an adenoma, except for small foci of capsule or capsular vascular invasion. These carcinomas are virtually always cured by ipsilateral lobectomy with recurrence rates approximating 1 per cent. Patients who have metastatic disease and poor prognosis fall into the frankly invasive category.

Follicular carcinoma metastasizes by the hematogenous route and uncommonly spreads to lymph nodes. It may produce lung, bone, liver, and cerebral metastases.

### Hürthle Cell Carcinoma

This particular variant of follicular carcinoma is noteworthy for the appearance of its epithelial cells. They have abundant granular cytoplasm containing a profusion of mitochondria as revealed by electron microscopy. The nuclei often are noticeably irregular in size and appear markedly hyperchromatic. The cells usually grow in solid sheets without the formation of follicular structures. The criteria for the diagnosis of malignancy are the same as those for ordinary follicular carcinoma. Grossly, these tumors appear well circumscribed and have a brownish color to their cut surface. Their prognosis is similar to that of follicular carcinoma.[21]

### Medullary Carcinoma

The carcinomas of papillary, follicular, and mixed papillary and follicular patterns share a common ancestor, the follicular epithelial cell. Medullary carcinomas arise from the parafollicular or C cell epithelium and are descendants of the dispersed neuroendocrine cells. This difference in lineage accounts for differences in clinical behavior, histology, and prognosis and also for some unique genetic relationships.

The genetic nature of medullary tumors is of key importance in understanding their behavior. They usually occur as an isolated or sporadic finding, but they may be a component of the multiple endocrine neoplasia (MEN) syndrome or familial medullary carcinoma.[3] Familial medullary carcinoma tends to be upper and lateral in the thyroid gland and is always multifocal. When one carcinoma is found in an afflicted familial case, evidence of preneoplastic C cell hyperplasia is found both in the ipsilateral and the contralateral side. The sporadic form of tumor is not associated with endocrine tumors of other sites.

The tumors appear grayish white and have a firm consistency. They are poorly delimited and often appear unencapsulated. Microscopically, they have a cellular and somewhat organoid appearance with acellular pink zones that often give positive histochemical reactions for amyloid (Fig. 4–11). Approximately 15 per cent of these carcinomas show at least foci of mucin secretion. Immunohistochemical stains for calcitonin or other hormonal peptides will be positive in the acellular zones of amyloid as well as in the cytoplasm of the tumor cells. Some of these carcinomas will not have recognizable amyloid so that the histologic appearance as well as the immunohistochemical reactions may be important for accurate diagnosis.

Recently, carcinomas composed of mixtures of the medullary and follicular types have been described.[21]

### Undifferentiated Carcinoma

Numerically, undifferentiated carcinoma forms only a small diagnostic category in

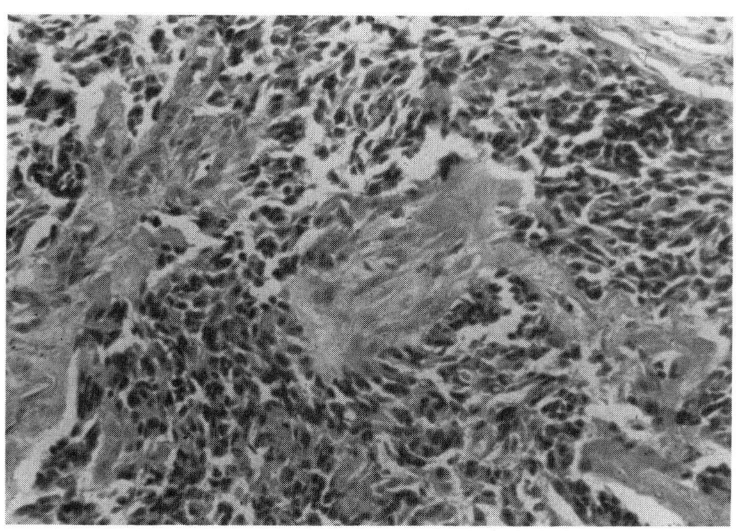

**FIGURE 4–11.** Typical medullary carcinoma. Acellular zones stain positively for amyloid and for calcitonin (hematoxylin & eosin; 100 ×).

thyroid tumors. These have been designated as small-cell undifferentiated and large-cell undifferentiated carcinoma.

Small-cell carcinoma occupies the most controversial niche in thyroid pathology.[21] Indeed, some hesitate to accord it a legitimate position in the nosology at all. On review, many of the cases formerly classified this way have now been recognized as some other form of thyroid cancer. Thus, many are classified as lymphoma or anaplastic versions of medullary carcinoma. However, evidence does exist that this entity is real but that strict diagnostic criteria should be employed. Proof rests with documentation by ultrastructural and immunohistochemical means.[4, 18]

Large-cell undifferentiated carcinoma is a well-recognized and highly lethal form of thyroid carcinoma. Its gross characteristics are those of a highly infiltrative bulky white-tan tumor often with foci of necrosis. It extends aggressively into surrounding structures, often compressing the trachea and the great vessels. Microscopically, it may take on a sarcomatoid appearance, frequently with the presence of multinucleated giant cells. It may otherwise consist of anaplastic large tumor cells with interspersed giant cells. These tumors are fatal in a short time period and are not amenable to surgical excision with rare exception. They can sometimes show a gratifying response to intensive radiation therapy.[24]

Another tumor category, insular carcinoma, falls somewhere between follicular and undifferentiated carcinoma in prognosis. These tumors are categorized by sheets of follicular cells that form follicles poorly.[21]

## Thyroid Lymphoma

Lymphoma may involve the thyroid gland as either a primary or secondary process.[11] These malignant tumors may arise spontaneously or as a long-term complication of chronic thyroiditis. Recognition of the possibility of this diagnosis may help to avoid misdiagnosis as either undifferentiated carcinoma or medullary carcinoma. In addition, the diagnosis of lymphoma can be made using fine needle aspiration biopsy, sometimes obviating the need for surgery, but the particular subtype characterization may require a biopsy or tissue specimen.

Grossly, these tumors appear as bulky tan masses with a homogeneous "fish-flesh" texture. They may involve the gland in a focal manner, afflicting a single lobe, or may diffusely replace the parenchyma. Microscopically, the tumor is classified in the same manner as extranodal lymphomas elsewhere with careful attention paid to the extent of disease, such as capsular invasion or regional nodal involvement (Fig. 4–12).

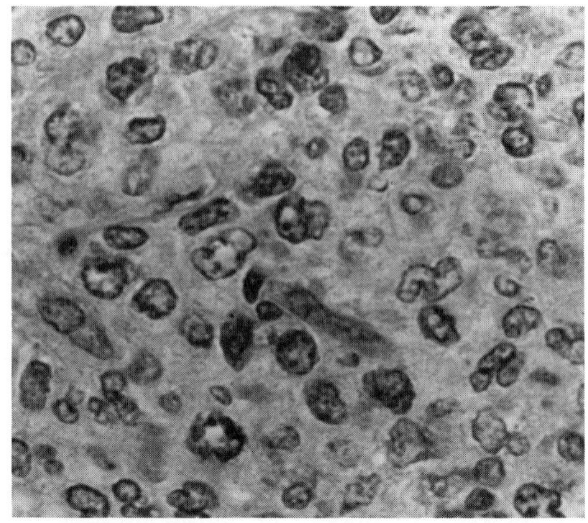

**FIGURE 4–12.** Thyroid lymphoma. Histology is the same as for lymphomas occurring elsewhere. Prognosis is determined by stage, with tumors confined to the gland associated with a more favorable outlook (hematoxylin & eosin; 400 ×).

The thyroid gland may also harbor malignant tumors of plasma cell origin (malignant plasmacytoma) as a primary event, but these are rare. The diagnosis should rest on careful scrutiny and adherence to criteria.[23]

## Squamous Cell Carcinoma

Primary squamous cell carcinoma of the thyroid is rare. Squamous carcinoma of the thyroid may be the result of direct extension from the pulmonary and digestive tracts or metastatic disease from a more distant site. Some of the cases reflect metaplastic change in an otherwise typical form of follicular carcinoma. The rare instances that occur have a histology similar to that seen in squamous carcinoma elsewhere and are associated with a poor prognosis.[15] Occasional mixed forms exist that have the same prognosis as the more ordinary forms of thyroid carcinoma.

## Metastatic Tumors

Metastatic disease may occasionally present as a thyroid mass lesion. Obviously, tumors of the neck region, such as of the larynx, may locally invade the gland and in the case of squamous tumors may actually be a source of confusion regarding the origin of a particular tumor. Any of the tumors that give rise to systemic metastasis have been seen in the thyroid, particularly at autopsy. However, lung, kidney, and breast carcinomas, melanoma, and malignant lymphoma are the most common culprits.

## PARATHYROID PATHOLOGY

Histologically, normal parathyroid glands consist of a variable admixture of chief cells (thought to be the active secretory cells), oxyphil cells (thought to represent senescent cells), water-clear cells (thought to represent a form of transitional cell), and adipose tissue. The proportion of adipose tissue to glandular epithelium is highly variable but in general increases with the age of the patient. The chief cells in the normal gland generally outnumber the oxyphil and water-clear cells.

The pathologic approach to parathyroid disease is different from the emphasis in thyroid pathology. The major interest in parathyroid pathology for the clinician relates to the surgical approach to hyperparathyroidism. Rarely is the identification of carcinoma a concern because it is an uncommon condition in the parathyroid glands.

### *Hyperparathyroidism*

Hyperparathyroidism may exist in primary, secondary, or, theoretically, tertiary forms. Primary hyperparathyroidism is the result of either diffuse glandular hyperplasia or, more commonly, a solitary adenoma. Secondary hyperplasia represents an increase in parathyroid mass and activity secondary to a metabolic state that loses calcium, such as chronic renal failure. Tertiary hyperparathyroidism reflects the emergence of an autonomous adenoma on the background of chronic secondary hyperplasia.[1]

### *Adenoma*

An adenoma is an expansion of a glandular mass in one or two glands. Commonly, there is a striking increase in the population of chief cells at the expense of the other elements. The amount of glandular adipose tissue is often decreased dramatically. Frequently, a rim of normal-appearing gland is seen to border the adenoma, a helpful but diagnostically unreliable sign (Fig. 4–13). An adenoma may have nests of oxyphil cells so their presence does not rule out adenoma as a diagnosis. Although the configuration histologically is usually that of a monotonous expansion of chief cells, a host of cellular organizations can be observed, including fibrous septa, acini, or even rosettes. Mitotic figures and foci of necrosis are almost uni-

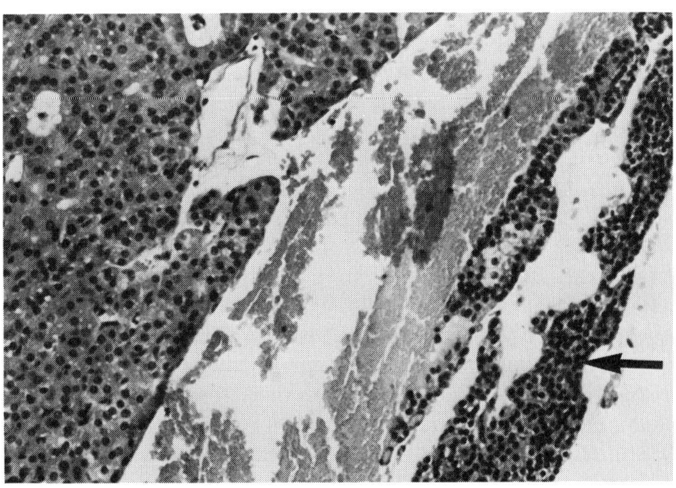

**FIGURE 4–13.** Typical parathyroid adenoma. The cell population displays uniformity with diminished adipose tissue. Note rim of normal tissue (*arrow*) (hematoxylin & eosin; 100 ×).

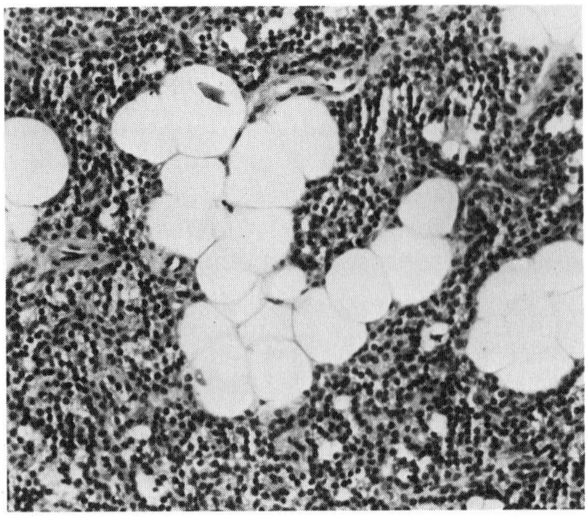

**FIGURE 4–14.** Hyperplastic parathyroid gland. Note the heterogeneous cell population. This is distinguished from adenoma by the examination of a separate normal gland (hematoxylin & eosin; 100 ×).

formly absent, and their presence should raise the possibility of carcinoma.

The most important criterion of adenoma as opposed to diffuse hyperplasia rests with the examination of more than one parathyroid gland. Adenoma usually involves only one gland. Therefore, the presence of a single histologically normal gland virtually assures the diagnosis of adenoma in a hyperparathyroid patient with a single enlarged gland. Thus, it becomes incumbent on the surgeon to provide at least a portion of normal gland to the pathologist for the diagnosis of adenoma; the pathologist should request such a tissue sample from the surgeon to be certain of the diagnosis.

A variant of adenoma, lipoadenoma, is a neoplastic lesion consisting of adipose tissue and chief cells. It may be responsible for clinical hyperparathyroidism and must be distinguished from hyperplasia.[2]

## *Diffuse Hyperplasia*

Diffuse hyperplasia is an enlargement of all four parathyroid glands. It may occur as the result of some chronic cause of hypocalcemia or hyperphosphatemia, such as chronic renal failure. It thus appears to be a reactive compensatory mechanism for restoring calcium equilibrium, albeit an imperfect one. Often, this can be appreciated grossly by the experienced surgeon. Histologically, hyperplasia is most easily recognized by the diminished amount of adipose tissue, although this particular judgment can be highly subjective. Occasionally, there will be an almost normal complement of fatty tissue, making careful observation of weight and measurement parameters vital. In general, the glands will be of fairly uniform size, a departure from the finding with adenoma. Nodular islands of chief cells with diminished adipose tissue are seen histologically (Fig. 4–14).

Occasionally, hyperplasia will closely resemble adenoma histologically. In these cases, there is a nodular increase in mass often with a pattern similar to that seen in adenoma. Careful attention to the presence of other parathyroid tissue that appears hyperplastic is the key to making the diagnosis of hyperplasia. Such nodular hyperplasia may provide significant problems for the surgeon if there is a discrepancy in gland size.

## *Parathyroid Carcinoma*

Although cases of parathyroid carcinoma are well documented in the literature, the exact criteria are less well agreed on. A constellation of clinical, gross, and microscopic findings is of help in making this diagnosis.

Often the level of parathormone measured preoperatively is much higher than the range encountered with the usual adenoma. In addition, the malignant gland may be palpable clinically, which is distinctly unusual for typical cases of hyperparathyroidism. The surgeon will often state that the nodule feels firmer and more adherent to neighboring structures than usual. The presence of local invasion into contiguous thyroid or soft tissue may be detected. Frozen section diagnosis can be of use in planning the appropriate extirpative therapy at the primary operation.

The pathologist will find that the nodule has a firm consistency compared with the ordinary adenoma. Often the cut surface will not bulge in the way that is customary for adenoma (Fig. 4–15).

Microscopically, the presence of dense fibrous bands that impart a distinctive lobularity will be noted. Zones of increased mitotic activity and necrosis may be seen (Fig. 4–16). Although there may be greater cellular pleomorphism than is usually seen with ade-

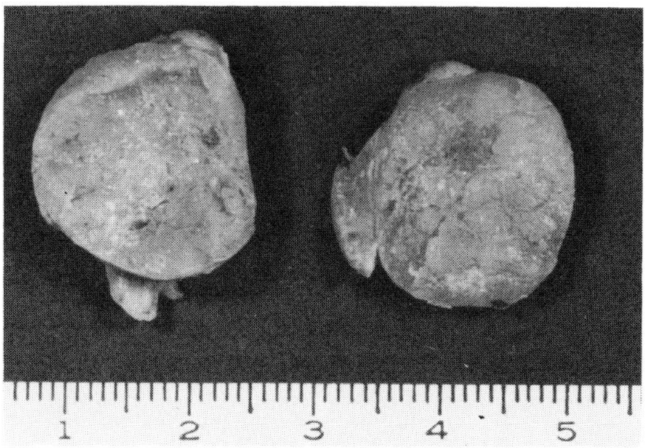

**FIGURE 4–15.** Parathyroid carcinoma. Note the hard edge to the cut surface. This is different from that expected in adenoma, which has a bulging appearance.

noma, this is not of diagnostic significance. The most useful diagnostic criterion is local invasion or distant metastases at the time of initial surgery. In such cases, invasion of the thyroid gland or neighboring soft tissue will be evident to the surgeon by the lack of clear dissection planes. The prognosis of patients without gross invasive tumor is good, with long survival times recorded.[9] Patients with metastatic disease often die of recalcitrant hypercalcemia.

### *Parathyroid Cyst*

Parathyroid tissue may take on a cystic morphology under a number of conditions and clinical states. Occasionally, cyst formation replaces an otherwise normal parathyroid gland. At other times, an adenoma may be primarily cystic. Patients with diffuse hyperplasia may have cyst formation as well. It is important that the surgeon understand the possibility of cyst formation in the process of neck exploration for hypercalcemia. Most often it merely represents an incidental finding.[6]

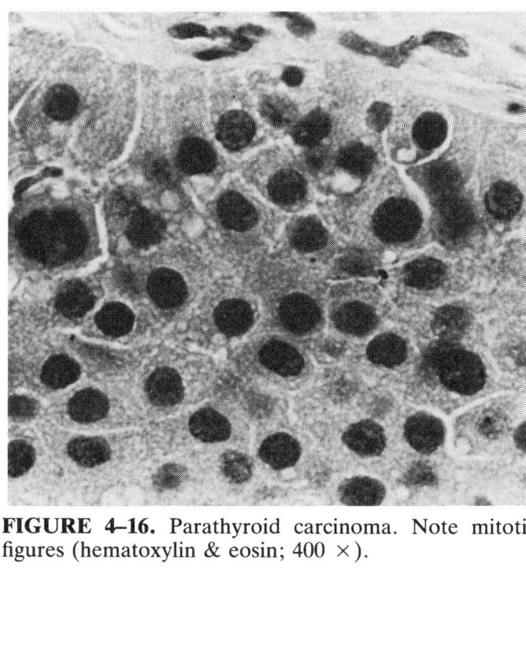

**FIGURE 4–16.** Parathyroid carcinoma. Note mitotic figures (hematoxylin & eosin; 400 ×).

## REFERENCES


1. Ackerman, L. V.: Ackerman's Surgical Pathology. Edition 6. St. Louis, C. V. Mosby, 1981, p. 342.
2. Allen, P. W.: Tumors and Proliferations of Adipose Tissue: A Clinicopathologic Approach. New York, Masson Publishing, U.S.A., 1981, p. 77.
3. Bloodworth, J. M. B., Jr. (ed.): Endocrine Pathology: General and Surgical. Edition 2. Baltimore, Williams & Wilkins, 1982.
4. Burt, A. D., Kerr, D. J., Brown, I. L., et al.: Lymphoid and epithelial markers in small cell anaplastic thyroid tumours. J. Clin. Pathol., *38*:893–896, 1985.
5. Cady, B., Sedgwick, C. E., Meissner, W. A., et al.: Changing clinical, pathologic, therapeutic, and survival patterns in differentiated thyroid carcinoma. Ann. Surg., *183*:541–553, 1976.
6. Castleman, B., and Roth, S. I.: Tumors of the parathyroid glands. *In* Atlas of Tumor Pathology. 2nd series, fascicle 14. Washington, D.C., Armed Forces Institute of Pathology, 1978.
7. Chan, J. K. C., and Saw, D.: The grooved nucleus: A useful diagnostic criterion of papillary carcinoma of the thyroid. Am. J. Surg. Pathol., *10*:672–679, 1986.
8. Chem, K. T., and Rosai, J.: Follicular variant of thyroid papillary carcinoma: A clinicopathologic study of six cases. Am. J. Surg. Pathol., *1*:123–130, 1977.
9. Cohn, K., Silverman, M., Corrado, J., et al.: Parathyroid carcinoma: The Lahey Clinic experience. Surgery, *98*:1095–1100, 1985.
10. Favus, M. J., Schneider, A. B., Stachura, M. E., et al.: Thyroid cancer occurring as a late consequence of head-and-neck irradiation: Evaluation of 1056 patients. N. Engl. J. Med., *294*:1019–1025, 1976.
11. Hamburger, J. I., Miller, J. M., and Kini, S. R.: Lymphoma of the thyroid. Ann. Intern. Med., *99*:685–693, 1983.
12. Hammer, M., Wortsman, J., and Folse, R.: Cancer in cystic lesions of the thyroid. Arch. Surg., *117*:1020–1023, 1982.
13. Hapke, M. R., and Dehner, L. P.: The optically clear nucleus: A reliable sign of papillary carcinoma of the thyroid? Am. J. Surg. Pathol., *3*:31–38, 1979.
14. Kahn, N. F., and Perzin, K. H.: Follicular carcinoma of the thyroid: An evaluation of the histologic criteria used for diagnosis. Pathol. Annu., *18*(Pt.1):221–253, 1983.

15. LiVolsi, V. A., and Merino, M. J.: Squamous cells in the human thyroid gland. Am. J. Surg. Pathol., *2*:133–140, 1978.
16. LiVolsi, V. A., Perzin, K. H., and Savetsky, L.: Carcinoma arising in median ectopic thyroid (including thyroglossal duct tissue). Cancer, *34*:1303–1315, 1974.
17. MacLeod, W. A. J., and Holloway, C. K.: Hyperparathyroid crisis: A collective review. Ann. Surg., *166*:1012–1015, 1967.
18. Mambo, N. C., and Irwin, S. M.: Anaplastic small cell neoplasms of the thyroid: An immunoperoxidase study. Hum. Pathol., *15*:55–60, 1984.
19. Meissner, W. A., and Warren, S.: Tumors of the thyroid gland. *In* Atlas of Tumor Pathology. 2nd series, fascicle 4. Washington, D.C., Armed Forces Institute of Pathology, 1969.
20. Meissner, W. A.: Follicular carcinoma of the thyroid. Am. J. Surg. Pathol., *1*:171–173, 1977.
21. Rosai, J., and Carcangiu, M. L.: Pathology of thyroid tumors: Some recent and old questions. Hum. Pathol., *15*:1008–1012, 1984.
22. Rossi, R. L., Cady, B., Silverman, M. L., et al.: Current results of conservative surgery for differentiated thyroid carcinoma. World J. Surg., *10*:612–622, 1986.
23. Shimaoka, K., Gailani, S., Tsukada, Y., et al.: Plasma cell neoplasm involving the thyroid. Cancer, *41*:1140–1146, 1978.
24. Simpson, W. J.: Anaplastic thyroid carcinoma: A new approach. Can. J. Surg., *23*:25–27, 1980.

# 5

# CYTOPATHOLOGY OF FINE NEEDLE ASPIRATION OF THYROID GLAND

*John M. Dugan, M.D.*

The accuracy and utility of fine needle aspiration biopsy of the thyroid are entirely dependent on the technical quality of the procedure. Multiple steps and multiple disciplines are involved so that problems at any stage can make the results of biopsy uninterpretable. Close cooperation among the physician, the aspirator, and the cytologist is essential to obtain optimal results. The steps involved are collection of the specimen; cytopreparation, which includes slide preparation, fixation, and staining; and cytopathologic interpretation.[25] The technical aspects of obtaining a fine needle aspiration biopsy specimen are detailed elsewhere in this text; only the second and third components of the process are discussed in this chapter.

## CYTOPREPARATION

### Slide Preparation

The first step in cytopreparation is slide preparation, which can be accomplished in two ways. Direct smears of the specimen can be made at the time of aspiration. This method is similar to the bone marrow aspiration technique, in which a drop of the aspirated material is expelled from the needle onto the slide. A second slide is then placed on top of the first, and a smear is made by gently pulling apart the top and bottom slides. For specimens diluted with blood or cyst fluid, a peripheral blood smear technique is used in which the edge of a second slide, or coverslip, is used to spread the material on the first slide.[30] Advantages of smears include their ease and low cost of preparation. In addition, rapid assessment of adequacy of the specimen is possible so that repeat aspirations can be performed immediately if necessary. Well-prepared smears often include tissue fragments, thus permitting assessment of architecture. The major disadvantage is that skill and experience are needed to prepare good smears because inexpertly handled smears may show excessive air-drying, crush artifact, or cell distortion that can hinder cytologic interpretation. Also, the smear technique may not be optimal for bloody specimens because the cells of interest are often obscured by erythrocytes.

The second method of cytopreparation involves immediate fixation of the specimen in a fixative, such as Carbowax (Lerner Laboratories, New Haven, CT), 2 per cent ethylene glycol in 50 per cent alcohol. The cellular material is retrieved by centrifugation, and cytocentrifuge or cell block preparations can be made. The advantages include immediate cell fixation without concern about air drying. The cytology laboratory is not dependent on the aspirator for smear technique or proper fixation. Thus, specimens can be collected anywhere and referred to the laboratory, and the need for an assistant to be present to prepare the smears during aspiration is obviated. Finally, cell blocks can be prepared, thereby expanding the spectrum of special studies that can be performed. Disadvantages include a longer time and greater cost for cytopreparation than with direct smears and nuclear shrinkage because of alcohol fixation. In addition, tissue fragments may lose their architectural features after centrifugation.

A supplemental technique that is useful with abundantly cellular specimens, particularly those with blood or cyst fluid, is rinsing the needle and syringe with alcohol fixative after direct smears are made. These specimens can be handled as outlined previously under the second method so that membrane filters, cell blocks, or cytocentrifuge specimens can be made. We have also applied this supplemental technique when direct smears are submitted in alcohol fixative because cells may be dislodged from the slides and fall into the fixative fluid. The fixative is centrifuged, and the cellular sediment can be processed by one of the previously mentioned methods.

### Fixation and Staining

The choices of fixation method and staining technique are usually made concurrently because use of the metachromatic stains requires air-dried unfixed preparations, and the Papanicolaou and hematoxylin and eosin methods of staining require fixation. The advantages of using air-dried smears with metachromatic stains, such as Romanovsky's, May-Grünwald-Giemsa, and Diff-Quick (Dade Diagnostic, Inc., Aguada, PR), are that they are performed quickly and simply, and fixation is not needed. These stains can be helpful in the diagnosis of lymphoma. A variety of intracellular and extracellular metachromatic substances can be recognized, such as colloid from thyroid follicles and intracytoplasmic eosinophilic granules in medullary carcinoma of the thyroid. Disadvantages include suboptimal nuclear detail, indistinct borders of most epithelial cells, inability to discern architectural features of tissue fragments, and difficulty in the recognition of functional differentiation of cytoplasm.

The most commonly used fixative is 95 per cent ethyl alcohol, either by immersion of the smears or as a spray fixative. Alcohol is readily available and reliable but causes hemolysis, resulting in granular debris that may obscure the cells of interest. Also, cellular material may fall off slides immersed in alcohol unless the slide is coated with albumin. On the other hand, albumin imparts a background eosinophilia to the smear, which can impair interpretation.

Spray fixation of smears is preferred by many laboratories because it provides optimal cytomorphology with excellent nuclear detail, demonstration of differentiation, and preservation of architectural features without red cell lysis or background staining. Either peroxidase-antiperoxidase or hematoxylin and eosin staining can be used with these fixation methods because both provide excellent cytomorphology with good nuclear detail, although colloid from thyroid follicles stains poorly. The Papanicolaou method of staining has the added advantage of enabling recognition of cytoplasmic differentiation.

The choice of cytopreparation method is largely a matter of personal preference and depends on the setting in which the cytopathology laboratory operates. Major determining factors include the aspirator, whether the specimen arrives in the laboratory in fixative or as prepared slides, cost constraints, and the background and training experience of the cytopathologist.

## CYTOPATHOLOGIC INTERPRETATION

The first step in cytopathologic interpretation is assessment of the adequacy of the biopsy. Although no firm criteria have been created, guidelines were established by several investigators. Kini and Purslow[25] recommended that, to be called satisfactory, a biopsy should demonstrate eight to ten cell groups or tissue fragments of well-preserved thyroid follicular epithelium on each of two separate slides. The presence of changes of cystic degeneration (histiocytes, acellular debris, and blood) without follicular epithelium is an inadequate biopsy and is interpreted as nondiagnostic. A brief description of the principal benign and malignant lesions identified by fine needle aspiration biopsy is provided.

### Nodular or Adenomatous Goiter

The most common lesion identified by aspiration biopsy is nodular or adenomatous goiter. These aspirates tend to be sparsely cellular, consisting of scattered cells and small clusters of uniform follicular epithelium. Abundant colloid is a useful feature in the diagnosis of goiter. Occasionally, tissue fragments are obtained that contain follicles of widely varying size lined by flattened or cuboidal epithelium. Evidence of cystic degeneration or old hemorrhage may be present (Fig. 5–1).[10, 11, 26, 29, 30]

### Thyroiditis

Acute suppurative thyroiditis resulting from bacterial infection is rare, and aspirates are highly cellular, consisting of neutrophils, macrophages, and cellular debris. Subacute thyroiditis (de Quervain's thyroiditis) has a characteristic clinical presentation.[29] Aspirates demonstrate lymphocytes, plasma cells, epithelioid histiocytes, and multinucleated giant cells. Clinical correlation is mandatory because this inflammatory pattern can also be seen with some papillary carcinomas.

Lymphocytic thyroiditis (Hashimoto's thyroiditis) is an autoimmune disease that can produce diffuse enlargement of the thyroid or can result in solitary or multiple nodules. Fine needle aspirates usually consist of numerous lymphocytes and plasma cells with follicular cells showing oncocytic features (Hürthle cells). Hürthle cells contain abundant dense granular cytoplasm and may possess hyperchromatic, highly atypical nuclei. The recognition of Hashimoto's thyroiditis can be difficult for the cytopathologist, especially when only the inflammatory or epithelial component is present. This difficulty can lead to a false-positive diagnosis of lymphoma or carcinoma, especially Hürthle cell tumor.[11, 12] To complicate the matter, patients with lymphocytic thyroiditis are at a higher risk for the development of both lymphoma[16, 21, 23, 33] and carcinoma.[18] Experienced cytopathologists[19] note that one of the most important missed diagnoses in thyroid cytology is lymphoma of the thyroid, which is often misdiagnosed as Hashimoto's thyroiditis (Fig. 5–2).[21]

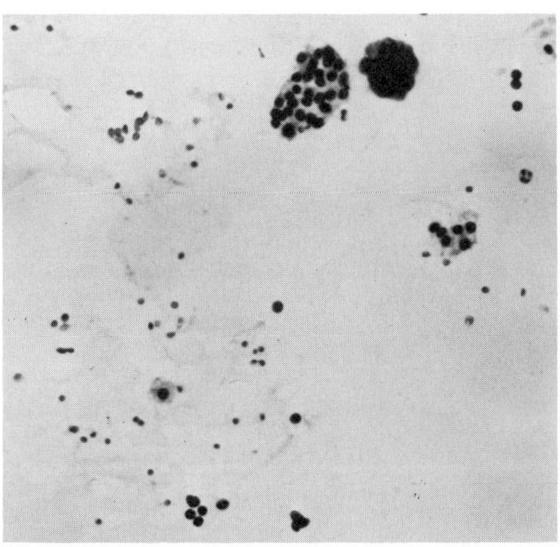

**FIGURE 5–1.** Fine needle aspirate of nodular or adenomatous goiter. Sparse benign follicular epithelium with abundant colloid, blood, and acellular debris (Papanicolaou stain; original magnification × 100).

### Toxic Hyperplasia

Findings on aspiration biopsy in patients with toxic hyperplasia (Graves' disease) include sheets and small clusters of follicular epithelium that may demonstrate wide variability in nuclear size. Some cells may have vacuolated cytoplasm. Colloid is scant, and blood may be abundant. Often, this appearance cannot be differentiated cytologically from a follicular adenoma, and radionuclide scan used in conjunction with clinical impression is invaluable because toxic nodules are almost always hot and follicular adenomas are almost always cold.[41]

### Cysts

Aspiration of thyroid cysts can be both diagnostic and therapeutic. When the nodule does not completely disappear after removal of cyst contents, the residual mass should be

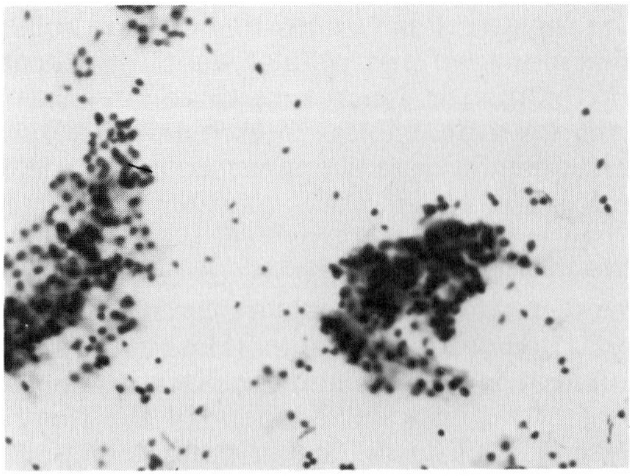

**FIGURE 5–2.** Fine needle aspirate of Hashimoto's thyroiditis. Follicular epithelium with Hürthle cell features admixed with a lymphocytic infiltrate (Papanicolaou stain; original magnification × 100).

reaspirated because malignant as well as benign processes may undergo cystic degeneration. About 3 per cent of cystic lesions were found to represent papillary carcinomas with cyst formation.[39] Cyst contents usually include foamy histiocytes, blood, and acellular debris. The presence of cyst contents without follicular epithelium must be interpreted as nondiagnostic cytologically because the epithelial component of the nodule cannot be evaluated.[29]

### Neoplasms

Papillary carcinoma is the most common malignant neoplasm of the thyroid. Diagnostic aspirates may contain three-dimensional papillary fronds, monolayered sheets, tissue fragments, intranuclear cytoplasmic inclusions, psammoma bodies, and multinucleated giant cells.[10, 24, 27, 29] Another helpful feature is the presence of "ground-glass" nuclei characterized by pale homogeneous staining of the nucleus with peripheral clumping of chromatin.[29] Additional features include nuclear grooves, micronucleoli, and metaplastic cytoplasm.[25] Caution must be exercised, however, in applying these criteria because each of these features may be found in benign lesions. This situation is especially problematic when the cytologic material is scanty (Fig. 5–3).[27, 29]

The diagnosis of follicular neoplasms, similar to the significant diagnostic difficulty it poses in histologic material, is perhaps the most difficult problem in thyroid cytopathology. The histologic diagnosis of follicular carcinoma requires the presence of capsular or extrathyroidal invasion, vascular invasion, and lymph node or distant metastasis.[8, 24] Well-differentiated carcinomas may be cytologically indistinguishable from follicular adenomas, and benign follicular lesions with marked cytologic atypia may mimic cancer. For these reasons, most investigators[3] have concluded that follicular adenomas and follicular carcinomas cannot be differentiated reliably by cytologic methods. Some authors[13, 14, 25, 29] contend, however, that cytologic atypia is helpful in the identification of follicular lesions with a greater probability of harboring carcinoma and report those lesions as such. Most cytopathologists do not attempt to separate these two lesions and give a diagnosis of "follicular neoplasm, adenoma or carcinoma" with the recommendation that surgical excision or further evaluation be performed.

Benign and malignant follicular neoplasms can assume several histologic patterns, and the needle aspirates reflect this variability. The specimens are usually extremely cellular with inconspicuous colloid. Often, sheets of epithelium are present, occasionally with "microfollicles" containing colloid. Nuclear atypia can be seen in both adenomas and carcinomas, although some authors[29] reported that crowding and overlapping of nuclei, coarsely granular chromatin, and prominent nucleoli are markers for malignancy (Fig. 5–4).

Medullary carcinoma is an uncommon tumor that arises from the parafollicular C cells

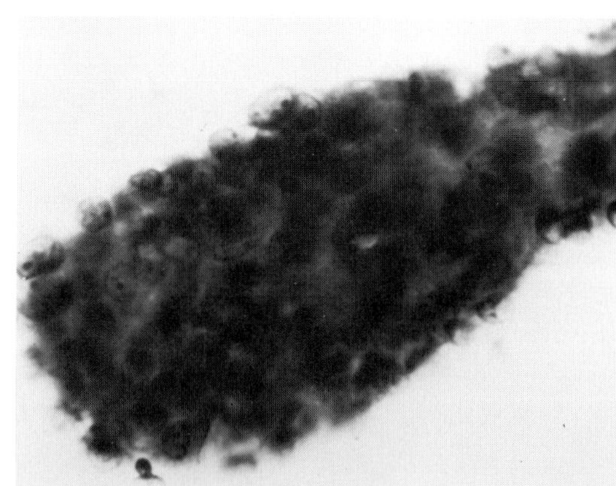

**FIGURE 5–3.** Fine needle aspirate of papillary carcinoma. Delicate papillary frond lined by cuboidal epithelium (Papanicolaou stain; original magnification × 400).

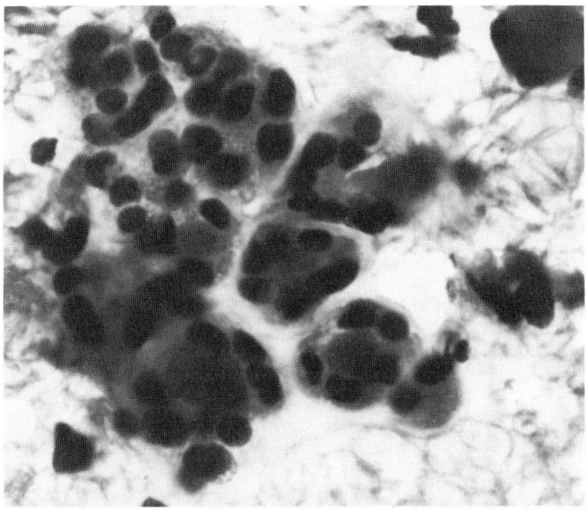

**FIGURE 5–4.** Fine needle aspirate of follicular neoplasm. Highly cellular smear with monotonous follicular cells, microfollicles, and scant amounts of colloid (Papanicolaou stain; original magnification × 400).

that produce calcitonin. Aspirates can contain polygonal, oval, or spindle-shaped cells with acellular deposits of amyloid.[13, 28, 37] Metachromatic stains reveal characteristic red-staining cytoplasmic granules apparently specific for medullary carcinoma.[37] Intranuclear cytoplasmic inclusions similar to those seen in papillary carcinoma may be present. Congo red staining for amyloid and immunoperoxidase staining for calcitonin can be diagnostic.[13] Correct diagnosis of this tumor is important because it is frequently associated with a familial multiple endocrine neoplasia syndrome (Sipple's syndrome), which includes pheochromocytoma. Recognition of medullary carcinoma of the thyroid enables preoperative evaluation of the patient for the presence of a pheochromocytoma. Despite these characteristic features, medullary carcinoma can easily be confused cytologically with other thyroid malignancies, particularly anaplastic carcinoma.[28]

Hürthle cell tumors are considered separately because controversy continues over their diagnosis, natural history, and management.[4, 7, 15, 17, 40, 42] The histologic criteria for benign and malignant Hürthle cell tumors are the same as those for follicular neoplasms, but some investigators[32] believe Hürthle cell tumors are not predictable on histologic grounds. Cytologically, these aspirates consist of a uniform population of Hürthle cells containing abundant granular densely staining cytoplasm with distinct cell borders and a variable degree of nuclear hyperchromatism and atypia. Controversy exists over the usefulness of cytologic atypia in the identification of malignant Hürthle cell neoplasms. A diagnostic pitfall is identification of a non-neoplastic Hürthle cell nodule in Hashimoto's thyroiditis as a Hürthle cell tumor. This can occur when few chronic inflammatory cells are present in an aspirate of thyroiditis.[29]

Undifferentiated (anaplastic) carcinoma of the thyroid is an uncommon highly malignant neoplasm with a characteristic clinical presentation.[29] Subtypes of anaplastic carcinoma include giant cell carcinoma and spindle cell carcinoma. Some authors[31] recognize a small cell variant of anaplastic carcinoma. This entity continues to be controversial, however, because other investigators[6] believe that all of these small cell neoplasms are lymphomas. Fine needle aspirates are usually diagnostic and contain numerous obviously malignant and often bizarre tumor cells. Fine needle aspiration biopsy is especially useful because a definitive diagnosis can be made without surgery.

An uncommon but important tumor is primary lymphoma of the thyroid, which includes most of the small cell undifferentiated tumors. Most of these patients have a background of Hashimoto's thyroiditis, and cytologic differentiation between lymphoma and lymphocytic thyroiditis can be exceedingly difficult.[21] The differentiation of lymphoma from small cell anaplastic carcinoma may be impossible cytologically and histologically, and definitive diagnosis may necessitate immunoperoxidase studies to characterize the epithelial or lymphoid nature of the neoplastic cells.[6, 31]

Other thyroid lesions include branchial cleft cyst, thyroglossal duct cyst, and, rarely, squamous cell carcinoma, sarcoma, and metastatic carcinoma.[29]

The cytopathologic report for thyroid fine needle aspiration biopsy typically includes a description of cytologic findings along with a diagnosis or differential diagnosis. In addition, a statement placing the biopsy result in one of several diagnostic categories is usually included. Use of these categories provides a degree of uniformity and standardization in biopsy diagnosis that helps guide the clinician in managing the patient. At the Lahey Clinic, five diagnostic categories are used.

The first category is "Nondiagnostic" or

"Unsatisfactory," and the criteria for this interpretation have been discussed previously. This diagnosis is rendered when insufficient numbers of well-preserved follicular cells are present or when excessive blood or artifactual degeneration obscures cellular detail. The presence of cyst contents without follicular epithelium is also nondiagnostic.

The second diagnostic heading, "No tumor cells found," is used with non-neoplastic diagnoses, such as nodular goiter, toxic hyperplasia, and thyroiditis (lymphocytic, subacute and acute). This finding supports a decision for conservative management if the clinical impression is that the nodule is benign and if nonoperative management of the nodule is clinically appropriate.

The third category is designated "Atypical." This usually refers to cellular aspirates with abundant follicular epithelium, frequently with scant amounts of colloid. Follicular neoplasms (adenomas and carcinomas) and Hürthle cell tumors comprise the majority of lesions in this category. Because "atypical" lesions include benign and malignant neoplasms, surgical removal of these nodules is suggested by this classification, if that course of action is appropriate on clinical grounds.

The final two categories are "Suspicious for malignancy" and "Diagnostic for malignancy." These categories are usually associated with papillary carcinomas, anaplastic carcinomas, and medullary carcinomas. Only rarely are follicular carcinomas included in these groups. Lymphomas may be included in these categories when the characteristic cytologic findings of cancer are apparent. Lymphomas of the thyroid may also be designated as "Atypical" when differentiation of neoplastic lymphocytes from reactive lymphocytes in a background of Hashimoto's thyroiditis is not possible. The difference between these final two categories is the cytopathologist's degree of certainty in the diagnosis. "Suspicious for malignancy" is used when some of the diagnostic criteria for malignancy are lacking. This phrase indicates that intraoperative confirmation of the diagnosis should be obtained before definitive radical surgery (e.g., total thyroidectomy) is performed. The category "Diagnostic for malignancy" is used when the cytopathologist is sufficiently confident in the diagnosis to permit initiation of definitive surgical or nonsurgical treatment without further tissue confirmation. Because of the implications of a definitive cytologic diagnosis, many cytopathologists insist that all diagnostic criteria of malignancy be present before a conclusive diagnosis is made.

Use of these "coded" diagnostic categories greatly facilitates communication between clinician and cytopathologist. They provide standardization of the cytologic diagnosis regardless of which pathologist interprets the slides. The categories also correspond to broad management schemes, thereby assisting the clinician in managing patients with a thyroid nodule.

## RESULTS

### Efficacy

Numerous studies have examined the efficacy of fine needle aspiration biopsy of the thyroid in both the United States and Europe (Table 5–1). In Europe, needle aspiration and cytopathologic interpretation are usually performed by the same person, most often with use of May-Grünwald-Giemsa metachromatic stain. On the other hand, in the United States needle aspiration and cytologic interpretation are frequently carried out by different individuals, and slides are fixed in alcohol and stained by the Papanicolaou method. In the latter instance, close communication between the aspirator and cytologist becomes critical.

About 15 to 20 per cent of operated nodules are found to be malignant when the decision for surgery is based solely on clinical grounds and the results of fine needle aspiration biopsy are not used (Table 5–1).[2, 32] Use of the information from fine needle aspiration biopsy in the preoperative evaluation increased the percentage of malignancies in operated lesions from 14 to 29 per cent and from 24 to 56 per cent in two large series.[20, 32] On the other hand, the percentage of excised benign nodules decreased from 36 to 9 per cent and from 85 to 68 per cent in these same studies.[20, 32]

In most studies, the rate of false-negative cytologic diagnoses with fine needle aspiration biopsy has been less than 3 per cent; false-positive diagnoses were observed in 10.4

**TABLE 5–1. Results of Fine Needle Aspiration Biopsy of Thyroid***

| | BENIGN | | | MALIGNANT OR SUSPICIOUS | | | | INSUFFICIENT | | | TOTAL | | |
|---|---|---|---|---|---|---|---|---|---|---|---|---|---|
| AUTHOR(S) | No. Cases | No. Operated | No. False-Negative | No. Cases | No. Operated | No. Malignant | No. False-Positive | No. Cases | No. Operated | No. Malignant | No. Cases | No. Operated | No. Malignant |
| Aretz et al.[1] | 76 | 25 | 2 | 9 | 9 | 6 | 3 | — | — | — | 85 | 34 | 8 |
| Ashcraft and Van Herle[2]† | 848 | 848 | 22 | 482 | 482 | 246 | 7 | 51 | 51 | 0 | 1381 | 1381 | 268 (19.4%)‡ |
| Ashcraft and Van Herle[2]§ | 8313 | 1520 | 36 | 1229 | 789 | 446 | 26 | 475 | 40 | 1 | 10,387 | 2355 | 483 |
| Fitz-Patrick et al.[9] | 148 | 2 | 0 | 16 | 16 | 11 | 5 | 36 | — | — | 200 | 18 | 11 |
| Hamberger et al.[20] | 74 | 6 | 0 | 40 | 38 | 12 | 26 | 10 | — | — | 124 | 46 | 12 |
| Miller et al.[32] | 741 | 62 | 1 | 334 | 269 | 170 | 99 | — | — | — | 1075 | 331 | 171 |
| Prinz et al.[34] | 39 | 39 | 1 | 39 | 39 | 30 | 9 | 31 | 31 | 2 | 109 | 109 | 33 |
| Russ et al.[35] | 77 | 21 | 3 | 8 | 8 | 8 | 0 | — | — | — | 85 | 29 | 11 |
| Stavric et al.[38] | 1479 | 37 | 4 | 57 | 38 | 35 | 3 | — | — | — | 1536 | 75 | 39 |
| Suen and Quenville[39] | 233 | 9 | 2 | 71 | 70 | 65 | 5 | 15 | 2 | 2 | 304 | 79 | 37 |
| TOTALS | 12,028 | 2569 | 71 (2.8%) | 2285 | 1758 | 1029 | 183 (10.4%) | 618 | 124 | 5 (4.0%) | 15,286 | 4457 | 1073 (24.1%)¶ |

*Adapted from Ashcraft, M. W., and Van Herle, A. J.: Management of thyroid nodules. II. Scanning techniques, thyroid suppressive therapy, and fine needle aspiration. Head Neck Surg., *3*:297–322, 1981.

†A collected series of reports in which all clinically identified thyroid nodules were surgically removed regardless of cytologic findings.

‡Percentage of malignant nodules at surgery when all nodules were removed regardless of cytologic findings.

§A collected series of reports in which only selected nodules were removed based on clinical and cytologic criteria. Percentage of false-negative or false-positive results or malignant nodules, respectively, using number of operated nodules as denominator.

¶Percentage of cancers found in this category.

per cent of patients. In reports of the outcome of unsatisfactory or insufficient aspirations, cancer was demonstrated in about 4 per cent of patients. This finding emphasizes the importance of establishing defined criteria for adequacy of an aspirate because a sparsely cellular specimen cannot be equated with benignity.

### Cost-Effectiveness

Several investigators have evaluated the cost-effectiveness of fine needle aspiration biopsy in the management of thyroid nodules. Miller and coworkers[32] showed that with the introduction of fine needle aspiration biopsy the number of patients undergoing operation was halved and the percentage of cancers discovered in surgically removed nodules was doubled. The number of patients with benign disease who underwent operation decreased by 75 per cent, and the total percentage of identified cancers remained about the same, thus indicating that cancers were probably not being missed by this management scheme. Miller and colleagues[32] estimated that about $750 was saved for each patient evaluated and treated. Similarly, Hamberger and colleagues[20] compared the cost of management of thyroid nodules before and after the introduction of fine needle aspiration biopsy at the Mayo Clinic and identified a cost savings of $400 (25 per cent) per patient with fine needle aspiration biopsy. The yield of cancers in surgical specimens was doubled, and the percentage of patients undergoing thyroid operations decreased from 67 per cent to 43 per cent. Suen and Quenville[39] noted an increase from 14 to 47 per cent in the percentage of cancers in surgically excised nodules after the introduction of fine needle aspiration biopsy.

Van Herle and associates[41] analyzed the cost effectiveness of various schemes for evaluation of thyroid nodules and compared the accuracy of fine needle aspiration biopsy, radionuclide scanning techniques, and ultrasonography. They stated that the most effective management strategy results in the fewest missed cancers and the fewest operations for benign conditions at the lowest cost. This goal is achieved by the test with the highest specificity and sensitivity in the selection of patients for surgery. Although the sensitivity of fine needle aspiration biopsy is similar to that of other commonly used screening techniques, its specificity is much greater. When both indicators are considered together, fine needle aspiration biopsy appears to be the most accurate screening technique. These authors[41] recommended an evaluation plan with fine needle aspiration biopsy as the initial screening test. Aspirates that are found to be positive for cancer result in a recommendation for surgery; suspicious aspirates lead to radionuclide scanning. Hot nodules on scans are managed nonsurgically, and the remainder are removed. This strategy produced the lowest average cost per nodule and the lowest average cost per correct diagnosis, and the number of missed cancers was comparable to that for the other evaluation plans.

### Relative Accuracy of Needle Biopsy Techniques

The accuracy of fine needle aspiration biopsy (using a 22- to 27-gauge needle) has been compared with the results of large needle (16 to 18 gauge) or cutting needle (14 gauge) biopsies. Ashcraft and Van Herle[2] reviewed several studies using these techniques and found no appreciable differences in the accuracy or yields of the three methods. Core needle biopsy using the Vim-Silverman needle results in a higher proportion of unsatisfactory aspirates. In addition, core needle biopsy carries a higher risk of complications, including hematoma, transient sweating and dizziness, and injury to the trachea, laryngeal nerve, or vascular structures. Large needle biopsy is associated with minimal risks, and complications resulting from fine needle aspiration are rare.[10] Silverman and colleagues[36] compared concurrent fine needle aspiration biopsy with large needle or core needle biopsy in 23 patients and found the diagnostic accuracy of the techniques to be comparable. However, large needle and core needle biopsies yielded unsatisfactory results in 15 per cent of patients. In addition, large needle and core needle biopsies can be performed only on lesions greater than 1.0 to 1.5 cm in diameter, thus further limiting their usefulness.

## DISCUSSION

Thyroid nodules are exceedingly common in the adult population, but malignant thyroid nodules are rare. Because surgical treatment of all nodules is impractical, an effective screening technique is needed to select those nodules that should be removed surgically. Although no screening tool is completely accurate, fine needle aspiration biopsy is currently the most sensitive and specific method available. Nevertheless, certain limitations and pitfalls must be kept in mind.

### Sampling Error

Sampling error is a major hazard in thyroid cytology. The rate of unsatisfactory aspirates reportedly ranges from 7.5 to 46 per cent.[39] Well-defined criteria for specimen adequacy should be established by each laboratory. Probably the most common instance of false-negative diagnoses involves the interpretation of inadequate specimens as benign. This problem diminishes with increased experience in both aspiration and cytologic interpretation. Therefore, a negative test result does not rule out the possibility of malignant disease, and a negative result should not deter further evaluation when other clinical findings suggest cancer. Similarly, aspiration of cyst contents without follicular epithelium is inadequate for cytologic interpretation and should be reported as nondiagnostic.

### Synchronous Thyroid Diseases

A second pitfall is encountered when more than one disease is present in the thyroid. This situation is particularly problematic in patients with chronic lymphocytic thyroiditis because synchronous malignant epithelial neoplasms have been reported in more than 10 per cent of patients with Hashimoto's thyroiditis.[18, 19] Specifically, recognition of primary lymphoma of the thyroid in a background of lymphocytic thyroiditis, with which this neoplasm is usually associated, can be extremely difficult.[21] Occult carcinomas can also be missed primarily because of limitations of sampling. Another possibility for error that arises in the setting of Hashimoto's thyroiditis is the overinterpretation of abundant follicular epithelium with oncocytic features as a Hürthle cell neoplasm.

### Follicular Neoplasms

Perhaps the most difficult problem in thyroid cytology is the characterization of follicular neoplasms. Most investigators agree that follicular adenomas cannot be distinguished consistently and reliably from follicular carcinomas by cytologic studies. When a cellular aspirate of follicular epithelium is obtained, most cytopathologists report this as "follicular neoplasm" and suggest surgical biopsy.[3] A follicular adenoma identified by biopsy after such a recommendation should not be construed as a false-positive cytologic result because adenomas represent benign neoplasms that can be distinguished from carcinoma only by thorough histologic evaluation. Hyperplastic nodular goiter can also mimic a follicular neoplasm, thus occasionally leading to a false-positive cytologic interpretation.

### Seeding of Tumor Along Needle Track

A concern that has impeded the implementation of fine needle aspiration biopsy in the United States is the fear of tumor implantation along the needle track. One instance of seeding was reported after biopsy with a Vim-Silverman needle, and an instance of implantation of a renal cell carcinoma metastatic to the thyroid occurred after Vim-Silverman needle biopsy.[2] A subcutaneous implant of thyroid carcinoma was detected six months after preoperative fine needle aspiration biopsy and surgical removal of a tumor, although the source of tumor implantation could not be determined with certainty.[5] No other instances of tumor implantation have been reported after fine needle aspiration biopsy of the thyroid despite extensive worldwide experience with this technique for 57 years. The risk of tumor implantation after core needle biopsy has been overestimated, and the risk after fine needle aspiration biopsy appears to be exceedingly small.[2]

### Cutoff Point to Discriminate between Positive and Negative Results

A fifth limitation is one that is inherent in all screening tests, i.e., error due to setting a cutoff point to discriminate between positive and negative test results.[22] In a practical sense, fine needle aspiration biopsy of the thyroid can produce two results: negative (observe the patient without surgical intervention) or positive (proceed to surgical removal of the nodule). The numbers of false-positive results, i.e., surgery recommended for benign disease, or false-negative results, i.e., observation recommended for malignant disease, depend on where the cutoff point is set. Although a small percentage of false-positive results may be acceptable to minimize the number of missed cancers, a useful screening test should produce few false-negative results. Miller and coworkers[32] stated that the minimal rate of false-positive findings is about 10 per cent if one wishes to avoid missing a diagnosis of cancer. Because of the qualitative rather than quantitative nature of this cutoff point, the diagnosis will be suspicious or equivocal in an estimated 30 per cent of patients.[22] Whether an investigator includes this equivocal category with the positive or the negative results markedly affects the nominal sensitivity, specificity, predictive values, and efficiency of the test (Table 5–2).[22]

Hajdu and Melamed[17, 18] reported that fine needle aspiration biopsy of the thyroid was "largely abandoned at Memorial Sloan-Kettering Cancer Center" because "aspiration cytology has a very limited role in the definitive diagnosis of primary neoplasms of the thyroid, and a negative report certainly should not be considered conclusive and diagnostic." This statement is based on their assumption that "aspiration cytology is a diagnostic and not a screening technique." It is true that fine needle aspiration biopsy of the thyroid is diagnostic in only a minority of circumstances. The technique can yield a definitive diagnosis in most instances of anaplastic or medullary carcinoma and in many instances of papillary carcinoma and Hashimoto's thyroiditis.[11, 13, 15, 27, 28, 29, 37] However, most cold nodules of the thyroid represent follicular lesions,[3] and fine needle aspiration biopsy is infrequently definitive in these instances. Nevertheless, it is the most effective screening method available and consistently provides useful information in the management of the thyroid nodule. The most important role of fine needle aspiration biopsy of the thyroid is as a preoperative screening procedure. With careful application of this method and close communication between the clinician and the cytopathologist, fine needle aspiration biopsy is a useful tool in

**TABLE 5–2. Variations in Sensitivity, Specificity, Positive Predictive Value, Negative Predictive Value, and Efficiency, Depending on Definition of Positive Test***

| AUTHOR(S) | NO. PATIENTS | SENSITIVITY† (%) | SPECIFICITY‡ (%) | POSITIVE PREDICTIVE VALUE§ (%) | NEGATIVE PREDICTIVE VALUE (%) | EFFICIENCY¶ |
|---|---|---|---|---|---|---|
| Ashcraft and Van Herle[2] | 1050 | | | | | |
| Narrow definition# | | 73 | 99 | 97 | 94 | 94 |
| Broad definition** | | 92 | 74 | 46 | 97 | 78 |
| Löwhagen et al.[30] | 412 | | | | | |
| Narrow definition# | | 66 | 100 | 100 | 91 | 92 |
| Broad definition** | | 91 | 69 | 47 | 96 | 74 |
| Prinz et al.[34] | 109 | | | | | |
| Broad definition** | | 88 | 80 | 77 | 90 | 83 |

*Adapted from Hoffman, W. H.: Diagnostic accuracy of fine-needle aspiration biopsy in the diagnosis of thyroid malignancy. Pathologist, *40*:9–14, 1986.

$$\dagger\text{Sensitivity} = \frac{\text{True positives}}{\text{True positives} + \text{false negatives}}$$

$$\ddagger\text{Specificity} = \frac{\text{True negatives}}{\text{True negatives} + \text{false positives}}$$

$$\S\text{Positive Predictive Value} = \frac{\text{True positives}}{\text{All positives}}$$

$$\text{Negative Predictive Value} = \frac{\text{True negatives}}{\text{All negatives}}$$

$$\P\text{Efficiency} = \frac{\text{True positives} + \text{true negatives}}{\text{All results}}$$

#Narrow definition includes only conclusive diagnoses of malignancy as positive tests.

**Broad definition includes both "suspicious for malignancy" and "conclusive for malignancy" among positive results. Inclusion of suspicious diagnoses in positive results (i.e., broad definition) improves sensitivity but worsens specificity, efficiency, and positive predictive value of the test.

the management of patients with thyroid nodules.

## REFERENCES


1. Aretz, H. T., Silverman, M. L., Kolodziejski, J. L., et al.: Fine-needle aspiration: Why it deserves another look. Postgrad. Med., *75*:49–56, 1984.
2. Ashcraft, M. W., and Van Herle, A. J.: Management of thyroid nodules. II. Scanning techniques, thyroid suppressive therapy, and fine needle aspiration. Head Neck Surg., *3*:297–322, 1981.
3. Atkinson, B., Ernst, C. S., and LiVolsi, V. A.: Cytologic diagnoses of follicular tumors of the thyroid. (Editorial) Diagn. Cytopathol., *2*:1–3, 1986.
4. Bauman, A., and Strawbridge, H. T. G.: Spontaneous disappearance of an atypical Hürthle cell adenoma. Am. J. Clin. Pathol., *80*:399–402, 1983.
5. Block, M. A., Miller, J. M., and Kini, S. R.: The potential impact of needle biopsy on surgery for thyroid nodules. World J. Surg., *4*:737–745, 1980.
6. Burt, A., Kerr, D. J., Brown, I. L., et al.: Lymphoid and epithelial markers in small cell anaplastic thyroid tumours. J. Clin. Pathol., *38*:893–896, 1985.
7. Caplan, R. H., Abellera, R. M., and Kisken, W. A.: Hürthle cell tumors of the thyroid gland: A clinicopathologic review and long-term follow-up. J.A.M.A., *251*:3114–3117, 1984.
8. Evans, H. L.: Follicular neoplasms of the thyroid: A study of 44 cases followed for a minimum of 10 years, with emphasis on differential diagnosis. Cancer, *54*:535–540, 1984.
9. Fitz-Patrick, D., Navin, J. J., and Fukunaga, B. N.: Fine-needle aspiration biopsy of thyroid nodules: A diagnostic method that minimizes the need for surgery. Postgrad. Med., *80*:62–68, 1986.
10. Frable, W. J.: Thin Needle Aspiration Biopsy. Philadelphia, W. B. Saunders Co., 1983, pp. 152–182.
11. Frable, W. J., and Frable, M. A.: Fine-needle aspiration biopsy of the thyroid: Histopathologic and clinical correlations. *In* Fenoglio, C. M., and Wolff, M. (eds.): Progress in Surgical Pathology. Volume 1. New York, Masson, 1980, pp. 105–118.
12. Friedman, M., Shimaoka, K., Rao, U., et al.: Diagnosis of chronic lymphocytic thyroiditis (nodular presentation) by needle aspiration. Acta Cytol., *25*:513–522, 1981.
13. Geddie, W. R., Bedard, Y. C., and Strawbridge, T. G.: Medullary carcinoma of the thyroid in fine-needle aspiration biopsies. Am. J. Clin. Pathol., *82*:552–558, 1984.
14. Gershengorn, M. C., McClung, M. R., Chu, E. W., et al.: Fine-needle aspiration cytology in the preoperative diagnosis of thyroid nodules. Ann. Intern. Med., *87*:265–269, 1977.
15. Gosain, A. K., and Clark, O. H.: Hürthle cell neoplasms: Malignant potential. Arch. Surg., *119*:515–519, 1984.
16. Guarda, L. A., and Baskin, H. J.: Inflammatory and lymphoid lesions of the thyroid gland: Cytopathology by fine-needle aspiration. Am. J. Clin. Pathol., *87*:14–22, 1987.
17. Gundry, S. R., Burney, R. E., Thompson, N. W., et al.: Total thyroidectomy for Hürthle cell neoplasm of the thyroid. Arch. Surg., *118*:529–532, 1983.
18. Hajdu, S. I., and Melamed, M. R.: Limitations of aspiration cytology in the diagnosis of primary neoplasms. Acta Cytol., *28*:337–345, 1984.
19. Hajdu, S. I., and Melamed, M. R.: Limitations of aspiration cytology in the diagnosis of primary neoplasms. (Letter) Acta Cytol., *29*:491–492, 1985.
20. Hamberger, B., Gharib, H., Melton, L. J., et al.: Fine-needle aspiration biopsy of thyroid nodules: Impact on thyroid practice and cost of care. Am. J. Med., *73*:381–384, 1982.
21. Hamburger, J. I., Miller, J. M., and Kini, S. R.: Lymphoma of the thyroid. Ann. Intern. Med., *99*:685–693, 1983.
22. Hoffman, W. H.: Diagnostic accuracy of fine needle aspiration biopsy in the diagnosis of thyroid malignancy. Pathologist, *40*:9–14, 1986.
23. Holm, L. E., Blomgren, H., and Löwhagen, T.: Cancer risks in patients with chronic lymphocytic thyroiditis. N. Engl. J. Med., *312*:601–604, 1985.
24. Iida, F.: Surgical significance of capsule invasion of adenoma of the thyroid. Surg. Gynecol. Obstet., *144*:710–712, 1977.
25. Kini, S. R.: Guides to Clinical Aspiration Biopsy: Thyroid. New York, Igaku-Shoin Medical Publishers, Inc., 1987.
26. Kini, S. R., Miller, J. M., and Hamburger, J. I.: Cytopathology of thyroid nodules. Henry Ford Hosp. Med. J., *30*:17–24, 1982.
27. Kini, S. R., Miller, J. M., Hamburger, J. I., et al.: Cytopathology of papillary carcinoma of the thyroid by fine needle aspiration. Acta Cytol., *24*:511–521, 1980.
28. Kini, S. R., Miller, J. M., Hamburger, J. I., et al.: Cytopathologic features of medullary carcinoma of the thyroid. Arch. Pathol. Lab. Med., *108*:156–159, 1984.
29. Koss, L. G., Woyke, S., and Olszewski, W.: Aspiration Biopsy: Cytologic Interpretation and Histologic Bases. New York, Igaku-Shoin, 1984, pp. 154–190.
30. Löwhagen, T., Granberg, P. O., Lundell, G., et al.: Aspiration biopsy cytology (ABC) in nodules of the thyroid gland suspected to be malignant. Surg. Clin. North Am., *59*:3–18, 1979.
31. Mambo, N. C., and Irwin, S. M.: Anaplastic small cell neoplasms of the thyroid: An immunoperoxidase study. Hum. Pathol., *15*:55–60, 1984.
32. Miller, J. M., Hamburger, J. I., and Kini, S. R.: The impact of needle biopsy on the preoperative diagnosis of thyroid nodules. Henry Ford Hosp. Med. J., *28*:145–148, 1980.
33. Noguchi, M., Mori, N., Kojima, M., et al.: A case report of malignant lymphoma with Hashimoto's thyroiditis. Am. J. Clin. Pathol., *83*:650–655, 1985.
34. Prinz, R. A., O'Morchoe, P. J., Barbato, A. L., et al.: Fine needle aspiration biopsy of thyroid nodules. Ann. Surg., *198*:70–73, 1983.
35. Russ, J. E., Scanlon, E. F., and Christ, M. A.: Aspiration cytology of head and neck masses. Am. J. Surg., *136*:342–347, 1978.
36. Silverman, J. F., West, R. L., Finley, J. L., et al.: Fine-needle aspiration versus large-needle biopsy

or cutting biopsy in evaluation of thyroid nodules. Diagn. Cytopathol., *2*:25–30, 1986.
37. Söderström, N., Telenius-Berg, M., and Ånkerman, M.: Diagnosis of medullary carcinoma of the thyroid by fine needle aspiration biopsy. Acta Med. Scand., *197*:71–76, 1975.
38. Stavric, G. D., Karanfilski, B. T., Kalamaras, A. K., et al.: Early diagnosis and detection of clinically non-suspected thyroid neoplasia by the cytologic method. Cancer, *45*:340–344, 1980.
39. Suen, K. C., and Quenville, N. F.: Fine needle aspiration biopsy of the thyroid gland: A study of 304 cases. J. Clin. Pathol., *36*:1036–1045, 1983.
40. Thompson, N. W., Dunn, E. L., Batsakis, J. G., and Nishiyama, R. H.: Hürthle cell lesions of the thyroid gland. Surg. Gynecol. Obstet., *139*:555–560, 1974.
41. Van Herle, A. J., Rich, P., Ljung, B. E., et al.: The thyroid nodule. Ann. Intern. Med., *96*:221–232, 1982.
42. Watson, R. G., Brennan, M. D., Goellner, J. R., et al.: Invasive Hürthle cell carcinoma of the thyroid: Natural history and management. Mayo Clin. Proc., *59*:851–855, 1984.

# 6

# THYROID PHYSIOLOGY AND FUNCTION TESTS

*Mary Beth Hodge, M.D.*

The thyroid gland synthesizes, stores, and secretes thyroid hormone, which is necessary for normal growth and development, and plays a vital role in numerous diverse metabolic processes.[4, 5]

## THYROID HORMONE SYNTHESIS

Iodine is crucial to the production of thyroid hormone. Dietary iodine is absorbed in the gastrointestinal tract and circulates in the bloodstream as inorganic iodide. Approximately 150 to 200 μg of iodine is required each day. In the United States, the average daily intake of iodine is approximately 500 μg/day but varies in different regions. Iodine is present in many foods and water, but it is also present in many medications, vitamins, and antiseptic solutions. Another source of iodine is that which is derived from the body's deiodination of monoiodotyrosine and diiodotyrosine. The iodide is recirculated and is trapped by the thyroid. Iodide in the plasma that is not trapped by the thyroid is removed through the salivary glands, kidney, and gastrointestinal tract. (Some may be reabsorbed and recirculated.)

Thyrotropin (TSH) secreted by the anterior pituitary gland enhances the ability of the thyroid to trap iodide. When iodide is trapped by the thyroid, it is oxidized by the peroxidase enzyme to form a higher valence form of iodine. After this oxidation step, the iodine is capable of iodinating tyrosine residues of the thyroglobulin molecule to form monoiodotyrosine and diiodotyrosine. This is known as the organification step.[5] Thyroglobulin is a large glycoprotein that is synthesized within the thyroid follicular cell and secreted into the lumen of the follicle.

After the formation of monoiodotyrosine and diiodotyrosine, a coupling enzyme unites two diiodotyrosine molecules to form tetraiodothyronine ($T_4$). The same coupling enzyme unites one molecule of diiodotyrosine with one molecule of monoiodotyrosine to form 3,3′,5′triiodothyronine ($T_3$).

The final step in thyroid hormone synthesis involves the release of $T_4$ and $T_3$ into the bloodstream. This is accomplished by proteolytic enzymes that cleave $T_4$ and $T_3$ from the thyroglobulin molecule. Thyroglobulin is too large to be transported across the thyroid follicular cell membrane and in general is only released into the circulation in large quantities after acute damage to the thyroid follicle, such as is seen with subacute thyroiditis or after radiation therapy. However, many patients with goiter and even some patients with no discernible thyroid disease will have a detectable level of thyroglobulin, but the level usually is not elevated.

The only source of endogenous $T_4$ is that produced by the thyroid gland. The thyroid produces much more $T_4$ than $T_3$. Only approximately 20 per cent of $T_3$ is produced by the thyroid gland. The remaining 80 per cent of $T_3$ is produced by peripheral conversion of $T_4$ to $T_3$.[5] This is accomplished by the enzyme 5′monodeiodinase, which removes the 5′iodine from the outer ring of $T_4$. This reaction takes place in the peripheral tissues, such as the liver, muscles, kidney, and anterior pituitary gland. However, in early primary hypothyroidism and in certain types of hyperthyroidism, such as Graves' disease and toxic nodular goiter, direct thyroid secretion of $T_3$ may account for a much larger proportion of $T_3$ production than occurs under normal circumstances.

Usually, the proportion of $T_4$ not converted to $T_3$ is instead converted to reverse $T_3$ by removal of the 5′iodine from the inner ring of $T_4$. Reverse $T_3$ is essentially metabolically inactive. In certain situations, both physiologic and pathologic, conversion of $T_4$ to $T_3$ and degradation of reverse $T_3$ are decreased (Table 6–1). Whether this results in hypothyroidism at the level of the peripheral tissues is not known. The amount of TSH is not increased, and this phenomenon may represent a method of energy conservation in critical illness and thus serve as an adaptive response.[3]

**TABLE 6–1. States Associated with Decreased Peripheral Conversion of $T_4$ to $T_3$**

| |
|---|
| Fetal and neonatal life |
| Starvation |
| Acute and chronic liver disease |
| Acute and chronic renal disease |
| Acute and chronic nonthyroidal illness (euthyroid sick syndrome) |
| Postoperative state |
| Drugs |
|   Propylthiouracil |
|   Propranolol |
|   Dexamethasone—Only in large doses |
|   Amiodarone—In standard doses |
| Iodinated radiocontrast agents |

Adapted from Ingbar, S.: Diseases of the thyroid. *In* Brunwald, E., Isselbacher, K. J., Petersdorf, R. G., et al. (eds.): Harrison's Principles of Internal Medicine. Edition 11. New York, McGraw-Hill Book Co., 1987, pp. 1732–1752.

Several substances can interfere with the normal production of thyroid hormone by blocking various enzymatic steps. Potentially, this could result in hypothyroidism and formation of a goiter by secondarily increasing TSH. Even iodine, when given in large enough doses, can acutely block the organification and coupling steps and prevent the release of thyroid hormone. This can lead to hypothyroidism, which is usually transient (Wolff-Chaikoff effect).[12] Most of the time, the normal thyroid gland can escape this inhibition and continue to produce hormone. An abnormal thyroid, such as is present in Hashimoto's thyroiditis, may not be able to escape and thus reduction of thyroid hormone production is sustained. Patients with active Graves' disease may be able to escape from this effect and that is why stable iodine is not an effective long-term treatment. However, patients with Graves' disease who were previously treated with radioactive iodine and who remain mildly hyperthyroid may have a sustained Wolff-Chaikoff effect when given stable iodine. It is unclear why these patients have a sustained sensitivity to stable iodine, but its cause may be related to a possible defect in hormone synthesis induced by radioactive iodine. The fetal thyroid gland is also sensitive to the inhibitory effects of large doses of iodine and can result in a large goiter and hypothyroidism.

Interestingly, large doses of iodine, such as given during intravenous radiocontrast examinations, can lead to the development of hyperthyroidism in patients with autonomously functioning thyroid tissue, such as in the presence of Graves' disease and multinodular goiter. This iodine-induced hyperthyroidism is known as jodbasedow effect and is usually a transient phenomenon.[2]

Lithium, which is used to treat manic depressive illness, has several effects on intrathyroidal iodine metabolism and can block the release of thyroid hormone and eventually can lead to the formation of a goiter and hypothyroidism.[11] Occasionally, lithium may cause hyperthyroidism, although the mechanism is unknown. Decadron can also block the release of thyroid hormone.

In the evaluation of a patient with a goiter or thyroid dysfunction, it is important to take a thorough history of all drugs used by the patient, including over-the-counter drugs, such as kelp, vitamins, and topical antiseptics, that often contain iodine and that patients do not consider medications because they are not prescribed by a physician.

## THYROID HORMONE TRANSPORT

When the thyroid hormones are released from the thyroid, they are bound to various thyroxine-binding proteins and are transported to the peripheral tissues. Approximately 75 per cent of $T_4$ is bound to thyroxine-binding globulin (TBG), 15 per cent of $T_4$ is bound to thyroxine-binding prealbumin, and 10 per cent of $T_4$ is bound to albumin. Triiodothyronine is less avidly bound to TBG and albumin. Thyroid hormone is metabolically inactive when bound to any one of the binding proteins. The much smaller fraction of unbound or free thyroid hormone is the metabolically active hormone (free $T_4$, free $T_3$). That $T_3$ is less avidly bound to proteins accounts for its rapid onset of action.

Various disturbances (physiologic, pathologic, or pharmacologic) of the serum-binding protein levels alter the total but not the free circulating $T_4$ and $T_3$ concentrations. Perhaps the most common disturbance seen is an elevated TBG caused by exogenous (oral contraceptive) or endogenous (pregnancy) estrogens (Table 6–2).

**TABLE 6–2. Conditions Associated with Altered Concentration of Thyroxine-Binding Globulin (TBG)**

| INCREASED TBG | DECREASED TBG |
|---|---|
| Pregnancy | Androgens |
| Oral contraceptives | Glucocorticoids |
| Estrogen replacement therapy | Severe systemic illness |
| | Acromegaly |
| Neonate | Nephrotic syndrome |
| Acute intermittent porphyria | Congenital TBG deficiency |
| | Chronic liver disease |
| Hepatitis | L-Asparaginase |
| Primary biliary cirrhosis | |
| Perphenazine; clofibrate | |
| Congenital TBG excess | |

Adapted from Ingbar, S.: Diseases of the thyroid. *In* Brunwald, E., Isselbacher, K. J., Petersdorf, R. G., et al. (eds.): Harrison's Principles of Internal Medicine. Edition 11. New York, McGraw-Hill Book Co., 1987, pp. 1732–1752.

## MECHANISM OF ACTION OF THYROID HORMONE

Interaction with a specific intracellular receptor initiates the effects of thyroid hormone. Considerable evidence indicates that $T_3$ is the active hormone because $T_3$ binds to nuclear receptors with greater affinity than $T_4$, and $T_3$ is two to four times as potent as $T_4$ in several biologic systems.

## REGULATION OF THYROID FUNCTION

The hypothalamus and pituitary gland are important in the regulation of thyroid function. In addition, an autoregulatory mechanism is found within the thyroid gland that serves to keep the pool of thyroid hormone stable.[4]

Thyrotropin, a glycoprotein secreted by the anterior pituitary gland, stimulates iodine trapping and the biosynthesis and secretion of $T_4$ and $T_3$. Thyrotropin also causes follicular cell hypertrophy and hyperplasia.

Thyrotropin secretion is regulated by thyrotropin-releasing hormone (TRH) and thyroid hormone ($T_4$ and $T_3$). Thyrotropin-releasing hormone is secreted by the hypothalamus and stimulates the synthesis and secretion of TSH in the anterior pituitary gland. Thyroid hormones $T_4$ and $T_3$ inhibit the action of TRH on the anterior pituitary gland, thus resulting in a decrease in the secretion of TSH. Of the two thyroid hormones, $T_4$ and $T_3$, $T_3$ is thought to play the larger role in the inhibition of TSH secretion by the pituitary gland. This occurs by way of the intrapituitary conversion of $T_4$ to $T_3$.[4] However, L-thyroxine rather than L-triiodothyronine is the drug of choice when attempting to suppress TSH because L-thyroxine has a longer half-life and is therefore a more stable hormone. Exogenous $T_4$, like endogenous $T_4$, will be converted to $T_3$ within the pituitary gland as well as elsewhere.

Intrathyroidal regulation of thyroid function involves the ability of various amounts of ingested iodine either to enhance or to suppress thyroid iodide trapping and subsequent thyroid hormone synthesis. When a large amount of iodine is ingested, the iodide trapping is decreased, and thus thyroid hormone synthesis is decreased. When a person is in a state of iodine depletion, iodide trapping is increased to attempt to increase thyroid hormone synthesis. These reciprocal changes in thyroid iodide trapping, depending on the amount of iodine available, serve to keep the thyroid hormone pool constant.[4]

## LABORATORY TESTS TO DETERMINE THYROID FUNCTION

Many laboratory tests are available to determine the functional status of the thyroid gland. A thorough understanding of these tests is important to utilize them properly. Symptoms and signs represent clinical manifestations of peripheral thyroid hormone action and may identify many patients, but the often subtle onset of and nonspecific manifestations of both hyperthyroidism and hypothyroidism make the history and physical examination alone unreliable.

### *Serum Total $T_4$*

The serum total $T_4$ concentration is measured by radioimmunoassay. This assay measures that portion of $T_4$ that is bound to the binding proteins (the most important of which is TBG) as well as the unbound $T_4$, known as free $T_4$. The level of total $T_4$ is elevated in the majority of patients with hyperthyroidism, but it is also elevated in euthyroid patients who have elevated TBG (pregnancy, estrogen use, congenital TBG excess). When the level of total $T_4$ is elevated, only by an estimation of the TBG concentration or by a determination of the free $T_4$ concentration can hyperthyroidism be distinguished from an elevated level of TBG. Patients who have an elevated level of total $T_4$ on the basis of an elevated level of TBG will have a normal free $T_4$ level.

### *Serum Free Thyroxine*

The serum free thyroxine (free $T_4$) concentration can now be measured directly by radioimmunoassay. The free $T_4$ assay has proved to be accurate and is useful to obtain when the levels of total $T_4$ and $T_3$ resin uptake are borderline abnormal and are suggestive of but not diagnostic of hyperthyroidism. An elevated level of free $T_4$ is firm evidence that the patient is hyperthyroid.

The free thyroxine index is a calculation using the total $T_4$ and the $T_3$ resin uptake, which provides information similar to but not as precise as the free $T_4$ test. When interpreting laboratory results, the clinician must be careful not to confuse the free $T_4$ with the free thyroxine index.

### *Triiodothyronine Resin Uptake Test*

The $T_3$ resin uptake is the best available test for the indirect measurement of serum TBG concentration. It is not a measure of total $T_3$ or free $T_3$ concentrations. Total $T_4$ and $T_3$ resin uptake test results are used in combination to distinguish $T_4$ production abnormalities from TBG alterations when the free $T_4$ test is not available.

When the levels of total $T_4$ and $T_3$ resin uptake are abnormal in the same direction, a true thyroid hormone production abnormality is present. When the levels of total $T_4$ and $T_3$ resin uptake are abnormal in opposite directions, usually a TBG abnormality is present (e.g., in true hypothyroidism, both total $T_4$ and $T_3$ resin uptakes are decreased; in TBG excess, total $T_4$ is increased, and $T_3$ resin uptake is decreased).

### *Serum Total $T_3$*

Like the serum total $T_4$, the total $T_3$ is measured by radioimmunoassay technique. The total $T_3$ consists of the $T_3$, which is bound to the binding proteins, plus the free fraction of $T_3$. The level of total $T_3$ is elevated in most patients with hyperthyroidism and is useful in patients who are suspected of having a toxic nodule or toxic multinodular goiter because in these two types of hyperthyroidism more $T_3$ than $T_4$ is often produced. The level of total $T_3$ will also be elevated in patients who have an elevated level of TBG.

Approximately 10 to 20 per cent of all patients with hyperthyroidism have $T_3$ toxicosis. In $T_3$ toxicosis, the level of total $T_3$ is elevated, and the level of total $T_4$ is usually in the upper range of normal.

The total $T_3$ is more useful than the total $T_4$ when early recurrent hyperthyroidism in Graves' disease is suspected.

Hypothyroidism is not accurately diagnosed by measurement of total $T_3$ because early increases in TSH result in preferential production of $T_3$ over $T_4$ such that $T_3$ remains in the normal range (usually in the low range of normal) until the hypothyroidism is of moderate severity.

The total $T_3$ is useful in detecting supraphysiologic levels of $T_3$ associated with the use of desiccated thyroid. This thyroid hormone preparation often has more $T_3$ than $T_4$ and patients can be hyperthyroid; the physician may be unaware of this fact when only the total $T_4$ is measured. The total $T_3$ is low in patients with the euthyroid sick syndrome because of decreased conversion of $T_4$ to $T_3$ in critically ill patients.

## *Protein-Bound Iodine*

The protein-bound iodine test is now obsolete, being replaced by the more specific radioimmunoassays for both total $T_4$ and total $T_3$.

## *Serum Thyrotropin-Stimulating Hormone*

The serum thyrotropin-stimulating hormone (TSH) concentration can be measured by radioimmunoassay with little cross-reactivity with the other pituitary glycoprotein hormones. The measurement of serum TSH is the most sensitive test to detect primary hypothyroidism and subclinical hypothyroidism. In the latter condition, the level of serum TSH is elevated as an early manifestation of inefficient thyroid hormone production at a time when the patient is still clinically euthyroid and the level of serum total $T_4$ is normal.

Measurement of serum TSH concentration enables one to distinguish untreated primary hypothyroidism (TSH greatly increased) from pituitary and hypothalamic hypothyroidism (TSH undetectable or in the normal range). In hyperthyroidism, the level of TSH is suppressed or undetectable except in the patient who is hyperthyroid because of a TSH-producing pituitary tumor (rare) and in the patient with pituitary resistance to thyroid hormone (extremely rare).

Measurement of TSH is also useful in the evaluation of a critically ill patient with a low level of total $T_4$. The test may help to distinguish between primary hypothyroidism (TSH elevated) and euthyroid sick syndrome (TSH normal).

The ultrasensitive immunoradiometric assay for TSH is performed by using monoclonal antibodies. In the future, it is possible that the ultrasensitive TSH assay may be used as a single screening test for thyroid disease in general, although this is still being debated.[7, 9]

## *Thyrotropin-Releasing Hormone Stimulation Test*

The TRH stimulation test is a study that not only permits determination of the functional status of the pituitary TSH secretory mechanism but it also permits determination of the presence of autonomous thyroid function as is seen in patients with a functioning thyroid nodule that may not yet have caused hyperthyroidism. The test is useful in determining whether TSH secretion is blunted in a patient with a pituitary tumor. It is also useful in a patient who is being evaluated for possible hyperthyroidism but in whom the results of thyroid function tests are "borderline high." In this situation, a blunted or flat TSH response to TRH will be apparent in the truly hyperthyroid patient. The ultrasensitive TSH assay probably replaces the need to carry out a TRH stimulation test in a patient with borderline high thyroid hormone levels.

Patients with untreated early primary hypothyroidism will have a supranormal TSH response to TRH. The TRH test may also be used to help distinguish between pituitary and hypothalamic hypothyroidism (flat response in the former and normal response in the latter).

The tendency was to perform a TRH stimulation test to determine the adequacy of TSH suppression by exogenous thyroid hormone in patients with thyroid carcinoma. The ultrasensitive TSH assay eliminates the need to perform a TRH stimulation test because normal persons as well as those with inadequate suppression by thyroid hormone will have a detectable level of TSH using the ultrasensitive TSH assay, but patients with adequate suppression will have an undetectable level of TSH.

The TRH stimulation test involves obtaining a baseline random TSH level. Then, TRH, 500 μg, is given intravenously, and TSH is assayed at 30 minutes and at 60 minutes. A normal response should yield a rise in the level of TSH of at least 6 μU/mL from the baseline level.

## Serum Thyroid Antibodies

Graves' disease and Hashimoto's thyroiditis are thought to represent autoimmune thyroid disorders. Approximately 80 to 90 per cent of patients with Hashimoto's thyroiditis will have detectable thyroid autoantibodies (antimicrosomal and antithyroglobulin). However, the frequency of either antibody alone is probably much less than 80 per cent. The antimicrosomal antibody is the more useful test because the result is frequently positive and occurs in higher titer than the antithyroglobulin antibody. Antimicrosomal and antithyroglobulin antibodies are also found in patients with Graves' disease, although with less frequency than is seen in patients with Hashimoto's thyroiditis.[4] The presence of antithyroid antibodies does not determine the functional status of the thyroid, but they usually provide a clue to the nature of the thyroid disorder.

The majority of patients with Graves' disease have detectable thyroid-stimulating immunoglobulins. These immunoglobulins are usually not seen in other forms of hyperthyroidism. It is not necessary to obtain this test in the patient with Graves' disease because their presence or absence does not necessarily alter the management of the patient. One situation in which the thyroid-stimulating immunoglobulin determination may be worthwhile is in the pregnant woman with a past or current history of Graves' disease. When the woman has an elevated thyroid-stimulating immunoglobulin titer, this immunoglobulin can cross the placenta and can potentially cause fetal or neonatal Graves' disease. Both of these are treatable conditions but can result in severe morbidity if not detected and treated.[8] Another indication for using the thyroid-stimulating immunoglobulin assay is in a patient who appears to have Graves' ophthalmopathy but is otherwise euthyroid (euthyroid Graves' ophthalmopathy). The level of thyroid-stimulating immunoglobulin is usually elevated in this disorder.

## Serum Thyroglobulin Assay

Several thyroid disorders release large amounts of thyroglobulin into the circulation. Noteworthy are destructive types of thyroid disorders, such as radiation injury, subacute thyroiditis, suppurative thyroiditis, large goiters, and Graves' disease.[6]

Differentiated thyroid carcinoma may also release thyroglobulin into the circulation. While the radioimmunoassay for serum thyroglobulin is a useless test in the diagnosis of thyroid carcinoma, it is useful in assessing the adequacy of the initial therapy and in monitoring the patient for recurrent or metastatic differentiated thyroid carcinoma, especially when the patient has had total thyroidectomy or subtotal thyroidectomy and ablation of the thyroid remnant with radioiodine. Measurement of the serum thyroglobulin complements radioactive iodine scanning in the detection of residual local or metastatic disease.[1, 10]

Serum thyroglobulin may also be useful in the differentiation of factitious thyrotoxicosis (surreptitious ingestion of thyroid hormone) from endogenous hyperthyroidism because the serum thyroglobulin is suppressed in the former and elevated in the latter.

## Radioactive Iodine Uptake Test

The serum thyroid function tests are the best direct measurements of the metabolic status, but the radioactive iodine uptake (RAIU) is a test that gives some indication of the thyroid gland's potential. This test involves oral administration of either $^{123}I$ or $^{131}I$; $^{123}I$ is preferred because less radiation exposure is possible than with $^{131}I$. The administered radioiodine mixes uniformly with the endogenous iodide within the extracellular fluid. The absorbed radioiodine is taken up by the thyroid or excreted by the kidneys. Some radioiodine is also taken up by the salivary glands. The RAIU test measures the percentage of iodine that is taken up by the thyroid. The RAIU is usually measured 24 hours after administration of the radioiodine because the uptake has reached a plateau by this time. The normal range for the 24-hour RAIU is approximately 5 to 30 per cent of the administered dose, but this varies in different regions of the United States.[5] This test does not distinguish between hypothyroidism and the euthyroid state, but values above 30 per cent often indicate thyroid hyperfunction. In some patients with severe hyperthyroidism, the RAIU may peak before 24 hours, and results of the test may be normal by 24 hours. Thus, the RAIU may need to be measured at 6 to 18 hours.

Administration of iodine either orally or intravenously, such as that contained in radiographic contrast agents, will blunt the RAIU for approximately 4 weeks and can result in misleading information when the RAIU test is performed less than 4 weeks after the patient received radiographic contrast material.

The RAIU test is useful in differentiating among the causes for hyperthyroidism. It should not be used as a primary test for diagnosing this disorder. The RAIU will be increased in patients with Graves' disease, toxic nodule, toxic multinodular goiter, iodine deficiency, and in patients who are euthyroid but in whom thyroid hormone is synthesized inefficiently because of a defect in the synthetic pathway for thyroid hormone. Many patients with toxic nodule or toxic multinodular goiter will have a normal RAIU. The RAIU will be decreased in patients with factitious thyrotoxicosis, hypothyroidism, the early phase of subacute thyroiditis, chronic painless thyroiditis with transient hyperthyroidism, ingestion of excessive iodine (kelp or such expectorants as supersaturated solution of potassium iodide), after intravenous administration of iodinated radiocontrast agents, and in those with ectopic thyroid tissue (struma ovarii, lingual thyroid).

The RAIU test is also used to calculate the therapeutic dose of $^{131}I$ in the treatment of patients with thyrotoxicosis.

Thyroid imaging techniques are discussed elsewhere in this book.

## SUMMARY

Many tests are available to measure thyroid function both directly and indirectly. This chapter helps clarify which tests should be ordered when various types of thyroid dysfunction are suspected. The clinician must be familiar with the limitations of each test and with the ability of various substances and nonthyroidal illnesses to interfere with the results.

## REFERENCES

1. Barsano, C. P., Skosey, C., DeGroot, L. J., and Refetoff, S.: Serum thyroglobulin in the management of patients with thyroid cancer. Arch. Intern. Med., *142*:763–767, 1982.
2. Braverman, L. E.: Iodine-induced thyroid disease. *In* Ingbar, S. H., and Braverman, L. E. (eds.): The Thyroid. Philadelphia, J. B. Lippincott Co., 1986, pp. 735–746.
3. Chopra, I. J., Hershman, J. M., Pardridge, W. M., and Nicoloff, J. T.: Thyroid function in nonthyroidal illnesses. Ann. Intern. Med., *98*:946–957, 1983.
4. Ingbar, S.: The thyroid gland. *In* Wilson, J. D., and Foster, D. W. (eds.): Williams Textbook of Endocrinology. Edition 7. Philadelphia, W. B. Saunders Co., 1985, pp. 682–815.
5. Ingbar, S.: Diseases of the thyroid. *In* Brunwald, E., Isselbacher, K. J., Petersdorf, R. G., et al. (eds.): Harrison's Principles of Internal Medicine. Edition 11. New York, McGraw-Hill Book Co., 1987, pp. 1732–1752.
6. LoGerfo, P., Colacchio, T., Colacchio, D., and Feind, C.: Thyroglobulin in benign and malignant thyroid disease. J.A.M.A., *241*:923–925, 1979.
7. Mardell, R. J., Gamlen, T. R., and Winton, M. R. J.: High sensitivity assay of thyroid stimulating hormone in patients receiving thyroxine for primary hypothyroidism and thyroid carcinoma. Br. Med. J., *290*:355–356, 1985.
8. Mestman, J. H.: Management of thyroid diseases in pregnancy. Clin. Perinatol., *7* (Pt. 2):371–385, 1980.
9. Ross, D. S.: New sensitive immunoradiometric assays for thyrotropin. Ann. Intern. Med., *104*:718–720, 1986.
10. Schneider, A. B., Line, B. R., Goldman, J. M., and Robbins, J.: Sequential serum thyroglobulin determinations, $^{131}I$ scans, and $^{131}I$ uptakes after triiodothyronine withdrawal in patients with thyroid cancer. J. Clin. Endocrinol. Metab., *53*:1199–1206, 1981.
11. Transbøl, I., Christiansen, C., and Baastrup, P. C.: Endocrine effects of lithium. I. Hypothyroidism: Its prevalence in long-term treated patients. Acta Endocrinol., *87*:759–767, 1978.
12. Wolff, J.: Iodide goiter and pharmacologic effects of excess iodide. Am. J. Med., *47*:101–124, 1969.

# 7

# IMAGING OF THYROID GLAND WITH RADIONUCLIDES

*Peter F. Winter, M.D.*

Radionuclide imaging continues to play an important role in the investigation of the thyroid gland. It is unique compared with other imaging methods in that it visualizes the thyroid gland by means of its intrinsic function, thus providing a functional image. All other imaging methods display an image of the thyroid gland by means of physical characteristics unrelated to thyroid function, such as reflection of sound as in ultrasonography, absorption of x-rays as in computed tomography, and density of protons as in magnetic resonance imaging.

## TECHNICAL CONSIDERATIONS

The radionuclides that can be employed for thyroid imaging are technetium and iodine. Technetium is available in the radioactive state as technetium 99m ($^{99m}$Tc), and for thyroid imaging, it is used in the chemical form of sodium pertechnetate ($NaTcO_4$). Iodine is available in a variety of isotopic states, but only the ionic forms of iodine 123 ($^{123}$I) and iodine 131 ($^{131}$I) are currently used for thyroid imaging.

$^{99m}$Tc decays with a half-life of 6 hours and emits gamma rays of 140 keV. Emission of beta particles and other gamma rays is negligible. Its chemical form of $NaTcO_4$ is obtained by eluting a $^{99}$Mo-$^{99m}$Tc generator with isotonic saline solution. $^{99}$Mo is a by-product of nuclear fission, and because of its half-life of 67 hours, it is a convenient source of $^{99m}$Tc pertechnetate, requiring only weekly replacement of the generator.

After the intravenous injection, $^{99m}$Tc pertechnetate is rapidly trapped in the thyroid gland. The uptake of $^{99m}$Tc pertechnetate by the thyroid is 0.3 to 3.0 per cent, which is reached approximately at 20 minutes and is transient.

$^{123}$I decays with a half-life of 13.2 hours and emits x-rays of 159 keV with negligible emission of beta particles and other gamma rays. $^{123}$I is produced in a cyclotron. $^{131}$I decays with a half-life of 8.1 days and emits a variety of beta and gamma rays. Only the gamma ray of 364 keV is used for imaging. $^{131}I$ is a by-product of nuclear fission.

After oral administration, iodide rapidly enters the bloodstream through gastric absorption and is subsequently trapped by the thyroid gland. Unlike $^{99m}Tc$ pertechnetate, it enters further into the organification process by which thyroid hormones are produced. The maximal uptake of iodide by the thyroid occurs at 4 hours when it reaches a plateau in the range of 5 to 30 per cent, which lasts well beyond 24 hours.

Although clinically useful images can be obtained with either $^{99m}Tc$ pertechnetate or radioiodide, accumulation of iodide can be considered a more specific indicator of functioning thyroid tissue. The selection of tracer is based on a variety of factors, such as the clinical findings to be investigated, availability, cost, radiation burden, and practicability.

$^{99m}Tc$ pertechnetate is readily available because of its preeminent position as a labeling tracer in nuclear medicine. It can be produced daily in the department or a nearby radiopharmacy by eluting the $^{99}Mo$-$^{99m}Tc$ generator, it is inexpensive, and its photon energy of 140 keV is optimal for scintigraphy with currently available gamma cameras. A thyroid study after intravenous injection of $^{99m}Tc$ pertechnetate can be completed in less than 1 hour and does not require a second patient visit.

$^{123}I$ as a cyclotron-produced isotope is expensive, and it must be delivered daily to the department. This is inconvenient and adds to the cost of the study. $^{123}I$ is given orally, and images are traditionally obtained at 4 or 24 hours. Both time intervals are inconvenient. As an advantage over $^{99m}Tc$ pertechnetate, it permits calculation of the global radioactive iodine uptake in the thyroid gland. This can provide useful information concerning thyroid function. In addition, $^{123}I$ delineates ectopic thyroid tissue, such as a retrosternal goiter, to better advantage[10] and might provide further information on palpable thyroid nodules not seen on a $^{99m}Tc$ pertechnetate image.[11]

$^{131}I$, of course, follows the biologic pathway of $^{123}I$, but its high proportion of beta radiation and long half-life result in a high radiation burden to the patient. In addition, its main gamma ray of 364 keV is suboptimal for imaging with currently available scintillation cameras, resulting in inferior images compared with $^{123}I$ or $^{99m}Tc$ pertechnetate. However, it remains the tracer of choice in the search for functioning metastatic thyroid tumor. Its long half-life permits imaging at 48 hours or 72 hours, with improved delineation of the usually faint uptake in functioning metastatic lesions because of almost complete clearance of tracer from the remaining tissues of the body at that time. Thus, $^{131}I$ outweighs all previously mentioned disadvantages for this specific clinical indication.

$^{131}I$ plays an important role as therapeutic agent in the treatment of patients with hyperthyroidism and functioning thyroid metastatic disease. Here, the desired effect is the tissue damage of its beta radiation.

## NORMAL RESULTS ON THYROID SCAN

### $^{99m}$*Tc Pertechnetate Scan*

Approximately 20 minutes after the intravenous injection of $^{99m}Tc$ pertechnetate, 1.0 to 2.0 mCi, anterior and both oblique images of the neck are obtained with the scintillation camera fitted with a pinhole collimator. A normal scintigraphic image displays uniformly accumulated tracer in both lobes, giving the thyroid gland the appearance of a butterfly. The thyroid lobes can be slightly asymmetric. The isthmus varies in size from barely visible to a wide band connecting both lobes. A pyramidal lobe is occasionally visualized, usually arising from the upper pole of the right lobe. A normal thyroid gland is shown in Figure 7–1. Oblique views are mandatory in all patients investigated for known or suspected nodules because even sizable nodules might be seen only on the oblique view.

Images of the neck can also be obtained with a rectilinear scanner. The advantage of a rectilinear scan is the 1:1 display, making it easy to mark a palpable finding on the scan for correlation. Disadvantages of this method are inferior resolution compared with that obtained by a camera image and unavailability of a rectilinear scanner in many nuclear medicine departments as of this writing.

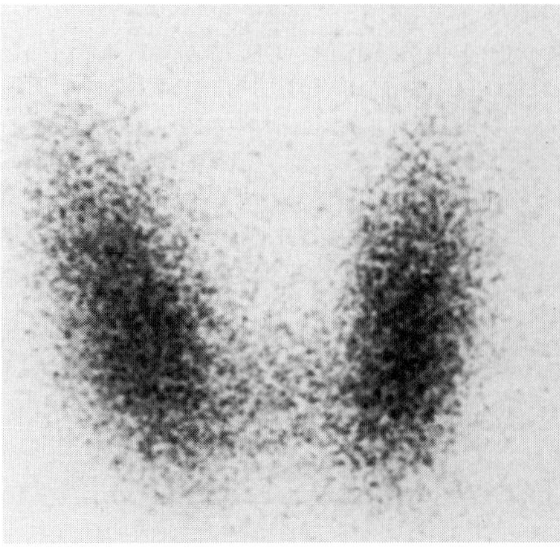

**FIGURE 7–1.** Normal gland. Anterior view, $^{99m}$Tc pertechnetate. The normal gland exhibits a lepidopterous configuration with uniform uptake in both "wings."

## $^{123}$*Iodide Scan*

After the oral administration of $^{123}$I, 300 μCi, images of the neck are obtained at 4 or 24 hours using the same technique described in conjunction with $^{99m}$Tc pertechnetate scintigraphy. The preferred interval is 24 hours, primarily for historical reasons. Compared with $^{99m}$Tc pertechnetate scintigraphy, $^{123}$I provides an image of higher target-to-background ratio. No other noticeable differences exist between the images of the normal thyroid gland. However, inflammatory and neoplastic disease processes might selectively affect organification without interfering with trapping of the radionuclide tracer, thus causing decreased $^{123}$I accumulation without corresponding defect on a $^{99m}$Tc pertechnetate scan.[11] Fortunately, this event is rare and probably does not justify preference of one tracer over the other in a routine clinical setting but warrants a $^{123}$I scan when the result of the $^{99m}$Tc pertechnetate scan does not explain the clinical findings.

In addition to obtaining an image of the thyroid gland, radioactive iodine permits assessment of thyroid function by measuring thyroid activity in the thyroid gland with a scintillation probe and the calculation of the relative radioactive iodine uptake. The normal values vary from geographic region and department. As a guideline, the normal value for the 24-hour radioactive iodine uptake in the United States at this time should fall between 5 and 30 per cent.[8]

Increased radioactive iodine uptake reflects hyperthyroidism but can be seen in glands recovering from thyroiditis. Decreased radioactive iodine uptake indicates primary or secondary hypothyroidism or thyroiditis in addition to the causes that are unrelated to thyroid function.

The radioactive iodine uptake can be depressed for a variety of extraneous reasons. The commonest cause is iodide overload from a recent radiographic study with injection of an iodide-containing contrast agent, such as in excretory urography, angiography, or computed tomography. The stable iodide dissociated from the contrast agent competes with the radioactive iodine for the thyroid binding sites, resulting in decreased radioactivity in the thyroid gland. Usually, an interval of 2 to 3 weeks is sufficient to reduce the stable iodide pool to a level that is no longer competitively inhibiting. Another frequently encountered cause is concurrent administration of a thyroid hormone, resulting in decreased radioactive iodine uptake from thyroid stimulating hormone suppression. Discontinuation of administration of the thyroid hormone before the scan rectifies this problem.

## $^{131}$*Iodide Scan*

The role of $^{131}$I as a diagnostic tracer is now confined to the evaluation of the patient with known follicular or papillary thyroid carcinoma after thyroidectomy. After the oral administration of $^{131}$I, 1 to 2 mCi, scintigraphic images of the neck and torso, including the proximal extremities, are obtained to search for residual thyroid tissue in the neck and for functioning metastatic disease in the body. The patient should discontinue taking any thyroid hormone replacement for $^{131}$I scintigraphy. The suggested interval before the study is 8 days for any $T_3$ preparation (for example, Cytomel) and 3 weeks for preparations containing $T_4$ (for example, Euthyroid, Thyroid USP). This interval permits adequate build-up of the patient's intrinsic thyroid stimulating hormone. Extrinsic administration of thyroid stimulating hormone does not appear to be necessary.

After complete surgical resection or radioactive iodine ablation of the thyroid gland, scintigraphy shows a variety of findings. First, findings in the neck are not necessarily silent.

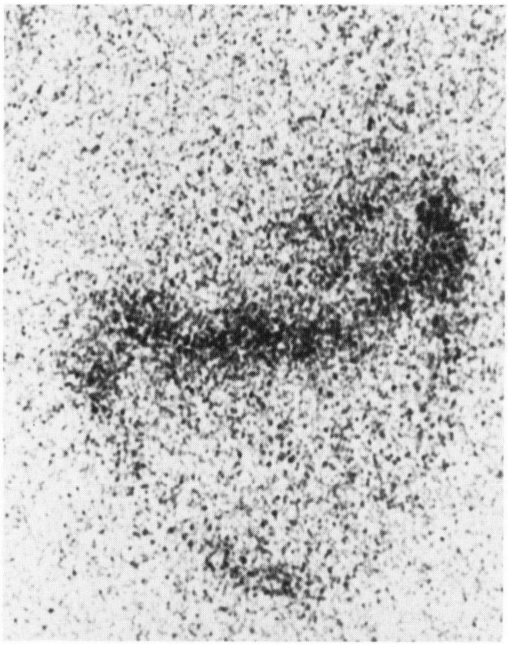

**FIGURE 7–2.** $^{131}I$ body scan. Anterior view of the torso obtained 48 hours after administration of $^{131}I$. Physiologic activity is seen in the stomach and colon only.

Although uptake in the thyroid gland is no longer identified, activity can be seen in the salivary glands, which should not be mistaken for functioning thyroid tissue (Fig. 7–2). Second, physiologic areas of accumulation of radioactive iodine are invariably seen in the stomach and colon (Fig. 7–2). Although the physiologic excretion of radioactive iodine is usually completed at the time of the scan, occasionally residual activity can be seen in the urinary bladder or in a hydronephrotic kidney.

Residual thyroid tissue in the neck is seen as areas of accumulation of tracer of various configurations and sizes, whereas residual functioning tumor cannot reliably be distinguished from functioning metastatic disease. Any activity outside the neck not clearly explained as physiologic must be considered metastatic disease. Occasionally, diffuse hepatic activity is encountered in a patient with a sizable amount of residual thyroid tissue. This activity is the result of physiologically degraded thyroid hormone that incorporated $^{131}I$ during its synthesis in the residual thyroid tissue and should not be mistaken for metastatic disease to the liver.

A large amount of residual thyroid tissue in the neck limits the search for distant functioning metastatic disease. Because of the greater avidity of normal thyroid tissue for iodide compared with carcinoma of the thyroid, it is conceivable that the amount of the administered $^{131}I$ available for the less avid metastatic tissue is inadequate for imaging. In this situation, the scan should be repeated after ablation of residual thyroid tissue with $^{131}I$.

## CLINICAL APPLICATIONS

Radionuclide thyroid scanning can provide useful and frequently unique information in the investigation of a clinical presentation suggestive of a thyroid condition, with the following clinical applications believed to be typical and common.

### *Evaluation of Enlarged Thyroid Gland*

The enlarged thyroid gland is imaged to determine whether the enlargement is caused by an increase in functioning or nonfunctioning tissue or both. A slightly enlarged gland with uniform tracer uptake is frequently encountered in young women and is probably of no clinical importance. Any diffusely enlarged gland, however, can be a manifestation of Graves' disease (Fig. 7–3) and mandates a functional evaluation by means of the

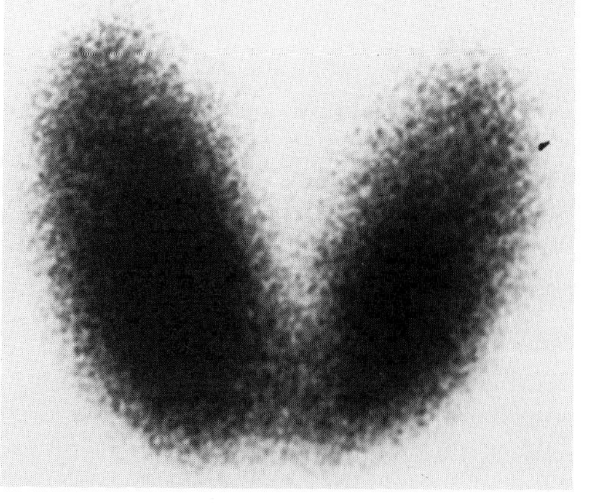

**FIGURE 7–3.** Graves' disease. Anterior view, $^{123}I$. The gland is diffusely enlarged, with the lateral margins exhibiting a convex rather than concave configuration.

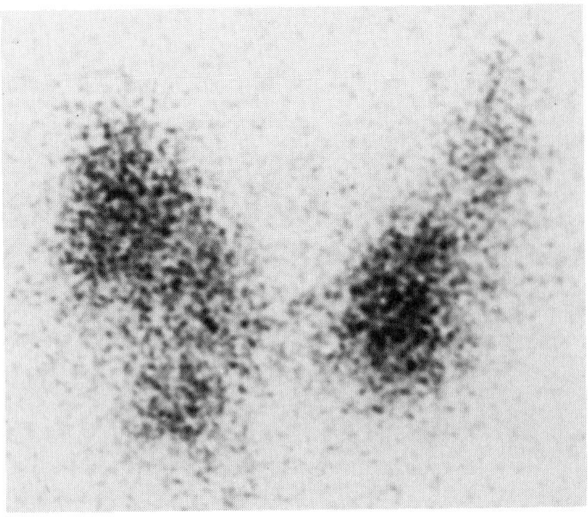

**FIGURE 7–4.** Multinodular goiter. Anterior view, $^{99m}Tc$ pertechnetate. The gland is enlarged and distorted with several areas of decreased uptake.

appropriate laboratory tests or a 4- or 24-hour radioactive iodine uptake. Elevated serum levels of thyroid hormone or an increased radioactive iodine uptake or both establish the diagnosis of Graves' disease.

An enlarged gland with areas of decreased activity (Fig. 7–4) reflects changes secondary to subacute or chronic thyroiditis or a multinodular goiter. From the scintigraphic point of view, no further evaluation can be offered except for determining the radioactive iodine uptake, which usually is within the normal range in multinodular goiter. A depressed radioactive iodine uptake would suggest subacute or chronic thyroiditis. The possibility of a neoplastic change in a gland with multiple cold areas can be considered so remote that, on the basis of the scintigraphic image alone, it does not have to be pursued. However, clinical reasons, such as an otherwise unexplained rapidly enlarging gland or previous external radiation therapy, might suggest the presence of a carcinoma of the thyroid.

One should approach a solitary nonfunctioning area in an enlarged gland like a palpable nonfunctioning nodule, as discussed later, whether it is palpable or not.

Focal areas of increased uptake in an enlarged gland represent either residual normal tissue within functionally impaired thyroid tissue or autonomous nodules. Further evaluation of this finding is discussed under evaluation of functioning nodule.

## *Evaluation of Palpable Nodule*

For the management of a patient with a palpable thyroid nodule, it is crucial to know whether the nodule is nonfunctioning or functioning. Consequently, to relate properly the palpable finding with the scintigraphic image, it is mandatory to mark the palpable nodule on at least one image.

***Nonfunctioning Nodule.*** A nonfunctioning nodule, colloquially referred to as a "cold" nodule, is displayed as an area of decreased activity compared with surrounding thyroid tissue (Fig. 7–5). A peripherally located nodule might be delineated only as a marginal indentation, often solely appreciated in the oblique view when the nodule is anterior or posterior rather than lateral in location.

The differential diagnosis of a solitary nonfunctioning nodule includes carcinoma, colloid nodule, and nonfunctioning adenoma and cyst, whereby the possibility of a carcinoma is the major concern. According to the literature,[2, 9] the incidence of carcinoma ranges from 5 to 20 per cent. This relatively high incidence is in part the result of a selection bias of cases included in published series, usually from referral centers, and it can be assumed that the real incidence of carcinoma in a uninodular gland is considerably lower. Nevertheless, because of the unacceptability of missing a thyroid carcinoma, a solitary nonfunctioning nodule demands

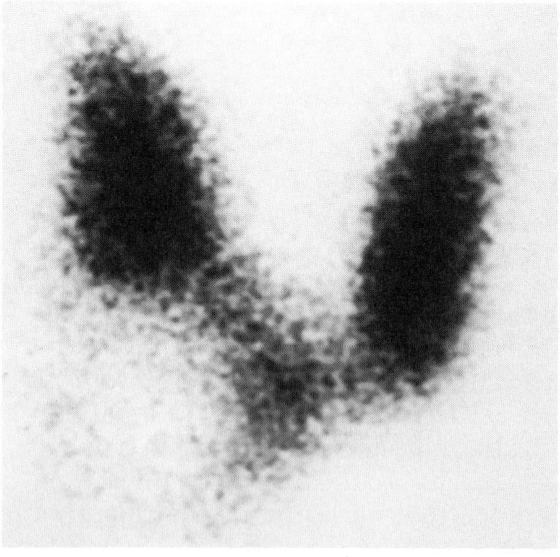

**FIGURE 7–5.** Solitary nonfunctioning nodule. Anterior view, $^{123}I$. The lower pole of the right lobe is expanded by a nonfunctioning area.

further evaluation. The different options, which have been discussed widely in the literature,[4, 7] range from observation with and without exogenous thyroid hormone for thyroid-stimulating hormone suppression to needle aspiration and excisional biopsy.

The number of patients who require further evaluation because of a solitary nonfunctioning nodule can be kept small by searching the thyroid scan for additional nonfunctioning areas. The detection of other nonfunctioning areas in addition to the palpable nodule places the gland in a low-risk group for carcinoma because, in the majority of patients, this combination of findings can be assumed to reflect a multinodular goiter with just a dominant nodule.

***Functioning Nodule.*** A functioning nodule, frequently referred to as a "hot" nodule, is seen as an area of increased activity (Fig. 7–6) and occurs considerably less frequently than nonfunctioning nodules. A discrete area of increased activity can be solitary (Fig. 7–6), which is usually found in a young patient with an otherwise normal thyroid gland, or multiple, which is typically found in an older patient having a multinodular goiter that exhibits areas of decreased activity as well. A solitary nodule can also arise in a multinodular goiter (Fig. 7–7).

The presence of solitary or multiple functioning nodules in the thyroid gland directs

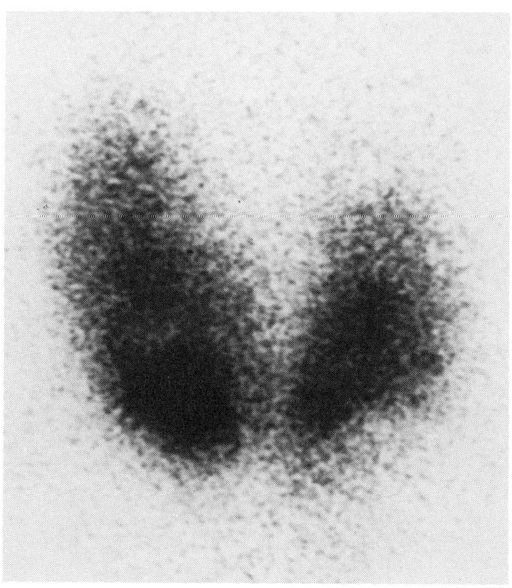

**FIGURE 7–6.** Solitary functioning nodule. Anterior view, $^{99m}Tc$ pertechnetate. The lower pole of the right lobe shows a small area of increased activity.

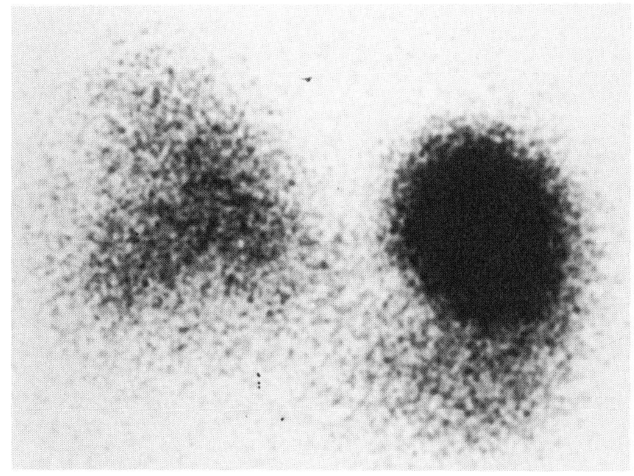

**FIGURE 7–7.** Plummer's disease. Anterior view, $^{99m}Tc$ pertechnetate. The gland is enlarged and distorted. In addition to areas of decreased activity, a large area of increased activity is identified in the expanded appearing left upper lobe.

the diagnostic work-up in a direction different from that of a thyroid gland with areas of decreased activity. In the evaluation of solitary or multiple functioning nodules, their thyroid-stimulating hormone dependence must be addressed. The majority of the few cases of carcinoma in hot nodules reported in the literature can be assumed to be coincidental, representing a scintigraphically silent carcinoma adjacent to a scintigraphically apparent functioning nodule.

A functioning nodule independent of thyroid-stimulating hormone, a so-called autonomous nodule, can be the cause of overt or subclinical hyperthyroidism, while a functioning nodule dependent on thyroid-stimulating hormone invariably represents regional hypertrophy of otherwise normally functioning tissue mediated by thyroid-stimulating hormone because of inflammatory or degenerative processes in the remaining thyroid gland. Thyroid-stimulating hormone dependence can be established by a repeat scan after a short course of oral administration of triiodothyronine (Cytomel, 25 μg 3 times a day for 5 days). Such a suppression scan shows persistent activity in the autonomous nodule and almost no uptake in a hypertrophic or reactive nodule (Fig. 7–8).

## *Search for Retrosternal Goiter*

A retrosternal goiter constitutes one of the commonest causes of widening of the superior mediastinum found on conventional pos-

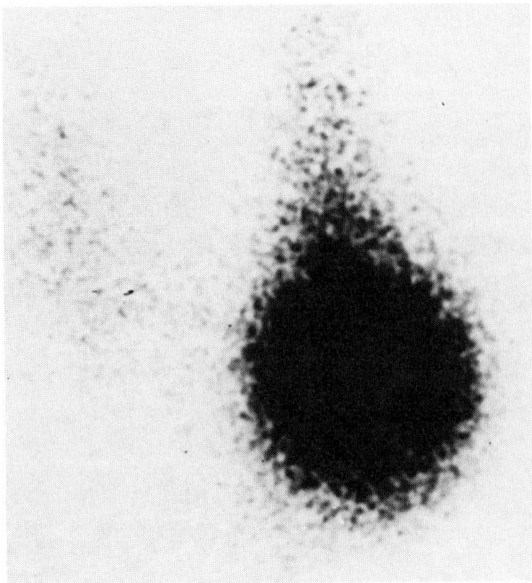

**FIGURE 7–8.** Autonomous nodule with suppression of remaining gland. Anterior view, $^{123}$I. The lower pole of the right lobe is expanded by an area of intense uptake representing the functioning nodule. The remaining gland is suppressed and shows only faint uptake, indicative of autonomy of the functioning nodule.

teroanterior radiography of the chest. The retrosternal thyroid tissue usually has adequate function to accumulate a detectable amount of $^{123}$I, and a thyroid scan with $^{123}$I can establish the presence of a retrosternal goiter in almost all patients.[10] A scan with $^{99m}$Tc pertechnetate is considered inadequate in these patients. Its inferior thyroid-to-soft tissue ratio leads to poor delineation of the thyroid tissue against the relatively high activity of the normal mediastinal structures. Furthermore, the blood pool activity in the aortic arch seen on the scan with $^{99m}$Tc pertechnetate can easily be mistaken for retrosternal thyroid tissue.

For correct interpretation of the findings, care must be taken to mark the suprasternal notch on the scan and to correlate the findings on the scan with the findings on radiography of the chest (Fig. 7–9).

## Evaluation of Hyperthyroidism

Thyroid scanning and calculation of radioactive iodine uptake can assist in the investigation of suspected hyperthyroidism. With the improvements in laboratory evaluation of the functional status of the thyroid gland, scintigraphic evaluation is rarely needed to establish the diagnosis of hyperthyroidism. Scintigraphic imaging today is primarily confined to distinguishing a diffuse toxic goiter (Fig. 7–3) as found in Graves' disease from a toxic nodular goiter (Fig. 7–7), also referred to as Plummer's disease, when the palpable evaluation is inconclusive. Determination of the radioactive iodine uptake supplements functional testing of the thyroid status in patients with borderline serum $T_4$ or $T_3$ val-

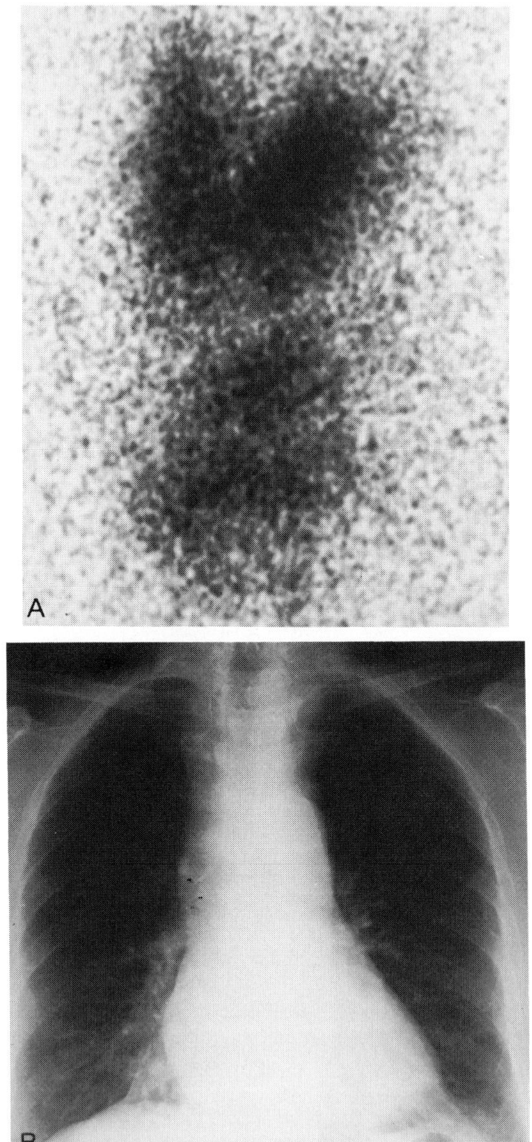


**FIGURE 7–9.** Retrosternal goiter. Anterior view of the neck and upper chest, $^{123}$I. *A,* The thyroid gland is enlarged, and the lower pole extends well below the suprasternal notch. *B,* The corresponding chest radiograph shows a widened mediastinum corresponding to the activity seen on the $^{123}$I scan.

ues, and, in conjunction with a suppression test, it can verify the diagnosis of so-called euthyroid Graves' disease.

The thyroid suppression test is usually performed by measuring the 24-hour radioactive iodine uptake before and after 1 week's course of triiodothyronine (Cytomel), 25 μg 3 times a day, with the second dose of $^{123}$I administered on the seventh day and the radioactive iodine uptake measured 24 hours later. A decline in the 24-hour radioactive iodine uptake of less than 50 per cent of the initial value suggests thyroid autonomy as found in Graves' disease, even in the absence of other functional abnormalities. In particular, the suppression test can be the only positive finding in euthyroid Graves' disease with infiltrative ophthalmopathy, which can present as unilateral or bilateral exophthalmos.

## *Search for Occult Thyroid Neoplasm*

Patients with increased risk for harboring thyroid carcinoma because of head and neck irradiation in childhood have been found to have more lesions detected by thyroid scanning with $^{99m}$Tc pertechnetate than by palpation. Not all lesions are malignant, however, and management of patients with scintigraphically detected "cold" nodules is still under discussion.[12]

## *Search for Thyroid Metastases*

After complete removal of the thyroid gland by total thyroidectomy or by subtotal thyroidectomy with subsequent ablation of the residual tissue with $^{131}$I, any accumulation of orally administered $^{131}$I that cannot be attributed to a physiologic site must be considered a functional carcinoma of the thyroid (Fig. 7–10). Lungs and bones are the most frequent sites of metastatic disease. Any thyroid carcinoma visualized by total body scan is suitable for therapy with $^{131}$I, 100 to 200 mCi.

The search for metastatic disease with $^{131}$I scanning is confined to follicular and papillary carcinoma. Metastatic disease from anaplastic and medullary carcinoma of the thyroid gland does not accumulate iodide and is neither detectable by scanning nor treatable with $^{131}$I.

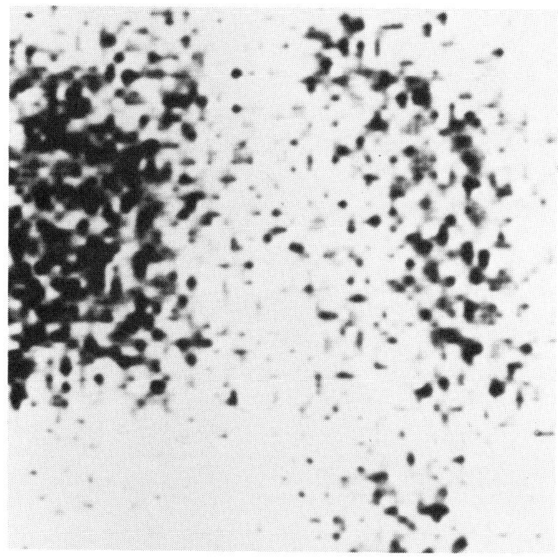

**FIGURE 7–10.** $^{131}$I body scan. An anterior view of the chest obtained 48 hours after administration of $^{131}$I. Activity in both lungs corresponds to functioning nodular metastatic disease throughout both lungs. Activity below the left lung base represents physiologic uptake in the stomach.

## *Search for Ectopic Thyroid Tissue*

Ectopic thyroid tissue can occur anywhere from the base of the tongue to the diaphragm because of arrested or extended migration of the thyroid anlage. In addition, ovarian dermoid tumors have been found to harbor thyroid tissue. The base of the tongue is the most frequent location of ectopic thyroid tissue, characteristically presenting as a localized bulge here. Usually, these patients do not have any thyroid tissue in the expected position in the anterior neck, and their euthyroid status depends on the ectopic thyroid tissue only. The diagnosis of a lingual thyroid gland is established when the $^{123}$I scan shows uptake in this region. $^{123}$I is clearly preferred for this indication because of the salivary activity found with $^{99m}$Tc pertechnetate (Fig. 7–11).

## *Evaluation of Thyroiditis*

The scintigraphic appearance of thyroiditis is diverse, depending on the nature and extent of the underlying inflammatory process and its stage at the time of the study. In subacute thyroiditis, a condition of uncertain etiology, trapping and organification of iodide are temporarily impaired, resulting in regionally or diffusely decreased to absent

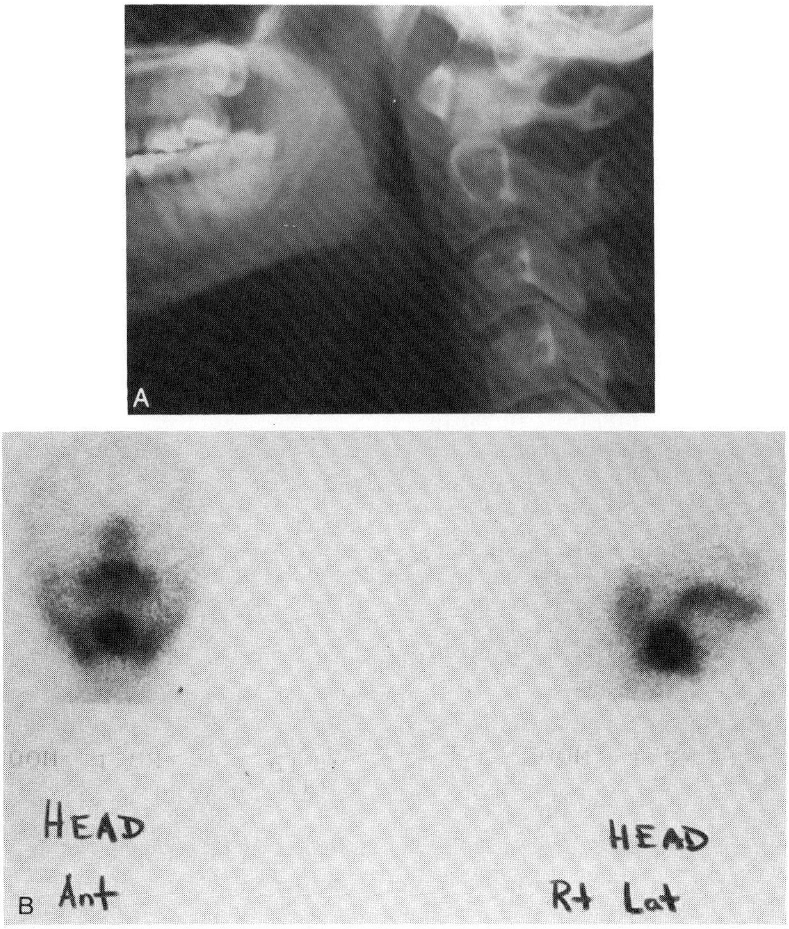


**FIGURE 7–11.** Lingual thyroid gland. *A,* Anterior and lateral views show a round area of intense uptake at the base of the tongue, representing the lingual thyroid gland. This scan was performed with $^{99m}$Tc pertechnetate as evidenced by activity in the salivary glands. It is preferable to use $^{123}$I for the search of a lingual thyroid gland to avoid the potentially interfering activity of the salivary gland found with $^{99m}$Tc pertechnetate. *B,* The corresponding lateral radiograph shows the lingual thyroid gland as a soft tissue bulge at the base of the tongue.

uptake of $^{99m}$Tc pertechnetate and $^{123}$I. Within weeks to months the thyroid function recovers, and the scan shows normal findings but can reveal persistent areas of decreased activity.

In Hashimoto's thyroiditis, also referred to as chronic or lymphocytic thyroiditis because of its protracted course and typical histologic findings, the thyroid scan shows a normal-sized or enlarged gland with various areas of decreased activity. The iodide metabolism is impaired in that the trapping mechanism frequently is less severely involved than the organification process and thus can lead to discrepant findings between a $^{99m}$Tc pertechnetate scan and a $^{123}$I scan, with the former showing normal uptake in areas in which the latter exhibits decreased or absent uptake. This dissociation between trapping and organification also gives rise to positive findings on a perchlorate discharge test.

A perchlorate discharge test can be used whenever defective thyroid organification of iodide is suspected. After determination of a baseline radioactive iodine uptake at 2 to 3 hours, an oral dose of potassium perchlorate (1 g) is administered, and the radioactive iodine uptake is measured again 1 hour later or, alternatively, sequential radioactive iodine uptakes are determined over a short period of time. In a normal thyroid gland, the radioactive iodine content remains constant, and the calculated radioactive iodine uptake is unchanged. A decrease in the radioactive iodine uptake of 20 per cent or more indicates an appreciable discharge of unorganified iodide as a manifestation of an organification defect.

In patients with subacute thyroiditis or Hashimoto's thyroiditis, the radioactive iodine uptake can be normal, decreased, or increased, frequently discordant with the serum levels of $T_3$ or $T_4$, which can be normal, decreased, or increased. Early in the disease, the radioactive iodine uptake can be low because of impaired organification of iodide, and the serum levels of $T_3$ or $T_4$ or both are high because of excessive release of stored hormones from the diseased gland. Later in the disease, the reverse is true. While the gland recovers, the radioactive iodine uptake is increasing, restoring the depleted intrathyroid hormone pool, and until this process is completed, the serum levels of $T_3$ and $T_4$ will remain low.

Other forms of thyroiditis, such as acute suppurative thyroiditis and Riedel's struma, are extremely rare and do not give rise to any specific scan pattern.

## OTHER IMAGING METHODS WITH RADIONUCLIDES

In a few clinical situations, tracers other than radioactive iodine and $^{99m}$Tc pertechnetate can provide useful imaging information. $^{131}$I metaiodobenzylguanidine (MIBG), an agent with an affinity for neuroectodermally derived tumors, has been found to localize in medullary carcinoma,[6] a carcinoma of ectodermal origin. The sensitivity of $^{131}$I MIBG imaging in this series[6] of nine medullary carcinomas was low, with tracer uptake found in three carcinomas only. $^{99m}$Tc dimercaptosuccinic acid (DMSA) has been found to visualize medullary carcinoma with a considerably better sensitivity, with eight of nine proved tumor sites showing tracer uptake in one series.[5] The mechanism of the uptake of $^{99m}$Tc pertechnetate by medullary carcinoma is not known.

Gallium-67 citrate can occasionally visualize thyroid conditions. Gallium-67 citrate accumulates in neoplastic and inflammatory disease processes and has been found to indicate lymphoma and carcinoma of the thyroid as well as Graves' disease and thyroiditis.[1, 3] The reported sensitivity of gallium-67 imaging for lymphoma is 85 per cent and that for carcinoma is 40 per cent, with most of the carcinomas being of the relatively rare anaplastic cell type.

## REFERENCES


1. Allard, J. C., Lee, V. W., and Franklin, P.: Thyroid uptake of gallium in Graves' disease. Clin. Nucl. Med., *13*:663–669, 1988.
2. Atkins, H. L.: The thyroid. *In* Freeman, L. (ed.): Freeman & Johnson's Clinical Radionuclide Imaging. 3rd ed. Orlando, Grune & Stratton, 1984, pp. 1275–1317.
3. Bekerman, C., Hoffer, P. B., and Bitran, J. D.: The role of gallium-67 in the clinical evaluation of cancer. Semin. Nucl. Med., *15*:72–103, 1985.
4. Blum, M., and Rothschild, M.: Improved nonoperative diagnosis of the solitary "cold" nodule: Surgical selection based on risk factors and three months of suppression. J.A.M.A., *243*:242–245, 1980.
5. Clarke, S. E., Lazarus, C. R., Wraight, P., et al.: Pentavalent [$^{99m}$Tc]DMSA, [$^{131}$I]MIBG, and [$^{99m}$Tc]MDP: An evaluation of three imaging techniques in patients with medullary carcinoma of the thyroid. J. Nucl. Med., *29*:33–38, 1988.
6. Clarke, S. E., Lazarus, C. R., Edwards, S., et al.: Scintigraphy and treatment of medullary carcinoma of the thyroid with iodine-131 metaiodobenzylguanidine. J. Nucl. Med., *28*:1820–1825, 1987.
7. Gharib, H., and Goellner, J. R.: Evaluation of nodular thyroid disease. Endocrinol. Metab. Clin. North Am., *17*:511–526, 1988.
8. Hooper, P. L., Turner, J. R., Conway, M. J., and Plymate, S. R.: Thyroid uptake of 123I in a normal population. Arch. Intern. Med., *140*:757–758, 1980.
9. Molitch, M. E., Beck, J. R., Dreisman, M., et al.: The cold thyroid nodule: An analysis of diagnostic and therapeutic options. Endocr. Rev., *5*:185–199, 1984.
10. Park, H. M., Tarver, R. D., Siddiqui, A. R., et al.: Efficacy of thyroid scintigraphy in the diagnosis of intrathoracic goiter. A. J. R., *148*:527–529, 1987.
11. Ryo, U. Y., Vaidya, P., Schneider, A., and Pinsky, S. M.: Histopathology of thyroid lesions that caused discrepant findings between Tc-99m scan and I-123 scan. Abstract. J. Nucl. Med., *20*:678, 1979.
12. Schneider, A. B., Pinsky, S., Bekerman, C., and Ryo, U. Y.: Characteristics of 108 thyroid cancers detected by screening in a population with a history of head and neck irradiation. Cancer, *46*:1218–1227, 1980.

# 8

# CROSS-SECTIONAL IMAGING OF THYROID GLAND

*Carl R. Larsen, M.D.*

In its superficial anatomic position in the neck, the thyroid gland is easily accessible for clinical evaluation, for several cross-sectional imaging modalities, and for surgery. Radionuclide studies offer the best method for delineation of physiologically active thyroid tissue.[14, 27] However, despite its role as the initial imaging technique, scintigraphy is unsatisfactory in the assessment of hypofunctioning thyroid tissue.[32] A poorly functioning area seen on scintigraphy is nonspecific and can represent possible benign adenoma, cyst, thyroiditis, hyperplasia, hemorrhage, carcinoma, or even extrinsic compression.[12] Ultrasonography, computed tomography, and magnetic resonance imaging provide meaningful evaluation of the size, shape, texture, and position of thyroid tissue. These cross-sectional imaging modalities offer the clinician an extension of the physical examination.

## ULTRASONOGRAPHY

Diagnostic ultrasonography is a simple, safe noninvasive imaging modality that employs a high-frequency sound wave with imaging dependent on differences in acoustic impedance of various tissues of the body. Sound waves are reflected, transmitted, or attenuated as they pass through the body. Reflections occur whenever a difference exists in the acoustic impedance of adjacent tissues, producing an image of the outline of organs and of their internal structure. The strength of the echo varies with the difference in acoustic properties.[17]

Ultrasonography offers an effective modality for differentiating solid from cystic lesions. Fluid-filled structures have well-demarcated echogenic borders, they lack internal echoes, and they demonstrate good transmission of sound waves through the lesion (Fig. 8–1). Solid structures, however, will have varying degrees of internal echogenicity, will cause attenuation of the sound wave resulting in the posterior margin of a mass being less clearly defined than the anterior aspect, and will transmit only a portion of the sound beam beyond the mass.[17]

Early imaging with static gray-scale ultrasonography was cumbersome and disappointing, which limited its routine use in evaluating

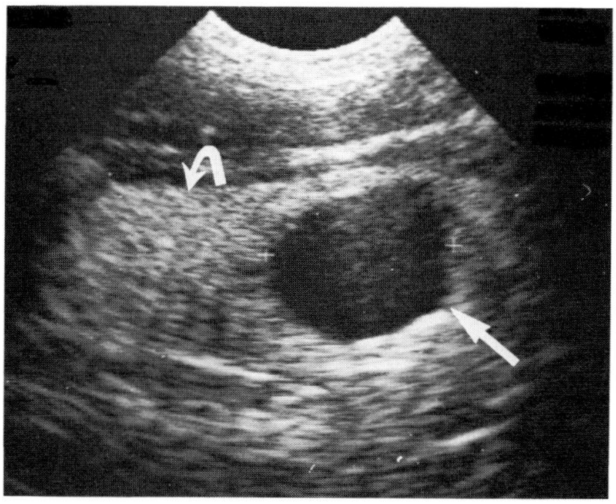

**FIGURE 8–1.** Ultrasonographic study of sagittal section demonstrating a cyst (*straight arrow*) in the lower pole of thyroid. Note strong echogenic texture of normal thyroid (*curved arrow*).

thyroid disease.[5, 15] With the availability of high-frequency real-time imaging, dramatic improvements in visualization of the thyroid gland have been realized. High-resolution imaging of superficially located structures can be obtained with either a 7.5 MHz or, optimally, a 10.0 MHz transducer. These high-resolution small parts scanners, capable of detecting 3 mm thyroid nodules,[6] have resulted in the demonstration of nonpalpable thyroid lesions of uncertain clinical importance. In one series[6] of 67 patients undergoing imaging of the extracranial carotid, the incidence of unsuspected thyroid nodules was 13.4 per cent.

## Indications

Use of ultrasonography to differentiate cystic from solid thyroid lesions is probably outdated. Even with high-resolution scanning, only one true cystic lesion was found in 100 surgically proved cases in more than 550 patients examined.[31] The static ultrasonography equipment was limited in being able to show small amounts of tissue in what appeared then to be cystic lesions. Current applications of high-resolution ultrasonography are primarily to detect a multinodular gland when only a single nodule is palpable and to determine occult thyroid carcinoma when metastatic disease is present elsewhere.[31] Other uses include determining the size and volume of a nodule, assessing response of a nodule to therapy, screening patients with a history of radiation to the head and neck area,[21] scanning the contralateral side when glands are suspected of being cancerous before surgery, evaluating possible recurrent disease,[29, 31] and for guiding fine needle biopsy.[20]

## Ultrasonographic Patterns of Disease

The sonographic features of thyroid disease are independent of thyroid function (hot versus cold nodules), and benign and malignant patterns overlap considerably.[24] Histopathologic specificity is lacking both with ultrasonography and computed tomography, and limited experience with magnetic resonance imaging has not allowed any criteria to be established. Although ultrasonography cannot distinguish with certainty between benign and malignant processes, unique echographic patterns of various pathologic conditions have been defined.

## Normal Thyroid

Normal thyroid parenchyma characteristically has a homogenous medium level echo pattern, which is greater than the echogenicity of the regional neck muscles. This uniform pattern of the thyroid facilitates detection of thyroid masses. Some asymmetry of the lobes may be apparent, but usually the lobes are of equal size. The air-filled trachea is identified as a curvilinear echo-free reflecting surface. Anterior to the thyroid gland are the muscle groups of the neck, including the sternocleidomastoid, sternohyoid, and sternothyroid, which appear as sonolucent bands.[5, 15] Posteriorly, the longus colli muscle is evident and is usually indistinguishable from the neurovascular bundle.[5] The esophagus with its echogenic mucosa is visualized medially adjacent to the trachea. The common carotid arteries lie immediately lateral to the lobes of the thyroid, serving as anatomic landmarks. The internal jugular veins are evident lateral to the arteries and vary in size and shape. Full distention of the veins of the neck may be obtained with the Valsalva maneuver.

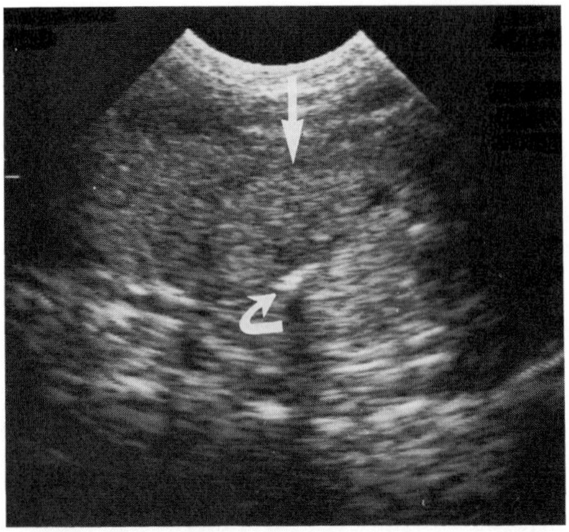

**FIGURE 8–2.** Ultrasonographic study of adenoma, which is hyperechoic (*straight arrow*) compared with normal thyroid tissue adjacent to it. Strong echoes with acoustic shadows represent calcification (*curved arrow*).

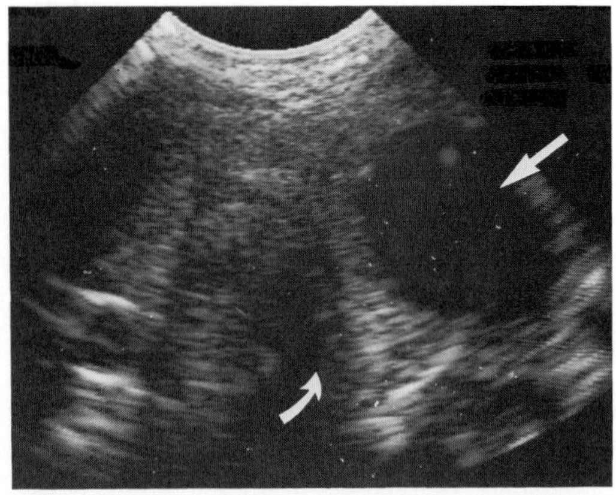

**FIGURE 8–4.** Ultrasonographic study of necrotic, almost entirely sonolucent, thyroid adenoma (*straight arrow*). Trachea is identified as echo-free area (*curved arrow*).

## *Follicular Adenoma*

A pattern characteristic of a solid simple adenoma without cystic degeneration is a high-amplitude group of echoes centrally surrounded by low-amplitude echogenicity (Fig. 8–2). The rim of low-level echoes usually surrounding the lesion corresponds histologically to the capsule of the tumor and its associated edema. This sonolucent rim or "halo" sign (Fig. 8–3) usually resembles a benign adenoma; however, occasionally it has also been reported to be associated with malignancy.[12] Simeone and associates[5, 31] found the halo sign in 45 patients, with a follicular adenoma present in 43 patients. The remaining two patients had papillary carcinoma. Thyroid adenomas can have a varied echo appearance, being hypoechoic (Fig. 8–4), hyperechoic, or isoechoic with or without the surrounding halo. Cystic degeneration (Fig. 8–5) may be present either as single or multiple foci.[21] The regional vasculature may be displaced if the nodule becomes large.

## *Colloid or Adenomatous Nodule*

Colloid or adenomatous nodules result from cycles of hyperplasia and involution

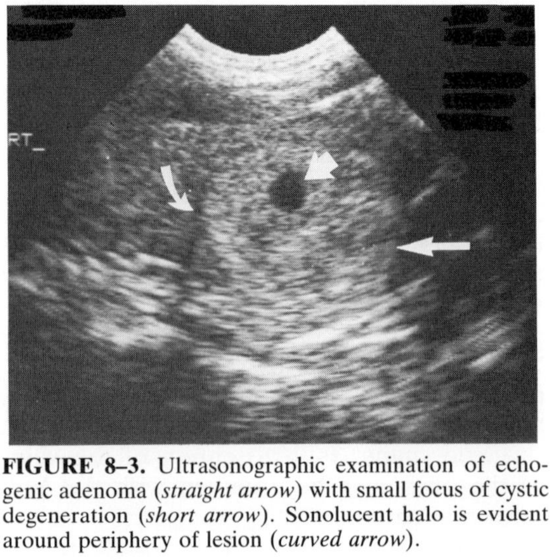


**FIGURE 8–3.** Ultrasonographic examination of echogenic adenoma (*straight arrow*) with small focus of cystic degeneration (*short arrow*). Sonolucent halo is evident around periphery of lesion (*curved arrow*).

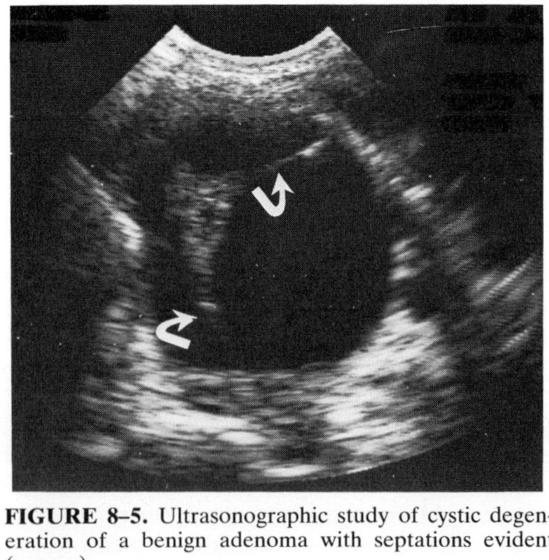

**FIGURE 8–5.** Ultrasonographic study of cystic degeneration of a benign adenoma with septations evident (*arrows*).

involving a thyroid lobule. They are not considered a true neoplasm and may be mistaken for a cyst when hemorrhage or necrosis is present.[15] A true cyst of the thyroid is uncommon. Dystrophic calcification may be present occasionally.

## *Hemorrhagic Cyst*

Hemorrhagic cysts most often result from spontaneous hemorrhage into a follicular adenoma (Fig. 8–6) but may result from blunt trauma to the neck.[5] Sonographically, the hemorrhagic cyst appears as a sonolucent or cystlike mass with irregular borders and multiple internal septations.[31] The septations may eventually disappear, and the borders become better defined. A fluid-fluid level may develop.[5]

## *Thyroid Cyst*

The frequency of the true thyroid cyst varies in the literature from 0.1 to 20 per cent.[24, 31] With the availability of high-frequency ultrasonography, it has become apparent that many of the cysts reported in the early literature were secondary cystic degeneration of a solid nodule. The group at Massachusetts General Hospital[5] identified only one true cyst in more than 1,000 patients. The thyroid cyst is echo free with a well-demarcated wall and excellent transmission of the sound wave through the cyst. Some authors[5, 20] believe the use of ultrasonography to show the rarely occurring true cyst is not clinically helpful, considering that both benign and malignant lesions can have cystic degeneration.

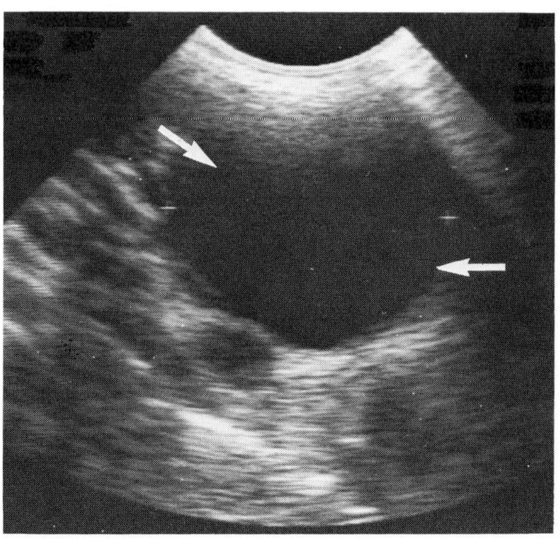

**FIGURE 8–6.** Ultrasonographic study of cystic degeneration of nodule of adenomatous goiter (*arrows*).

## *Diffuse Thyroid Enlargement*

Conditions producing diffuse enlargement of the thyroid gland include Graves' disease, infection, iodine deficiency, and Hashimoto's and other varieties of thyroiditis.

Ultrasonography may be indicated in the diagnosis of goiter only when the underlying disease process causes asymmetric thyroid enlargement.[15] Patients with multinodular goiter have generalized distortion of the overall glandular structure.[16] The texture of the thyroid gland can be diffusely inhomogenous without recognizable thyroid tissue or normal thyroid tissue may be interspersed with multiple discrete nodules. Coarse fibrous tissue may separate the nodules.[5, 15, 18] Asymmetric enlargement of both lobes is frequently evident, and calcification, when present, will produce strong echoes, casting acoustic shadows. Pathologically, the nodules of multinodular goiter are colloid or adenomatous and are not regarded as true neoplasms but are a result of hyperplasia and involution of a thyroid lobule. Hemorrhage and cystic degeneration are frequently evident.[5, 15, 18, 29]

Thyroiditis has a typical but nonspecific sonographic appearance. Diffuse enlargement will be present with a coarse echo pattern and low-amplitude echoes.[2, 3, 28] Usually, no normal parenchyma is identified. Discrete nodules and occasional calcification have been reported[5, 31] in 30 per cent of patients. Frequently, the ultrasonographic picture is similar to that of multinodular goiter, requiring differentiation by laboratory and clinical methods.[5]

## *Malignant Thyroid Disease*

Carcinoma of the thyroid accounts for 1 per cent of all clinically important cancers[5] but for approximately 10 to 25 per cent of all solitary nodules.[4, 29, 31] The risk of a nodule of multinodular goiter being cancerous is less than 1 per cent.[4] Currently, sonographic differentiation between benign and malignant lesions is not possible. The sonographic appearance of a malignant thyroid process (papillary, follicular, medullary, anaplastic, or metastatic) is variable, but thyroid carcinoma typically has an irregular margin that usually is hypoechoic relative to the normal thyroid parenchyma. Lesions may vary from having a solid appearance to having an almost cystic appearance, and occasionally they have the same echo texture as normal thyroid tissue.[32] Nodules that exhibit a hyperechoic texture relative to the normal thyroid gland are frequently benign. A sonolucent halo usually associated with benign follicular adenoma may be present infrequently. When clinically indicated, echography can be used as a guide in the performance of aspiration biopsy of a suspicious thyroid nodule.

### Needle Aspiration Biopsy

Fine needle aspiration of thyroid nodules with echographic guidance offers a simple and safe technique with an accuracy approaching 95 per cent for solid lesions and 88 per cent for predominantly cystic masses.[20] Needle biopsy is least effective with the degenerative nodule. In one series,[20] a false-negative rate of 45 per cent for cystic papillary carcinoma was obtained; however, this was thought to be a sampling error rather than cytologic misdiagnosis. Needle aspiration with echographic guidance permits sampling of solid tissue rather than degenerative debris.

### Limitations of Ultrasonography

Although ultrasonography can demonstrate lesions as small as 2 mm, it offers no information on the functioning of the thyroid gland. The ultrasonographic patterns of both benign and malignant diseases overlap considerably, and ultrasonography cannot fully evaluate a multinodular goiter that has extended intrathoracically.

## COMPUTED TOMOGRAPHY

Computed tomography is a technique that involves the acquisition of x-ray attenuation data, its integration in mathematical terms by a computer, and the conversion of these data into a cross-sectional image of varying shades of gray.[33] Since 1972, computed tomography has been an extremely valuable modality in the preoperative assessment of the location of a neck mass and its effect on nearby structures and in evaluating coexistence of lymph node disease. Although ultrasonography is the primary imaging technique of the thyroid gland and radionuclide scans provide functional information, computed tomography plays a selective role in evaluating thyroid problems.

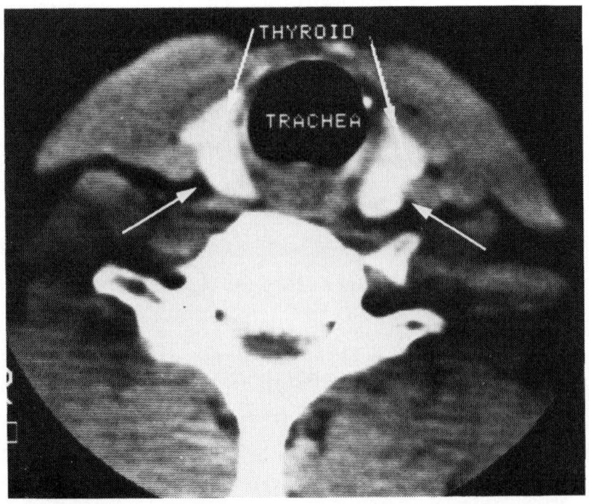


**FIGURE 8–7.** Computed tomographic scan of neck with the normal thyroid (*arrows*) having high density compared with normal soft tissues of neck.

The thyroid gland is readily identified on computed tomography (Fig. 8–7) because of its high density compared with the rest of the soft tissue structures of the neck. The biologic concentration of iodine in the thyroid gland accounts for this greater attenuation. Most normal thyroid glands have attenuation values in the range of 70 to 120 Hounsfield units with proportionate increase of these values compared with adjacent soft tissues after the use of iodinated intravenous contrast agents.[21, 30] The usefulness of computed tomography in the evaluation of thyroid disease is limited, particularly in differentiating benign from malignant disease. Thyroid tumors, whether benign (Fig. 8–8) or malignant, may be hypodense, hyperdense, or isodense compared with normal thyroid tissue.[25, 26] Malignant tumors (Fig. 8–9) may be inhomogenous with irregular margins, but they also appear as a homogenous mass and may have a cystic presentation.[21] Cystlike lesions can be identified by their lower density with computed

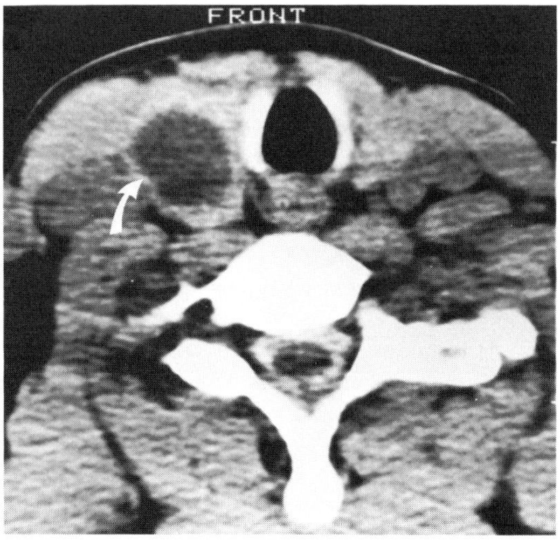


**FIGURE 8–8.** Computed tomographic scan of neck showing cystic degeneration of an adenoma in right lobe of thyroid (*arrow*).

tomography values approaching the attenuation value of water. However, the presence of iodine in the fluid of the cyst may raise the density of the cyst considerably, making an accurate diagnosis impossible. A true cyst will have a smooth well-defined margin and occasionally be calcified, similar to the ultrasonographic presentation.[31]

Computed tomography provides useful clinical information regarding the presence and extent of a substernal goiter, the degree of airway compression and vascular displacement associated with a thyroid mass, the presence of lymphadenopathy, the assessment of the integrity of fascial planes and fatty compartments of the neck, and the presence of the thyroid tissue in an ectopic location.[5, 24, 26] The probability of malignancy is increased with evidence of invasion of regional structures, nodal disease, and destruction of cartilage.[25, 30]

Mediastinal goiters constitute 5 to 11 per cent of mediastinal masses resected at thoracotomy.[11] Although radionuclide scanning is a standard modality used in evaluating whether thyroid tissue accounts for a mediastinal mass, negative results have been reported in the presence of a mediastinal goiter when little or no functioning tissue is present.[1, 23] In most instances, substernal thyroid tissue (Fig. 8–10) is secondary to direct extension of a goitrous thyroid and rarely the occurrence of totally ectopic thyroid tissue. The continuity of the extension can be appreciated on computed tomography evaluation and not with radionuclide studies when the connection is by thin extension of tissue.[11] Computed tomography can image in the axial plane and in the coronal plane with a reformatted reconstruction to confirm continuity of thyroid tissue extending into the chest. Computed tomography may also demonstrate punctate, coarse, or ringlike calcifications (Fig. 8–11) and nonhomogeneity of tissue with minimal or nonenhancing foci. Because of its higher attenuation values compared with adjacent structures, substernal thyroid

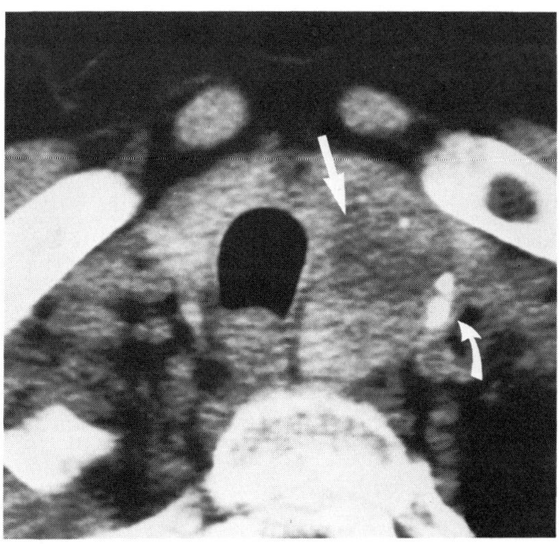

**FIGURE 8–9.** Computed tomographic scan of thyroid carcinoma in enlarged left lobe of thyroid with cystic degeneration (*straight arrow*) and calcification (*curved arrow*).

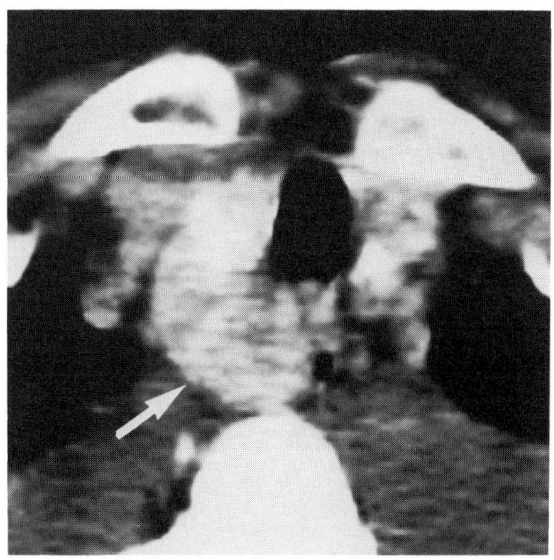

**FIGURE 8–10.** Computed tomographic scan of retrosternal goiter with large retrotracheal right lobe (*arrow*). High densities in both lobes are secondary to calcification.

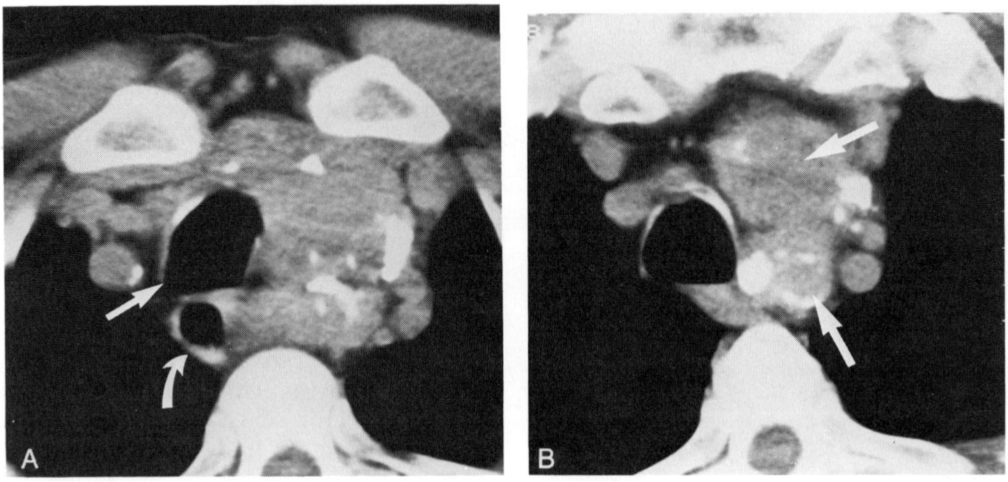


**FIGURE 8–11.** *A,* Computed tomographic scan of retrosternal goiter displacing air-filled esophagus (*curved arrow*) and trachea (*straight arrow*). Calcifications are present. *B,* More caudal section showing retrosternal extension of goiter (*arrows*).

tissue can easily be identified, and computed tomography can provide assistance in the evaluation of the pattern of extension of the goiter into the chest.[1, 11]

## MAGNETIC RESONANCE IMAGING

With the emergence of magnetic resonance imaging (Fig. 8–12) as a new technique during the past few years, considerable enthusiasm regarding its potential as a superlative diagnostic imaging modality has been created. Although it does not yet compare with computed tomography in spatial resolution, magnetic resonance imaging gives superior contrast resolution.[22] An advantage of magnetic resonance imaging is direct imaging in any plane, and, unlike computed tomography, magnetic resonance imaging can provide high contrast images without the need for contrast agents or ionizing radiation.[34] Magnetic resonance imaging will continue to follow a course of development similar to that of computed tomography, undergoing major improvements in design.

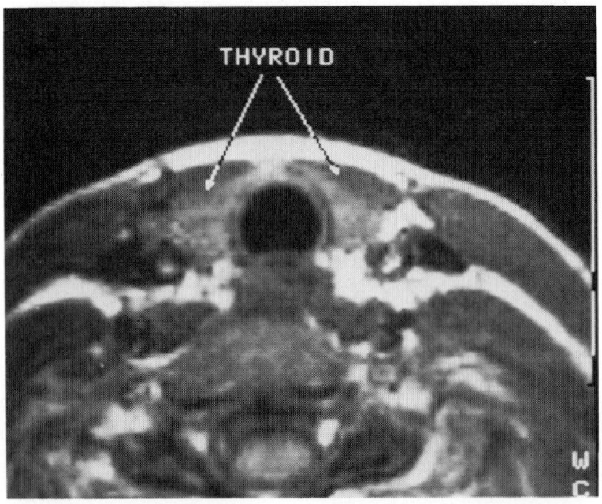


**FIGURE 8–12.** Magnetic resonance image of neck showing normal thyroid (*arrows*) with mildly increased signal intensity on either side of trachea.

Magnetic resonance imaging relies on the interaction of magnetic properties of certain atomic nuclei with an external magnetic field. When these nuclei are placed in a magnetic field, they align themselves in the direction of the external magnetic field. When a second magnetic field is applied perpendicular to the direction of the aligned nuclei, this will induce them to tip their axis of rotation. After the second energy source is switched off, the nuclei revert to a lower energy state. The excess energy emitted is identified and used to create cross-sectional images in any plane. Various tissues will emit signals comparable to their intrinsic physical properties.

Magnetic resonance imaging is in its infancy, and its role in evaluation of the thyroid gland has not yet been established (Fig. 8–13). It appears to be similar to that of computed tomography and of value in assessing Graves' disease,[7] mediastinal extent of thy-

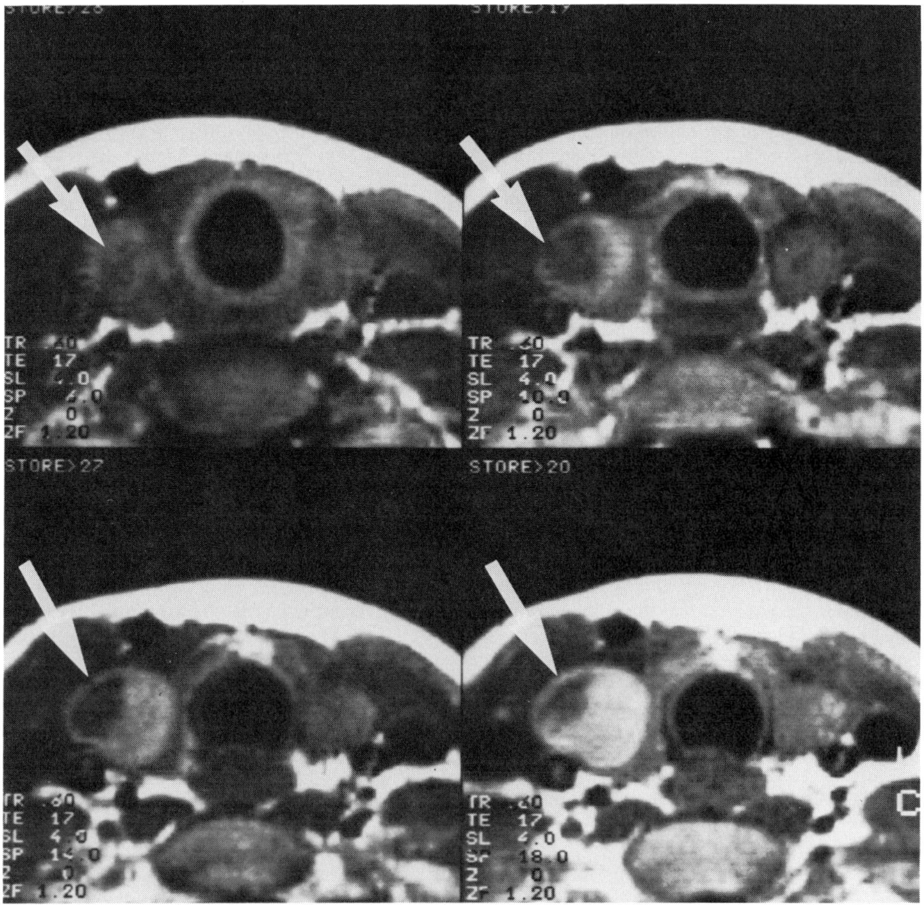

**FIGURE 8–13.** Magnetic resonance image of four contiguous sections of the neck showing incidentally found adenoma in right lobe of thyroid having varying signal intensities (*arrows*).

roid disease,[9, 22] and the extent and invasiveness of thyroid carcinoma.[19] Magnetic resonance imaging has the advantage of direct coronal imaging for evaluation of substernal thyroid enlargement[13] and offers excellent contrast between tumor and adjacent muscles and vessels so that local invasion can be assessed.[8, 10] Currently, magnetic resonance imaging is competing with fourth-generation computed tomography, and, if the technology of magnetic resonance imaging progresses as quickly as it did for computed tomography, the potential for its use may be unlimited.

## REFERENCES


1. Bashist, B., Ellis, K., and Gold, R. P.: Computed tomography of intrathoracic goiters. A.J.R., *140*:455–460, 1983.
2. Blum, M., and Passalaqua, A. M.: Managing the solitary thyroid nodule: Echography's role. Hosp. Pract., *13*:65–72, 1978.
3. Blum, M., Passalaqua, A. M., Sackler, J. P., and Pudlowski, R.: Thyroid echography of subacute thyroiditis. Radiology, *125*:795–798, 1977.
4. Brown, C. L.: Pathology of the cold nodule. Clin. Endocrinol. Metab., *10*:235–245, 1981.
5. Butch, R. J., Simeone, J. F., and Mueller, P. R.: Thyroid and parathyroid ultrasonography. Radiol. Clin. North Am., *23*:57–71, 1985.
6. Carroll, B. A.: Asymptomatic thyroid nodules: Incidental sonographic detection. A.J.R., *138*:499–501, 1982.
7. Charkes, N. D., Maurer, A. H., Siegel, J. A., et al.: MR imaging in thyroid disorders: Correlation of signal intensity with Graves disease activity. Radiology, *164*:491–494, 1987.
8. Epstein, D. M., Kressel, H., Gefter, W., et al.: MR imaging of the mediastinum: A retrospective comparison with computed tomography. J. Comput. Assist. Tomogr., *8*:670–676, 1984.
9. Gamsu, G., Stark, D. D., Webb, W. R., et al.: Magnetic resonance imaging of benign mediastinal masses. Radiology, *151*:709–713, 1984.
10. Gefter, W. B., Spritzer, C. E., Eisenberg, B., et

al.: Thyroid imaging with high-field-strength surface-coil MR. Radiology, *164*:483–490, 1987.

11. Glazer, G. M., Axel, L., and Moss, A. A.: CT diagnosis of mediastinal thyroid. A.J.R., *138*:495–498, 1982.
12. Hassani, N.: Ultrasonic investigation of solid thyroid tumors with gray-scale and real-time scanning: The halo sign. Appl. Radiol., *6*:165–177, 1977.
13. Higgins, C. B., McNamara, M. T., Fisher, M. R., and Clark, O. H.: MR imaging of the thyroid. A.J.R., *147*:1255–1261, 1986.
14. Hoffer, P. B., Gottschalk, A., and Quinn, J., III: Thyroid in vivo studies. *In* Gottschalk, A., and Potchen, E. J. (eds.): Diagnostic Nuclear Medicine. Baltimore, Williams & Wilkins, 1976, pp. 255–277.
15. James, E. M., and Charboneau, J. W.: High-frequency (10 MHz) thyroid ultrasonography. Semin. Ultr. C.T. M.R., *6*:294–309, 1985.
16. Katz, J. F., Kane, R. A., Reyes, J., et al.: Thyroid nodules: Sonographic-pathologic correlation. Radiology, *151*:741–745, 1984.
17. Laffey, P. A.: Ultrasound techniques. *In* Teplick, J. G., and Haskin, M. E. (eds.): Surgical Radiology: A Complement in Radiology and Imaging to the Sabiston-Davis-Christopher Textbook of Surgery, Volume 1. Philadelphia, W.B. Saunders Co., 1981, pp. 55–58 and 108–109.
18. Miskin, M., Rosen, I. B., and Walfish, P. G.: Ultrasonography of the thyroid gland. Radiol. Clin. North Am., *13*:479–492, 1975.
19. Mountz, J. M., Glazer, G. M., Dmuchowski, C., and Sisson, J. C.: MR imaging of the thyroid: Comparison with scintigraphy in the normal and diseased gland. J. Comput. Assist. Tomogr., *11*:612–619, 1987.
20. Müller, N., Cooperberg, P. L., Suen, K. C., and Thorson, S. C.: Needle aspiration biopsy in cystic papillary carcinoma of the thyroid. A.J.R., *144*:251–253, 1985.
21. Noyek, A. M., Greyson, N.D., Steinhardt, M. I., et al.: Thyroid tumor imaging. Arch. Otolaryngol., *109*:205–224, 1983.
22. Noma, S., Nishimura, K., Togashi, K., et al.: Thyroid gland: MR imaging. Radiology, *164*:495–499, 1987.
23. Park, H. M., Tarver, R. D., Siddiqui, A. R., et al.: Efficacy of thyroid scintigraphy in the diagnosis of intrathoracic goiter. A.J.R., *148*:527–529, 1987.
24. Radecki, P. D., Arger, P. H., Arenson, R. L., et al.: Thyroid imaging: Comparison of high-resolution real-time ultrasound and computed tomography. Radiology, *153*:145–147, 1984.
25. Reede, D. L., and Bergeron, R. T.: The CT evaluation of the normal and diseased neck. Semin. Ultr. C.T. M.R., *7*:181–201, 1986.
26. Reede, D. L., Whelan, M. A., and Bergeron, R. T.: CT of the soft tissue structures of the neck. Radiol. Clin. North Am., *22*:239–250, 1984.
27. Refetoff, S.: Tests of thyroid function. *In* Gottschalk, A., and Potchen, E. J. (eds.): Diagnostic Nuclear Medicine. Baltimore, Williams & Wilkins, 1976, pp. 237–253.
28. Sackler, J. P., Passalaqua, A. M., Blum, M., and Amorocho, L.: A spectrum of diseases of the thyroid gland as imaged by gray scale water bath sonography. Radiology, *125*:467–472, 1977.
29. Scheible, W., Leopold, G. R., Woo, V. L., and Gosink, B. B.: High-resolution real-time ultrasonography of thyroid nodules. Radiology, *133*:413–417, 1979.
30. Silverman, P. M., Newman, G. E., Korobkin, M., et al.: Computed tomography in the evaluation of thyroid disease. A.J.R., *142*:897–902, 1984.
31. Simeone, J. F., Daniels, G. H.., Mueller, P. R., et al.: High-resolution real-time sonography of the thyroid. Radiology, *145*:431–435, 1982.
32. Solbiati, L., Volterrani, L., Rizzatto, G., et al.: The thyroid gland with low uptake lesions: Evaluation by ultrasound. Radiology, *155*:187–191, 1985.
33. Stanley, R. J., and Sagel, S. S.: Computed tomography in the diagnosis of surgical disorders. *In* Teplick, J. G., and Haskin, M. E. (eds.): Surgical Radiology: A Complement in Radiology and Imaging to the Sabiston-Davis-Christopher Textbook of Surgery, Volume 1. Philadelphia, W.B. Saunders Co., 1981, pp. 125–127.
34. Von Schulthess, G. K., McMurdo, K., Tscholakoff, D., et al.: Mediastinal masses: MR imaging. Radiology, *158*:289–296, 1986.

# 9

# EVALUATION OF THYROID NODULES

*Marvin S. Wool, M.D.*

Although 10 million United States citizens are estimated to have a nodular goiter, less than 10,000 persons in any given year will have surgical excision of a thyroid carcinoma. The selection of patients for whom surgery is recommended challenges the art as well as the science of medicine inasmuch as no single foolproof diagnostic test is yet available. Even with careful application of history, physical examination, serum testing, radioisotope scanning, ultrasound examination of the thyroid, and the use of thyroid suppressive therapy, only 20 per cent of operations in the past yielded thyroid carcinoma. In the 1980s, however, with the rediscovery of the utility of the fine needle aspiration biopsy, evaluation of the thyroid nodule has undergone a near revolution. Increasing technical skill in obtaining and interpreting diagnostic biopsy material has doubled the yield of thyroid carcinoma at operation. Although it has become the single most important diagnostic test, needle biopsy continues to have important limitations when employed as the sole preoperative diagnostic test.

## HISTORY

Evaluation of the patient with a goiter who is suspected of having carcinoma of the thyroid begins with a carefully taken history. Undoubtedly, the most important element is exposure to external irradiation therapy to the head or neck area between infancy and early adulthood. In 25 per cent of patients with such exposure, a goiter will develop within three decades, and 25 per cent of these goiters will harbor a malignant lesion, although frequently that will be a microscopic focus of doubtful clinical significance.

Although thyroid carcinoma is two to three times more common among women than men, the prevalence of benign goiters is many times higher in women. Therefore, any goiter in a man should be regarded with great suspicion. Additionally, a family history of differentiated thyroid carcinoma (papillary or follicular) infers a somewhat greater likelihood that a carcinoma will develop. Finally, a family history of the rarer bilateral medullary carcinoma is important because this disease has an autosomal dominant inheritance pattern. Similarly, a personal or family history of hyperparathyroidism or pheochromocytoma raises the question of a multiple endocrine neoplasia syndrome type II, which includes medullary carcinoma in its clinical triad.

## PHYSICAL EXAMINATION

The presence of an apparently solitary thyroid nodule is the most important physical sign raising a question of carcinoma, although many such nodules may actually be found to be part of a multinodular gland on pathologic examination. Despite this dichotomy, Veith et al.[23] found that 17 of 31 differentiated carcinomas that originated in thyroid glands were proved uninodular after pathologic examination. Another study[21] found that four fifths of differentiated and two thirds of anaplastic carcinomas originated in uninodular glands. Nevertheless, a large minority of carcinomas originate in multinodular glands, most often in the dominant nodule, which have been considered multinodular by physical examination, ultrasonography, or radioisotope study. Such dominant nodules, therefore, should be evaluated with vigor for carcinoma. In patients who have had exposure to irradiation, investigation of a multinodular goiter with or without a dominant nodule should be pursued aggressively because such glands often reveal multiple histologic variations, including carcinoma in smaller nodules.

Rapid painless enlargement of a preexistent nodule is suggestive of carcinoma, as is the appearance of a new solitary or predominant nodule not present on previous examination. Painful rapid enlargement of a thyroid nodule may be associated with subacute thyroiditis or commonly hemorrhage into a preexistent nodule. Statistically, such hemorrhages are more likely to occur in benign nodules, but reexamination a number of weeks later is essential to confirm resolution of the hemorrhage, and further investigation is indicated when a palpable lesion remains. The subjective consistency of a thyroid nodule has some relationship to the presence of carcinoma, although only about half of thyroid carcinomas have been felt to be hard on clinical examination. The sensitivity of this finding is clearly low. Conversely, Kendall and Condon[13] found that 10 per cent of benign tumors had been characterized as hard on physical examination, rendering such a finding less specific as well.

Fixation of a goiter to contiguous structures of the trachea or to strap muscles is a much more useful finding because this occurs only with thyroid carcinoma and the rare Riedel's struma.

Although the presence of unilateral vocal cord paralysis secondary to recurrent nerve pressure or invasion had been thought to be a reliable indicator of carcinoma, Cerise et al.[6] found that four of 10 patients with such a finding had a benign thyroid lesion. Compression symptoms affecting the trachea (dyspnea while lying on either side) or esophagus (dysphagia) or the superior vena cava syndrome is related more to the size and location of a nodule than to the pathologic state and are, therefore, neither sensitive nor specific findings.

The presence of unilateral cervical adenopathy provides an important suggestion of papillary carcinoma. In young persons, not infrequently, the initial presentation of this disease is with one or more enlarged cervical lymph nodes, sometimes present for years, without clinically apparent nodules in the thyroid bed itself. In fact, more than one third of 662 papillary tumors in a Mayo Clinic series[24] presented in this manner, as was the case in 25 per cent of our[5] patients. Pretracheal and paratracheal lymph nodes usually are involved initially with medial lesions, followed by deep anterior and lower lateral cervical nodes, and finally by upper cervical and submandibular lymph nodes.

## SERUM TESTS

Twenty years ago, the thyroid protein thyroglobulin was first detected in the sera of patients with Graves' disease and nontoxic goiter. Shortly afterward, with more sensitive assays, the protein was also detected in the sera of 75 per cent of patients without thyroid disease, albeit in lower concentration than in patients with a goiter. Because the serum levels of thyroglobulin appeared to correlate with size of the goiter, consideration of such measurements as a screening procedure for carcinoma arose.

Schneider et al.[19] investigated more than 900 patients with a prior history of head or neck irradiation and found disappointing results. Patients with a palpable goiter had higher levels than patients without a goiter on average, but much overlap was apparent. Patients with carcinoma had similar mean thyroglobulin levels as patients with benign disease, and the levels correlated neither with the size of the malignant lesion nor with its histologic type or invasiveness. Therefore, the test is of no value in predicting the initial presence of carcinoma, but it does have utility in early detection of recurrent disease in patients who have had operations and radioactive iodine therapy for follicular carcinoma.

Measurements of serum calcitonin have been useful in screening kindreds of patients with medullary carcinoma. In one such kindred with 76 family members, 14 were found to have medullary carcinoma;[12] only six of the 14 had a palpable goiter, but all 14 had elevated levels of calcitonin. Of the eight patients with a nonpalpable goiter, two had basal elevated levels while the other six had normal levels, which rose after provocation with intravenously administered calcium. This calcium infusion test, however, is cumbersome, and alternative stimulating tests using glucagon and pentagastrin have been evaluated.[20] The latter is simpler to administer and is as reliable as the former. The basal unstimulated calcitonin level is also useful for surveillance for recurrence of disease in patients treated after established diagnosis.

Antithyroglobulin antibody measurements are of no value in screening for carcinoma, having a similar prevalence in patients with exposure to irradiation in childhood in whom a benign or malignant goiter ultimately developed.[19]

Serum levels of thyroxine ($T_4$) and triiodothyronine ($T_3$) are likewise of little value,[19] although ratios of $T_3$ to $T_4$ are said to be higher on average in patients with carcinoma. Elevated $T_3$ or $T_4$ levels in the presence of a solitary nodule are suggestive of autonomy of the nodule, in which case the likelihood of carcinoma is low. Conversely, low levels of serum hormones are found commonly in patients with the benign condition of Hashimoto's thyroiditis and rarely in patients with the unusual anaplastic carcinoma, which is destructive of a majority of normal thyroid tissue. Low levels, however, are not found in patients with the common types of papillary or follicular carcinoma who do not have underlying Hashimoto's disease.

## SENSITIVITY, SPECIFICITY, AND ACCURACY

Any diagnostic test must be evaluated in terms of its sensitivity and specificity. A tabular depiction of this concept is provided in Table 9–1. Actual disease, as confirmed by pathologic examination, can be defined as the presence of carcinoma. Results of diagnostic tests from top to bottom are categorized as positive or negative. Percentage of false negatives and false positives is defined by the numbers in those categories divided by the total number of patients studied, in our example 2 per cent and 20 per cent, respectively. Sensitivity is defined as the number of true positives divided by the number of true positives plus false negatives and represents that fraction of patients with true disease who will be identified correctly by the diagnostic test in question (e.g., 18 of 20 or 90 per cent). Specificity is defined as true negatives over false positives plus true negatives and indicates that fraction of patients correctly identified as not having the disease by criteria of the test (e.g., 60 of 80 patients or 75 per cent). Accuracy is defined by dividing the true positives and true negatives by the total number of patients studied (e.g., 78 of 100 or 78 per cent).

The ideal diagnostic test, of course, would yield 100 per cent sensitivity, specificity, and accuracy and zero false negatives and false positives. When the definition of a positive diagnostic test is broadened, the sensitivity of the test will be increased (i.e., a larger percentage of patients with true disease will be identified) while the specificity will be decreased (i.e., a smaller proportion of patients *without* disease will be identified by the test), in our example not spared operation. Conversely, when the criteria for a positive test are narrowed, the sensitivity of the test will be decreased (i.e., fewer patients with true disease will be identified) while the spec-

**TABLE 9–1. Example of Analysis of a Diagnostic Test***

| | CARCINOMA | NO CARCINOMA |
|---|---|---|
| Positive test | True positive (TP) (18)† | False positive (FP) (20) |
| Negative test | False negative (FN) (2) | True negative (TN) (60) |

$$\text{Sensitivity} = \frac{TP}{TP + FN} = \frac{18}{20} \text{ or 90 per cent}$$

$$\text{Specificity} = \frac{TN}{FP + TN} = \frac{60}{80} \text{ or 75 per cent}$$

$$\text{Accuracy} = \frac{TP + TN}{TP + FN + FP + TN} = \frac{78}{100} \text{ or 78 per cent}$$

False negative = 2 per cent
False positive = 20 per cent

*For research purposes beyond the scope of this discussion, more extensive evaluation of interobserver bias and test power can be obtained by statistical analysis of Receiver Characteristic Curves (ROC analysis) from data of this type.

†Arbitrary example of number of tests in TP category.

ificity will be increased (i.e., fewer of those patients without disease will be subjected to surgery).

## ULTRASONOGRAPHY

Ultrasound examination provides anatomic information about the thyroid gland. Specific nodules are usually described as cystic, mixed cystic and solid, or pure solid. Ashcraft and Van Herle[1] reviewed 16 series in which 69 per cent of nodules were solid, 19 per cent were cystic, and 12 per cent were mixed. Although patients with solid lesions coming to operation showed the highest prevalence of carcinoma at 21 per cent and although 12 per cent of mixed lesions also proved to be carcinoma, the finding of a pure cystic lesion did not exclude the presence of carcinoma. In 30 series, including almost 2,300 thyroid cysts, patients with 229 cysts were operated on, yielding 21 carcinomas, representing 1 per cent of the total cysts and 10 per cent of cysts operated on. Only eight of the 21 carcinomas were identified by preoperative examination of aspirated fluid. Van Herle et al.[22] reviewed published series, including nearly 700 patients who had a variety of preoperative tests and ultimately came to operation. They found that when ultrasonography gave a positive result, the lesion was broadly defined as solid or mixed; the sensitivity was 90 per cent (i.e., nine of 10 carcinomas were detected by the test), but the specificity was only 18 per cent (more than four benign nodules were removed for each carcinoma). Narrowing the criteria for a positive result on ultrasonography to solid lesions only improved the specificity to 33 per cent but decreased the sensitivity to 85 per cent.

Therefore, we believe ultrasonography has no role as a primary diagnostic test for the thyroid nodule. Ultrasonography may however be of use in patients who have had aspiration of a thyroid cyst with a remaining palpable nodule, enabling characterization anatomically of the remaining lesion.

## RADIOISOTOPE SCANNING OF THYROID

Radioisotope scanning provides a measure of the functional activity of the thyroid gland or a map for correlation with palpable physical findings. The technique has been a diagnostic mainstay for more than 30 years since Dobyns et al.[7] determined that carcinomatous tissue concentrated less radioactive iodine than did normal thyroid tissue. Clinically, Perlmutter and associates[15, 16] first demonstrated its utility by finding only a single carcinoma among 40 hyperfunctioning thyroid nodules while finding 23 carcinomas in 99 nonfunctional nodules. Although $^{131}I$ was the original isotope employed, it has subsequently been replaced by $^{123}I$ and technetium

99m pertechnetate, which expose the thyroid to less radiation. The latter isotope at first was thought to have a theoretic advantage over $^{123}I$ because its imaging merely required trapping in the thyroid gland and not the more sophisticated function of organification. The theory held that certain carcinomas could trap technetium and be visualized on scan but were not able to organify iodine and therefore appeared cold on iodine scan. This theoretic advantage, however, has not been borne out, and Ashcraft and Van Herle,[1] in a review of six series using technetium scanning, have shown a similar prevalence of carcinoma in nodules classified identically by iodine and technetium.

They further reviewed 22 series involving more than 5,000 patients who came to operation after thyroid scans with various isotopes.[1] Nodules were classified as cold in 84 per cent (i.e., trapping no isotope), warm in 10.5 per cent (i.e., trapping isotope in equal concentration to the rest of the gland), and hot (i.e., trapping all the isotope) in 5.5 per cent. Carcinomas were found in 16 per cent of the cold nodules, 9 per cent of the warm nodules, and only 4 per cent of the hot nodules. Therefore, when the scan showed "positive" results and the nodule was classified broadly as either cold or warm, the test used alone had a sensitivity of 96 per cent, missing only 4 per cent of thyroid carcinomas. The specificity, however, was only 17 per cent, therefore requiring five operations on benign nodules to yield a single thyroid carcinoma. Limiting the criterion of "positive" results to a cold nodule increased the specificity to 30 per cent requiring operation on only two benign nodules for each carcinoma. The sensitivity with this narrower criterion, however, was reduced to 87 per cent; thereby 13 per cent of true carcinomas were missed.

## NEEDLE BIOPSY

Although needle biopsy was first used in this country 60 years ago and attained popularity in Scandinavian countries in the interim, interest in it was revived in the United States only in the 1970s. Interest was initially directed both toward large needle core biopsy and fine needle aspiration, but use of the former has waned. Its theoretic advantage of providing a larger amount of tissue for a histologic rather than cytologic examination and therefore producing a greater yield of diagnostic material has not been confirmed. Ashcraft and Van Herle,[1] examining series of patients undergoing fine needle aspiration, found a cumulative false-negative rate of 2.5 per cent compared with 1.1 per cent in series of large needle core biopsies. Interestingly, the false-positive rates with the large needle biopsy were 6 per cent or twice that with fine needle aspiration, and surprisingly, 14 per cent of the large needle core biopsies yielded insufficient material, while only about 5 per cent of results of fine needle aspirations were unsatisfactory.

### *Classification of Fine Needle Aspiration Cytology*

Although varying criteria for cytologic classification of needle aspiration biopsy are used, four classes can usually be delineated: 0, unsatisfactory specimen for interpretation; 1, frankly benign; 2, suspicious; and 3, frankly malignant.

The smears of benign lesions have sparsely cellular components and uniform thyroid cells with regular nuclei and have a moderate amount of extracellular colloid. Suspicious aspirates are more cellular and have lesser amounts of colloid, more variability in cell and nuclear size, and some degree of mitotic activity. Approximately 30 per cent of cytologic specimens fall into this classification,[17] and 15 to 40 per cent of these specimens proved to have true carcinoma at operation,[17] usually the follicular or Hürthle cell type. Frankly malignant aspirates have cytologic criteria, including papillary fragment cells with intranuclear intrusions (so-called Little Orphan Annie eye nuclei), psammoma bodies, or cellular aspirates with a high degree of mitoses and absence of extracellular colloid.

### *Use of Fine Needle Aspiration*

Ashcraft and Van Herle[1] have provided the fullest documentation of the use of fine needle aspiration. They reviewed eight series of 13,071 patients, all of whom came to operation; 848 patients had benign cytologic findings with only 22 of those patients ultimately found to have carcinoma at operation for a 2.6 per cent false-negative rate. Of 484 patients with lesions suspected or proved malignant who came to operation, 246 carcinomas were found with only seven false positives. A survey of an additional 20 series, including more than 10,000 patients, not all of whom came to operation, revealed a similar false-negative rate of 2.4 per cent and a false-positive rate of 3.3 per cent. Van Herle et al.,[22] analyzing the same series, calculated a sensitivity of 92 per cent and a specificity of 74 per cent for fine needle aspiration. When the definition of a positive result on biopsy was narrowed to definite carcinoma only, the specificity rose to 99 per cent (i.e., almost no patients would be operated on for benign disease), but the sensitivity fell to 73 per cent, with 27 per cent of carcinomas missed, most of which would have been found in the "suspicious" group.

Asp et al.[2] analyzed the use of fine needle aspiration according to histologic cell type. In 37 patients who came to operation after fine needle aspiration, 28 had lesions classified as malignant or suspicious, and nine had lesions classified as benign by cytology. Using the broader criterion of malignant plus suspicious as a positive result, they found 100 per cent sensitivity of the test.[2] Overall, the specificity for 11 patients having papillary carcinoma was 100 per cent (i.e., all were true positive), but the specificity for follicular lesions was only 47 per cent because the seven instances of follicular carcinoma were balanced by 11 follicular adenomas in the suspicious cytology group, which proved to be benign. Rojeski and Gharib,[17] who reviewed additional series, have calculated a 90 per cent sensitivity for fine needle aspiration considered positive by frank malignancy or suspicious findings. In 102 patients, Norton et al.[14] reported a sensitivity of 90 per cent and a specificity of 77 per cent.

Van Herle et al.[22] concluded that by use of a broad "positive" fine needle aspiration criterion of frank malignancy plus suspicion, the yield of thyroid carcinoma at operation would be 45 per cent, with only 2.5 per cent missed carcinomas. Hamberger et al.,[10] comparing groups of patients before and after availability of fine needle aspiration, showed an increased yield at operation from 14 per cent to 29 per cent. Al-Sayer et al.,[18] by employing fine needle aspiration, showed an increase in the yield of carcinoma to 50 per cent from 31 per cent, and Asp et al.[2] demonstrated a yield of 64 per cent among 28 patients who had undergone preoperative fine needle aspiration versus 26 per cent in 35 patients who had not undergone aspiration.

## *Limitations of Fine Needle Aspiration*

Nearly 5 per cent of fine needle aspirations produce unsatisfactory cytologic specimens. Although this number may be reduced by repeat fine needle aspiration or subsequent large needle biopsy, a remaining small percentage of nodules will not yield diagnostic material. Nodules less than 1 cm present difficult biopsy targets, and, conversely, nodules of 4 cm or larger readily yield diagnostic material but are subject to inadequate sampling. Equally important as the skill of the biopsy technician is that of the cytologist examiner. In recent years, however, more dissemination of both types of skills is apparent. Asp et al.[2] examined results of fine needle aspiration in an institution where only 50 biopsies per year were performed and reported sensitivity, specificity, and accuracy of diagnosis equivalent to those in much larger reported series.

Of great concern is the reproducibility of fine needle aspiration. Hamburger[11] reported on 247 nodules that had required repeat aspiration. Of interest were 181 patients who had repeat fine needle cytology in which 22 or 12 per cent had a change in diagnosis. Of greater concern were six patients with biopsies initially classified benign who on repeat biopsy were shown to have frankly malignant lesions. Twelve other patients with initial benign biopsies were, on repeat, thought to have suspicious results; five patients came to operation with one having a nodule actually proving to contain carcinoma. Although the 181 patients studied represented only a small fraction of all biopsies performed in Hamburger's clinic over an 8-year period and although they may have been selected for rebiopsy because of other clinical indications, the nonreproducibility or change of diagnosis in the 12 per cent of resampled nodules is of concern.

A major continuing dilemma is that of those nodules classified as "suspicious," or suspected of being cancerous. Gharib et al.,[9] in a series of 1,970 biopsies at the Mayo Clinic from 1980 to 1982, found 17 per cent suspicious cytologic examinations. They reviewed eight additional series representing 2,500 cases in which the incidence of suspicious or indeterminate cytology ranged from 15 to 30 per cent and in which the ultimate incidence of carcinoma in such nodules proved to be between 10 and 50 per cent. In their own series of nearly 2,000 biopsies, 17 per cent were classified as suspicious, 253 patients came to operation, and 25 per cent were proved to have carcinoma. These investigators[9] did not believe other factors were helpful prognostically. They considered that the thyroid scan was not helpful inasmuch as 83 per cent of patients with suspicious lesions who had scans had hypofunctional nodules (cold nodules). Further, two carcinomas were found in patients who had hot nodules.

Block et al.[4] found 18 suspicious biopsies among 120 performed from 1980 to 1982 with two of 11 coming to operation being malignant. Twenty of Hamburger's patients who had suspicious findings on initial biopsy underwent rebiopsy.[11] Nine repeat biopsies remained suspicious. Three patients were operated on and had benign lesions. Eleven other nodules were considered benign on repeat fine needle aspiration, and two of these were confirmed at operation. The subject of needle biopsy of the thyroid is addressed more completely in the excellent chapter by the Doctors Hamburger.

## THYROID SUPPRESSIVE THERAPY

Thyroid hormone suppression is an additional therapeutic and diagnostic tool for nodules considered benign by clinical criteria, including fine needle aspiration, or in patients who refuse operation. The rationale for such therapy is that benign lesions are thought to be more likely responsive to stimulation by circulating thyroid-stimulating hormone (TSH), and therefore suppression of that pituitary hormone might lead to shrinkage. Conversely, it appears that at least in a small portion of patients, thyroid carcinoma responds to suppressive therapy.[3, 8]

Evaluation of this therapeutic diagnostic test is difficult. Even with an acknowledgment of accurate measurement of a nodule by physical examination, criteria for response to suppressive therapy vary in different series from no measurable growth of the nodule to various percentages of shrinkage or disappearance. Further false assurances may be provided by shrinkage of surrounding normal tissue with carcinoma in the remaining nodule. Evaluation of this technique is further hampered by the varying doses of thyroid hormone employed in different series and by the fact that most patients undergoing hormone suppression are not operated on. Nevertheless, Ashcraft and Van Herle[1] reviewed 10 series of 164 patients with solitary nodules who were thought to show complete or partial response to hormone suppression. Thirty of these patients were operated on, and two were found to have carcinoma. In 446 other patients, no change or enlargement was observed in the nodule with thyroid suppression; 165 patients underwent operation, and 23 had carcinoma. Using the broader definition of a positive test as no change or growth of the nodule, Van Herle et al.[22] calculated a sensitivity of the suppressive therapy tests of 83 per cent, with a specificity of only 33 per cent. When the definition of a positive result was narrowed to growth of the nodule during suppressive therapy, it became highly specific at 96 per cent, although the sensitivity fell to 33 per cent.

## PLANS FOR MANAGEMENT

With the resurrection of fine needle aspiration and widening expertise in its use, this technique has assumed a preeminent position in the evaluation of the thyroid nodule. This popularity has been achieved despite shortcomings, including a small incidence of unsatisfactory specimens, sampling errors, a lack of reproducibility, and a significant proportion of cytologic examinations thought to be indicative of but not diagnostic of carcinoma.

Various protocols have been advocated for

evaluation of the thyroid nodule, including three put forth by Van Herle et al.[22] The first two of these protocols involve the thyroid scan as an initial test while the third recommends fine needle aspiration as the initial test followed by scan in certain circumstances. The latter variation has achieved much popularity, and Rojeski and Gharib[17] recommend fine needle aspiration as the initial diagnostic test. For nodules indeterminate or suspicious by cytologic examination, they would proceed to thyroid scan, with further selection for immediate operation, thyroid suppression, or periodic examination being determined by the nature of the thyroid scan.

## *Lahey Clinic Plan*

No single diagnostic test has yet achieved 100 per cent sensitivity and specificity, but fine needle aspiration has achieved the greatest degree of specificity, and scanning with $^{123}I$ has achieved great sensitivity. Therefore, we favor an approach including both techniques. This plan includes a scan with $^{123}I$ as the initial diagnostic test, with nodules proving nonfunctional or hypofunctional by scan being submitted to needle aspiration biopsy. Patients with indeterminate, suspicious, or malignant findings on aspiration cytology are referred for operation. Patients with frankly benign changes are examined periodically in follow-up studies. Thyroid hormone suppression is not recommended for this group of patients unless the serum TSH is detectable.

Patients with warm nodules (i.e., scanning characteristics of the nodule indistinguishable from the rest of the gland) are given a trial of suppressive therapy, and fine needle aspiration is recommended unless the nodule completely disappears within 6 months. Patients with hot or hyperfunctioning nodules are not subjected to aspiration biopsy initially. Suppressive therapy in this group is not of benefit inasmuch as these nodules function autonomously of TSH. Early needle aspiration biopsy for warm or hot nodules is not recommended because of the likelihood of false-positive biopsy results in such patients and because submission to unnecessary operation is far greater than the likelihood of a false-negative clinical assessment. Some of these patients may require operation if hyperthyroidism develops.

In patients found to have cysts at the time of fine needle aspiration, no further diagnostic tests or treatment is recommended if the cyst disappears entirely and remains nonpalpable 6 months later. When a residual palpable nodule remains, the evaluation proceeds as with nonfunctional nodules with fine needle aspiration and further recommendations based on the cytologic findings.

No rigid protocol, even one relying on sensitive scanning techniques and specific fine needle aspiration, negates consideration of other potentially overriding factors. A history of radiation exposure, a family history of thyroid carcinoma, recent rapid painless growth of a nodule, apparent adherence of the nodule to adjacent structures, presence of cervical adenopathy, and vocal cord paralysis are all signals for consideration of surgical resection.

## REFERENCES


1. Ashcraft, M. W., and Van Herle, A. J.: Management of thyroid nodules. I. History and physical examination, blood tests, X-ray tests, and ultrasonography. II. Scanning techniques, thyroid suppressive therapy, and fine needle aspiration. Head Neck Surg., *3*:216–230 and 297–322, 1981.
2. Asp, A. A., Georgitis, W., Waldron, E. J., et al.: Fine needle aspiration of the thyroid: Use in an average health care facility. Am. J. Med., *83*:489–493, 1987.
3. Balme, H. W.: Metastatic carcinoma of the thyroid successfully treated with thyroxine. Lancet, *1*:812–813, 1954.
4. Block, M. A., Daily, G. E., and Robb, J. A.: Thyroid nodules indeterminate by needle biopsy. Am. J. Surg., *146*:72–78, 1983.
5. Cady, B., Sedgwick, C. E., Meissner, W. A., et al.: Changing clinical, pathologic, therapeutic, and survival patterns in differentiated thyroid carcinoma. Ann. Surg., *183*:541–553, 1976.
6. Cerise, E. J., Randall, S., and Ochsner, A.: Carcinoma of the thyroid and nontoxic nodular goiter. Surgery, *31*:552–561, 1952.
7. Dobyns, B. M., Skanse, B., and Maloof, F.: Method for preoperative estimation of function in thyroid tumors: Its significance in diagnosis and treatment. J. Clin. Endocrinol., *9*:1171–1184, 1949.
8. Dunhill, T.: Surgery of thyroid gland. Trans. Med. Soc. (London) *60*:234–282, 1937.
9. Gharib, H., Goellner, J. R., Zinsmeister, A. R., et al.: Fine needle aspiration biopsy of the thyroid: The problem of suspicious cytologic findings. Ann. Intern. Med., *101*:25–28, 1984.
10. Hamberger, B., Gharib, H., Melton, L. J., 3d, et al.: Fine-needle aspiration biopsy of thyroid nodules: Impact on thyroid practice and cost of care. Am. J. Med., *73*:381–384, 1982.
11. Hamburger, J. I.: Consistency of sequential needle

biopsy findings for thyroid nodules: Management implications. Arch. Intern. Med., *147*:97–99, 1987.
12. Jackson, C. E., Tashjian, A. H., Jr., and Block, M. A.: Detection of medullary thyroid cancer by calcitonin assay in families. Ann. Intern. Med., *78*:845–852, 1973.
13. Kendall, L. W., and Condon, R. E.: Prediction of malignancy in solitary thyroid nodules. Lancet, *1*:1071–1073, 1969.
14. Norton, L. W., Wangensteen, S. L., Davis, J. R., et al.: Utility of thyroid aspiration biopsy. Surgery, *92*:700–705, 1982.
15. Perlmutter, M., and Slater, S. L.: Which nodular goiters should be removed? Physiologic plan for diagnosis and treatment of nodular goiter. N. Engl. J. Med., *255*:65–71, 1956.
16. Perlmutter, M., Slater, S. L., and Attie, J.: Method for preoperative differentiation between benign and possibly malignant solitary nontoxic thyroid nodule. J. Clin. Endocrinol., *14*:672–673, 1954.
17. Rojeski, M. T., and Gharib, H.: Nodular thyroid disease: Evaluation and management. N. Engl. J. Med., *313*:428–436, 1985.
18. Al-Sayer, H. M., Krukowski, Z. H., Williams, V. M., and Matheson, N. A.: Fine needle aspiration cytology in isolated thyroid swellings: A prospective two year evaluation. Br. Med. J., *18*:1490–1492, 1985.
19. Schneider, A. B., Favus, M. J., Stachura, M. E., et al.: Plasma thyroglobulin in detecting thyroid carcinoma after childhood head and neck irradiation. Ann. Intern. Med., *86*:29–34, 1977.
20. Sizemore, G. W., and Go, V. L. W.: Stimulation tests for diagnosis of medullary thyroid carcinoma. Mayo Clin. Proc., *50*:53–56, 1975.
21. Staunton, M. D., and Greening, W. P.: Clinical diagnosis of thyroid cancer. Br. Med. J., *4*:532–535, 1973.
22. Van Herle, A. J., Rich, P., Ljung, B.-E., et al.: Thyroid nodule. Ann. Intern. Med., *96*:221–232, 1982.
23. Veith, F. J., Brooks, J. R., Grigsby, W. P., and Selenkow, H. A.: Nodular thyroid gland and cancer: A practical approach to the problem. N. Engl. J. Med., *270*:431–436, 1964.
24. Woolner, L. B., Beahrs, O. H., Black, B. M., et al.: Thyroid carcinoma: General considerations and follow-up data on 1181 cases. *In* Young, S., and Inman, D. R. (eds.): Thyroid Neoplasia. New York, Academic Press, 1968, pp 51–79.

# 10

# USE OF NEEDLE BIOPSY DATA IN DIAGNOSIS AND MANAGEMENT OF THYROID NODULES

*Joel I. Hamburger, M.D., and Stuart W. Hamburger, M.D.*

The thyroid nodule is one of the commonest of human abnormalities. More than 90 per cent of them are benign. For a small minority of patients with thyroid carcinoma, the history and physical findings are virtually diagnostic. For example, a diagnosis of papillary carcinoma in a young patient with a progressively enlarging mass accompanied by prominent adjacent lymph nodes does not require great perspicacity. A woman in her 70s with a hard, rapidly growing mass probably has carcinoma, possibly a lymphoma of the thyroid, or an undifferentiated carcinoma. A family history of medullary carcinoma makes that diagnosis likely for another member of that family with a thyroid nodule. However, for most patients with thyroid nodules, no decisive clinical findings distinguish malignant lesions from the more common benign ones. Prevailing opinion calls for surgical treatment of thyroid carcinomas and observation for benign thyroid nodules.

The first useful laboratory test for the diagnosis of thyroid nodules was the thyroid image (scan). Nodules with increased function ("hot" nodules), especially if autonomously functioning, can safely be considered benign. Unfortunately, more than 90 per cent of thyroid nodules have reduced function ("cold" nodules), a finding compatible with thyroid carcinoma but more often associated with benign disease. Although echography can distinguish between solid and cystic nodules, neither finding confirms or excludes carcinoma.[1, 25]

Currently, primary reliance for the diagnosis of thyroid nodules is placed on needle biopsy. Needle biopsy was first reported by Martin in 1930.[58] Using large needle aspiration biopsy, he showed that histologic diagnoses could be made. Subsequently, others[15, 55, 87] favored biopsy of material collected by large needle cutting methods using the Silverman or TruCut needle. The popular fine needle biopsy technique, introduced in the 1950s by Scandinavian workers,[17, 53, 65, 67, 78] provides specimens for cytologic diagnoses. Between 1930 and the middle 1970s, despite sporadic reports[14, 21, 22, 42, 44, 51, 71, 86] advocating needle biopsy for the diagnosis of thyroid nodules, widespread use was curtailed for several reasons.

It was usually appreciated that the differentiation of benign from malignant thyroid nodules could be exceedingly difficult, even for an experienced thyroid pathologist working with the entire surgical specimen. Hence, many general pathologists were reluctant to accept the concept that reliable diagnoses could be made on small needle biopsy samples. In retrospect, it is surprising how readily physicians accepted the logical fallacy that because the diagnosis of carcinoma is difficult in a minority of thyroid nodules, one should not rely on needle biopsy to establish or exclude that diagnosis for any thyroid nodules.

One report[15] of seeding carcinoma in the needle track so dampened enthusiasm for needle biopsy that an entire generation of patients with thyroid nodules was denied the benefit of the improved diagnostic precision of needle biopsy.

In 1958, Frazell and Foote[20] (curiously also at Memorial Hospital in New York where Martin's pioneering work with large needle aspiration biopsy was performed) found a 26.4 per cent rate of false-negative diagnoses in patients with papillary carcinoma. They concluded that needle biopsy diagnoses were unreliable. It is hard to reconcile their experience with the current consensus that papillary carcinoma is one of the easiest diagnoses to make by needle biopsy.

To use needle biopsy, physicians first had to learn how to secure the specimens and how to interpret them. Before 1979, no ready reference was available to assist in acquiring either skill.

Between 1976 and 1979, a series of reports from North American centers[16, 18, 22, 38, 59, 87] gave impetus for more extensive study of needle biopsy. Because large needle techniques provide tissue for conventional histologic examination, some physicians thought that pathologists, experienced with the histologic study of surgical specimens, could more easily make the diagnosis on large needle biopsy samples than learn the newer techniques of cytologic diagnosis. However, large needle biopsy is a more formidable procedure than fine needle biopsy, with a greater potential for complication. Also, large needle biopsy is usually restricted to nodules larger than 2.5 cm, while fine needle biopsy can be used for nodules as small as 0.5 cm if favorably placed. Most thyroid nodules are detected on routine examination at the 1 cm to 2 cm size, for which only fine needle biopsy is practical.

As cytology experience increased, the accuracy of fine needle biopsy diagnoses so improved that the need for large needle technique has greatly diminished. Furthermore, even with the large nodules for which large needle biopsy specimens can easily be obtained, the fine needle technique has an important advantage. The ease and simplicity of fine needle collection permit the acquisition of biopsy specimens from multiple sites within the lesion to ensure adequacy of sampling. Although malignant nodules are no doubt malignant throughout, features indicative of carcinoma may be more evident in some portions of a tumor than in others. Hence, the fine needle technique has become the biopsy collection method of choice in most clinics. The principal continuing indication for large needle biopsy, especially the simpler large needle aspiration biopsy, is its use in the event of fine needle biopsy failure, common in loosely organized, partially degenerated nodules. Here, the fine needle method tends to produce specimens with few or no thyroid epithelial cells because the degeneration fluid is more readily aspirated than the sparse epithelial tissue. The size of the needle and more vigorous suction of large needle aspiration may produce useful tissue fragments.

The increase in precision of diagnosis on the basis of needle biopsy compared with diagnoses made by conventional clinical methods was easily established.[59] In our practice, diagnosis using needle biopsy led to a substantial reduction in the number of patients sent to operation, with no loss in cancer yield compared with that for a similar size population we had previously selected for operation without needle biopsy.[30]

## NEEDLE BIOPSY METHODS

We will briefly describe the large needle aspiration biopsy method and provide a detailed discussion of the more widely used fine needle biopsy method, emphasizing the avoidance of pitfalls. Large cutting needle procedures are seldom needed and will not be described here. The interested reader can review the technique in an earlier publication.[38]

## *Large Needle Aspiration Biopsy Technique*

For large needle aspiration biopsy, we employ a 1.5-inch 16-gauge disposable hypodermic needle. An 18-gauge needle may be used for smaller nodules. The patient is placed in the recumbent position with a pillow under the shoulders so the neck is hyperextended. Hyperextension should be limited in older patients to avoid occlusion of the vertebral arteries. The skin is cleaned with alcohol and infiltrated with 0.05 per cent lidocaine (Xylocaine). The needle, attached to a 20-ml disposable syringe containing an anticoagulant, is inserted into the nodule in a direction perpendicular to the anterior surface of the skin (Fig. 10–1*A*). Suction is applied, and the barrel of the syringe is rotated through 360 degrees. With this maneuver, the sharp bevel of the needle is turned through the tissue, severing small fragments that are aspirated into the syringe (Fig. 10–1*B*). While suction is maintained, the needle is withdrawn to the capsule of the nodule and reinserted in different directions, with the rotational maneuver repeated each time; 3 to 5 ml or more of bloody fluid is obtained.

After the last aspiration, the needle is retracted to the capsule, suction is released, and the needle is withdrawn. A few milliliters of saline solution is aspirated into the syringe to ensure that all tissue is within the barrel of the syringe. The syringe is upended and the plunger is withdrawn, pouring the specimen out of the proximal end of the syringe onto a filter paper. This technique protects the specimen from fragmentation that might be caused if the aspirate were forced out through the needle. As the fluid passes through the filter, the tissue is readily visible on the paper (Fig. 10–2). Using an anticoagulant and filtering the specimen ensures that tissue rather than just a blood clot will be sent to the pathologist. Also, the physician can judge the adequacy of the tissue obtained and repeat the biopsy if the tissue seems insufficient. The tissue is picked up by the needle and placed in Bouin's solution for fixation. Direct formalin fixation of these small tissue fragments is less satisfactory because finer nuclear anatomy will thereby be obscured.[38] Pressure is maintained on the biopsy site for 20 min to control bleeding, and the patient may then be released.

Large needle aspiration biopsy can be performed immediately after fine needle biopsy, but the tissue disruption and bleeding induced by large needle aspiration biopsy preclude the performance of a subsequent fine needle biopsy for a few weeks.

## *Fine Needle Biopsy Technique*

Patient positioning and preparation are the same as for large needle aspiration biopsy. Some physicians say that local anesthesia is unnecessary because the discomfort of administering the anesthesia is similar to that associated with the procedure.[29, 57, 79, 86] We

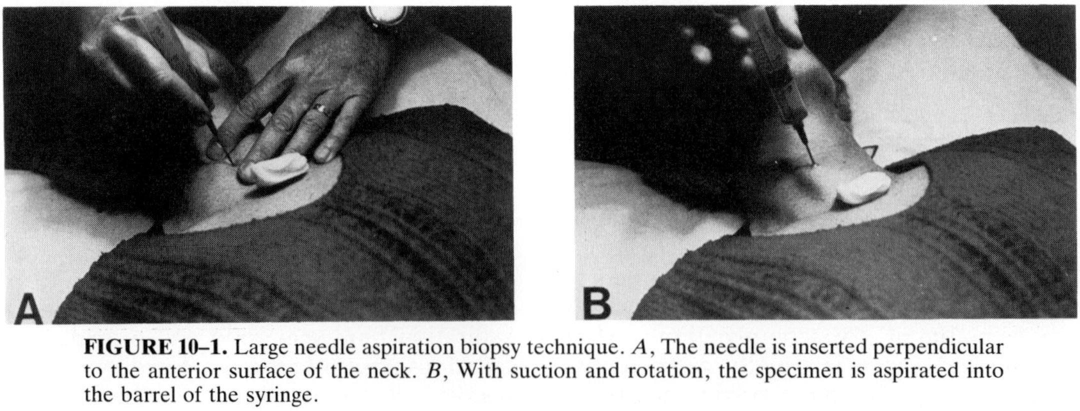


**FIGURE 10–1.** Large needle aspiration biopsy technique. *A*, The needle is inserted perpendicular to the anterior surface of the neck. *B*, With suction and rotation, the specimen is aspirated into the barrel of the syringe.

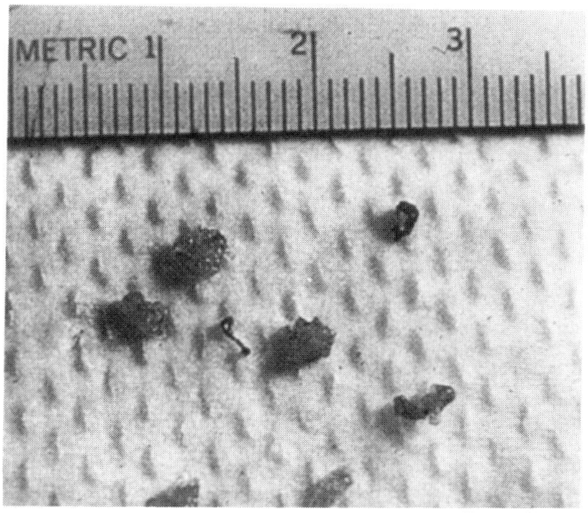


**FIGURE 10–2.** Large needle aspiration biopsy specimen. Tissue fragments remain on filter paper after the fluid portion of the specimen has drained through.

disagree. We emphasize the importance of multiple aspirates, at least six, to ensure adequate sampling. In some patients, 12 to 15 punctures are needed to secure six samples that appear promising on macroscopic inspection. Local anesthesia ensures patient tolerance and cooperation. Also, the unanesthetized patient may involuntarily contract the cervical musculature as the needle penetrates the skin. This makes it more difficult to palpate smaller nodules for accurate needle placement. The argument that the infiltrate of local anesthesia obscures the nodule is specious. A moment's gentle massage readily disperses the fluid. For the occasional patient who is sensitive to local anesthetics, continuous reassurance and distracting conversation will help maintain cooperation.

The 1.5-inch 25-gauge disposable needle is ideal for fine needle biopsy. Finer needles are too flexible, and larger needles often cause excessive bleeding that so dilutes the specimens that too few follicular cells are present for reliable diagnosis. The needle is attached to a 10-ml disposable syringe and inserted into the nodule in a direction perpendicular to the anterior surface of the neck. The nodule is fixed by the opposite hand as the needle is inserted (Fig. 10–3*A*). When the needle is in place, the opposite hand holds the syringe; the hand that inserted the needle withdraws the plunger to create suction (Fig. 10–3*B*). The opposite hand again fixes the nodule for the rest of the procedure. We do not use the metal syringe holder[19, 57] that permits continuous one-hand operation of the syringe-needle assembly. We have found it awkward, and with it the biopsy hand must be kept an additional distance from the end of the needle and the nodule, with loss of tactile sense.[28] It adds an unnecessarily complicated step to the procedure, not to mention the added expense of the instrument.

The novice will insert the needle directly into the most accessible point, the center of the nodule. However, this is the portion of the nodule most likely to have undergone degeneration and therefore least likely to provide diagnostically useful material. A better technique calls for insertion of the needle circumferentially at the periphery of the nodule. The obvious risk is that one may miss the nodule and sample adjacent tissue. However, with reasonable experience this is not a problem. For nodules 1 cm or less, it may be impractical to aim for anything other than the center of the nodule, but these smaller nodules are less likely to have undergone much degeneration. Degeneration is more common and more extensive in the larger nodules for which peripheral aspiration is easy.

After the needle is inserted, some method of gentle tissue disruption is necessary to dislodge the specimen. The method employed depends on the consistency of the nodule. For some nodules, insertion of the needle alone is enough. The application of suction is followed promptly by the appearance of blood-tinged fluid in the hub of the needle. When this happens, suction is released, the needle is withdrawn, and the specimen will be in the needle. One does not want so voluminous a specimen that it will enter the barrel of the syringe because it will be too dilute and not recoverable.

When the nodule is dense, inserting the needle alone will not cause enough tissue disruption to dislodge a specimen. The needle is moved in and out through a vertical depth of 1 to 2 mm while suction is maintained.[57] As soon as material is visible in the hub of the needle, the maneuver is stopped, suction is released, and the needle is withdrawn. In hard dry dense nodules, occasionally papillary carcinomas, the in and out movement is not enough, and the rotational maneuver described for large needle aspiration biopsy may be used. However, this is seldom necessary.

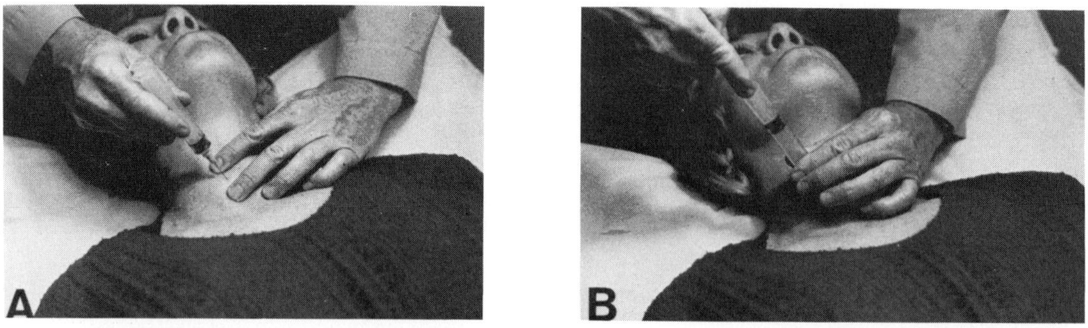


**FIGURE 10–3.** Fine needle aspiration biopsy technique. *A*, The needle is inserted perpendicular to the anterior surface of the neck. *B*, Suction and in and out movement produce a specimen in the needle.

When the needle strikes calcium, one should not be deterred from proceeding. Often the nodule can be penetrated between calcifications to obtain specimens, which occasionally produce a diagnosis of papillary carcinoma.[33] It is common to experience a gritty sensation as the needle is inserted in a papillary carcinoma because these lesions often contain fine calcific deposits. This finding, however, is nonspecific.

After the needle has been withdrawn from the nodule, it is detached from the syringe, a few milliliters of air is aspirated into the syringe, the needle is reattached, and the air is expressed through the needle to expel the specimen onto a glass slide. The specimen is inspected to assess its suitability for cytologic evaluation. The specimen desired consists of a drop or two of red-orange fluid (Fig. 10–4). A larger bloody specimen will usually not be useful. These bloody samples can be salvaged by absorbing the excess fluid, thereby concentrating the specimen.[28, 89] We seldom use this method because it is time consuming. In an anesthetized patient, it is simpler to sample another site. Thin green-colored or brown-colored degeneration fluid is useless. Similarly useless is the less frequently encountered cheesy white or thick oily fluid. In the final analysis, a fundamental limitation for fine needle biopsy is that nothing other than that which is contained within the nodule can be aspirated. When the nodule has undergone extensive degeneration or fibrosis, enough useful cellular material may not be obtained no matter how many aspirations are performed. Furthermore, neither degeneration nor fibrosis excludes carcinoma.

After the specimen has been expressed onto a glass slide, it is smeared. The frequently used technique of approximating the edge of a second slide at a 45-degree angle, permitting the fluid to flow along the edge of the top slide and then drawing the specimen out over the bottom slide produces thick uneven smears. A better technique is to place the top slide flat on the specimen and with the index finger press down and slide the top slide over the bottom slide (Fig. 10–5). This

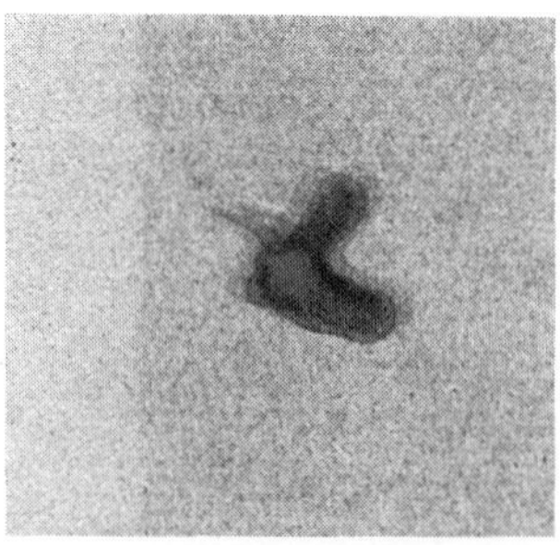

**FIGURE 10–4.** Fine needle aspiration biopsy specimen. A single drop of red-orange fluid.

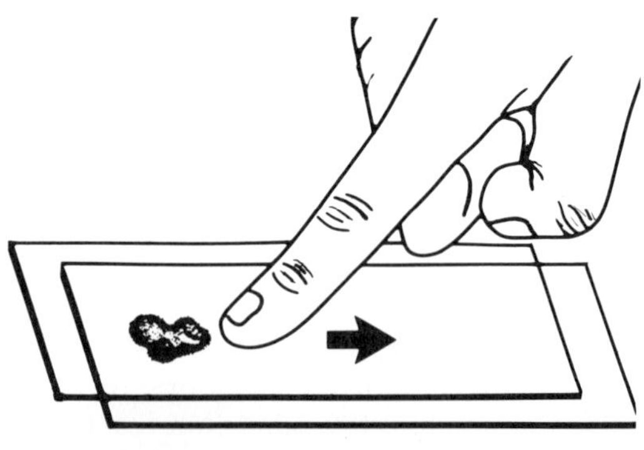

**FIGURE 10–5.** Smearing the fine needle biopsy specimen. A second slide is placed flat over the specimen, pressure is applied by the index finger, and the top slide is pulled over the bottom slide to prepare a uniform flat smear.

produces a thin, evenly dispersed smear that is ideal for cytologic evaluation.

The smear should be fixed immediately. Air drying will produce a loss of the nuclear detail so important for the cytologic evaluation of Papanicolaou-stained preparations. The air-dried smears stained with Giemsa stain favored by European cytopathologists are inferior in nuclear detail.

## FINE NEEDLE BIOPSY INTERPRETATION

### *Adequacy of the Specimen*

The first critical judgment is whether enough cells are present to make any diagnosis. How much is enough depends on which diagnosis one is attempting to make. A few clusters of malignant cells may be enough to make a diagnosis of carcinoma, even of the specific type of carcinoma. Malignant cells can come only from a malignant lesion. However, a similar number of benign cells is completely inadequate to exclude carcinoma. Every thyroid gland has benign cells. Benign cells are always in close approximation to a malignant nodule—on either side or perhaps in front of or behind it if the nodule is small. Also, within a malignant lesion the morphology may be highly pleomorphic, with some areas composed of tissue that may appear benign.

The issue of pleomorphism is illustrated by the findings on study of a 62-year-old woman who had three large needle biopsies between 1981 and 1985. The initial finding was nodular goiter, the second large needle biopsy diagnosis was follicular adenoma, and the third large needle biopsy diagnosis was follicular carcinoma (Fig. 10–6). The surgical specimens (Fig. 10–6) showed areas that closely resembled each of the biopsy specimens. The results of fine needle biopsy studies performed concurrently with the large needle biopsies were consistently indicative of a follicular neoplasm. The therapeutic implications of the fine needle biopsy diagnoses were ignored by physicians managing the patient until the third large needle biopsy; they thought that the large needle specimens might be more reliable. The tumor, although malignant, did not enlarge perceptibly during the 3 years of observation. We have seen similar cases involving older patients with large pleomorphic follicular carcinomas in whom large needle biopsy gave a false-negative diagnosis.

Needle biopsy has been advocated as a way to reduce unnecessary surgery in which only benign nodules are removed. The principal objective, therefore, was to identify those nodules that could safely be left in situ, that is, to exclude carcinoma. It should have been clear from the beginning that the exclusion of carcinoma would require more stringent criteria for adequacy of sampling than were needed to establish a diagnosis of carcinoma. Unfortunately, we learned this lesson only after making a number of false-negative diagnoses based on too few benign-appearing cells. Consequently, we established criteria for adequacy of sampling designed to reduce sharply the potential for false-negative diagnoses.

First, we obtain at least six aspirates that appear promising on macroscopic inspection. If this requires 12 to 15 aspirates, so be it. We may retain and submit smears of specimens that seem too bloody or composed of degeneration fluid just in case they contain follicular cells too, but we do not count them. Also, multiple aspirates reduce the possibility of missing the portion of a pleomorphic nodule most likely to contain malignant cells.

To exclude carcinoma, we now require at least six clusters of benign epithelium on each of at least two of the six smears. Of course, malignant cells must not be present. The physician in charge of management decisions should relate the cellular content of the samples to the size of the nodule sampled. To do this, the physician must know how many clusters of cells were present on each of the slides studied. This information should be provided by the cytopathologist. The common practice of offering only a diagnosis with no description of the cellular content is an inadequate performance. When the nodule is only 1 cm and the cellular content just meets the criterion of six clusters on each of two slides, that should be enough. When the nodule is 3 cm or larger, more than six aspirates should be taken, and more cellular material must be present. Otherwise, it is prudent to repeat the fine needle biopsy in the hope of obtaining more cells. Whenever

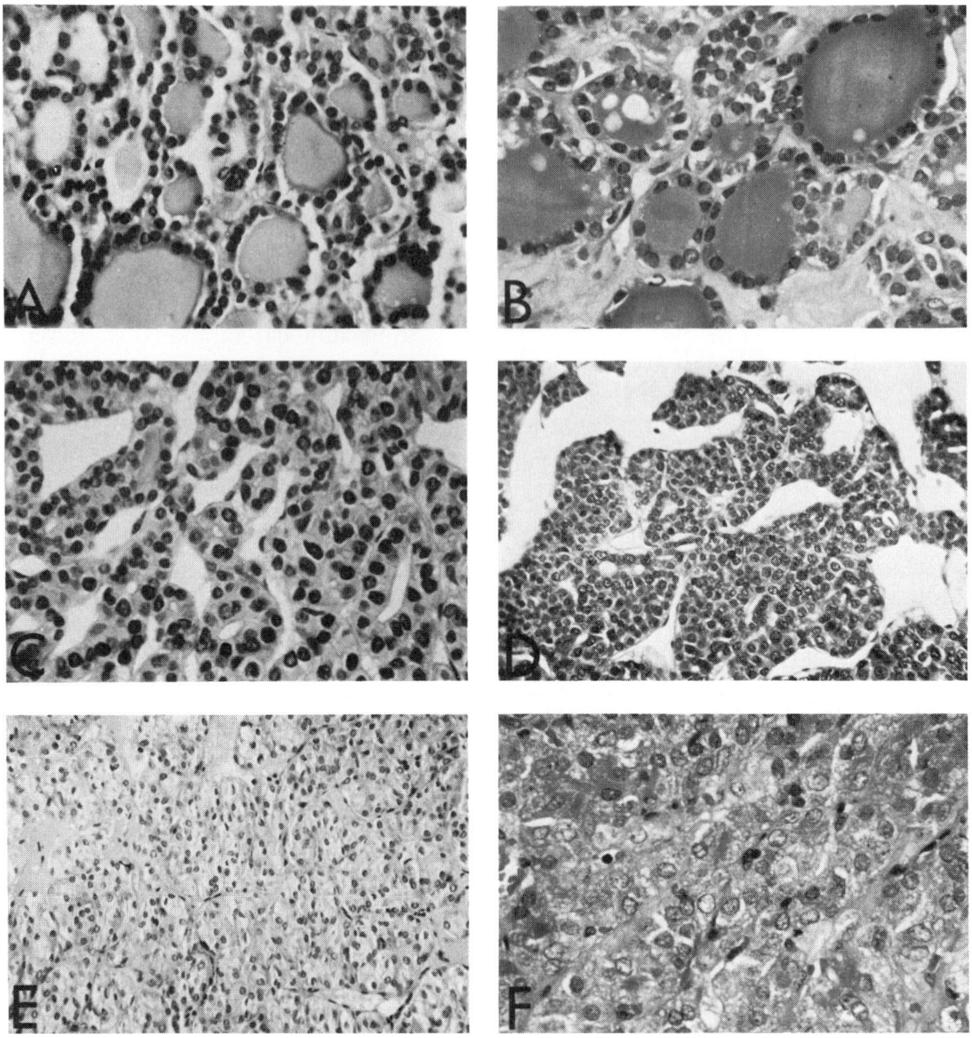


**FIGURE 10–6.** Comparison of large needle biopsy specimens with corresponding areas of the surgical specimen. *A*, The initial large needle biopsy (1981) showed a macrofollicular pattern. *B*, A section from the surgical specimen showing a similar histologic pattern. *C*, The second large needle biopsy (1985) showed a trabecular pattern. *D*, A section from the surgical specimen showing a similar histologic pattern. *E*, The third large needle biopsy (1986) showed a solid pattern with nuclear atypia interpreted as indicative of follicular carcinoma. *F*, A section from the surgical specimen showing a similar histologic pattern.

fine needle biopsy is repeated because of inadequate cellular material on the first biopsy, at least eight and often more aspirates are obtained, depending on the appearance of the samples. Benign cells on only one slide—even multiple clusters—is inadequate to exclude carcinoma.

Between 1985 and 1987, we prospectively evaluated criteria in 888 patients of whom 159 had surgery. The fine needle biopsy diagnoses made by our cytopathologist and the surgical findings, when available, are given in Table 10–1. Operation was performed for various reasons on 33 patients despite fine needle biopsy diagnoses of benign disease or Hashimoto's thyroiditis, and all of the lesions were benign. An additional nine patients whose fine needle biopsy diagnosis of benign disease was obtained before 1985 underwent another biopsy procedure and again had a fine needle biopsy diagnosis of benign disease. They also had benign nodules at operation. We are not so naive as to conclude from this favorable experience that our criteria will eliminate false-negative fine needle biopsy diagnoses. However, these results rep-

**TABLE 10–1. Fine Needle Biopsy Diagnosis Compared with Surgical Diagnoses (888 Patients Studied Between 1985 and 1987)**

| | | | | SURGICAL DIAGNOSIS | | | | |
|---|---|---|---|---|---|---|---|---|
| FINE NEEDLE BIOPSY DIAGNOSIS | NO. | PER CENT | NO. EXCISED | Benign | Papillary Carcinoma | Follicular Carcinoma | Hürthle Cell Carcinoma | Other Cancers |
| Benign* | 445 | 50 | 30 | 30 | — | — | — | — |
| Hashimoto's thyroiditis | 126 | 14 | 3 | 3 | — | — | — | — |
| Granulomatous thyroiditis | 4 | — | 0 | — | — | — | — | — |
| Cellular adenoma† | 38 | 4 | 25 | 22 | — | 3 | — | — |
| Hürthle cell adenoma | 19 | 2 | 10 | 9 | — | — | 1 | — |
| Suspected papillary carcinoma | 8 | 1 | 7 | 4 | 2 | 1 | — | — |
| Papillary carcinoma | 54 | 6 | 53 | 1 | 52 | — | — | — |
| Follicular carcinoma | 1 | — | 1 | — | 1 | — | — | — |
| Metastatic carcinoma to thyroid | 2 | — | 2 | — | — | — | — | 2 |
| Medullary carcinoma | 1 | — | 1 | — | — | — | — | 1 |
| Lymphoma | 2 | — | 2 | — | — | — | — | 2 |
| Inadequate | 136 | 15 | 15 | 10 | 4 | 1 | — | — |
| Acellular | 52 | 6 | 10 | 8 | — | — | — | 1‡ |
| Total | 888 | | 159 (18 per cent) | 87 | 59 | 5 | 1 | 6 |

*Includes nodular goiter and macrofollicular adenomas.
†Includes microfollicular and mixed microfollicular and macrofollicular adenomas.
‡C cell hyperplasia.

resent a great improvement over our initial experience in which 10 per cent of 89 patients with a fine needle biopsy diagnosis of benign disease who were nevertheless operated on had cancer.[61] Similarly, high rates of false-negative diagnoses have been reported by others on the basis of limited experience. Those experiences do not represent the best that fine needle biopsy can do, and they do not justify such conclusions as "only positive (for cancer) findings give real information, with negative reports leaving the matter unsettled."[27]

## *Cytologic Diagnoses*

To permit a relatively direct comparison of the accuracy of needle biopsy diagnoses with those we had made previously by clinical methods,[30] initially we categorized biopsy diagnoses into three groups that had management implications: probably malignant, possibly malignant, and benign.[59] For probably malignant lesions, curative surgery is usually attempted (except for metastatic carcinoma to the thyroid, some lymphomas, and many undifferentiated carcinomas). Nodules with diagnoses of benign disease are ordinarily observed. If possibly malignant nodules include only lesions with a low probability of low-grade cancer, operation may be advised for young healthy patients. However, for the older and infirm, observation may be preferable. A word of caution is in order. Others have employed categories that might appear to be similar to ours but in reality differ greatly. For example, the intermediate category called "suspicious" at the Mayo Clinic is different from our intermediate possibly malignant category. Nearly 25 per cent of their suspicious lesions were malignant, and some of the malignancies were high grade.[23] This discrepancy is not the result of any difference in the cytologic features observed but rather is a consequence of different philosophies on which the diagnostic categories were structured. At the Mayo Clinic, only lesions for which a diagnosis of carcinoma was certain were called malignant. Highly suspect lesions were assigned to the suspicious category. The investigators wanted to eliminate false-positive diagnoses of malignancy. Hence, they recommend routine surgery for patients with a fine needle biopsy diagnosis of malignant and for patients with a diagnosis of "suspicious." They could just as well have had only two categories: "operate" and "observe." Because the approach to the categorization of fine needle biopsy diagnosis has not been standardized, it is difficult to compare data from different institutions. Hence, it is preferable to report fine needle biopsy findings in terms of the specific cytologic diagnoses that experience permits (Table 10–1). Figures 10–7 and 10–8 show representative cytologic presentations for the principal nodular lesions of the thyroid.

## *Avoiding False-Negative Fine Needle Biopsy Diagnoses*

The commonest cause of false-negative fine needle biopsy diagnoses is inadequate sampling. Our strict criteria for adequacy of sampling have led to a 21 per cent rate of unsatisfactory fine needle biopsy evaluations (Table 10–1). For 28 per cent of these patients (6 per cent of the entire series), the specimens contained no thyroid follicular cells. However, 72 per cent of the specimens contained benign-appearing follicular cells on one or more of the slides but not enough to fulfill our criteria for adequacy. Other clinicians might make a diagnosis of benign disease on such samples, but this would lead to false-negative diagnoses. The importance of recognizing that these specimens were inadequate rather than indicative of benign disease was shown by a review of the surgical findings on 8 of these patients who had cancer (Table 10–2). Three cancers had inadequate numbers of benign-appearing cells on the initial fine needle biopsy, but a diagnosis of papillary carcinoma was readily made on a

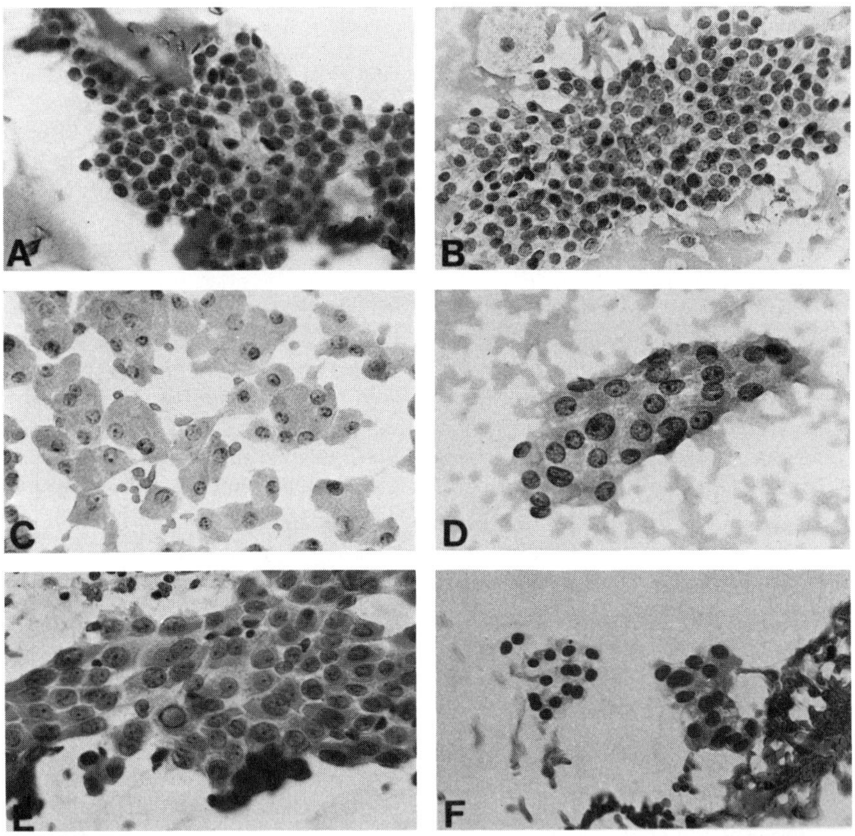


**FIGURE 10–7.** Representative fine needle biopsy specimens. *A*, Benign nodular goiter. Cells are uniform with smooth nuclear borders and finely granular nuclear chromatin. Regularly spaced nuclei without overlapping present a honeycomb appearance. *B*, Follicular adenoma. Nuclei, although relatively uniform, are slightly enlarged with overlapping. *C*, Hürthle cell tumor. Large polygonal cells with distinct cell borders, eccentric nuclei, and prominent nucleoli. *D*, Hürthle cell carcinoma. Cell borders are lacking, and nuclei are large and pleomorphic. *E*, Papillary carcinoma. A sheet of large nuclei with prominent nucleoli and a large clear intranuclear cytoplasmic inclusion. *F*, Follicular carcinoma. To the left are small benign-appearing nuclei and to the right are larger pleomorphic nuclei. (From Hamburger, J. I., Miller, J. M., and Kini, S. R.: Clinical-Pathological Diagnosis of Thyroid Nodules: Handbook and Atlas. Southfield, Michigan, private publication by Hamburger, J. I., 1979, with permission.)

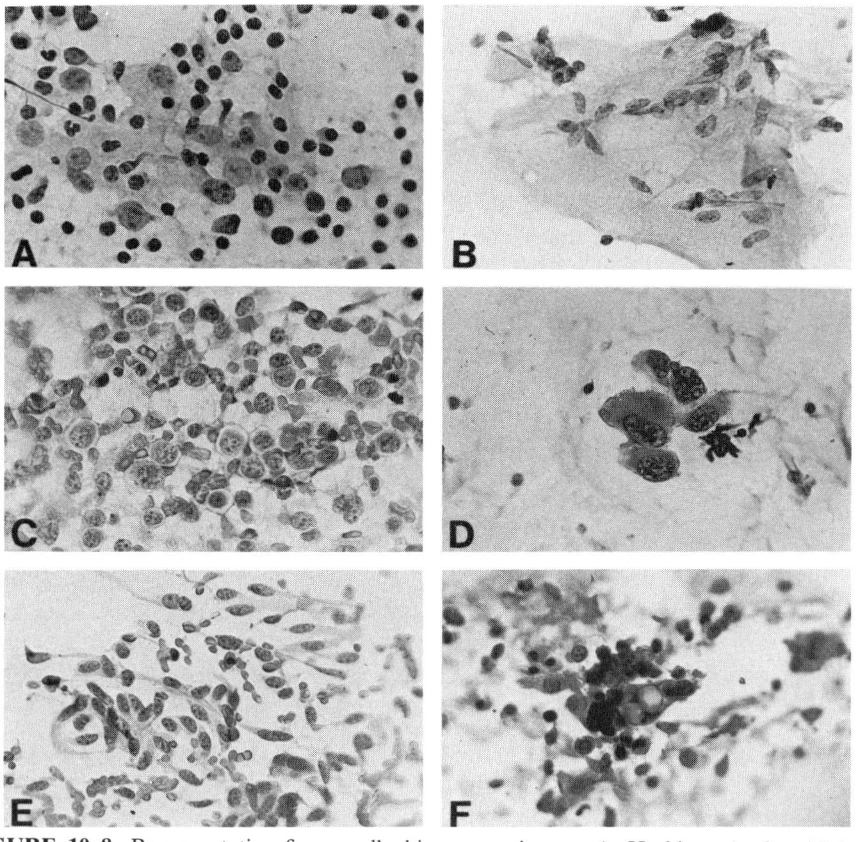


**FIGURE 10–8.** Representative fine needle biopsy specimens. *A*, Hashimoto's thyroiditis. A mixture of atypical follicular cells, lymphocytes, plasma cells, and transforming lymphocytes. *B*, Granulomatous thyroiditis. A multinucleated giant cell. *C*, Lymphoma of the thyroid. A monotonous pattern of large malignant cells with large nuclei, coarse chromatin, and prominent nucleoli. *D*, Undifferentiated carcinoma. Large noncoherent irregular cells with pleomorphic bizarre nuclei, clumped chromatin, and multiple nucleoli. *E*, Medullary carcinoma. A loose group of spindle-shaped cells with large oval hyperchromatic pleomorphic nuclei with prominent nucleoli. *F*, Metastatic colon carcinoma to the thyroid. A centrally located large carcinoma cell with large secretory vacuoles. (From Hamburger, J. I., Miller, J. M., and Kini, S. R.: Clinical-Pathological Diagnosis of Thyroid Nodules: Handbook and Atlas. Southfield, Michigan, private publication by Hamburger, J. I., 1979, with permission.)

second fine needle biopsy. Responsible use of fine needle biopsy data requires an appreciation that an inadequate biopsy has the same management implications as if no biopsy were done.

Recognizing lymphoma of the thyroid in the presence of Hashimoto's thyroiditis may present difficulties. Although lymphoma usually occurs in a background of Hashimoto's thyroiditis, Hashimoto's thyroiditis is much more common. Hence, cytopathologists must beware of making the "obvious" diagnosis of Hashimoto's thyroiditis rather than the unusual diagnosis of lymphoma. Indeed, an alert cytopathologist will search for features of lymphoma routinely whenever fine needle biopsy findings are compatible with Hashimoto's thyroiditis.[26, 39]

Recognition of the lymphomatous implications of a monomorphic cell population without epithelial cells and germinal centers should permit the diagnosis to be made or at least suspected with relative ease in most patients. The conditions of the two patients with lymphoma cited in Table 10–1 were diagnosed by fine needle biopsy without difficulty. The false-negative diagnoses made early in our experience were directly attributable to a failure to consider a diagnosis of lymphoma despite suggestive cytologic features. Because lymphoma of the thyroid seems to be on the increase,[26, 39, 43] an in-

**TABLE 10–2. Findings on Eight Patients with Malignant Nodules Who Had Fine Needle Biopsy Specimens with Inadequate Cells for Diagnosis**

| | | FINE NEEDLE BIOPSY 1 | | FINE NEEDLE BIOPSY 2 | | |
|---|---|---|---|---|---|---|
| CASE Age/Sex | NODULE Size, cm | No. Aspirations | No. Clusters | No. Aspirations | No. Clusters | SURGICAL DIAGNOSIS |
| 1 60/M | 1.25 | 6 | 1 Slide, 6 Microfollicular | — | — | Papillary carcinoma, follicular variant |
| 2 42/F | 0.75 | 6 | 2 Slides, 2 | — | — | Papillary carcinoma |
| 3 39/F | 4.0 | 6 | Acellular | 8 | 1 Slide, 6 3 Slides, few isolated cells | Follicular carcinoma |
| 4 36/F | 3.0 | 6 | 1 Slide, 1 | 6 | Acellular | Papillary carcinoma, follicular variant |
| 5 43/F | 4.0 | 6 | 1 Slide, 6 2 Slides, 3 | 10 | 1 Slide, 4 | Papillary carcinoma |
| 6 23/F | 1.5 | 8 | 1 Slide, 2 1 Slide, 1 | 10 | Papillary carcinoma | Papillary carcinoma |
| 7 36/F | 0.5 | 10 | Acellular | 8 | Papillary carcinoma | Papillary carcinoma |
| 8 49/F | 1.0 | 6 | Acellular | 8 | Papillary carcinoma | Papillary carcinoma |

creased level of suspicion is important. Clinical findings that suggest lymphoma, in addition to evidence of Hashimoto's thyroiditis, include an enlarging nodule or goiter, especially if painful and associated with hoarseness and decreased function on imaging.[39] Enlargement despite treatment with thyroid hormone is particularly ominous.[39]

The major continuing problem that needle biopsy cannot fully address is the exclusion of carcinoma in follicular neoplasms. Most follicular neoplasms, especially the macrofollicular lesions, are benign. Malignant follicular lesions are sometimes easily identified by fine needle biopsy.[50] Willems and Löwhagen[89] observed an increased nuclear size in cells from follicular carcinomas, a finding that Kini et al.[50] utilize in assessment of the probabilities that follicular neoplasms are malignant. The usual fine needle biopsy pattern is that of a mixed microfollicular and macrofollicular tumor for which the possibility of carcinoma cannot be excluded for two reasons. First, follicular carcinomas are often highly pleomorphic. Much of the tissue may be indistinguishable microscopically from normal thyroid tissue. Only the identification of capsular or vascular invasion reveals the malignant process, and these features are not available for evaluation by fine needle biopsy or even by large needle biopsy in most instances. Second, we must consider the less obvious issue of the future behavior of a follicular neoplasm that, if excised, might not show evidence of carcinoma even on serial section. Can we safely conclude that such a neoplasm would not have become malignant if left in situ for the life of the patient? Suen and Quenville[79] cite three references from older literature that support their idea that occasional adenomas can evolve into carcinomas. Lo Gerfo et al.[56] believe that follicular carcinomas are malignant from their onset, although they acknowledge that the concept is difficult to prove. Actually, that statement begs the question. Even when follicular carcinomas are malignant from their onset, it is possible that they do not exhibit the cytologic and histologic features that pathologists recognize as indicative of malignancy until they reach a critical level of maturity.

The risk of false-negative diagnoses is inherent in any method of evaluation of thyroid nodules that leaves most nodules in situ for observation. Nevertheless, selective surgery for patients with thyroid nodules is the prevailing treatment. No responsible voice is calling for excision of all these lesions. Therefore, concern for false-negative fine needle biopsy diagnoses really means concern that the reduction in surgery that fine needle biopsy permits might lead to a corresponding decrease in the number of carcinomas that are detected compared with the cancer yield when nodules are selected for surgery by conventional clinical methods.

In our hands, the improved specificity and sensitivity of fine needle biopsy over conventional methods were readily demonstrated.[38, 59] Our results were compared with those from a number of other centers[5, 6, 11, 18, 23, 28, 30, 38, 66, 68, 76, 79, 86] to see what proportion of patients studied had cancer detected and to determine whether the number of cancers detected was related to the proportion of patients operated on (Table 10–3). As standards for comparison, we provide our current data (from Table 10–1) and our data on 1,094 patients studied before we used needle biopsy when selection for operation was based on conventional clinical methods.[30] With the exception of one report with a low prevalence of carcinoma and another with an unusually high prevalence (18 per cent), both of which were from relatively small series (and will be disregarded in the further analysis), the concentration of values within the narrow range of 7 to 12 per cent is striking. These figures are remarkably similar to the 12 per cent prevalence of carcinoma in our series of patients evaluated clinically, especially when it is appreciated that about 10 per cent of those carcinomas were microscopic lesions that are excluded from consideration in the evaluation of the results of fine needle biopsy. (Obviously they would not have undergone biopsy.) Physicians who operated on many of their patients, 41 to 60 per cent, detected carcinoma in 10 per cent of the 979 patients evaluated. Physicians who operated on only 15 to 28 per cent of their patients detected carcinoma in 9 per cent of the 4,827 patients evaluated. By chi square analysis, this small difference is statistically significant ($p < 0.01$), assuming the populations studied were comparable. However, an even greater difference in the detection of carcinoma is seen between our 1979 report (11 per cent) and our current series studied between 1985 and 1987 (8 per cent). We attribute this difference to the lesser selectivity of referrals we currently receive because the physician community has become increasingly aware of the availability of fine needle biopsy and is convinced of its value and prudence. This conclusion is consistent with the observation that a lower rate of carcinoma is seen in reports with the largest numbers of patients (Table 10–3). Also, in the centers operating on a high percentage of patients, only 21 per cent of the patients had carcinoma whereas in centers where surgery was more selective, 42 per cent of patients operated on had carcinoma.

This analysis provides limited assurance that the more selective surgery permitted by greater experience with fine needle biopsy is not likely to be unacceptably costly in terms of overlooked carcinomas. Less selective surgery negates the principal value of fine needle

**TABLE 10–3. Cancer Yield in Thyroid Nodules Studied by Fine Needle Biopsy**

| | | | EXCISED | | MALIGNANT | | PER CENT MALIGNANCY IN SURGICAL SPECIMENS |
|---|---|---|---|---|---|---|---|
| AUTHOR | YEAR | NO. CASES | No. | Per Cent | No. | Per Cent* | |
| Hamburger[30] | 1978 | 1,094 | 582 | 53 | 128 | 12 | 22† |
| Walfish et al.[86] | 1977 | 150 | 90 | 60 | 17 | 11 | 19 |
| Esselstyn and Crile[18] | 1978 | 460 | 67 | 15 | 31‡ | 7 | 46 |
| Hamburger et al.[38] | 1979 | 1,023 | 286 | 28 | 116 | 11 | 41 |
| Collacchio et al.[11] | 1980 | 300 | 80 | 27 | 23 | 8 | 29 |
| Norton et al.[66] | 1982 | 102 | 21 | 21 | 10 | 10 | 48 |
| Suen and Quenville[79] | 1983 | 304 | 79 | 26 | 37 | 12 | 47 |
| Hamaker et al.[28] | 1983 | 116 | 41 | 35 | 21 | 18 | 51 |
| Gharib et al.[23] | 1984 | 1,970 | 364 | 18 | 158 | 9 | 43 |
| Ramacciotti et al.[68] | 1984 | 221 | 126 | 57 | 25 | 11 | 20 |
| Brauer and Silver[6] | 1984 | 224 | 134 | 60 | 26 | 12 | 19 |
| Boey et al.[5] | 1984 | 384 | 157 | 41 | 37 | 10 | 24 |
| Silverman et al.[76] | 1986 | 309 | 60 | 19 | 8 | 3 | 13 |
| Hamburger (Table 1) | 1987 | 888 | 159 | 18 | 71 | 8 | 45 |

*Percentage of the total number evaluated for which carcinoma was detected.

†These patients selected for operation by clinical methods before the use of fine needle biopsy.

‡Includes 9 patients with carcinomas that were not excised (1 follicular carcinoma, 2 metastatic carcinomas to the thyroid, 2 lymphomas, and 4 undifferentiated carcinomas).

biopsy, that is, avoidance of unecessary surgery, without a corresponding benefit in cancer detection and elimination. Although fine needle biopsy clearly has the potential for eliminating much unnecessary surgery, obviously it is less decisive than routine surgery in the detection of all carcinomas. Patients who are observed on the basis of fine needle biopsy diagnoses of benign disease should be apprised of the small risk of a false-negative diagnosis so that informed consent for medical management is obtained. Those who prefer the greater diagnostic certainty that excision permits and are willing to accept the costs and risks of operation provide us with an ongoing control of the risk of false-negative fine needle biopsy diagnoses.

## *Avoiding False-Positive Errors*

With experience, false-positive diagnoses become less frequent. Table 10–1 shows that only five of 66 patients (8 per cent) operated on after fine needle biopsy diagnoses of suspected or definite carcinomas had benign disease. Three of the five had atypical adenomas. Only one false-positive fine needle biopsy diagnosis was recorded in 59 patients operated on who had fine needle biopsy diagnoses of definite carcinoma. However, 31 of 35 patients (84 per cent) operated on because of fine needle biopsy diagnoses of cellular or Hürthle cell adenomas had benign disease. From a practical standpoint, these too were false-positive diagnoses, that is, operation was advised for possible carcinoma when the lesions were benign. If these patients are included, 36 of 101 patients (36 per cent) operated on for a fine needle biopsy diagnosis of carcinoma or suspected carcinoma or for a fine needle biopsy diagnosis that could not exclude carcinoma had a false-positive fine needle biopsy diagnosis. To ensure that carcinomas will not be missed, these false-positive diagnoses are unavoidable. This will not be discouraging for clinicians because they are used to making false-positive diagnoses on thyroid nodules. Before fine needle biopsy was employed for the diagnosis of thyroid nodules, about 75 per cent of the patients operated on for possible thyroid carcinoma had benign lesions.[30] Therefore, the false-positive rate of 36 per cent that fine needle biopsy permits represents an important reduction in this unnecessary surgery.[59]

Nevertheless, certain elementary errors can be avoided. Benign papillary fronds or inspissated colloid seen in nodular goiter only superficially resemble papillations or psammoma bodies of papillary carcinoma.[61] The Hürthle cell change of Hashimoto's thyroiditis or nodular goiter usually can be differentiated from the Hürthle cells of Hürthle cell neoplasms.[48] Spindle-shaped stromal cells should not be confused with spindle cells of undifferentiated carcinoma.[61] Finally, the atypical follicular cells common in Hashimoto's thyroiditis should not be considered suggestive of follicular carcinoma, a tumor rarely encountered in association with Hashimoto's thyroiditis.[47]

## *Follow-up of Patients with Fine Needle Biopsy Diagnosis of Benign Disease*

A fine needle biopsy diagnosis of benign disease is not a guarantee that carcinoma is not present. With reasonable experience, fine needle biopsy diagnoses of benign disease can achieve better than 95 per cent reliability for the exclusion of carcinoma. However, 100 per cent accuracy is not going to be possible with present technology. Hence, these patients require lifelong follow-up. Thyroid hormone may produce some regression in the nodules. When regression happens it is reassuring, but most of the time the response to this treatment is not substantial.[68]

In considering what should be done, some advise routine surgery.[3, 68] This course seems too aggressive to us because few nodules diagnosed with fine needle biopsy as benign turn out to be malignant. Furthermore, in accord with this advice, 50 per cent of the patients of Ramacciotti et al.[68] had surgery. This is the same proportion that we operated on before we used needle biopsy when selection for operation was made on the basis of clinical evaluation.[30] Now, only 18 per cent of our patients have surgery. Less than 25 per cent of the nodules Ramacciotti's group excised were malignant, the same prevalence of malignancy we reported before using needle biopsy.[30] They had 9 per cent false-negative diagnoses. This high figure suggests inadequate sampling. Also, the fine needle biopsy technique might have been suboptimal because 12 physicians shared in the 28 fine needle biopsies performed annually, thus diluting the experience.

We[34] and others[29] have advised a repeat fine needle biopsy after 1 to 2 years for nodules that do not regress during treatment with thyroxine. Fine needle biopsy might be performed even sooner for the infrequent occurrence of a nodule that enlarges despite administration of thyroxine therapy. A review of the records of 198 patients who had repeat fine needle biopsy after earlier diagnoses of benign disease (before we had rigidly applied our current criteria for adequacy) revealed a 3 per cent incidence of findings indicative of carcinoma.[34] As of this writing, all patients who have had surgery despite two fine needle biopsy diagnoses of benign disease have had benign nodules. Assuming that second fine needle biopsies, performed after initial fine needle biopsy diagnoses of benign disease, produce a small yield of cancers, would third, fourth, and more fine needle biopsies continue to be productive? No cancers have as yet been detected in a limited number of patients who have had three fine needle biopsies, and so it seems unlikely that more than two fine needle biopsy procedures will be cost-effective routinely. It might be preferable to limit additional fine needle biopsies to nodules that are enlarging or exhibit some other suspicious alteration in their physical characteristics.

## *Use of Fine Needle Biopsy Data for Surgical Planning*

Fine needle biopsy is usually thought of as a procedure to select patients with thyroid nodules for operation or observation. However, when the decision to operate is made, the surgeon must determine the procedure. Before the advent of fine needle biopsy, conventional surgical practice commonly was to inform the patient as follows: The operation is for possible cancer. The initial procedure will be a lobectomy-isthmectomy. A frozen section will be performed on the lesion. If a diagnosis of malignancy is confirmed, the operation will be extended to total or near total thyroidectomy (unless the lesion is a minimal cancer).[68] Unfortunately, this strategy was frequently frustrated by frozen section findings that were useless or misleading. For many patients, the surgical pathologist defers the diagnosis until after study of permanent sections. For others, false-negative frozen section diagnoses are made. False-positive diagnoses are made less often. As a result, some patients are faced with the unpleasant prospect of undergoing a second surgical procedure when a delayed diagnosis of carcinoma is made, while others have been subjected inappropriately to the additional risks of cancer operations when lesions were benign.

Such experiences suggested to us that fine needle biopsy data might be used for surgical planning as well as for surgical selection. After all, the data were available because all of our patients having surgery for thyroid nodules have preoperative fine needle biopsy diagnoses. The question that had to be answered was whether fine needle biopsy data could be as reliable, or preferably more reliable, than frozen section data. If this were the case, three benefits might accrue. First, the patient could be informed preoperatively of the extent of the operation to be performed rather than finding out after the fact.[74] Second, the frozen section procedure could be eliminated, saving pathology charges and reducing the duration of the operation as well. Finally, the knowledge that a thyroid carcinoma is being treated permits both patient and attending physician to select a surgeon skilled in dealing with that disease.

With these considerations in mind, we compared the reliability of fine needle biopsy diagnoses with those of frozen section in predicting the final diagnoses on permanent sections from surgical specimens for 359 patients.[35] Overall, fine needle biopsy diagnoses were more reliable than frozen section diagnoses, especially for malignant lesions, a finding with which others concur.[25, 69, 76] In fairness, it must be acknowledged that the fine needle biopsy diagnoses were made by cytopathologists with special interest and expertise in thyroid cytopathology, while the frozen section diagnoses were made by surgical pathologists in various hospitals, most of whom had no special training in thyroid disease. False-positive diagnoses of carcinoma were more common by fine needle biopsy; false-negative diagnoses were more frequent by frozen section. Surgical pathologists try hard to avoid false-positive frozen section diagnoses that can lead to unnecessary cancer surgery, but false-negative frozen section diagnoses only delay a needed cancer operation by a few days.

The most difficult problem involving fine needle biopsy was the differentiation of benign from malignant follicular or Hürthle cell tumors when suspicious cytologic features were observed. Frozen section was equally unreliable.[35] For these patients, surgical planning must be based on advance discussion between surgeon and patient of the advantages and disadvantages of a primary cancer operation as opposed to a limited primary operation that may have to be followed by a second surgical procedure if the lesion is malignant.

For lower risk lesions, that is, fine needle biopsy diagnoses of benign disease or Hürthle cell or follicular lesions without features of malignancy, surgery limited to a diagnostic lobectomy (with or without the isthmus) would have been adequate for at least 90 per cent of patients. Altering that plan on the basis of frozen section findings would not have been beneficial. Four of eight frozen section diagnoses of carcinoma were erroneous, six carcinomas were called benign, and for five carcinomas, the frozen section diagnosis was deferred.[35]

Surgical plans based on fine needle biopsy diagnoses suggesting probably malignant lesions would have led to appropriate surgery in 135 of 144 patients (94 per cent). Reliance on frozen section would have been substantially less efficient. Reported were 18 false-negative diagnoses, two false-positive diagnoses, and 23 deferred diagnoses on cancers.[35] The only clear-cut indications for frozen section were to investigate enlarged lymph nodes in patients with low-risk lesions and to diagnose nodules discovered at operation that had not been found preoperatively. Bugis et al.[7] found more favorable results with frozen section. Fine needle biopsy detected only 43 per cent of cancers in their study compared with 64 per cent by frozen section, no false-positive frozen section diagnoses but 5 per cent by fine needle biopsy, and 8.5 per cent false-negative diagnoses by fine needle biopsy compared with 5 per cent by frozen section. Because they studied only 198 patients with fine needle biopsy, we are confident that after they have more experience with fine needle biopsy their findings will more closely resemble ours, in which 81 per cent of cancers were diagnosed as definitely malignant by fine needle biopsy with no (or perhaps few) false-negative diagnoses (Table 10–1).

## *How Difficult Is It to Acquire Expertise in Fine Needle Biopsy Cytopathology?*

We still receive feedback from physicians in the United States and abroad who want to use fine needle biopsy but fear that their cytopathologists might not provide reliable diagnoses. Naturally, we, too, had this concern when we first studied the procedure in 1976. Little in the way of didactic or illustrative material was available to assist physicians and cytopathologists to learn how to perform the biopsies and how to interpret them. However, since 1979 considerable instructive material has been published,[38, 46–50, 61] with a corresponding increase in the number of active thyroid biopsy teams. We believe that any qualified and interested cytopathologist can do this work well after studying the literature and initially obtaining consultation on problem cases. The volume of specimens should be adequate, say five per week, to permit the acquisition of reasonable experience and confidence in the diagnoses.

The surgical specimens should be studied when lesions are excised to ensure quality control. Our practice is to have the patient sign a release for the pathology report at the time the biopsy is taken. When surgery is advised and we have not received the pathology report within 60 days, we contact the patient to find out whether surgery was performed and where. Then, we can obtain the pathology report and the slides if necessary. Only by this kind of regular self-assessment can the biopsy team develop the understanding that leads to confidence in making specific fine needle biopsy diagnoses. Also, those who are not obtaining reliable diagnoses can look into the reasons for their lack of success. False-negative and false-positive fine needle biopsy diagnoses should be reviewed to establish whether the specimens really contained an adequate number and type of cells and whether the error was in the interpretation or sampling.

We tested our hypothesis that skills in cytopathology diagnoses on thyroid nodules were transferable when in 1985 we began to utilize the cytopathologists at Sinai Hospital of Detroit rather than those at the Henry Ford Hospital. We anticipated that this change might have an unfavorable impact on the reliability of our fine needle biopsy diagnoses and that consultation would be needed by the Sinai Hospital cytopathologists for many patients initially. Neither of these concerns materialized. A comparison of fine needle biopsy diagnoses at Sinai Hospital with those made on the first 2,000 patients studied at Henry Ford Hospital[61] showed remarkable similarities. Diagnoses of benign disease were made on 67 per cent of the fine needle biopsy specimens evaluated at Henry Ford Hospital and on 64 per cent of those evaluated at Sinai Hospital (Table 10–1). Carcinomas were diagnosed for 11 per cent of the specimens evaluated at Henry Ford Hospital and for 8 per cent of the specimens evaluated at Sinai Hospital. However, results showed 19 per cent false-positive diagnoses at Henry Ford Hospital and only 8 per cent at Sinai Hospital. A 10 per cent incidence of false-negative fine needle biopsy diagnoses was encountered at Henry Ford Hospital. As of this writing, only one false-negative fine needle biopsy diagnosis has been identified in patients studied at Sinai Hospital (subsequent to the compilation of the data in Table 10–1). That diagnosis was a well-differentiated follicular carcinoma. However, the Sinai Hospital cytopathologists had the advantage of having reviewed the Henry Ford Hospital errors and the reasons for them, and thus avoided making the elementary false-negative diagnoses that the pioneering Henry Ford Hospital cytopathologists made while they were mastering the method but also no longer make. Thus, after careful study of the published Henry Ford Hospital experiences and guidelines, the Sinai Hospital cytopathologists were able to start making fine needle biopsy diagnoses with a higher level of accuracy than was possible for the Henry Ford Hospital cytopathologists during a similar stage in their experience. These findings served to confirm our belief that expertise in fine needle biopsy diagnosis is transferable given the willingness and determination to acquire the skill.

## *Does Fine Needle Biopsy Eliminate the Need for Thyroid Images (Scans)?*

This question relates to a matter of great current concern. As the cost of medical care escalates, physicians must look critically at procedures, diagnostic and therapeutic, to make sure that the benefits justify the costs. Some physicians believe that an initial fine needle biopsy will obviate the need for most thyroid images.[7, 13, 84] We must ask what is lost for the sake of what might be gained? The element that is lost is an appreciation of the overall anatomy of the thyroid gland that may be more comprehensive than that obtainable by palpation alone. The value of this information is inversely related to the physician's examination skills. The diagnosis of a nontoxic autonomous nodule will surely be missed. This may be less important when the fine needle biopsy diagnosis is benign disease. However, when the fine needle biopsy suggests a cellular or follicular adenoma, without imaging one might advise operation. An initial image showing an autonomous nodule would obviate the need for the fine needle biopsy and the operation. The situation could be salvaged by use of an image obtained after the fine needle biopsy. However, because about 15 per cent of fine needle biopsy diagnoses suggest macrofollicular, cellular, or microfollicular neoplasms, those patients would still require imaging studies. If 5 to 10 per cent of solitary nodules are autonomous,[32] at least that proportion of fine needle biopsies will be unnecessary.

When operation is performed for probable or possible carcinoma, is it useful to have an image before operation to define the location and extent of tumor involvement for comparison with postoperative imaging when radioiodine therapy might be useful? For whatever portion of those patients the answer is yes, preoperative imaging will still be needed.

When the fine needle biopsy diagnosis is benign disease, is imaging indicated to rule out autonomous function before treatment with thyroxine? Is it adequate to give the treatment and reserve imaging for those who subsequently have clinical or laboratory evidence of overdosage? When the latter approach is taken, because the dose of thyroxine that can be tolerated without inducing elevated in vitro thyroid tests varies considerably, one would have to anticipate the necessity of imaging in a substantial proportion of patients treated with thyroxine. Otherwise, avoidable extra thyroid function tests also must be anticipated for patients who happen to have autonomously functioning nodules.

Thus, depending on attitudes of the responsible physicians and subsequent developments, the number of images avoided may be less than expected, and the price is a 5 to 10 per cent increase in fine needle biopsies. Because the cost of a fine needle biopsy (in our facility) is about 150 per cent of the cost of a thyroid image study, the savings of performing an immediate fine needle biopsy without imaging may be illusory.

Nevertheless, immediate fine needle biopsy is a viable option that some day may be mandated as regulation of standards of medical care increases. We perform images before fine needle biopsy because we like to know what kind of nodule we are putting a needle into before the biopsy. Also, from the patient's perspective, imaging is a less intimidating procedure than fine needle biopsy, so we are happy to spare them the fine needle biopsy whenever possible.

## MANAGEMENT OF THE CYSTIC THYROID NODULE

Most thyroid cysts are degenerated preexisting nodules. In 1918, Goetsch[24] showed that the blood vessels penetrating to the interior of thyroid nodules are thin walled and lack connective tissue support. Consequently, they are prone to rupture and produce central hemorrhagic degeneration. Capsular blood supply is richer and more viable so that a rind of preserved parenchyma surrounding a central cystic cavity is commonly found. The thin-walled, purely cystic lesion is much less common. Hemorrhagic degeneration is usually silent and slowly progressive. However, on occasion, hemorrhage is sudden in onset. Patients commonly report lumps that "popped out" overnight. These lesions are usually painless unless tension on the capsule is considerable. Pain and tenderness can be relieved promptly by aspiration. Autonomously functioning nodules are especially prone to central hemorrhagic degeneration. When the process is acute, the attendant follicular disruption may discharge thyroid hormone stores into the circulation, causing transient and spontaneously resolving hyperthyroidism.[36]

Clark,[9] reviewing the literature, reported that thyroid nodules are cystic 6 to 25 per cent of the time. This broad range probably reflects differences in definition rather than in the prevalence of cystic nodules. When the diagnosis is limited to lesions that are entirely cystic or nearly so, the lower figure would be applicable. When nodules with any degree of cystic degeneration are included—even those that are predominantly solid—the higher figure would be obtained. In a systematic examination of 341 specimens from patients operated on for thyroid nodules, 35 per cent of the nodules had fluid-filled cavities larger than 1 cm.[40] Of course, most of these nodules had a solid component, and many were predominantly solid lesions.

Predominantly cystic nodules may be recognized by physical examination because they are round, smooth, and feel tense or resilient on palpation. Echography and needle biopsy have greatly enhanced the ability to identify cystic thyroid nodules without operation. B-mode echography is not uniformly reliable. In one report[40] in which all lesions were excised, 32 per cent false-positive diagnoses of cysts and 29 per cent false-negative diagnoses were obtained. Ultrasonographers may do better with newer instruments, but is the information worth the effort? Fine needle biopsy reliably distinguishes between cystic and solid nodules and will be performed in either case. In cystic lesions, aspiration is carried out to provide fluid for cytology and, probably more important, to try to eliminate the lesions. For solid nodules, fine needle biopsy is performed for diagnosis. Because fine needle biopsy would be performed regardless of whether the echographic diagnosis is cystic or solid and because fine needle biopsy will reliably (perhaps more reliably) differentiate between cysts, partially cystic lesions, and solid lesions, echography would seem to be redundant and not cost-effective.[1, 25]

Early reports suggested that cystic lesions are benign. Blum[4] said that the chance of carcinoma occurring in a thyroid cyst is no greater than the chance of an occult carcinoma occurring elsewhere in the thyroid. Concern for the large amount of unnecessary surgery that was being performed for benign thyroid nodules prompted Crile[12] and Miller et al.[62] to treat patients with cystic lesions by aspiration. Success in 69 to 94 per cent of patients was claimed after one or two aspirations.[10, 12, 62] Others[60] have reported failures in up to 60 per cent of patients, especially in those having larger cysts. Consequently, injection of a sclerosing solution was suggested for recalcitrant cystic lesions. Kessler et al.[45] remind us that the instillation of tincture of iodine was effective in 1861. Recently, sodium tetradecyl[80] or tetracycline[82] has been used. Ryan[72] thought that tetracycline might be safer because sodium tetradecyl may cause pain and sloughing of the tissue if the solution extravasates. However, he[73] soon found that tetracycline can cause local pain severe enough to require morphine or meperidine for relief. He suggested that this complication might be avoided by only partly evacuating the cyst and then instilling a mixture of lidocaine and tetracycline. In response, Treece[81] reported that one of his patients also experienced severe pain, and in another patient vocal cord paralysis developed 22 months after administration of tetracycline. Exploration of the neck revealed fibrosis involving the recurrent laryngeal nerve adjacent to the nodule that had been injected. This report, following a number of treatment failures and several patients who complained of the pain's severity, led us to abandon the treatment in favor of excision for cysts that recur despite two or three aspirations. Surgery often may be performed under regional block anesthesia with low risk and minimal morbidity.

Our attitude reflects observations that thyroid cysts are not uniformly benign.[64, 70] The uncommon purely cystic thin-walled lesion that responds best to needle aspiration is almost never malignant. However, in one careful study,[40] the frequency of cystic degeneration was no different in benign or malignant nodules. Carcinoma was found in 23 and 32 per cent of cystic nodules excised principally because of failure to respond to needle aspiration[60, 70] and in some patients because examination of the cyst fluid suggested carcinoma.[70] To be sure, those were selected patients from a population depleted of the benign lesions that responded to aspiration. The prevalence of carcinoma in cystic thyroid lesions overall is much less. Unfortunately, most of the time examination of cyst fluid reveals no thyroid follicular epithelia whether the lesion is benign or malignant.[62] Although examination of cyst fluid for malignant cells is probably not cost-effective, it may be prudent from the medicolegal standpoint because of the occasional positive findings.

Lo Gerfo and Ting[54] advocated biopsy of the cyst wall using the TruCut needle. Although they obtained specimens on all 25 lesions, carcinoma was not evident. Probably this technique would produce a useful specimen in a degenerated carcinoma. Nevertheless, because a substantial proportion of carcinomas in cysts are isolated foci in the cyst wall, false-negative large needle biopsies must be anticipated. Also, as Lo Gerfo and Ting[54] observed, the procedure carries a risk of serious complications. It is simpler and safer to perform fine needle biopsy on any palpable solid residual mass after aspiration of the cyst. Success with fine needle biopsy in these circumstances, however, may not be achieved more than 50 per cent of the time,[70] and one must be careful about conclusions on specimens with inadequate numbers of cells. Whether fine needle biopsy with ultrasound guidance will improve results is unknown. Further study of this technique may be appropriate in centers with expertise in fine needle biopsy and echography and also with an ample supply of patients.

## MANAGEMENT OF NODULES IN IRRADIATED PATIENTS

By now, it is widely known that patients who have been exposed to therapeutic external beam radiation for conditions in the upper body have an increased risk for the subsequent development of thyroid carcinoma. Usually these tumors have been detected 10 to 20 years after the radiation exposure. Both malignant and benign thyroid tumors are more common in these irradiated persons. A high proportion of the carcinomas are low-risk occult papillary carcinomas or microcancers[16] often remote from the lesion for which operation was performed.[83] Also, for any given nodule, the probability of carcinoma occurring may be no different whether radiation had been given or not.[16, 37] In 1981, we[37] reported a comparison of the prevalence of carcinoma in surgical specimens from nonirradiated and irradiated patients. We operated on 25 per cent of nodules in nonirradiated patients and found carcinoma in 37 per cent. In irradiated patients, we operated on a higher proportion, 40 per cent—no doubt influenced by the histories of radiation therapy to take a more aggressive stance. However, this aggressiveness was rewarded with a correspondingly reduced cancer yield of only 27 per cent.

Nevertheless, some physicians[4, 68] still give more weight to a history of radiation than to a fine needle biopsy diagnosis of benign disease when advising treatment for patients with thyroid nodules. Some believe that virtually all such nodules should be excised. Because the incidence of carcinoma in irradiated nodules has been low in most reports,[16, 83] we agree with those who evaluate nodules in irradiated patients exactly as they would nodules in all other patients. We operate when fine needle biopsy findings are slightly or very indicative of carcinoma. If benign diagnoses are obtained, we treat with thyroid hormone (barring contraindication) and observe. Failure of the nodules to regress while the patient is taking thyroxine is an indication for repeat fine needle biopsy.[34] When the findings are still benign, we continue to observe. When the findings are more suspicious or the nodule undergoes otherwise unexplained enlargement during thyroxine therapy, we advise surgery. However, few of our patients with fine needle biopsy findings of benign disease have experienced these changes. Hence, we are content with an attitude of conservatism.

## USING NEEDLE BIOPSY DATA IN PATIENT MANAGEMENT

Needle biopsy diagnosis of thyroid nodules has been championed by internists whose primary concern was to reduce unnecessary thyroid surgery. In this endeavor, the primary role of needle biopsy is not to identify high-risk lesions that require excision but to identify low-risk lesions that may safely be left in situ for the remainder of the patient's anticipated life expectancy. Physicians who use and advocate needle biopsy are less concerned about false-positive diagnoses. No current method of evaluating a thyroid nodule with high sensitivity for detection of thyroid carcinoma is free of the risk of false-positive diagnoses. However, when nodules are selectively excised, that risk is much less with needle biopsy than without it.[59] Physicians are more concerned about false-negative diagnoses. That risk is small for most thyroid carcinomas if adequate samples are obtained. Clinical judgment is important in establishing a strategy that will minimize the risk to the patient of false-negative fine needle biopsy diagnoses. This strategy must be founded on an appreciation of the limitations of fine needle biopsy and, indeed, the limitations of our knowledge about the long-term biologic behavior of thyroid neoplasms, benign and malignant.

If clinical judgment is important to the proper use of fine needle biopsy in the management of patients with thyroid nodules, under what circumstances should surgery be advised despite a fine needle biopsy diagnosis of benign disease? We do not like large nodules—for example, more than 3 cm—especially if they are hard and irregular and especially in patients in the 50s and 60s. Even multiple fine needle biopsy samples cannot be expected to exclude follicular carcinoma. Nodules this large almost never respond to thyroxine, and thyroxine may be poorly tolerated in older patients because thyroid function is often incompletely suppressible. Also, in older patients, thyroid carcinoma may become more aggressive, occasionally seeming to convert from a sluggish differentiated to an aggressive undifferentiated lesion.[2] If fine needle biopsy shows a follicular neoplasm with no evidence of obvious carcinoma, if it is a carcinoma, it will probably be a low-grade lesion for which lobectomy may provide a cure. The risk of a lobectomy (assuming the patient has no important medical problem) should be low, and we advise it.

We share the concern of Lo Gerfo et al.[55] for nodules that enlarge despite treatment with thyroxine. However, we do not agree that all such lesions should be excised. Most of these nodules are not malignant. Nodules enlarge most commonly because of central hemorrhage. With needle aspiration, the diagnosis can be made and the swelling will regress. Nodules also may enlarge because of autonomous function. Some physicians perform fine needle biopsy without imaging[84] and may not realize that a nodule is functioning autonomously. Also, a preliminary image that shows reduced nodule function may not preclude the subsequent demonstration of autonomous function. A case in point is a 28-year-old woman who had a 3-cm nodule in the left lobe of the thyroid. Imaging (Fig. 10–9*A*) showed irregularly reduced tracer uptake in the nodule. The fine needle biopsy diagnosis was benign nodular goiter. She was treated with levothyroxine, 0.1 mg daily. Three months later, she had mild symptoms of hyperthyroidism. The nodule had enlarged to 3.5 cm. The level of serum free thyroxine was elevated at 2.5 ng/dl (normal range, 0.6 to 2.2). Suppression imaging[31] while the patient continued taking thyroxine (Fig. 10–9*B*) showed localized zones of increased tracer uptake in the nodule with less uptake than previously noted in the contralateral (right) lobe. This was an autonomous nodule that had undergone partial hemorrhagic degeneration. Recovering autonomous function led to the induction of mild hyperthyroidism because of the summation effects of endogenous and exogenous thyroid hormone.

Local swelling during thyroxine therapy may result from inflammatory disease, especially subacute thyroiditis. Pain and tenderness is characteristic, but sometimes the pain is minimal.

Of course, carcinoma is the most important differential diagnostic consideration. We believe that reliance can be placed on fine needle biopsy to clarify the diagnosis and to provide guidance as to the appropriate surgical procedure. When even limited findings of a follicular or Hürthle cell lesion are present or when fully adequate fine needle biopsy specimens are not obtained, we advise prompt surgery.

Finally, we are unhappy with discrete firm nodules larger than 2 cm in young persons that do not respond to thyroxine therapy and for which fine needle biopsy suggests findings of follicular adenoma, even macrofollicular adenoma. It is not that we expect the nodule to be malignant. Rather, we do not look forward to the prospect of watching such a lesion for 30 to 50 years, seeing the patient annually, and at each visit having to consider repeating the fine needle biopsy (perhaps every 3 to 5 years).[5, 29, 34] Also, the patient would have to be informed of the small risk of fine needle biopsy error and carry that low-level burden of concern for life. We believe that a frank and full discussion should be held with the patient of the risks and advantages of observation versus those of prompt lobectomy. After such a discussion, about half of our patients prefer the certainty and simplified follow-up that surgery permits.

## CRITICISMS OF FINE NEEDLE BIOPSY

Since our 1979 report,[59] numerous confirmatory studies have shown that fine needle biopsy improved on the accuracy of clinical diagnoses on patients with thyroid nodules, reducing the proportion undergoing unnec-

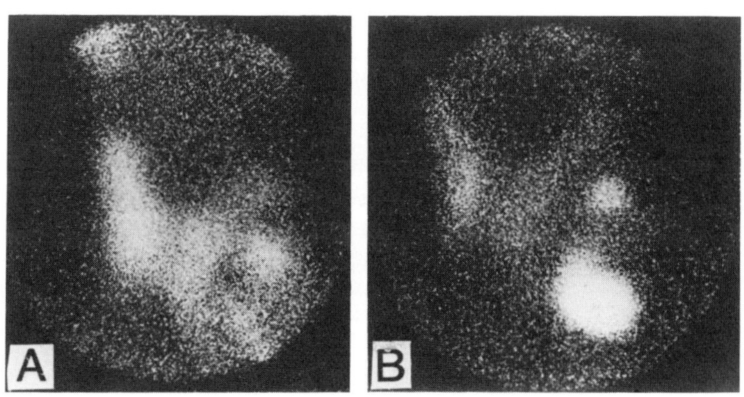


**FIGURE 10–9.** A degenerated autonomously functioning nodule presenting as a hypofunctional nodule. *A*, Imaging of the thyroid shows irregularly reduced activity in the left lobe nodule. *B*, A repeat image while the patient was taking levothyroxine (a suppression image) shows a relative increase in tracer uptake by the nodule compared with that by extranodular tissue.

essary surgery, while at the same time identified carcinomas that otherwise, at least initially, would have been overlooked. However, some opinions on fine needle biopsy are less favorable. Physicians from major academic centers have said that fine needle biopsy is inconclusive for the exclusion of carcinoma, that fine needle biopsy does not improve the prognosis for patients with thyroid nodules, and that large needle biopsy is more accurate than fine needle biopsy. We shall examine these criticisms on their own merits and from the perspective of our experience and that of others.

## *Is Fine Needle Biopsy Inconclusive for the Exclusion of Malignancy?*

Hajdu and Melamed[27] said that fine needle biopsy has a "very limited role in the definitive diagnosis of primary neoplasms of the thyroid, and a negative report certainly should not be conclusive." Although they agree that fine needle biopsy will confirm "clinically obvious cancer,"[77, 88] during the 1950s, "after some 30 years' experience with needle aspirates of the thyroid, this procedure was largely abandoned." They support their argument by citing a 27 per cent false-negative rate for fine needle biopsy in the series of follicular neoplasms reported by Lang et al.[52] However, those authors clearly stated that false-negative diagnoses were "almost always caused by insufficient material or puncture at the wrong site in the thyroid." It may be difficult to make definite diagnoses in many follicular carcinomas. Nevertheless, for most of them, experienced cytopathologists report fine needle biopsy impressions of follicular neoplasms, lesions for which malignancy cannot be excluded.[18, 50] The lesions are not called benign. A fine needle biopsy diagnosis of benign disease implies that operation is unnecessary. A fine needle biopsy diagnosis of follicular neoplasm, which of course does not exclude carcinoma, suggests that surgery might be preferable for young healthy patients while observation may be suitable for older and infirm patients. Although fine needle biopsy diagnoses of follicular neoplasm may correctly be called inconclusive, that does not mean that the information is useless. Furthermore, only about 6 per cent of our most recent patients (Table 10–1) had a diagnosis of cellular (follicular) neoplasms (including Hürthle cell but excluding macrofollicular nodules without features suspicious for malignancy).

Similarly misleading is their reading of the report of Kini et al.[47] in which three patients with lymphoma had a fine needle biopsy diagnosis of Hashimoto's thyroiditis. Kini et al.[47] clearly stated that these errors were caused by inexperience and not by a lack of cytologic findings adequate to diagnose or suspect lymphoma. The uncritical acceptance by Hajdu and Melamed[27] of the egregious statement that 10 per cent of patients with Hashimoto's thyroiditis have associated thyroid carcinoma raises questions of credulity as well as credibility. A recent review[43] showed that only 2 of 829 patients with Hashimoto's thyroiditis had thyroid carcinoma.

Hajdu and Melamed[27] even doubt that papillary carcinomas can be diagnosed reliably by fine needle biopsy. This opinion harkens back to the 1958 report from their institution by Frazell and Foote[20] in which 26.4 per cent false-negative diagnoses were made by needle biopsy on patients with papillary carcinoma. After such a poor result, it is understandable why they "largely abandoned the procedure." But nowadays cytologic criteria for the diagnoses of papillary carcinoma have been refined substantially. In our recent series (Table 10–1), 52 of 53 patients operated on for fine needle biopsy diagnoses of papillary carcinoma had the disease. One additional patient was erroneously diagnosed as having follicular carcinoma. The diagnosis of suspected papillary carcinoma was less specific but necessary to maintain a high sensitivity for fine needle biopsy detection of those lesions. Four patients who had inadequate fine needle biopsy samples for any reliable diagnosis had papillary carcinoma, but no patient with papillary carcinoma has as yet had a fine needle biopsy diagnosis of benign disease. This experience is compatible with the extensive current literature indicating that papillary carcinoma is one of the easiest fine needle biopsy diagnoses to make or at least suspect.

The 30 years' experience to which Hajdu and Melamed[27] refer, having been acquired before 1960, may correctly be attributed to their institution, but it is unlikely that they were active participants in those studies.

Being pathologists, Hajdu and Melamed[27] are not immediately confronted with the clinical consequences of their recommendation that fine needle biopsy be abandoned. They do not have to make the management decisions that determine which thyroid nodules will come to pathologists for study. If they do not advise fine needle biopsy, what method do they recommend to determine which thyroid nodules should be excised and which can safely be observed? Do they seriously believe that physicians should revert to less sensitive and specific clinical methods of selection? Do they advise surgery for all thyroid nodules, for none, or only for those that are obviously malignant? On this issue, critical for clinicians, they are mute.

## *Does Fine Needle Biopsy Improve the Prognosis for Patients with Thyroid Nodules?*

Molitch et al.[63] said that decision analysis indicates no difference in the prognosis of these patients regardless of whether fine needle biopsy is used, the nodules are routinely excised, or the patients are treated with thyroxine. This nihilistic notion, published in the prestigious *Endocrine Reviews*[63] presumably after peer review and editorial approval, surely must have caused some distress to surgeons who thought they were improving the prognosis for their patients by skillfully excising thyroid cancers. Those who might have intuitive reservations about the conclusion of Molitch et al.[63] or enough experience with fine needle biopsy to object to their findings are referred to the 1982 report of Norton et al.[66] who found (also using decision analysis) that fine needle biopsy is "a reasonable first step in the evaluation of thyroid nodules." These disparate findings may reflect decisions made by the authors rather than the technique of decision analysis per se. For example, Norton et al.[66] analyzed their own data. Molitch et al.[63] either had no experience to analyze or chose not to be influenced by personal experience and thus confined their analysis to the data of others. The sources for the data they used had widely differing findings, but those authors dealt with that problem by averaging, a totally objective attitude no doubt based on the democratic principle that all published papers are equivalent in validity. When the average value did not suit their ideas of what the correct value should be, they simply picked a number more to their liking. For example, from data in 11 reports they determined that the average probability of a positive fine needle biopsy diagnosis on a malignant nodule was 69.8 per cent, ranging from 0 to 98 per cent. The numbers of cases of cancer in those reports ranged from 2 to 137. They relied on averaging to compensate for differences in fine needle biopsy experience, geographic differences, and probably technologic differences. On the other hand, 23 papers gave a prevalence of carcinoma from 1.5 to 38.1 per cent, an average 16.9 per cent. That average they did not like, so they substituted an "estimated" value of 10 per cent, a value that presumably fit their preconception of what the "correct" number ought to be.

We did not think we could ignore a report published in such an authoritative journal from an important academic institution. Neither do we wish to comment at greater length other than to suggest that those who set out to tell others that fine needle biopsy is irrelevant, despite a vast literature to the contrary, ought to try fine needle biopsy themselves first. If they then fail to obtain good results, they should make an honest effort to find out why.

## *Is Large Needle Biopsy Better Than Fine Needle Biopsy?*

Most current reports deal with fine needle biopsy because the procedure is simpler, safer, and applicable to the smaller tumors that constitute the preponderance of clinically detectable nodules. Esselstyn and Crile,[18] early proponents of large needle biopsy, have recently favored fine needle biopsy. When we were first learning to perform needle biopsy, we, too, relied heavily on large needle biopsy as a backup procedure, short of surgery, to clarify equivocal fine needle biopsy diagnoses. Indeed, large needle biopsy corrected a number of our early false-negative fine needle biopsy diagnoses. In our first 500 patients, 50 per cent had large needle biopsy.[59] This figure dropped to 39 per cent in our next report[61] dealing with 1,222 patients. After experience with 5,000 patients, we now use large needle biopsy after fine needle biopsy failure or when fine needle biopsy produces unpromising material from larger degenerated nodules. The increasing skill of our cytopathologists and the avoidance of fine needle biopsy failures by obtaining multiple aspirates circumferentially at the periphery of the nodules have reduced the percentage of patients requiring large needle biopsy to about 5 per cent. We use the simpler and safer large needle aspiration biopsy technique rather than those involving TruCut or Silverman needles, which could be hazardous. (One of our patients had a temporary recurrent nerve palsy after a cutting needle biopsy.) Boey et al.[5] reported a fibrotic reaction in the needle track interfering with subsequent surgery.

In a limited series of 164 patients, Schwartz et al.[75] found that large needle biopsy corrected two false-negative fine needle biopsy diagnoses, one on a lymphoma and the second on a follicular variant of papillary carcinoma. However, the descriptions of the fine needle biopsy specimens suggest inadequate cytologic material for diagnosis.

In a prospective study of 405 patients, Boey et al.[5] noted little difference in the accuracy of cancer detection by fine needle biopsy (87 per cent) and large needle biopsy (92 per cent). However, the combined use of the two procedures improved accuracy to 97 per cent. Once again, it remains to be seen whether greater experience will permit better fine needle biopsy results by these workers.

Lo Gerfo et al.[11, 55, 56] have three publications on the use of needle biopsy. Instead of progressing from large needle biopsy to fine needle biopsy, they have gone in the opposite direction. In their 1980 report[11] on 300 patients studied by fine needle biopsy, they concluded that the procedure "will greatly decrease the number of unnecessary thyroid resections." In 1982,[55] they found no difference in the cancer yield of the two methods, but large needle biopsy (TruCut) was better able to exclude carcinoma in adenomatous hyperplasia and therefore had greater potential than fine needle biopsy to aid in eliminating unnecessary surgery. However, only 69 per cent of the nodules in their study were large enough for large needle biopsy. In their 1985 paper[56] dealing with 922 patients, these workers rejected their 1980 endorsement of fine needle biopsy. They showed that the incidence of carcinoma in surgical specimens of nodules selected for surgery before fine needle biopsy was 28 per cent. After fine needle biopsy, it was 27 per cent—that is, no improvement. Patients selected for operation on the basis of large needle biopsy had a 41 per cent incidence of carcinoma. However, using fine needle biopsy alone, 45 per cent of the nodules we excised were malignant, and the figure is 56 per cent if patients who had operation despite a fine needle biopsy diagnosis of benign disease are excluded. Our experience is not unusual. Results of 41 to 51 per cent carcinoma were achieved with fine needle biopsy at five other institutions (Table 10–3). Whether the low yield of carcinoma in the patients of Lo Gerfo et al. and others studied by fine needle biopsy alone relates to inexperience, inadequate sampling, or a different patient population is unclear. Regardless of the reason, those poorer results are not indicative of the best that can be achieved with fine needle biopsy.

Hawkins et al.[41] showed that the prevalence of carcinoma in surgical specimens from patients studied by fine needle biopsy from 1981 to 1985 increased each year from a low of 8.3 per cent in 1981 to the final value of 37.3 per cent in 1985. This improvement in diagnostic accuracy was not related to any important improvement in the diagnosis of cancer but rather was achieved because of a corresponding fall in the proportion of patients operated on from the 1981 high of 61 per cent to the 1985 low of 14.9 per cent. That this reduction in surgery was a reduction in surgery for benign disease is evident from the finding that the proportion of the total number of patients evaluated for whom carcinoma was detected remained virtually constant at about 6 per cent for each year of the study. This relatively low value of 6 per cent is a consequence of the fact that only 80 per cent of their 1,399 patients had nodular goiter.

The learning curve these physicians experienced is typical for the acquisition of fine needle biopsy expertise. We suspect that with additional experience they probably will note a cancer prevalence in their surgical specimens in the 40 to 50 per cent range. Certainly, we were still learning important lessons after treating more than 2,000 cases. Careful study of the literature may shorten the learning process. However, to expect to do the best work possible after only a few hundred cases seems unrealistic. We found that the most useful factor in acquisition of fine needle biopsy expertise was rigorous and ongoing self-criticism.

As Vickery[85] said "it is astonishing that it has taken so long to gain popular recognition for a diagnostic method of proven value and safety for one of the most prevalent problems in clinical medicine."

***Acknowledgment***: Dr. Mujtaba Husain, Director of Cytopathology, Sinai Hospital of Detroit, provided Figure 10–6, a composite including large needle biopsy specimens provided by Dr. Sudha R. Kini, Department of Pathology, Henry Ford Hospital, and sections from the surgical specimen obtained at Sinai Hospital of Detroit.

## REFERENCES

1. Abdel-Nabi, H., Falko, J. M., Olsen, J. O., and Freimanis, A. K.: Solitary cold thyroid nodule: Cost-ineffectiveness of ultrasonography. South. Med. J., *77*:1146–1148, 1984.
2. Aldinger, K. A., Samann, N. A., Ibanez, M., and Hill, C. S., Jr.: Anaplastic carcinoma of the thyroid: A review of 84 cases of spindle and giant cell carcinoma of the thyroid. Cancer, *41*:2267–2275, 1978.
3. Blum, M.: The diagnosis of the thyroid nodule using aspiration biopsy and cytology. Arch. Intern. Med., *144*:1140–1142, 1984.
4. Blum, M., Goldman, A. B., Herskovic, A., and Hernberg, J.: Clinical applications of thyroid echography. N. Engl. J. Med., *287*:1164–1199, 1972.
5. Boey, J., Hsu, C., Collins, R. J., and Wong, J.: A prospective controlled study of fine-needle aspiration and TruCut needle biopsy of dominant thyroid nodules. World J. Surg., *8*:458–465, 1984.
6. Brauer, R. J., and Silver, C. E.: Needle aspiration biopsy of thyroid nodules. Laryngoscope, *94*:38–42, 1984.
7. Bugis, S. P., Young, J. E. M., Archibald, S. D., and Chen, V. S. M.: Diagnostic accuracy of fine-needle aspiration biopsy versus frozen section in solitary thyroid nodules. Am. J. Surg., *152*:411–416, 1986.
8. Cady, B.: Surgery of thyroid cancer. World J. Surg., *5*:3–14, 1981.
9. Clark, O.: Commentary. *In* Hamburger, J. I., and Miller, J. M. (eds.): Controversies in Clinical Thyroidology. New York, Springer-Verlag, 1981, pp. 218–225.
10. Clark, O. H., Okerlund, M. D., Cavalieri, R. R., and Greenspan, F. S.: Diagnosis and treatment of thyroid, parathyroid, and thyroglossal duct cysts. J. Clin. Endocrinol. Metab., *48*:983–988, 1979.
11. Colacchio, T. A., Lo Gerfo, P., and Feind, C. R.: Fine needle cytologic diagnosis of thyroid nodules: Review and report of 300 cases. Am. J. Surg., *140*:568–571, 1980.
12. Crile, G., Jr.: Treatment of thyroid cysts by aspiration. Surgery, *59*:210–212, 1966.
13. Crile, G., Jr.: Needle biopsy of the thyroid. Clin. Nucl. Med., *2*:422, 1977.
14. Crile, G., Jr., and Hawk, W. A., Jr.: Aspiration biopsy of thyroid nodules. Surg. Gynecol. Obstet., *136*:241–245, 1973.
15. Crile, G., Jr., and Vickery, A. L.: Special uses of the Silverman biopsy needle in office practice and and at operation. Am. J. Surg., *83*:83–85, 1952.
16. Crile, G., Jr., Esselstyn, C. B., Jr., and Hawk, W. A.: Needle biopsy in the diagnosis of thyroid nodules appearing after radiation. N. Engl. J. Med., *301*:997–999, 1979.
17. Einhorn, J., and Franzen, S.: Thin-needle biopsy in the diagnosis of thyroid disease. Acta Radiol., *58*:321–336, 1962.
18. Esselstyn, C. B., Jr., and Crile, G., Jr.: Needle aspiration and needle biopsy of the thyroid. World J. Surg., *2*:321–329, 1978.
19. Frable, W. J.: The treatment of thyroid cancer: The role of fine-needle aspiration cytology. Arch. Otolaryngol. Head Neck Surg., *112*:1200–1203, 1986.
20. Frazell, E. L., and Foote, F. W., Jr.: Papillary cancer of the thyroid: A review of 25 years of experience. Cancer, *11*:895–922, 1958.
21. Galvan, G.: Thin needle aspiration biopsy and cytological examination of hypofunctional, "cold" thyroid nodules in routine clinical work. Clin. Nucl. Med., *2*:413–421, 1977.
22. Gershengorn, M. C., McClung, M. R., Chu, E. W., et al.: Fine-needle aspiration cytology in the preoperative diagnosis of thyroid nodules. Ann. Intern. Med., *87*:265–269, 1977.
23. Gharib, H., Goellner, J. R., Zinsmeister, A. R., et al.: Fine-needle aspiration biopsy of the thyroid: The problem of suspicious cytologic findings. Ann. Intern. Med., *101*:25–28, 1984.
24. Goetsch, E.: Newer methods in the diagnosis of thyroid disorders: Pathological and clinical. N. Y. State J. Med., *18*:259–267, 1918.
25. Goldfarb, W. B., Bigos, T. S., Eastman, R. C., et al.: Needle biopsy in the assessment and management of hypofunctioning thyroid nodules. Am. J. Surg., *143*:409–412, 1982.
26. Guarda, L. A., and Baskin, H. J.: Inflammatory and lymphoid lesions of the thyroid gland: Cytopathology by fine-needle aspiration. Am. J. Clin. Pathol., *87*:14–22, 1987.
27. Hajdu, S. I., and Melamed, M. R.: Limitations of aspiration cytology in the diagnosis of primary neoplasms. Acta Cytol., *28*:337–345, 1984.
28. Hamaker, R. C., Singer, M. I., DeRossi, R. V., and Shockley, W. W.: Role of needle biopsy in thyroid nodules. Arch. Otolaryngol., *109*:225–228, 1983.
29. Hamberger, B., Gharib, H., Melton, L. J., III, et al.: Fine-needle aspiration biopsy of thyroid nodules: Impact on thyroid practice and cost of care. Am. J. Med., *73*:381–384, 1982.
30. Hamburger, J. I.: Clinical Exercises in Internal Medicine. Vol. 1: Thyroid Disease. Philadelphia, W. B. Saunders Co., 1978, pp. 221–222.
31. Hamburger, J. I.: The contribution of suppression scanning to the evaluation of thyroid nodules for cancer. *In* McReady, V. R., Taylor, D. M., Troth,

N. G., et al. (eds.): Radioactive Isotopes in the Localization of Tumours. London, Heinemann, 1979, pp. 107–113.
32. Hamburger, J. I.: Evolution of toxicity in solitary nontoxic autonomously functioning thyroid nodules. J. Clin. Endocrinol. Metab., *50*:1089–1093, 1980.
33. Hamburger, J. I.: Management of Thyroid Patients. Southfield, Michigan, private publication by Hamburger, J. I., 1985, pp. 136–137.
34. Hamburger, J. I.: Consistency of sequential needle biopsy findings for thyroid nodules: Management implications. Arch. Intern. Med., *147*:97–99, 1987.
35. Hamburger, J. I., and Hamburger, S. W.: Declining role of frozen section in surgical planning for thyroid nodules. Surgery, *98*:307–312, 1985.
36. Hamburger, J. I., and Taylor, C. I.: Transient thyrotoxicosis associated with acute hemorrhagic infarction of autonomously functioning thyroid nodules. Ann. Intern. Med., *91*:406–409, 1979.
37. Hamburger, J. I., Miller, J. M., and Garcia, M.: Do all nodules appearing in patients subsequent to radiation therapy to the head and neck areas require excision? *In* Hamburger, J. I., and Miller, J. M. (eds.): Controversies in Clinical Thyroidology. New York, Springer-Verlag, 1981, pp. 237–266.
38. Hamburger, J. I., Miller, J. M., and Kini, S. R.: Clinical-Pathological Diagnosis of Thyroid Nodules: Handbook and Atlas. Southfield, Michigan, private publication by Hamburger, J. I., 1979, pp. 14–17, 74–86.
39. Hamburger, J. I., Miller, J. M., and Kini, S. R.: Lymphoma of the thyroid. Ann. Intern. Med., *99*:685–693, 1983.
40. Hammer, M., Wortsman, J., and Folse, R.: Cancer in cystic lesions of the thyroid. Arch. Surg., *117*:1020–1023, 1982.
41. Hawkins, F., Bellido, D., Bernal, C., et al.: Fine needle aspiration biopsy in the diagnosis of thyroid cancer and thyroid disease. Cancer, *59*:1206–1209, 1987.
42. Heimann, P.: Needle aspiration biopsy for thyroid cancer (Letter). Arch. Surg., *110*:1517–1518, 1975.
43. Holm, L.-E., Blomgren, H., and Löwhagen, T.: Cancer risks in patients with chronic lymphocytic thyroiditis. N. Engl. J. Med., *312*:601–604, 1985.
44. Junginger, T., Finsterer, H., Pichlmaier, H.: Die Punktionsdiagnostik von Schilddrüsenerkrankungen. Munch. Med. Wochenschr., *115*:306–310, 1973.
45. Kessler, R. K., Kessler, W. B., Constantine, J., et al.: Sclerosis of thyroid cysts (Letter). Arch. Intern. Med., *144*:1693, 1697, 1984.
46. Kini, S. R., Miller, J. M., Hamburger, J. I., and Smith, M. J.: Cytopathology of papillary carcinoma of the thyroid by fine needle aspiration. Acta Cytol., *24*:511–521, 1980.
47. Kini, S. R., Miller, J. M., and Hamburger, J. I.: Problems in the cytologic diagnosis of the "cold" thyroid nodule in patients with lymphocytic thyroiditis. Acta Cytol., *25*:506–512, 1981.
48. Kini, S. R., Miller, J. M., and Hamburger, J. I.: Cytopathology of Hürthle cell lesions of the thyroid gland by fine needle aspiration. Acta Cytol., *25*:647–652, 1981.
49. Kini, S. R., Miller, J. M., Hamburger, J. I., and Smith, M. J.: Cytopathologic features of medullary carcinoma of the thyroid. Arch. Pathol. Lab. Med., *108*:156–159, 1984.
50. Kini, S. R., Miller, J. M., Hamburger, J. I., and Smith-Purslow, M. J.: Cytopathology of follicular lesions of the thyroid gland. Diagn. Cytopathol., *1*:123–132, 1985.
51. Kirstaedter, H. J., Engel, W., Gehrmann, C.: Cytodiagnostik kalter Schilddrusenknoten. Verh. Dtsch. Ges. Inn. Med., *76*:492–495, 1970.
52. Lang, W., Atay, Z., and Georgii, A.: Die cytologische Unterscheidung follikulärer Tumoren in der Schilddrüse. Virchows Arch. (Pathol. Anat.), *378*:199–211, 1978.
53. Ljungberg, O.: Cytological diagnosis of medullary carcinoma of the thyroid gland with special regard to the demonstration of amyloid in smears of fine needle aspirates. Acta Cytol., *16*:253–255, 1972.
54. Lo Gerfo, P., and Ting, W.: Method for biopsy of the wall of a thyroid cyst. Am. J. Surg., *146*:383–384, 1983.
55. Lo Gerfo, P., Colacchio, T., Caushaj, F., et al.: Comparison of fine-needle and coarse-needle biopsies in evaluating thyroid nodules. Surgery, 92:835–838, 1982.
56. Lo Gerfo, P., Starker, P., Weber, C., et al.: Incidence of cancer in surgically treated thyroid nodules based on method of selection. Surgery, *98*:1197–1201, 1985.
57. Löwhagen, T., Willems, J.-S., Lundell, G., et al.: Aspiration biopsy cytology in diagnosis of thyroid cancer. World J. Surg., *5*:61–73, 1981.
58. Martin, H. E., and Ellis, E. B.: Biopsy by needle puncture and aspiration. Ann. Surg., *92*:169–181, 1930.
59. Miller, J. M., Hamburger, J. I., and Kini, S.: Diagnosis of thyroid nodules: Use of fine-needle aspiration and needle biopsy. J.A.M.A., *241*:481–484, 1979.
60. Miller, J. M., Hamburger, J. I., and Taylor, C. I.: Needle aspiration of the cystic thyroid nodule: Effective and safe treatment? *In* Hamburger, J. I., and Miller, J. M. (eds.): Controversies in Clinical Thyroidology. New York, Springer-Verlag, 1981, pp. 209–217.
61. Miller, J. M., Kini, S. R., and Hamburger, J. I.: Needle Biopsy of the Thyroid. New York, Praeger Publishers, 1983, pp. 86, 94, 176, 182–185.
62. Miller, J. M., Zafar, S. U., and Karo, J. J.: The cystic thyroid nodule: Recognition and management. Radiology, *110*:257–261, 1974.
63. Molitch, M. E., Beck, J. R., Dreisman, M., et al.: The cold thyroid nodule: An analysis of diagnostic and therapeutic options. Endocr. Rev., *5*:185–199, 1984.
64. Müller, N., Cooperberg, P. L., Suen, K. C., and Thorson, S. C.: Needle aspiration biopsy in cystic papillary carcinoma of the thyroid. A.J.R., *144*:251–253, 1985.
65. Nilsson, L. R., and Persson, P. S.: Cytological aspiration biopsy in adolescent goitre. Acta Pediatr., *53*:333–338, 1964.
66. Norton, L. W., Wangensteen, S. L., Davis, J. R., et al.: Utility of thyroid aspiration biopsy. Surgery, *92*:700–705, 1982.
67. Persson, P. S.: Cytodiagnosis of thyroiditis: A comparative study of cytological, histological, immu-

nological and clinical findings in thyroiditis, particularly in diffuse lymphoid thyroiditis. Acta Med. Scand., *182* (Suppl. 483):7–25, 1967.
68. Ramacciotti, C. E., Pretorius, H. T., Chu, E. W., et al.: Diagnostic accuracy and use of aspiration biopsy in the management of thyroid nodules. Arch. Intern. Med., *144*:1169–1173, 1984.
69. Rosen, I. B., and Maitland, A.: Changing the operative strategy for thyroid cancer by node sampling. Am. J. Surg., *146*:504–508, 1983.
70. Rosen, I. B., Provias, J. P., and Walfish, P. G.: Pathologic nature of cystic thyroid nodules selected for surgery by needle aspiration biopsy. Surgery, *100*:606–613, 1986.
71. Rudowski, W.: Critical evaluation of aspiration biopsy in the diagnosis of tumours of the thyroid. Am. J. Surg., *95*:40–44, 1958.
72. Ryan, W. G.: Needling the thyroid (and thyroid surgeons?) (Editorial). Arch. Intern. Med., *143*:2249, 1983.
73. Ryan, W. G., and Dwarakanathan, A.: Minor complication of thyroid cyst sclerosis with tetracycline (Letter). Arch. Intern. Med., *146*:201–202, 1986.
74. Schnürer, L. B., and Widström, A.: Fine-needle biopsy of the thyroid gland: A cytohistological comparison in cases of goiter. Ann. Otol. Rhinol. Laryngol., *87* (2 Pt 1):224–227, 1978.
75. Schwartz, A. E., Nieburgs, H. E., Davies, T. F., et al.: The place of fine needle biopsy in the diagnosis of nodules of the thyroid. Surg. Gynecol. Obstet., *155*:54–58, 1982.
76. Silverman, J. F., West, R. L., Larkin, E. W., et al.: The role of fine-needle aspiration biopsy in the rapid diagnosis and management of thyroid neoplasms. Cancer, 57:1164–1170, 1986.
77. Smith, S. A., Gharib, H., and Goellner, J. R.: Fine-needle aspiration: Usefulness for diagnosis and management of metastatic carcinoma to the thyroid. Arch. Intern. Med., *147*:311–312, 1987.
78. Söderström, N.: Puncture of goiters for aspiration biopsy: A preliminary report. Acta Med. Scand., *144*:235–244, 1952.
79. Suen, K. C., and Quenville, N. F.: Fine-needle aspiration biopsy of thyroid gland: A study of 304 cases. J. Clin. Pathol., *36*:1036–1045, 1983.
80. Sykes, D.: The solitary thyroid nodule. Br. J. Surg., *68*:510–512, 1981.
81. Treece, G. L.: In reply (Letter). Arch. Intern. Med., *146*:202, 1986.
82. Treece, G. L., Georgitis, W. J., and Hofeldt, F. D.: Resolution of recurrent thyroid cysts with tetracycline instillation. Arch. Intern. Med., *143*:2285–2287, 1983.
83. Utiger, R. D.: Is external irradiation a risk factor for thyroid disease and thyroid carcinoma? (Editorial). J.A.M.A., *242*:2702, 1979.
84. Van Herle, A. J., Rich, P., Ljung, B.-M., et al.: The thyroid nodule. Ann. Intern. Med., *96*:221–232, 1982.
85. Vickery, A. L.: Needle biopsy pathology. Clin. Endocrinol. Metab., *10*:275–292, 1981.
86. Walfish, P. G., Hazani, E., Strawbridge, H. T., et al.: Combined ultrasound and needle aspiration cytology in the assessment and management of hypofunctioning thyroid nodule. Ann. Intern. Med., *87*:270–274, 1977.
87. Wang, C., Vickery, A. L., Jr., and Maloof, F.: Needle biopsy of the thyroid. Surg. Gynecol. Obstet., *143*:365–368, 1976.
88. Watts, N. B.: Carcinoma metastatic to the thyroid: Prevalence and diagnosis by fine-needle aspiration cytology. Am. J. Med. Sci., *291*:13–17, 1987.
89. Willems, J. S., and Löwhagen, T.: Fine-needle aspiration cytology in thyroid disease. Clin. Endocrinol. Metab., *10*:247–266, 1981.

# Commentary

*Blake Cady, M. D.*

This extraordinarily comprehensive and thorough review of the subject of needle biopsy in the diagnosis and management of thyroid nodules is an excellent analysis of the world's literature and an expression of the authors' own considerable experience. This chapter is recommended for close reading.

My preference for needle aspiration of a thyroid nodule is to fix and localize the nodule in the thyroid gland with the fingers of my left hand while aspirating the nodule with a one-handed syringe holder and an ordinary disposable large bore needle of size No. 18 or 19 held in the right hand. I use a 50-ml disposable syringe, which provides ample vacuum. The tip of the needle is moved back and forth through the nodule under direct control with the opposite palpating fingers. In this way, accurate location of the tip of the needle can be achieved, and the complications of the large core cutting needle methods, such as excessive bleeding, are avoided. The advantage of use of the large aspirating needle is that small fragments of tissue are removed from the nodule, which gives the pathologist not only cytologic tissue but micropathologic tissue that can be viewed in terms of organization and arrangement of clusters of cells.

Another technical point I use in obtaining material for a thyroid needle biopsy is to approach the nodule from above, aiming downward toward the feet rather than directly from the side. When the needle is bent, the syringe can be held at a more natural angle, thus avoiding possible penetration of the trachea and injury to the recurrent laryngeal nerves and providing a run through normal tissues before entering the nodule for more secure needle placement. While the needle is in the nodule, strong vacuum is placed on the syringe, and the tip of the needle is moved back and forth through a distance of about 1 cm to break up cells within the nodule. Vacuum is then released, the needle is withdrawn, and the cells are squirted onto cytology slides, smeared against each other, and immediately placed in Papanicolaou fixative.

Of utmost importance in the useful interpretation of thyroid needle biopsy is the understanding of what can be achieved by the results of the test. Unfortunately, many physicians and frequent reports in the literature indicate that an exact diagnosis of thyroid carcinoma can usually be achieved. As the Hamburgers point out, much discussion among authors occurs regarding the importance of the finding of "suspicious cells." If it is kept in mind that the major role of thyroid needle biopsy is to help make a decision whether or not to operate and *not* to provide an exact diagnosis, the histologic information can be used more meaningfully. Ascertaining whether the lesion is a follicular nodule in an adenomatous goiter, follicular adenoma, or follicular adenocarcinoma is difficult, even for the pathologist with the entire lesion or nodule removed at operation. The diagnosis of follicular adenocarcinoma depends on visualizing cells in the capsule or pseudocapsule of the thyroid tumor or in the blood vessels within and around the thyroid nodule. The diagnosis of cancer is not a histologic diagnosis because the histopathology of benign and malignant endocrine tumors is infrequently distinguishable. As in islet cell tumors of the pancreas, accurate diagnosis is achieved by visualizing cells outside the primary tumor in other tissues. Thus, specific diagnoses of carcinoma in follicular lesions by needle aspiration of the thyroid is neither necessary nor readily achievable. Papillary carcinoma of the thyroid can frequently be diagnosed specifically by aspiration cytology, but any follicular lesion should be removed surgically because the discrimination between benign and malignant lesions is frequently impossible short of an operation. In reality, the only purpose of needle biopsy of the thyroid is to eliminate from surgical consideration the patient with an obvious adenomatous goiter, accurately depicted on cytologic aspiration, and thyroiditis in which the possibility of cancer or lymphoma is not a clinical concern.

Patients with a large bulky benign goiter that needs surgical removal for cosmetic reasons are little served by aspiration biopsy beforehand, which merely confirms the clinical impression of colloid goiter. When patients who have clinical indications for thyroidectomy are eliminated, the thyroid nodules that are of diagnostic concern are small, and the accuracy of needle biopsy may be reduced considerably. I estimate that less than 50 per cent of patients with small nodules of some concern by physical examination can be spared surgical resection by means of needle aspiration cytology, which reveals a clearly benign process with colloid and a macrofollicular pattern to cells or thyroiditis. All other lesions should be removed surgically. Institutions with reports in the literature that indicate as great as an 80 per cent incidence of cancer in nodules operated on are clearly not subjecting enough patients to surgery and will be missing some cancers because of too rigid criteria for suspicious or positive aspiration cytology. Clinically, large nodules that are unsightly, disfiguring, or causing symptoms should be removed regardless of the results of aspiration cytology. Patients are sometimes rejected for thyroidectomy because of an aspiration biopsy diagnosis of benign disease despite the fact that the large nodule is unsightly and causing the patient some discomfort. Such patients need to have thyroid surgery for cosmetic and symptomatic relief and do not need needle biopsy.

Fear of thyroid surgery is largely unfounded. Thyroid operations can be performed without deaths, and the morbidity is extremely low. As long as the surgical resection performed is conservative, the major complications of hypoparathyroidism and injury to the recurrent laryngeal nerves can be reduced to an absolute minimum. The concern of endocrinologists and physicians today is that total thyroidectomy might result in hypoparathyroidism and injury to the recurrent laryngeal nerves. The best philosophic approach to the surgical management of a patient with a thyroid nodule is to be liberal with indications for surgery but conservative with removal of tissue during the operation. Unfortunately, the general philosophy among academic endocrine surgeons is the opposite: they may be extremely conservative in indications for surgery, but they are unnecessarily radical in the amount of tissue resected, resorting to total thyroidectomy for diseases that are largely benign in biologic behavior and require only partial removal of the thyroid gland. We are even reading about the absurd notion that a patient with an adenomatous goiter, Graves' disease, and Hashimoto's thyroiditis should have total thyroidectomy!

Thyroid cysts, which are aspirated either primarily or after their diagnosis with the aid of ultrasonography, create problems in decision making. In my experience, less than one half of thyroid cystic lesions are ultimately controlled nonoperatively with repeated aspiration. Papillary carcinoma frequently has a cystic component; thus, whenever a thyroid cyst is aspirated, the material should be sent for cytologic examination on the chance that a papillary carcinoma might be discovered. When a cyst recurs after three aspirations a month or more apart, the patient should be urged to have surgical removal of the cyst to prevent recurrence and to rule out a more serious problem. Thyroid cysts, when aspirated, usually reveal turgid, muddy, bloody, or dark fluid. When clear fluid is obtained in aspirating a cyst in the thyroid area, it is a parathyroid cyst, and the fluid should be analyzed for parathormone assay level. Not all parathyroid cysts are associated with hyperparathyroidism despite the presence of large amounts of parathyroid-rich material within the fluid of the cyst. A parathyroid cyst can usually be controlled by aspiration.

If one were to devise the most inexpensive and rapid diagnostic test sequence for evaluation of a clinically palpable thyroid nodule, a persuasive argument could be made for use of thyroid needle biopsy first. A cystic lesion will be discovered on aspiration. Solid material can be aspirated for cytology to decide whether this nodule needs to be removed surgically. Because palpable nodules suspected of being malignant are not associated with functional problems, thyroid function tests are of no help in making initial decisions regarding surgery. When the thyroid needle aspiration diagnosis is benign colloid goiter or thyroiditis, the patient may undergo a radioactive scan of the thyroid, thyroid function tests of the serum to outline the functional aspects of the thyroid and antibodies, and echography to complete the evaluation if necessary. Such a sequence of tests would greatly reduce the number of laboratory tests that are of little or no help in making surgical decisions and speed up the process of a diagnostic workup. The cost of this approach might also be considerably less.

As of this writing, the role of diagnostic

thyroid needle biopsy is well established, but the real test of effectiveness and usefulness of this procedure has not been addressed in the critical group of patients. The true test of this procedure will be its accuracy and reliability in detecting the nature of small nodules, less than 1.5 cm or 2 cm in diameter. It is with these small nodules, which would not require surgery from a clinical point of view because they cause no cosmetic or symptomatic distress, that decision making is most obscure. The accuracy of cutting needle biopsy or aspiration cytology in such small nodules is considerably less than stated in typical reports in the literature. Such nodules were usually being operated on by clinical criteria under any circumstances. In the future, the role of thyroid needle biopsy may become more modest after the recent initial enthusiasm, but it will remain the most direct assessment of the nature of nodules of the thyroid gland short of surgical resection.

# 11

# HYPERTHYROIDISM

*Marvin S. Wool, M.D.*

In the 10 years since the previous edition of this book, the indications for surgical treatment of patients with hyperthyroidism have dramatically narrowed. In a 1984 poll of 54 thyroidologists[8] regarding their initial choice of therapy for a 19-year-old patient with Graves' disease, it was found that two thirds chose antithyroid drugs, one quarter selected radioactive iodine, and a scant 9 per cent preferred surgery. Surgery as initial therapy for a 29-year-old patient was even less popular, with 47 per cent choosing antithyroid drugs, 47 per cent selecting radioactive iodine, and only 6 per cent preferring surgery. Furthermore, for patients whose initial course of antithyroid drug therapy failed, only one third considered surgery as second-line therapy. The remainder resorted to a second course of medical therapy or radioactive iodine.

Disillusionment with surgery has resulted from both increased comfort with alternative modes of therapy and greater concerns with surgery itself. Antithyroid drug therapy has enjoyed resurgence, with reports of higher remission rates and with suggestions that it provides therapy of hypermetabolism and attacks the basic immunologic cause of Graves' disease. Radioactive iodine therapy has been employed more liberally in patients of childbearing age as well as in adolescents and children because earlier concerns regarding genetic and long-term effects have waned. These developments have insidiously compounded concerns about surgery by surgeons and their medical colleagues inasmuch as it has long been recognized that the incidence of serious complications of this procedure are inversely related to the current and accumulated experience of the surgeon. Historical reports[11, 36] from large centers with extensive experience indicate low complication rates, but as the frequency of thyroid surgery has decreased, a greater recognition of early complications has been appreciated. Furthermore, as studies have expanded, an increased awareness of longer term complications has resulted.

This report focuses on the diagnosis of hyperthyroidism, its causes, the differential diagnoses, and the current place of various treatment modalities. The emphasis is on Graves' disease, the most common cause of hyperthyroidism. Medical therapy is explored from the perspective of the cause of Graves' disease, remission rates to be anticipated, pretreatment prognostic factors, and intratherapy prognostic indicators. The techniques of therapy, including choice of drug, dose levels, and frequency and duration of administration, are discussed with regard to anticipated remission rates of hyperthyroidism and the underlying immunologic process. Radioactive iodine therapy is considered from the perspective of remission and recurrence rates, complications of hypothyroidism, mutagenesis, and genetic effects with particular attention to dose levels. The remaining indications for surgical therapy of hyperthyroidism are reviewed with emphasis on preoperative preparation regimens, results, and complications of treatment.

## ETIOLOGY OF HYPERTHYROIDISM

Graves' disease in a patient with a diffuse goiter is the most common cause of hyperthyroidism in the United States. A variant may occur in a patient with a preexistent multinodular goiter. In still other patients, usually older, hyperthyroidism may develop from excess hormone production by a solitary toxic adenoma, although Hashimoto's thyroiditis, an immunologic relative of Graves' disease, may also produce transient hyperthyroidism. Subacute (de Quervain's) thyroiditis is a viral illness that may also become manifest with toxicity. Silent thyroiditis occurring in the postpartum period and sporadically in the general population of the Midwest is a disease of limited duration but histologically akin to chronic thyroiditis. Patients with a multinodular goiter and occasional others with a diffuse goiter may have hyperthyroidism induced by ingestion of iodides in the form of contrast media, therapeutic iodides, or the new cardiac drug amiodarone (Cordarone). Exogenous thyroid hormone either iatrogenically or self-administered can produce toxicity, and rarely, thyroid-stimulating hormone (TSH) secreting pituitary tumors are at fault.

## DIAGNOSIS

The two active thyroid hormones are L-thyroxine ($LT_4$) and L-triiodothyronine ($LT_3$), with circulating concentrations of each being about equally responsible for the metabolic state. The former is produced exclusively by the thyroid gland and is 99.5 per cent bound by serum proteins; its unbound or free portion accounts for metabolic activity. L-Triiodothyronine is produced by the thyroid gland and by peripheral degradation of circulating $LT_4$. Although it is present in lower total concentrations in serum, $LT_3$ is more potent and less tightly bound to serum proteins with a higher proportion available in the free active state.

The current diagnostic test of choice for hyperthyroidism is the serum free $T_4$ test, which is more useful than the older total $T_4$ test by radioimmunoassay. The latter, as its name indicates, measures total rather than metabolically active free $T_4$ and is therefore subject to variations of serum proteins and attendant anomalous results. The total $T_3$ test by radioimmunoassay is useful in a small proportion of patients who have normal levels of free $T_4$ but have so-called $T_3$ toxicosis. The serum TSH by traditional radioimmunoassay is not helpful in the diagnosis of hyperthyroidism inasmuch as a significant minority of normal persons as well as patients with toxicity will have undetectable levels. The emerging availability of the so-called sensitive TSH assay, however, may assume an important role in the diagnosis of hyperthyroidism inasmuch as early studies have shown that normal persons have detectable levels of TSH by this technique while those with active hyperthyroidism have undetectable levels.

A useful adjunctive test in equivocal situations is the thyrotropin-releasing hormone (TRH) test. A standard dose of this synthetic hypothalamic factor is given intravenously, with serum TSH levels measured before and after administration. Normal persons will have a rise of the serum TSH level while those with toxicity will not. Finally, the 24-hr radioactive iodine 123 uptake test (24-hr RAIU) is useful in all patients with suspected hyperthyroidism to confirm the diagnosis and to differentiate among the various causes of toxicity.

## DIFFERENTIAL DIAGNOSIS

Graves' disease affects primarily women, occurs at any age, is more prevalent in the young, and is characterized by the presence of a diffuse goiter, which may be small and not clinically apparent in older patients. Characteristically, the serum free $T_4$ level is elevated, but in early stages, only the total $T_3$ level may rise. Results of the 24-hr RAIU test are elevated, and thyroid scan reveals a diffuse pattern of uptake. Associated findings may include ophthalmopathy and pretibial myxedema. Toxic multinodular goiter is probably a variant of Graves' disease, also occurring more commonly in women and usually in older patients who have a sizable multinodular goiter. The free $T_4$ level is usually elevated, but only the total $T_3$ level may be increased in some instances. Results of the 24-hr RAIU test may be in the high normal range or only slightly elevated, and scans may show uptake in one or more nodules or in the interstitium. Toxic thyroid adenomas occur in both sexes in older age groups, usually with the presence of a solitary thyroid nodule greater than 2.5 cm. The free $T_4$ level is elevated in the majority of instances, but not infrequently only the total $T_3$ level is elevated. Results of the 24-hr RAIU test are often in the normal range.

Hashimoto's thyroiditis with hyperthyroidism occurs with a female preponderance and is characterized by the presence of a multinodular goiter, an elevated level of free $T_4$ and total $T_3$, and usually an increased 24-hr RAIU (although occasionally the uptake is low). Subacute thyroiditis, a presumed viral illness, occurs with equal frequency in the two sexes and presents with a tender enlargement of one or both lobes of the thyroid, elevation of the free $T_4$ and total $T_3$ levels, an increase in the sedimentation rate to the range of 100 mm/hr, and a decreased to absent 24-hr RAIU. Silent thyroiditis occurs primarily in women and is characterized by the presence of a small nontender goiter, elevation of the level of serum thyroid hormones, and a normal 24-hr RAIU. Iatrogenic or self-induced hyperthyroidism is suspected in patients who have symptoms of hypermetabolism, have no goiter, and have elevation of the free $T_4$ or total $T_3$ level with a totally suppressed 24-hr RAIU level. Finally, patients with hyperthyroidism and either a diffuse or nodular goiter may have iodide-induced hyperthyroidism with increases in the levels of free $T_4$ and total $T_3$. Patients exposed to large doses of exogenous iodide may have depressed RAIU values while those receiving smaller doses may have a normal to elevated uptake.

## ETIOLOGY OF GRAVES' DISEASE

Although the precise cause of Graves' disease is unknown, it is clearly an autoimmune disorder closely akin to Hashimoto's thyroiditis. It is characterized by the presence of TSH receptor antibody of the immunoglobulin G (IgG) and perhaps immunoglobulin M (IgM) type.[3] Various antigens, mainly in thyroid membranes, may be responsible for production of these antibodies, which is enhanced by a defect of an antigen-specific lymphocyte suppressor cell. These stimulating antibodies act through TSH receptors to increase production of cyclic AMP by thyroid cells as well as by increasing iodide uptake, resulting in increased production and secretion of $LT_4$ and $LT_3$. Furthermore, these antibodies may have other target organ effects specifically in the eye, influencing the course of Graves' ophthalmopathy, and in the skin, producing dermopathy, usually pretibial myxedema.

Such antibodies have two potential areas of practical import. First, their presence or absence in varying concentration over time may have prognostic implications. Unfortunately, no current commercially available assay with sufficient specificity and sensitivity permits such use. The therapeutic modalities of surgery and radioactive iodine have the potential only of excising or destroying a portion of the thyroid gland but leaving in place the remainder of that organ that permits not only continued production of hormones but also continued antigenic stimulation of antibody production with adverse effects on the thyroid gland as well as on other target organs. Antithyroid drug therapy with propylthiouracil or methimazole, although not destroying thyroid gland tissue, interrupts the production of thyroid hormone while increasing evidence suggests that these drugs also interfere with the immunopathologic process.

Second, TSH receptor antibodies may be transmitted from the sera of pregnant women across the placenta and may potentially identify neonates at risk for the development of hyperthyroidism even when the mother is euthyroid.

## THIOCARBAMIDES

Thiocarbamide drug therapy for hyperthyroidism has been in clinical use since the 1940s. Such treatment was originally reported to induce metabolic remission in 50 to 70 per cent of patients with Graves' disease, but its popularity plummeted when Wartofsky[42] in 1973 reported a remission rate of only 13.6 per cent.

We,[40] however, found a remission rate of 40 per cent in patients treated between 1968 and 1974, the same period covered by Wartofsky's study. The past decade has been marked by new studies showing improving remission rates of 34 per cent,[37] 38 per cent,[20] 49 per cent,[1] 52 per cent,[41] and 57 per cent.[6] In a 1987 report, Wartofsky's group[33] also found a remission rate of 51 per cent of 69 patients treated with long-term antithyroid therapy between 1973 and 1986 and attributed these more optimistic results to decreasing amounts of iodide in the American diet in the later years.

Some studies have linked these remission rates with thiocarbamide treatment to its effect on the immunologic processes of Graves' disease. Various groups[5, 16, 24] have assessed the relative merits of propylthiouracil and methimazole, dose schedules, and duration of therapy as affecting remission, and others[1, 6, 37, 44, 45] have examined pretreatment and intratreatment prognostic factors.

Weetman et al.[43] summarized well the potential influence of antithyroid drugs on the immunologic basis of Graves' disease versus their direct effects of eliminating the symptoms of hyperthyroidism and their effects of lowering circulating thyroid hormone levels. Regimens employing the beta-blocker propranolol (Inderal) alone, which alleviates symptoms without changing thyroid hormones, produced an average remission rate of 24 per cent while those employing antithyroid drugs with the additional immunologic effect had average remission rates of 46 per cent. Weetman et al.[43] argued that this effect, as measured by suppression of RAIU, was independent of alterations of thyroid hormone levels and decreased levels of TSH receptor antibodies. He suggested that these effects were maximized by both high-dose antithyroid drug therapy as demonstrated by Romaldini et al.,[24] who achieved 75 per cent remission rates compared with 42 per cent rates with lower dose therapy, as well as by duration of therapy as shown by Sugrue et al.,[36] who noted remission rates of 10 per cent with 1 year of therapy versus 51 per cent at 2 years. Tamai et al.[38] also achieved remission rates of 31 per cent after 6 months of therapy and 82 per cent after 2 years of therapy.

After comparing the pharmacology of propylthiouracil and methimazole, Cooper[5] concluded that the latter deserves consideration as the drug of choice in most situations. He pointed out that although similar remission rates are achieved by both drugs and although they are equally effective in lowering serum $T_4$ levels, the half-life of 6 to 8 hours for methimazole versus that of 30 minutes for propylthiouracil permits a once-a-day dose. Furthermore, although both drugs produce a similar 5 per cent rate of minor toxicity, such as rash, fever, and arthralgias, the rarer more severe reactions of hepatic dysfunction and potentially lethal agranulocytosis appear to be less frequent at lower doses of methimazole.

Because of its tighter binding to serum proteins, propylthiouracil would be favored in the treatment of pregnant or lactating women. It is also theoretically more effective in severe hyperthyroidism or thyroid storm because in high doses it also inhibits peripheral $T_4$ to $T_3$ conversion, thereby decreasing serum $T_3$ levels more rapidly.

Greer and colleagues[16] first demonstrated in 1977 that a single daily dose of methimazole was effective in inducing and maintaining the euthyroid state. Shiroozu et al.[32] showed further that once-a-day low-dose methimazole (15 mg) was as effective as a once-a-day higher dose (30 mg) or a divided dose (30 mg) of methimazole in inducing fall of serum thyroid hormone levels. Romaldini et al.[24] demonstrated the effectiveness of higher doses and longer duration of therapy. Sixty-five patients given a high dose of methimazole (60 mg) or propylthiouracil (700 mg) supplemented by liothyronine sodium (Cytomel) for a duration of 12 to 18 months sustained a dramatic remission rate of 75 per cent as opposed to a second group of 48 patients who received a lower dose of methimazole (15 mg) or propylthiouracil (180 mg) a day for a similar duration who sustained a remission rate of only 42 per cent.

Although many patients with Graves' disease will undergo remission with antithyroid therapy, it is clear that many will not, prompting the evaluation of various pretreatment prognostic factors. Our study[40] suggested that relative gland size was a factor with patients having an estimated goiter size of less than 30 g more likely to experience remission. In addition, moderate chemical severity as measured by total $T_4$ was also a factor, with two thirds of patients undergoing remission having serum $T_4$ levels less than 50 per cent above the upper normal range. Takamatsu et al.[37] found that a high pretreatment $T_3$ to $T_4$ ratio was an important prognosticator. Of 36 patients, 21 with high ratios experienced a relapse as opposed to only two of ten with lower $T_3$ to $T_4$ ratios. Allanic et al.[1] evaluated the prognostic value of HLA haplotypes in patients undergoing prolonged antithyroid therapy. Of 40 patients with a positive HLA value, 20 experienced a relapse nearly identical to the 53 per cent of patients with a negative HLA value whose therapy failed, and they concluded that this was not an accurate prognosticator.

In the past decade, interest has continued in the evaluation of changing factors during therapy as a prognostic guide. Although no single factor has emerged, a number of studies[20, 24, 37, 44] have considered a constellation of changes. Romaldini et al.[24] achieved 75 per cent remission rates with high-dose antithyroid therapy and found that depression of the serum $T_4$ below normal levels during therapy was a positive factor, as was a fall in the microsomal antibody titer. Conversely, changes in levels of thyroid-stimulating antibodies during therapy were not predictive, although patients achieving remission had, on average, lower antibody titers at the end of therapy. They did not find that achievement of suppressibility of RAIU by exogenous $T_3$ during therapy was useful. Most studies, however, have found that return of suppressibility of RAIU by thyroid hormone is a favorable prognostic indicator. Yamada et al.[44] found that such suppressibility developed in 65 of 115 patients, with depressed $T_4$ levels also resulting in 43 patients. No patient who met both criteria experienced a relapse. They further found that fall of microsomal antibody titers during therapy correlated with remission. Kawamura et al.[20] noted that return of suppression of RAIU as well as decrease in the size of the goiter during therapy correlated with remission. Changes in serum thyroglobulin levels, although usually paralleling changes in the size of the goiter, proved not to be an independent predictor. Dahlberg et al.[6] achieved a 74 per cent remission rate in patients who had return of suppressibility during therapy as measured by TRH tests compared with only 29 per cent remission in patients whose TRH tests did not revert to normal levels. Finally, Takamatsu et al.[37] confirmed that return to a normal $T_3$ to $T_4$ ratio during therapy was an important predictor of potential response. Of 30 patients having a fall of the $T_3$ to $T_4$ ratio during treatment, 50 per cent entered remission while 80 per cent of ten patients who had normal $T_3$ to $T_4$ ratios initially sustained remission.

## *Selection of the Patient for Medical Therapy*

Despite improving remission rates, a noteworthy minority of patients will not undergo remission even with prolonged therapy, such as the 8-year average course employed by Yamamoto et al.[45] in which one third of patients experienced a relapse. It is, therefore, crucial to determine the best subset of patients for whom to consider such therapy. This group would include patients with a relatively small goiter and moderate severity of disease as measured by free $T_4$ levels and $T_3$ to $T_4$ ratios of less than 20. Treatment may be with a single daily dose of methimazole or divided doses of propylthiouracil or with larger doses of either that are supplemented by thyroid hormone and should be sustained for 12 to 18 months. Patients manifesting return of normal thyroid suppressibility by virtue of an appreciable fall of serum $T_4$, decreasing $T_3$ to $T_4$ ratio, normal results on TRH test, or suppressibility of RAIU can have a tapering of and ultimate discontinuance of treatment in anticipation of permanent remission. Patients whose disease is not controlled by therapy or who experience relapse on tapering or discontinuance of drugs are considered for alternative therapy with radioactive iodine or surgery.

## RADIOACTIVE IODINE TREATMENT

Radioactive iodine therapy, available for 45 years, has proved to be an effective treatment for patients with Graves' disease. It is also of value in the treatment of patients with hyperthyroidism associated with a multinodular goiter or with a single toxic adenoma. Concerns regarding its complications have focused on the well-documented one of hypothyroidism and the potential ones of carcinogenesis and mutagenesis.

### *Graves' Disease*

By the early 1960s, longitudinal studies[9] demonstrated a striking incidence of hypothyroidism of some 20 per cent during the first 2 years increasing at 2 to 3 per cent a year thereafter to more than 50 per cent by 15 years when conventional doses of radioactive iodine were employed (120 μc of $^{131}$I delivered per estimated gram of thyroid tissue). Therefore, in the 1960s, "low-dose $^{131}$ I therapy," averaging half previous doses, was initiated, and Hagen et al.[18] reported encouragingly low incidences of hypothyroidism in early years after radioactive iodine therapy. Subsequently, however, the same group[4] noted more pessimistic results with less adequate control of hyperthyroidism in the early post-treatment period and increasing incidences of hypothyroidism in later years approaching those incurred with higher treatment doses. Glennon et al.[13] reported similar results with even smaller doses of radioactive iodine. With these experiences in mind, Roudebush et al.[27] employed a technique referred to as compensated low-dose radioactive iodine therapy in which patients with small thyroid glands were given lower relative doses of radioactive iodine, that is, as little as 40 μg/g for normal-sized glands and up to 100 μg/g for huge glands. Despite their initial optimism, subsequent reports[14, 34] utilizing this technique have been discouraging. Sridama et al.[34] found only 12 per cent hypothyroidism at the end of 1 year but noted a cumulative incidence of 76 per cent by the 11th year. Likewise, Goolden and Stewart[14] also noted only 10 per cent hypothyroidism at 1 year but a cumulative incidence of 53 per cent by 15 years. Furthermore, 20 per cent of their patients required post-treatment antithyroid therapy until achieving remission, and 17 per cent of their patients required a second course of radioactive iodine therapy.

Schimmel and Utiger[30] suggested that treatment with stable potassium iodide immediately after radioactive iodine therapy produced only a transient decrease in serum $T_4$ to the hypothyroid ranges as well as inducing prompt control of toxicity. Ross et al.[26] employed this technique in one half of patients treated with radioactive iodine between 1968 and 1981. Although they thought that adjuvant stable iodide therapy effected control more rapidly, they found a higher incidence of transient hypothyroidism early and ultimately a high long-term incidence of hypothyroidism.

Although permanent hypometabolism may be anticipated in a majority of patients, Sawers et al.[29] and we[17] have cautioned that an appreciable number of patients in whom hypothyroidism developed within 4 months of therapy will ultimately spontaneously revert to the euthyroid state. Therefore, such patients should be reassessed for the necessity of permanent hormone replacement.

The risk of carcinogenesis was evaluated in a cooperative study[7] involving 35,000 adult patients treated for hyperthyroidism between 1946 and 1968; 25,000 patients with Graves' disease without a palpable thyroid nodule were included. Of these, two thirds were treated with radioactive iodine, nearly one third with surgery, and only a small percentage with antithyroid drugs alone. As anticipated, more thyroid carcinomas were discovered within 1 year of operation in the surgically treated group, but most of these carcinomas were occult lesions. Patients treated with radioactive iodine were followed up for up to 22 years, and the occurrence of thyroid carcinoma in this group was no higher than predicted from the experience with the surgical group. In fact, the incidence was only 1 per 1,200 compared with 2 per 1,000 in the surgically and medically treated groups. Studies[12, 28, 31] have shown no higher incidence of thyroid carcinoma in adolescents and children treated with radioactive iodine. Hamburger's[19] report of 262 children and adolescents treated between 1961 and 1984 has solidified a place for radioactive iodine therapy in young persons. Less than one quarter of 182 patients originally treated with medical therapy remained in remission for more than 2 years; 72 had initial treatment with radioactive iodine, and an additional 118 had radioactive iodine as secondary therapy. Of 53 pregnancies occurring subsequently in patients so treated, 49 resulted in a normal delivery and only two in spontaneous abortion. One hydrocephalic child and one hyperactive child were born to mothers in this group.

Graham and Burman[15] have extensively reviewed the teratogenic risks of radioactive iodine therapy. They emphasized that such damage may occur only after the tenth week of pregnancy at which point the fetal thyroid gland is able to trap iodine. Regarding the potential for genetic damage, they pointed out that an estimated gonadal dose of 3 cGy from an average treatment was likely to be no higher than that received in the course of a barium enema study or intravenous pyelography. Stoffer and Hamburger[35] reported a survey of 182 patients inadvertently treated during pregnancy with radioactive iodine. Two pregnancies terminated in spontaneous abortion and two others in stillbirth, and two infants were born with appreciable anomalies. The rates of these complications were no greater than anticipated in normal pregnancy. They pointed out, however, that six of 178 of the neonates were born with hypothyroidism. Therefore, radioactive iodine therapy is considered contraindicated during pregnancy, and pregnancy is best deferred when possible for 6 months after such therapy.

### *Toxic Adenoma*

Toxic thyroid adenomas usually are larger than 2.5 cm, and although the smallest among them had always been considered amenable to radioactive iodine therapy, it had been thought that larger ones would be responsive only to large doses of radioactive iodine and were often best treated by surgical excision. Ross et al.[25] reported that of 45 patients with toxic nodules treated between 1968 and 1980 with relatively low doses (5 to 15 μc) of radioactive iodine, most patients had residual small nodules, and 91 per cent were euthyroid by 6 months and 93 per cent by 1 year, with only three of the 45 requiring second treatments. Clinical hypothyroidism did not develop during a follow-up period of 1 to 9 years.

At the Lahey clinic, the initial treatment of choice for patients with a toxic adenoma is with a fuller dose of 30 μc of radioactive iodine ($^{131}I$), which we believe minimizes the possibility of a residual functional nodule without increased risk of hypothyroidism. Surgical excision is reserved for huge toxic nodules or rare nodules resistant to radioactive iodine.

## SURGICAL TREATMENT

### *Preoperative Preparation*

Until 20 years ago, the traditional preoperative preparation for surgery included a minimum of 6 weeks of thiocarbamide antithyroid therapy with a 10-day course of potassium iodide immediately before operation to reduce vascularity of the gland. Disadvantages of this regimen included the long preparation time and the potential continued vascularity of the gland from the antithyroid drug therapy.

With the availability of the short-acting beta-blocker propranolol in the late 1960s, that drug was employed as a sole pharmacologic preoperative treatment by a number of groups.[3, 21, 39] Such a regimen had the advantage of a shorter preparation time of approximately 3 weeks and decreased vascularity of the gland at operation with less resultant blood loss. Problems included the requirement of frequent administration of the short-acting propranolol and the variable doses required for the control of the pulse rate. Furthermore, patients coming to operation still had elevated free $T_4$ levels, although $T_3$ levels were reduced somewhat by the drug's inhibition of peripheral $T_4$ to $T_3$ conversion. This, of course, resulted in less stable metabolic status in the perioperative time frame. Feek et al.[10] and Michie et al.[22] pretreated patients with a 3-week course of propranolol as well as a 10-day course of potassium iodide. This schedule had the added advantage of lowering the $T_4$ level to normal range by the time of operation but was still subject to the poor predictability of the appropriate dose of propranolol. Overdoses led to hypoglycemia, impaired stress cortisol response, and bradycardia. Undertreatment resulted in continuing tachycardia.

Peden et al.[23] treated one group of patients with 3 weeks of propranolol alone, a second with propranolol and potassium iodide for 10 days, and the third with nadolol, a long-acting beta-adrenergic antagonist for 3 weeks as well as with potassium iodide for 10 days. The third group[23] had a consistent normalizing of the heart rate with a predictable dose of 160 mg/d as well as a normalizing of the $T_4$ and $T_3$ levels preoperatively and a smooth postoperative course. This latter regimen, therefore, is currently the preparation of choice for patients undergoing thyroidectomy as a primary treatment modality.

Patients whose primary therapy with antithyroid drugs has failed may best be prepared by an increase of drug to attain the euthyroid state and the preoperative addition of potassium iodide for 10 days.

## *Complications of Thyroidectomy for Graves' Disease*

Hypothyroidism represents the most frequent complication of thyroidectomy. Although it has been reported in incidences up to 49 per cent with linear increases over time, the true frequency in experienced hands is probably lower. Sridama et al.[34] reported 19 per cent hypothyroidism rates after 1 year rising to only 27 per cent at 11 years. They thought that this continuing increase was likely to occur in glands affected by a destructive immunologic process, possibly coexistent Hashimoto's thyroiditis, after they noted a 41 per cent incidence of hypometabolism in patients with positive thyroglobulin antibodies as opposed to a 25 per cent incidence in patients with a negative titer. Similarly, hypothyroidism developed in 30 per cent of their patients with a positive microsomal antibody titer. Bradley and Liechty,[2] in an attempt to decrease the frequency of this complication, employed modified subtotal thyroidectomy leaving an estimated 5-g thyroid remnant as opposed to standard procedures leaving 1 to 3 g. They found a 6 per cent incidence of recurrent hyperthyroidism but only a 2 per cent incidence of hypothyroidism after an average follow-up of 5 years.

Relapse or recurrent hyperthyroidism after operation is much less frequent, with reported incidences of 1 to 12 per cent. The frequency of other important permanent complications has been estimated by Foster et al.,[11] with hypoparathyroidism occurring in up to 3.5 per cent of patients and vocal cord paralysis in 0.2 per cent. Perioperative mortality, although rare, occurs as a result of anesthesia or operative mishap.

## *Place of Surgery in the Treatment of Hyperthyroidism*

In summary, the use of surgery for patients with hyperthyroidism has declined in recent years. For Graves' disease, its use is mainly limited to children and adolescents whose antithyroid therapy has failed, although it must be cautioned that complications of thyroid surgery in this younger age group are more frequent than in older patients. It may also be required in the second trimester of pregnancy for patients whose hyperthyroidism cannot be controlled with low doses of antithyroid drugs. In the older age group with Graves' disease, surgical indications are limited to patients with a coexistent nodule that is hypofunctional by scan and to patients whose antithyroid drug therapy has failed or who refuse radioactive iodine. Surgical therapy of a patient with a toxic multinodular goiter is likewise limited to patients whose radioactive iodine therapy has failed or who have a suspicious hypofunctional nodule. The role of surgical therapy of a solitary toxic adenoma has also diminished since the recent discovery of the efficacy of smaller doses of radioactive iodine in treating this condition.

Finally, before considering surgery, care must be exercised in excluding causes of hyperthyroidism that are responsive to conservative therapy, such as Hashimoto's thyroiditis, subacute thyroiditis, or painless or postpartum thyroiditis.

## REFERENCES

1. Allanic, H., Fauchet, R., Lorcy, Y., et al.: A prospective study of the relationship between relapse of hyperthyroid Graves' disease after antithyroid drugs and HLA haplotype. J. Clin. Endocrinol. Metab., 57:719–722, 1983.
2. Bradley, E. L., III, and Liechty, R. D.: Modified

subtotal thyroidectomy for Graves' disease: A two-institution study. Surgery, *94*:955–958, 1983.
3. Burman, K. D., and Baker, J. R., Jr.: Immune mechanisms in Graves' disease. Endocr. Rev., *6*:183–232, 1985.
4. Cevallos, J. L., Hagen, G. A., Maloof, F., and Chapman, E. M.: Low-dosage 131-I therapy of thyrotoxicosis (diffuse goiters): A five year follow-up study. N. Engl. J. Med., *290*:141–143, 1974.
5. Cooper, D. S.: Which anti-thyroid drug? Am. J. Med., *80*:1165–1168, 1986.
6. Dahlberg, P. A., Karlsson, F. A., Jansson, R., and Wide, L.: Thyrotropin-releasing hormone testing during antithyroid drug treatment of Graves' disease as an indicator of remission. J. Clin. Endocrinol. Metab., *61*:1100–1104, 1985.
7. Dobyns, B. M., Sheline, G. E., Workman, J. B., et al.: Malignant and benign neoplasms of the thyroid in patients treated for hyperthyroidism: A report of the cooperative thyrotoxicosis therapy follow-up study. J. Clin. Endocrinol. Metab., *38*:976–998, 1974.
8. Dunn, J. T.: Choice of therapy in young adults with hyperthyroidism of Graves' disease: A brief, case-directed poll of 54 thyroidologists. Ann. Intern. Med., *100*:891–893, 1984.
9. Dunn, J. T., and Chapman, E. M.: Rising incidence of hypothyroidism after radioactive-iodine therapy in thyrotoxicosis. N. Engl. J. Med., *271*:1037–1042, 1964.
10. Feek, C. M., Sawers, J. S., Irvine, W. J., et al.: Combination of potassium iodide and propranolol in preparation of patients with Graves' disease for thyroid surgery. N. Engl. J. Med., *302*:883–885, 1980.
11. Foster, R. S., Jr.: Morbidity and mortality after thyroidectomy. Surg. Gynecol. Obstet., *146*:423–429, 1978.
12. Fretas, J. E., Swanson, D. P., Gross, M. D., and Sisson, J. C.: Iodine-131: Optimal therapy for hyperthyroidism in children and adolescents? J. Nucl. Med., *20*:847–850, 1979.
13. Glennon, J. A., Gordon, E. S., and Sawin, C. T.: Hypothyroidism after low-dose $^{131}$I treatment of hyperthyroidism. Ann. Intern. Med., *76*:721–723, 1972.
14. Goolden, A. W., and Stewart, J. S.: Long-term results from graded low dose radioactive iodine therapy for thyrotoxicosis. Clin. Endocrinol., *24*:217–222, 1986.
15. Graham, G. D., and Burman, K. D.: Radioiodine treatment of Graves' disease: An assessment of its potential risks. Ann. Intern. Med., *105*:900–905, 1986.
16. Greer, M. A., Kammer, H., and Bouma, D. J.: Short-term antithyroid-drug therapy for the thyrotoxicosis of Graves' disease. N. Engl. J. Med., *297*:173–176, 1977.
17. Gresham, D. G., and Wool, M. S.: Hypothyroidism after radioiodine therapy for Graves' disease: Is its incidence increasing? Postgrad. Med., *75*:299–305, 1984.
18. Hagen, G. A., Ouellette, R. P., and Chapman, E. M.: Comparison of high and low dosage levels of 131-I in the treatment of thyrotoxicosis. N. Engl. J. Med., *277*:559–562, 1967.
19. Hamburger, J. I.: Management of hyperthyroidism in children and adolescents. J. Clin. Endocrinol. Metab., *60*:1019–1024, 1985.
20. Kawamura, S., Kishino, B., Tajima, K., et al.: Serum thyroglobulin changes in patients with Graves' disease treated with long term antithyroid drug therapy. J. Clin. Endocrinol. Metab., *56*:507–512, 1983.
21. Lee, T. C., Coffey, R. J., Mackin, J., et al.: The use of propranolol in the surgical treatment of thyrotoxic patients. Ann. Surg., *177*:643–647, 1973.
22. Michie, W., Hamer-Hodges, D. W., Pegg, C. A. S., et al.: Beta-blockade and partial thyroidectomy for thyrotoxicosis. Lancet, *1*:1009–1011, 1974.
23. Peden, N. R., Browning, M. C., Feely, J., et al.: The clinical and metabolic responses to early surgical treatment for hyperthyroid Graves' disease: A comparison of three pre-operative treatment regimes. Q. J. Med., *56*:579–591, 1985.
24. Romaldini, J. H., Bromberg, N., Werner, R. S., et al.: Comparison of effects of high and low dosage regimens of antithyroid drugs in the management of Graves' hyperthyroidism. J. Clin. Endocrinol. Metab., *57*:563–570, 1983.
25. Ross, D. S., Ridgway, E. C., and Daniels, G. H.: Successful treatment of solitary toxic thyroid nodules with relatively low-dose iodine-131 with low prevalence of hypothyroidism. Ann. Intern. Med., *101*:488–490, 1984.
26. Ross, D. S., Daniels, G. H., De Stephano, P., et al.: Use of adjunctive potassium iodide after radioactive iodine ($^{131}$I) treatment of Graves' hyperthyroidism. J. Clin. Endocrinol. Metab., *57*:250–253, 1983.
27. Roudebush, C. P., Hoye, K. E., and DeGroot, L. J.: Compensated low-dose $^{131}$I therapy of Graves' disease. Ann. Intern. Med., *87*:441–443, 1977.
28. Safa, A. M., Schumacher, O. P., and Rodriguez-Antunez, A.: Long-term follow-up results in children and adolescents treated with radioactive iodine (131I) for hyperthyroidism. N. Engl. J. Med., *292*:167–171, 1975.
29. Sawer, J. S., Toft, A. D., Irvine, W. J., et al.: Transient hypothyroidism after iodine-131 treatment of thyrotoxicosis. J. Clin. Endocrinol. Metab., *50*:226–229, 1980.
30. Schimmel, M., and Utiger, R. D.: Acute effect of inorganic iodide after 131I therapy for hyperthyroidism. Clin. Endocrinol., *6*:329–332, 1977.
31. Sheline, G. E., Lindsay, S., and Bell, H. G.: Occurrence of thyroid nodules in children following therapy with radioiodine for hyperthyroidism. J. Clin. Endocrinol. Metab., *19*:127–137, 1959.
32. Shiroozu, A., Okamura, K., Ikenoue, H., et al.: Treatment of hyperthyroidism with a small single daily dose of methimazole. J. Clin. Endocrinol. Metab., *63*:125–128, 1986.
33. Solomon, B. L., Evaul, J. E., Burman, K. D., and Wartofsky, L.: Remission rates with antithyroid drug therapy: Continuing influence of iodine uptake? Ann. Intern. Med., *107*:510–512, 1987.
34. Sridama, V., McCormack, M., Kaplan, E. L., et al.: Long-term follow-up study of compensated low-dose 131I therapy for Graves' disease. N. Engl. J. Med., *311*:426–432, 1984.
35. Stoffer, S. S., and Hamburger, J. I.: Inadvertent 131I therapy for hyperthyroidism in the first trimester of pregnancy. J. Nucl. Med., *17*:146–149, 1976.

36. Sugrue, D., McEvoy, M., Feely, J., and Drury, M. I.: Hyperthyroidism in the land of Graves: Results of treatment by surgery, radio-iodine and carbimazole in 837 cases. Q. J. Med., *49*:51–61, 1980.
37. Takamatsu, J., Kuma, K., and Mozai, T.: Serum triiodothyronine to thyroxine ratio: A newly recognized predictor of the outcome of hyperthyroidism due to Graves' disease. J. Clin. Endocrinol. Metab., *62*:980–983, 1986.
38. Tamai, H., Nakagawa, T., Fukino, O., et al.: Thionamide therapy in Graves' disease: Relation of relapse rate to duration of therapy. Ann. Intern. Med., *92*:488–490, 1980.
39. Toft, A. D., Irvine, W. J., McIntosh, D., et al.: Temporary hypothyroidism after surgical treatment of thyrotoxicosis. Lancet, *2*:817–818, 1976.
40. Totten, M. A., and Wool, M. S.: Medical treatment of hyperthyroidism. Med. Clin. North Am., *63*:321–328, 1979.
41. van Ouwerkerk, B. M., Krenning, E. P., Docter, R., et al.: Cellular and humoral immunity in patients with hyperthyroid Graves' disease before, during and after antithyroid drug treatment. Clin. Endocrinol., *26*:385–394, 1987.
42. Wartofsky, L.: Low remission after therapy for Graves disease: Possible relation of dietary iodine with antithyroid therapy results. J.A.M.A., *226*:1083–1088, 1973.
43. Weetman, A. P., McGregor, A. M., and Hall, R.: Evidence for an effect of antithyroid drugs on the natural history of Graves' disease. Clin. Endocrinol., *21*:163–172, 1984.
44. Yamada, T., Koizumi, Y., Sato, A., et al.: Reappraisal of the 3,5,3′-triiodothyronine-suppression test and the prediction of long term outcome of antithyroid drug therapy in patients with hyperthyroid Graves' disease. J. Clin. Endocrinol. Metab., *58*:676–680, 1984.
45. Yamamoto, M., Totsuka, Y., Kojima, I., et al.: Outcome of patients with Graves' disease after long-term medical treatment guided by triiodothyronine ($T_3$) suppression test. Clin. Endocrinol., *19*:467–476, 1983.

# 12

# NONTOXIC MULTINODULAR GOITER AND MEDIASTINAL GOITER

*Laura E. Sanders, M.D., and Ricardo L. Rossi, M.D.*

With the increasing use of new diagnostic tools, such as ultrasonography of small parts of the neck, nontoxic multinodular goiter is an increasingly common diagnosis. The two major indications for surgery are for suspected carcinoma and for the possible effects of local compression, particularly in goiters that extend into the mediastinum.

## ETIOLOGY

Nontoxic goiter may be endemic or sporadic. Although endemic goiter can result from iodine deficiency, this is becoming less common with dietary supplements. The traditionally accepted cause of sporadic goiter is a defect in hormone manufacture leading to overstimulation of the gland,[6] but the normal thyroid-stimulating hormone (TSH) level in most patients with goiter argues against this theory. Radiation to the head or neck in childhood increases the incidence of both benign and malignant nodules. Other explanations that have been suggested are a thyroid growth immunoglobulin and occasional extrinsic goitrogens, such as lithium or iodides.[6] None of these theories explain the development of nodularity in long-standing nontoxic goiter, which has usually been attributed to developing areas of hyperplasia with involution or atrophy of the remaining gland.[6]

## CLINICAL PRESENTATION

Nodular goiter is more common in women than in men. Palpable nodules can be found in 4 to 7 per cent of American adults, although ultrasonography can identify nodules in up to 50 per cent of adults more than 50 years of age.[4] Symptoms of nontoxic goiter are related to compression and depend on location. In the neck, they can create cosmetic problems or a feeling of tightness. In the mediastinum, goiters may cause dyspnea, chest pain, stridor, or dysphagia, often worse with recumbency. Patients may be asymptomatic even with considerable compression of the airway. Superior vena cava syndrome and even (albeit rarely) Horner's syndrome resulting from a benign goiter have been reported.[13]

In the neck, a goiter of any size is clinically apparent. A mediastinal goiter is sometimes noted on radiography of the chest as the incidental finding of a mass displacing the hyoid, trachea, and larynx and compressing the trachea or esophagus or both. Sometimes calcifications are present. Computed tomography of the chest will further define the mass and its location relative to other mediastinal structures.[14] Radioactive iodine scanning may be helpful only when results are positive. Mediastinal thyroid tissue may not concentrate the tracer as will thyroid tissue in the neck. Although the radioactive iodine scan may not show an abnormality, intrathoracic goiter cannot be ruled out.[13, 14] Pulmonary function tests often may confirm an obstructive deficit caused by tracheal compression.[7]

## DIFFERENTIAL DIAGNOSIS

In the evaluation of patients with a multinodular goiter, the burden of proof rests on the clinician to rule out carcinoma. In a study[11] comparing the incidence of carcinoma and solitary cold nodules versus multinodular goiter, it was found that in both groups the incidence of carcinoma was similar—13 and 17 per cent. In other studies,[14] the rates ranged from 1 to 16 per cent.

For accessible nodules in the euthyroid patient, fine needle aspiration biopsy is becoming accepted as the initial diagnostic study. Any palpable nodule, especially the dominant nodule or one increasing in size, should undergo needle aspiration.[12] Although thyroid scans are no longer being performed routinely, they can be useful for showing whether a nodule in a hyperthyroid patient is autonomous and thus is suppressing the rest of the gland. Ultrasonography can be used to check the size of a nodule or to locate a nonpalpable nodule on follow-up study.

## TREATMENT

The treatments currently in use for a patient with a multinodular nontoxic goiter that is not thought to be malignant are hormone suppression, radioactive iodine, and surgery. When given, radioactive iodine may induce hyperthyroidism (jodbasedow).[6] Suppressive thyroid therapy has been used widely in an attempt to control growth of a nodule but is not clearly useful for this purpose. A study[4] showed that 6 months of thyroid suppression did not shrink thyroid nodules appreciably as seen on serial ultrasonography. Moreover, physical examination can be misleading in determining the size of a nodule because shrinkage of tissue around a nodule can mimic shrinkage of the nodule itself. The rationale for this treatment had been based on the conjecture that multinodular goiter arises from the action of TSH acting on a gland that is defective in the manufacture of the hormone, a theory that has fallen from favor.[6]

Use of radioactive iodine has gained some support,[5, 8] and it has been shown to shrink a goiter and relieve symptoms, with the occasional complication of hypothyroidism. This treatment is particularly appropriate in the patient who has a strong medical contraindication to surgery or has a recurrent goiter. It is less effective for a mediastinal goiter because, especially in the elderly patient, radioactive iodine can produce an acute inflammatory reaction with obstruction of the airway.

The surgical indications for a patient with a nontoxic goiter are for cosmetic reasons, for suspicion of carcinoma, for respiratory symptoms, and for substernal goiter. Our usual treatment for patients with a multinodular goiter is bilateral subtotal thyroidectomy with meticulous protection of recurrent laryngeal nerves, superior laryngeal nerves, and parathyroid glands. All patients should receive thyroid hormone replacement therapy after operation, both in an attempt to prevent further enlargement of the gland (although the effectiveness of this practice is not clear[3]) and to avert hypothyroidism after thyroidectomy.

## MEDIASTINAL GOITER

The mediastinal goiter presents a separate set of surgical issues because of its inaccessibility to biopsy and the compressive effect of an expanding mass within the confined space of the chest. An intrathoracic goiter almost always arises from intrathoracic extension of the surgical gland. Lahey[9, 10] described the boundaries of the thyroid: superiorly, the thyroid and hyoid cartilages; anteriorly, the sternocleidomastoid muscle and strap muscles; and posteriorly, the trachea and prevertebral fascia. The path of least resistance is downward into the chest pulled by gravity and by the motions of swallowing and respiration.

Lahey[9, 10] believed that all intrathoracic goiters originated in a cervical gland. An occasional report[2] has described an ectopic thyroid arising primarily in the chest with an intrathoracic vascular pedicle, although this finding is extremely unusual.

The incidence of mediastinal goiter ranges from 1 to 20 per cent.[1, 14] For a totally intrathoracic goiter, the incidence is less than 1 per cent.[14] Of these goiters, 75 to 94 per cent are anterior to the recurrent laryngeal nerves and to the subclavian innominate vessels. Posterior mediastinal goiter, making up another 10 to 25 per cent, may descend behind the innominate vein, carotid artery, innominate and subclavian arteries, recurrent laryngeal nerve, and inferior thyroid arteries and is more often on the right side than on the left side. Occasionally a goiter may cross to the contralateral side even behind the esophagus.[14] A substantial number of patients (one fifth in one series[7]) have had previous thyroid surgery.

Most patients with an intrathoracic goiter are symptomatic because of compression of structures within the chest. Dyspnea, cough, neck swelling, stridor, and choking with recumbency are common. Patients may also have dysphagia, pain, superior vena cava syndrome, or Horner's syndrome. Rarely, abscess, hemorrhage, or venous distention may occur. The cervical part of the gland may not be palpably enlarged, even with a large intrathoracic goiter.[14]

The diagnosis of a mediastinal goiter can often (90 per cent[7]) be made from radiography of the chest showing a mass and tracheal displacement. The size of the goiter and its relation to other chest structures can be delineated further by computed tomography of the chest and by barium swallow. Scans after administration of radioactive iodine, as explained earlier, are so insensitive for thyroid tissue within the chest that they are useful only when results are positive. Pulmonary function tests may confirm respiratory compromise.

In patients without strong medical contraindications to surgery, a mediastinal goiter should be removed surgically. The natural history of these goiters is progressive expansion, making surgery increasingly difficult, with the possibility of a sudden expansion from hemorrhage causing respiratory compromise. Carcinoma occurs in 1 to 16 per cent of these goiters, just as it does in cervical glands, but they are not accessible to needle biopsy.[14]

Because of the cervical location of the vascular pedicle of the goiter, almost all intrathoracic glands can be removed through a collar incision. A partial or complete median sternotomy is occasionally necessary when the gland is large or fixed by inflammatory response. Consultation with a thoracic surgeon preoperatively is helpful in case this assistance is needed. After the cervical portion of the gland has been mobilized and the recurrent laryngeal nerves and parathyroid glands have been identified (the inferior gland can be displaced by a large goiter), the thoracic component can often be mobilized and delivered through the thoracic inlet. Lahey[9, 10] suggested fragmentation (morcellation) of the large gland that is difficult to deliver. When removal of the gland from the neck is prohibitively difficult, especially when the recurrent laryngeal nerve and parathyroid glands are at risk and the gland cannot be mobilized readily, partial or complete median sternotomy should be performed.[13] For the contralateral retrotracheal or retroesophageal posterior mediastinal goiter, a combined cervical and thoracic approach is recommended to permit optimal control of cervical and mediastinal vessels and protection of the recurrent laryngeal nerves.[14]

## REFERENCES


1. deSouza, F. M., and Smith, P. E.: Retrosternal goiter. J. Otolaryngol., *12*:393–396, 1983.
2. Falor, W. H., Kelly, T. R., and Jackson, J. B.: Intrathoracic goiter. Surg. Gynecol. Obstet., *117*:604–610, 1963.
3. Gerdsen, J. P., and Frølund, L.: Recurrence of nontoxic goitre with and without postoperative

thyroxine medication. Clin. Endocrinol., *21*:529–533, 1984.
4. Gharib, H., James, E. M., Charboneau, J. W., et al.: Suppressive therapy with levothyroxine for solitary thyroid nodules: A double-blind controlled clinical study. N. Engl. J. Med., *317*:70–75, 1987.
5. Hegedüs, L., Hansen, B. M., Knudsen, N., and Hansen, J. M.: Reduction of size of thyroid with radioactive iodine in multinodular non-toxic goitre. Br. Med. J., *297*:661–662, 1988.
6. Ingbar, S. H.: The thyroid gland. *In* Wilson, J. D., and Foster, D. W. (eds.): Williams Textbook of Endocrinology. 7th edition. Philadelphia, W. B. Saunders Co., 1985, pp. 682–815.
7. Katlic, M. R., Grillo, H. C., and Wang, C-A.: Substernal goiter: Analysis of 80 patients from Massachusetts General Hospital. Am. J. Surg., *149*:283–287, 1985.
8. Kay, T. W. H., d'Emden, M. C., Andrews, J. T., and Martin, F. I. R.: Treatment of non-toxic multinodular goiter with radioactive iodine. Am. J. Med., *84*:19–22, 1988.
9. Lahey, F. H.: Intrathoracic goiters. Surg. Clin. North Am., *25*:609–618, 1945.
10. Lahey, F. H., and Swinton, N. W.: Intrathoracic goiter. Surg. Gynecol. Obstet., *59*:627–637, 1934.
11. McCall, A., Jarosz, H., Lawrence, A. M., and Paloyan, E.: The incidence of thyroid carcinoma in solitary cold nodules and in multinodular goiters. Surgery, *100*:1128–1131, 1986.
12. Reeves, T.: Multinodular goiter. *In* Kempczinski, R. (ed.): Common Problems in Endocrine Surgery. Chicago, Year Book Medical Publishers, Inc., 1989, pp. 114–118.
13. Sand, M. E., Laws, H. L., and McElvein, R. B.: Substernal and intrathoracic goiter: Reconsideration of surgical approach. Am. Surg., *49*:196–202, 1983.
14. Shahian, D. M., and Rossi, R. L.: Posterior mediastinal goiter. Chest, *94*:599–602, 1988.

# 13

# THYROIDITIS

*Marvin S. Wool, M.D.*

The spectrum of the five types of thyroiditis is characterized by heterogeneous causes and variable prevalences. In only two of the conditions is surgical intervention indicated with any frequency, but acquaintance with the syndromes of all five types is important in the differential diagnosis.

## CHRONIC LYMPHOCYTIC (HASHIMOTO'S) THYROIDITIS

Although Hashimoto's thyroiditis was first described 68 years ago,[6] only in the last 30 years has its prevalence been appreciated. A member of the family of autoimmune diseases, it is characterized by goiter, often with hypothyroidism, and may also be associated with Addison's disease, primary gonadal failure, pernicious anemia, and diabetes mellitus. The disease occurs primarily in women and rarely in men, with a strong familial prevalence of thyroid disorders.

Initial presentation is usually with the discovery of a painless goiter, which is bilateral, with a finely nodular and occasionally nodular consistency. Cervical lymphadenopathy and systemic symptoms are rare unless concurrent hypothyroidism or rarely hyperthyroidism is present.

The most characteristic laboratory finding in 50 to 90 per cent of patients is that of thyroid antibodies in sera, often in titers of greater than 1/1600. The microsomal antibody test is the most sensitive test, and little indication exists for use of the less sensitive thyroglobulin antibody assay. Most often the serum free $T_4$ level is in the normal range, but in a large minority of patients, it is depressed. Rarely, the free $T_4$ level is elevated, producing the transient condition of Hashimoto's toxicosis. In patients whose free $T_4$ level is normal, the serum thyroid-stimulating hormone (TSH) level is modestly elevated, helping to confirm the diagnosis.

Therefore, the presence of a bilateral goiter with serum tests indicating a low free $T_4$ level and an elevated TSH level, a normal free $T_4$ level and an elevated TSH level, or normal free $T_4$ and TSH levels with a high microsomal antibody titer is sufficient to establish the diagnosis without fine needle aspiration biopsy. The latter is indicated only when a predominant nodule, which proves hypofunctional by thyroid scan, is present or there is cervical adenopathy and a diagnosis of carcinoma or lymphoma is suspected.

The initial and most often only required therapy is oral thyroid hormone (L-thyroxine), which serves as replacement therapy in hypothyroidism and for suppression of serum

TSH stimulation of the thyroid, which often accomplishes shrinkage of the goiter. Occasionally, the goiter is unchanged and may even increase diffusely in size, possibly because of the presence of thyroid growth-stimulating immunoglobulins.[14] In such instances, subtotal thyroidectomy may be indicated when signs and symptoms of mechanical obstruction occur. Signs include deviation and narrowing of the trachea and evidence of venous distention. Symptoms include postural dyspnea (occurring when the patient is supine or lies on one side or the other), less commonly dysphagia for dry foods or meat, and rarely persistent hoarseness because of compression of a recurrent laryngeal nerve.

A second indication for surgery is suspicion of coexistent thyroid carcinoma or intrathyroidal lymphoma. Questions of a higher prevalence of thyroid carcinoma in chronic thyroiditis were elicited by a retrospective study by Hirabayashi and Lindsay,[8] who reviewed the histology of 9,000 thyroidectomies performed between 1920 and 1963 and found that 22 per cent of glands with histologic evidence of thyroiditis manifested coexistent carcinoma while only 2.5 per cent of glands without thyroiditis harbored carcinoma. Dailey et al.[2] and Woolner et al.[15] studied 600 thyroid glands surgically removed from 1930 to 1936 with a diagnosis of lymphocytic thyroiditis. They found that only 3 per cent had coexistent carcinoma and that all patients had only focal thyroiditis rather than diffuse thyroiditis, suggesting that the inflammatory histologic reaction was secondary to the tumor rather than the cause. An important finding was a 2 per cent incidence of lymphoma.

Holm et al.[9] definitively showed that although the incidence of thyroid carcinoma was no higher in chronic lymphocytic thyroiditis goiters than in colloid goiters, the incidence of malignant lymphoma was clearly higher. Between 1959 and 1978, 829 patients with chronic lymphocytic thyroiditis and an equal number with colloid goiter as proved by needle biopsy were followed up through 1981. Thyroid carcinoma developed in only two patients in each group, a threefold increase over what was predicted in the general population. On the other hand, in 12 patients in the thyroiditis group, a myeloproliferative disorder developed, including four malignant lymphomas of the thyroid gland, which represented a relative risk of these types of malignant lesions 67-fold greater than the general population. These lymphomas became manifest between 17 and 145 months after the initial diagnosis of goiter.

Therefore, patients with a goiter from chronic lymphocytic thyroiditis who present with a dominant hypofunctional nodule or in whom such a nodule develops while the patient is taking thyroid hormone therapy should be considered at low risk for the development of thyroid carcinoma but at an importantly greater risk for the development of lymphoma. They should be considered for needle aspiration biopsy and possible thyroidectomy.

## SUBACUTE GRANULOMATOUS THYROIDITIS

Subacute granulomatous thyroiditis is a self-limited disease thought to be of viral etiology occurring equally in men and women without familial prevalence. It presents no true indication for surgical intervention but occasionally may be confused with goiters requiring surgical therapy during one of its three clinical phases.[5]

Initially, the goiter is preceded by systemic symptoms of upper respiratory infection and flulike syndrome. The gland is tender and usually bilaterally enlarged, but occasionally one lobe is affected first, suggesting a unilateral neoplasm. The serum free $T_4$ level is often elevated with mild symptoms of hyperthyroidism, but the radioactive iodine uptake is completely suppressed, and the sedimentation rate is elevated to a range of 100 mm/hr. Over weeks, the condition evolves to a second stage in which the goiter is still present but less tender and may be asymmetric and hard, again suggesting the possibility of carcinoma. Serum tests usually reveal a normal free $T_4$ level and radioactive iodine uptake, which has recovered into the normal range, with a sedimentation rate only mildly elevated. With such a presentation, the true diagnosis can be discerned mainly by eliciting a preceding history compatible with the first phase. Over further weeks, the goiter shrinks and becomes nontender, and the free $T_4$ level becomes transiently depressed with a concurrent elevation of serum TSH level and radioactive iodine uptake. Symptoms of hypothyroidism are not prominent, however, and spontaneous recovery to the euthyroid state without goiter is the rule. Restraint must be employed so that surgery is avoided during the first two phases.

## SUBACUTE LYMPHOCYTIC (PAINLESS) THYROIDITIS

In the mid 1970s, a syndrome of painless thyroiditis with hyperthyroidism attracted attention.[4, 12] By 1977, Nikolai and colleagues (unpublished data) suggested that in perhaps 25 per cent of patients, hyperthyroidism was the result of subacute lymphocytic thyroiditis, which presents with a small, usually nontender goiter. The serum free $T_4$ level is elevated, while in contradistinction to Graves' disease, the radioactive iodine uptake is depressed. The sedimentation rate is only modestly elevated, and, if present, microsomal antibodies are in low titer. A report by Vitug and Goldman[13] suggested that the syndrome is much less common in areas other than the midwestern United States. Only a single definite and three possible instances of silent thyroiditis were found among 86 consecutive patients with hyperthyroidism living in Brooklyn, New York.

Of continuing interest, however, is a variant of postpartum lymphocytic thyroiditis occurring 6 to 12 weeks after delivery. Again, the prevalence appears to be highest in the Great Lakes region of the United States. Nikolai et al.[11] found that 11 per cent of patients had evidence of some form of thyroid disease after delivery. Most patients had a small goiter and mild hyperthyroidism, others had a small nontoxic goiter, and still others had only elevated levels of microsomal antibody titer without a goiter. Amino et al.[1] from Japan and Jansson et al.[10] from Sweden reported incidences of this syndrome of 5.5 to 6.5 per cent, although Freeman et al.[3] from New York found only 2 per cent of patients with thyroid dysfunction during the 3-month postpartum period.

The general agreement is that most patients respond with spontaneous improvement, although scattered instances of persistent thyroid disease remain. The new presentation of a goiter in the immediate postpartum period should elicit clinical evaluation with therapeutic restraint, and only the persistence of a suspicious goiter 6 months after delivery should suggest more vigorous pursuit.

## RIEDEL'S INVASIVE FIBROUS THYROIDITIS

Riedel's thyroiditis is an extraordinarily rare condition, with only 37 cases noted on pathology studies involved in 56,700 thyroidectomies at the Mayo Clinic between 1920 and 1984.[7] It presents as a stony hard, ill-defined enlargement in the thyroid bed, which lacks discernible outline, and appears contiguous with the trachea and strap muscles. Serum tests are of little benefit in diagnosis, with thyroid function being normal and only occasionally low because of glandular invasion. The important differential diagnosis is among poorly differentiated follicular carcinoma, anaplastic carcinoma of the thyroid, and lymphoma. The stony hard nature of the goiter may preclude fine needle biopsy, and often an open biopsy is indicated. Although the disease is most often progressive, occasionally spontaneous regression occurs. When the mechanical symptoms, as described for chronic lymphocytic thyroiditis, are present, a decompressive surgical procedure is indicated with removal of the midline portion of the goiter to break the encircling arch of thyroid gland. More lateral and wider excision is hazardous because of the infiltrative nature of the process into the contiguous structures of the trachea, parathyroid glands, and recurrent laryngeal nerves.

## ACUTE SUPPURATIVE THYROIDITIS

Acute suppurative thyroiditis, a pyogenic infection of the thyroid gland, has virtually disappeared. Historically, it was related to a traumatic puncture wound of the thyroid, and in the postantibiotic era, it rarely is the result of seeding from a distant infection. Usually an afebrile systemic reaction occurs with a painful tender thyroid gland with overlying heat and redness. Treatment is with systemic antibiotics. Surgical drainage is indicated only for abscess formation.

## REFERENCES

1. Amino, N., Mori, A., Iwatani, Y., et al.: High prevalence of transient post-partum thyrotoxicosis and hypothyroidism. N. Engl. J. Med., *306*:849–852, 1982.
2. Dailey, M. E., Lindsay, S., and Skahen, R.: Relation of thyroid neoplasms to Hashimoto disease of the thyroid gland. Arch. Surg., *70*:291–297, 1955.
3. Freeman, R., Rosen, H., and Thysen, B.: Incidence of thyroid dysfunction in an unselected postpartum population. Arch. Intern. Med., *146*:1361–1364, 1986.
4. Gorman, C. A., Duick, D. S., Woolner, L. B., and Wahner, H. W.: Transient hyperthyroidism in patients with lymphocytic thyroiditis. Mayo Clin. Proc., *53*:359–365, 1978.
5. Greene, J. N.: Subacute thyroiditis. Am. J. Med., *51*:97–108, 1971.
6. Hashimoto, H: Zur Kenntniss der lymphomatösen Veränderung der Schilddrüse (struma lymphomatosa). Arch. Klin. Chir., *97*:219–248, 1912.
7. Hay, I. D.: Thyroiditis: A clinical update. Mayo Clin. Proc., *60*:836–843, 1985.
8. Hirabayashi, R. N., and Lindsay, S.: The relation of thyroid carcinoma and chronic thyroiditis. Surg. Gynecol. Obstet., *121*:243–252, 1965.
9. Holm, L. E., Blomgren, H., and Löwhagen, T.: Cancer risks in patients with chronic lymphocytic thyroiditis. N. Engl. J. Med., *312*:601–604, 1985.
10. Jansson, R., Bernander, S., Karlsson, A., et al.: Autoimmune thyroid dysfunction in the postpartum period. J. Clin. Endocrinol. Metab., *58*:681–687, 1984.
11. Nikolai, T. F., Turney, S. L., and Roberts, R. C.: Postpartum lymphocytic thyroiditis: Prevalence, clinical course, and long-term follow-up. Arch. Intern. Med., *147*:221–224, 1987.
12. Papapetrou, P. D., and Jackson, I. M.: Thyrotoxicosis due to "silent" thyroiditis. Lancet, *1*:361–363, 1975.
13. Vitug, A. C., and Goldman, J. M.: Silent (painless) thyroiditis: Evidence of a geographic variation in frequency. Arch. Intern. Med., *145*:473–475, 1985.
14. Weetman, A. P., and McGregor, A. M.: Autoimmune thyroid disease: Developments in our understanding. Endocr. Rev., *5*:309–355, 1984.
15. Woolner, L. B., McConahey, W. M., and Beahrs, O. H.: Struma lymphomatosa (Hashimoto's thyroiditis) and related thyroid disorders. J. Clin. Endocrinol. Metab., *19*:53–83, 1959.

# 14

# DIFFERENTIATED CARCINOMA OF THYROID GLAND

*Ricardo L. Rossi, M.D., and Blake Cady, M.D.*

Although occurring infrequently, thyroid carcinoma is the most commonly found endocrine carcinoma.[40] In the United States, more than 11,000 patients or between 25 and 40 individuals per 1,000,000 of the population are treated yearly for carcinoma of the thyroid,[10] and approximately 1,050 patients die yearly[6, 40] from this disease. Although the incidence of carcinoma of the thyroid does not vary appreciably among countries, one author[17] has suggested that the incidence is higher in areas of endemic goiter. The low incidence of carcinoma of the thyroid appreciated clinically contrasts with the high incidence found on autopsy studies (4.5 to 24 per cent),[7, 27, 38] suggesting that microscopic carcinoma is rarely of clinical importance.

The cause of carcinoma of the thyroid is not completely established. Low-dose radiation is one of the known factors in the cause of this disease.[18] Independent familial risk factors have also been suggested.[31] Whether these are genetic or environmental factors remains to be determined, but iodine deficiency may be associated with a higher incidence.

The relative infrequency of this carcinoma and the prolonged survival of patients with differentiated thyroid carcinoma explain why it is difficult to determine and compare the value of different therapeutic modalities. Therefore, controversies remain in papillary and follicular differentiated thyroid carcinomas with regard to the necessary extent of surgical treatment, the indications for use of radioactive iodine, and to a lesser degree the use of thyroid suppression. We present different aspects of our retrospective experience with 940 patients operated on between 1931 and 1980 and review the literature to elaborate on the factors that affect prognosis and discuss the biologic characteristics that could influence therapeutic decisions. In this chapter, we will address follicular and papillary carcinomas of the thyroid.

## MATERIALS AND METHODS

Records of patients with papillary and follicular carcinoma operated on at the Lahey Clinic between 1931 and 1980 were analyzed.

This review included a first study of 631 patients operated on between 1931 and 1960 with complete follow-up in 98 per cent of the patients and collected in 1975[13] with a minimum follow-up time of 15 years and a maximum follow-up time of 45 years. A second study group included 309 patients operated on between 1961 and 1980 and reported in 1985[34] with 100 per cent follow-up and a median follow-up time of 13 years (5 to 24 years). To eliminate favorable biases, the "dead of disease" category included patients who died of thyroid carcinoma, patients who were last seen with disease present, patients who died of other causes but with disease present, and postoperative deaths. The rest of the patients were classified as alive without carcinoma and dead of other causes but free of thyroid carcinoma with a minimum follow-up time of 5 years.

The histopathologic material was revised and reclassified by Meissner and Silverman according to the definitions of the Armed Forces Institute of Pathology,[29] World Health Organization,[25] and American Joint Committee for Cancer Staging and End-Results Reporting.[1] Follicular carcinoma included tumors with follicular elements only and tumors with oxyphilic cells (Hürthle cells). Any tumor with papillary elements was classified as papillary carcinoma because mixed papillary and follicular tumors and pure papillary tumors behave in a biologically similar manner.[13] Minimal capsular invasion was defined as minimal extension of the tumor into the tumor capsule without evidence of extracapsular extension. Major capsular invasion included extensive involvement of the tumor capsule or extension to perithyroidal soft tissues. The diameter of the tumor used for analysis was the maximum diameter described by the pathologist. Extraglandular invasion was defined as that detected at operation or on pathologic study and involved trachea, esophagus, prethyroid musculature, recurrent laryngeal nerves, and soft tissues.

Clinically occult carcinoma was defined as carcinoma not suspected before the pathologic report. These patients may not have had a discrete thyroid nodule, and they were operated on for presumed benign disease, such as hyperthyroidism or adenomatous goiter.

Surgically incurable carcinoma was defined as carcinoma with distant metastatic disease, extensive local disease that was not resectable, and macroscopic residual tumor at the conclusion of the operation.

Recurrent disease was defined as local recurrent disease when carcinoma occurred in the thyroid bed or soft tissues of the neck, nodal when carcinoma recurred in lymph nodes of the neck or mediastinum, and distant metastatic disease when carcinoma occurred outside the neck.

The statistical differences for recurrent disease and mortality were defined by the Miettinen modification of the Fisher exact test.[36] Studies that involved contingency tables larger than 2 × 2 tables were analyzed by the chi-square test with Yates correction. Analysis of linear tendencies was made with the Rothman and Boice[36] method. The correlation of recurrent disease and mortality with the size of the tumor was made by one-way analysis of variance. All P values were two-tailed. We considered P values of less than 0.05 as significant with calculation of exact values to indicate possible proximity to significance.

## RESULTS

### *Trends in Disease Presentation*

Of the 940 patients, 684 (73 per cent) had a papillary carcinoma and 256 (27 per cent) had a follicular carcinoma.[9, 13, 14, 33, 34] Although carcinoma of the thyroid is more frequent in women, the number of men with carcinoma of the thyroid has increased through the decades. From 1931 to 1950, from 1951 to 1960, and from 1961 to 1980, the proportion of men represented 19 per cent, 24 per cent, and 32 per cent of all patients, respectively. From 1961 to 1980, the number of men and women was similar for patients more than 50 years of age.

Carcinoma of the thyroid is being diagnosed at an earlier stage. The incidence of major capsular invasion has diminished. From 1931 to 1950, 1951 to 1960, and 1961 to 1980, it was present in 70 per cent, 51 per cent, and 25 per cent of patients in each group. Similarly, the incidence of histologic vascular invasion has decreased: 54 per cent, 38 per cent, and 25 per cent in the same time periods. Soft tissue extraglandular invasion was present in 20 per cent of patients treated between 1951 and 1960 and in only 11 per cent of patients treated between 1961 and 1980. Between 1931 and 1940, only 33 per cent of patients had an intraglandular tumor. However, between 1961 and 1980, 89 per cent of patients had intraglandular disease. The size of the carcinoma at diagnosis is smaller: in the 1961 to 1980 group, 62 per cent of patients in the low-risk group and 58 per cent of patients in the high-risk group presented with carcinomas of less than 2 cm. Distant metastatic disease was present in 2.4 per cent of patients initially diagnosed between 1931 and 1960 but in only 0.7 per cent of patients treated between 1961 and 1980.

## *Mortality*

For all patients with papillary carcinoma treated between 1931 and 1960, the recurrence rate was 20 per cent, and the mortality rate for patients with thyroid carcinoma was 11 per cent. These figures were 10 per cent and 6 per cent, respectively, for patients treated between 1961 and 1980. For patients with follicular tumors treated between 1931 and 1960, the recurrence rate was 32 per cent and the mortality rate was 24 per cent. For patients treated between 1961 and 1980, the recurrence rate was 11 per cent and the mortality rate was 14 per cent.

Analysis of patients treated between 1931 and 1960[13] with a follow-up time of 15 to 45 years showed that 55 per cent of papillary carcinomas that recurred did so within the first 5 years, 83 per cent within the first 10 years, 97 per cent within the first 15 years, and 100 per cent within 25 years of initial therapy. Of deaths from papillary thyroid carcinoma, 48 per cent occurred within 5 years, 62 per cent within 10 years, 83 per cent within 15 years, 90 per cent within 20 years, and all patients who died were dead by 30 years. For patients with follicular carcinoma, 61 per cent of the recurrent tumors occurred within 5 years of therapy, 85 per cent within 10 years, 94 per cent within 15 years, and 100 per cent within 20 years. Of the deaths, 49 per cent occurred within 5 years, 76 per cent within 10 years, 86 per cent within 15 years, 94 per cent within 20 years, and all patients who died were dead by 25 years. These findings suggest that with a median follow-up time of 13 years for patients treated between 1961 and 1980, the vast majority of recurrent tumors (about 80 per cent) and carcinomas causing death (about 70 per cent) would have been detected.[34] The lower recurrence and mortality rates of this second group could partly be explained by the shorter follow-up time and higher number of patients with less advanced disease.

## *Prognostic Factors*

### Histologic Type

The recurrence and mortality rates associated with thyroid carcinoma in patients with papillary and follicular tumors are listed in Table 14–1. The mortality rate for patients with follicular carcinoma was approximately twice that of patients with papillary tumors. However, as will be shown later, this is largely the result of the effect of age of the patient on presentation rather than on histology.

Some of the distinctive biologic features of papillary and follicular carcinoma are presented in Table 14–2. However, many of these differences are highly correlated with sex and age (risk group), the most important prognostic factors. Older patients tend to have more follicular carcinomas than papillary carcinomas. The histologic type appears

**TABLE 14–1. Recurrence and Mortality Rates According to Histologic Type of Carcinoma**

| | 1931–1960* | | | 1961–1980† | | |
|---|---|---|---|---|---|---|
| **TYPE** | **No.** | **Recurred** | **Dead of Disease** | **No.** | **Recurred** | **Dead of Disease** |
| Follicular | 178 | 57 (32%) | 48 (27%) | 66 | 9 (14%) | 7 (11%) |
| Papillary | 423 | 86 (12%) | 52 (12%) | 243 | 24 (10%) | 14 ( 6%) |
| | | P = 0.003 | P <0.0001 | | P = 0.39 | P = 0.19 |

*Follow-up: 15 to 45 years.
†Median follow-up: 13 years (5 to 24 years).

**TABLE 14–2. Major Differences, 1931–1970**

| FACTOR CONSIDERED | PAPILLARY AND MIXED | FOLLICULAR |
|---|---|---|
| Incidence of sex | | |
| Male incidence | 22% | 35% |
| Size | | |
| <2 cm | 49% | 34% |
| 2–4 cm | 38% | 43% |
| >4 cm | 15% | 23% |
| Surgically occult primary cancer | 34% | 51% |
| Lymph node metastases | 35% | 13% |
| Blood vessel invasion | 40% | 60% |
| Recurrence rate | 19% | 29% |
| Patients with recurrence who died of disease | 61% | 84% |
| Eventual overall mortality rate | 11% | 24% |
| Location of recurrent cancer | | |
| Distant metastases | 45% | 75% |
| Nodal metastases | 34% | 12% |
| Local recurrences | 20% | 12% |

to have a lesser effect on survival than age and sex.

## Local Extension of Tumor

Recurrence and mortality rates with regard to local extent of disease at the time of operation are listed in Table 14–3. Tumors with extraglandular involvement were associated with significantly higher recurrence and mortality rates primarily in older patients. Only one patient (0.3 per cent) with an occult carcinoma died of disease.

In patients operated on between 1961 and 1980 (Table 14–4),[34] major capsular invasion was associated with a recurrence rate of 22 per cent and minimal or no capsular invasion with a recurrence rate of 6 per cent (P = 0.0003). The mortality rates were 16 and 4 per cent, respectively (P = 0.001). For patients with and without vascular invasion, the recurrence rates were 24 and 6 per cent, respectively (P = 0.0001), and the mortality rates were 16 and 4 per cent, respectively (P = 0.001).

The recurrence and mortality rates for patients with carcinoma of the thyroid correlated with the size of the tumor in older patients (P = 0.002 and P = 0.005, respectively). In older patients in the high-risk group, the recurrence and mortality rates for patients with carcinomas less than 1 cm were 5 and 1 per cent, respectively; for tumors of 1 to 1.9 cm, the rates were 5 and 5 per cent; for tumors of 2 to 2.9 cm, the rates were 10 and 7 per cent; for tumors of 3 to 3.9 cm, the rates were 29 and 21 per cent; and for tumors 4 cm or more, the rates were 91 and 64 per cent. Even in older patients, tumors less than 2 cm were associated with low recurrence and mortality rates. The recurrence rates associated with multifocal and unifocal tumors were 15 and 10 per cent (P = 0.39); the mortality rates were 6 and 7 per cent (P = 0.92).

## Lymph Node Metastasis

Lymph node metastases are common in papillary thyroid carcinoma. Noguchi et al.,[30] studying specimens from prophylactic neck dissection in patients with papillary carcinoma, found occult micrometastasis in approximately 80 per cent of patients. Attie et al.[2] reported micrometastasis in 68 per cent of specimens from prophylactic neck dissections. Lymph node metastases were found far less commonly in the older age groups. Conversely, patients with lymph node metastasis tend to be in the younger age group.[13] In our series, among patients less than 30 years of age who had neck dissection, 90 per cent had lymph node metastasis. The most

**TABLE 14–3. Recurrence and Mortality Rates According to Extent of Disease**

| | 1931–1960* | | | 1961–1980† | | |
|---|---|---|---|---|---|---|
| TYPE | No. | Recurred | Dead of Disease | No. | Recurred | Dead of Disease |
| Intraglandular | 502 | 77 (15%) | 45 ( 9%) | 276 | 16 ( 6%) | 8 ( 3%) |
| Extraglandular‡ | 95 | 36 (38%) | 27 (28%) | 33 | 17 (52%) | 13 (39%) |
| | | P <0.0001 | P <0.0001 | | P <0.0001 | P <0.0001 |

*Follow-up: 15 to 45 years.
†Median follow-up: 13 years (5 to 24 years).
‡In 1931–1960 study, patients with residual tumor at operation were excluded. However, they were included in the table of patients operated on between 1961 and 1980.

**TABLE 14–4. Pathologic Features and Outcome, 1961–1980***

| PATHOLOGIC FINDING | NO. | OUTCOME | |
|---|---|---|---|
| | | Recurred | Patient Died of Disease |
| Follicular | 66 | 9 (14%) | 7 (11%) |
| Papillary | 243 | 24 (10%) | 14 ( 6%) |
| | | P = 0.39 | P = 0.19 |
| Blood vessel invasion | 76 | 18 (24%) | 12 (16%) |
| No blood vessel invasion | 233 | 15 ( 6%) | 9 ( 4%) |
| | | P = 0.0001 | P = 0.001 |
| Major capsular invasion | 77 | 17 (22%) | 12 (16%) |
| Minor or no capsular invasion | 232 | 15 ( 6%) | 9 ( 4%) |
| Size, cm† | | P = 0.0003 | P = 0.001 |
| <1 | 76 | 4 ( 5%) | 1 ( 1%) |
| 1–1.9 | 97 | 5 ( 5%) | 5 ( 5%) |
| 2–2.9 | 60 | 6 (10%) | 4 ( 7%) |
| 3–3.9 | 14 | 4 (29%) | 3 (21%) |
| >4 | 11 | 10 (91%) | 7 (64%) |
| Unknown | 51 | 4 ( 8%) | 1 ( 2%) |
| Positive nodes | 88 | 16 (18%) | 7 ( 8%) |
| Negative nodes | 221 | 17 ( 8%) | 14 ( 6%) |
| | | P = 0.01 | P = 0.61 |
| Multifocal | 33 | 5 (15%) | 2 ( 6%) |
| Unifocal | 276 | 28 (10%) | 19 ( 7%) |
| | | P = 0.39 | P = 0.92 |

*From Rossi, R. L., Cady, B., Silverman, M. L., et al.: Current results of conservative surgery for differentiated thyroid carcinoma. World J. Surg., *10*:615, 1986, with permission.

†Incidences of recurrence and death correlated exponentially with tumor size to significance levels of P = 0.002 and P = 0.005, respectively.

common pattern of nodal metastasis included a high incidence of positive central nodes (paratracheal, pretracheal, and paraglandular nodes) and midjugular and inferior jugular nodes.[32] Superior cervical nodes are involved less frequently, and submaxillary nodes are involved uncommonly.

Histologically proved lymph node metastasis did not affect survival in our two study periods. For patients operated on between 1931 and 1960, death from papillary thyroid carcinoma occurred in 11 per cent of patients with negative nodes and in 8 per cent of patients with positive nodes. For patients with follicular carcinoma, the mortality rate was 27 per cent for patients with negative nodes and 13 per cent for those with positive nodes in the few patients with lymph node metastases. For patients operated on between 1960 and 1980, the mortality rate for patients with differentiated carcinoma and negative nodes was 6 per cent, and for patients with positive nodes, the mortality rate was 8 per cent (P = 0.61). Recurrent lymph node metastases were more frequent (18 versus 8 per cent; P = 0.011) in patients with initially positive nodes than in those with negative nodes but did not affect long-term survival.

Our results regarding pathologic findings and extent of disease at operation are summarized in Tables 14–4 and 14–5.

## *Age and Sex*

Age at the time of diagnosis and primary therapy is the critical factor in the prognosis of patients with differentiated thyroid carcinoma and is more important than histologic type and extent of disease.[9, 13, 14, 33, 34] In our first study group, only 2 per cent of patients

**TABLE 14–5. Extent of Tumor at Operation and Outcome, 1961–1980***

| EXTENT OF TUMOR | NO. | OUTCOME | |
|---|---|---|---|
| | | Recurred | Patient Died of Disease |
| Occult | 75 | 1 ( 1%) | 1 ( 1%) |
| Apparent | 234 | 32 (14%) | 20 ( 9%) |
| | | P = 0.0008 | P = 0.02 |
| Intraglandular | 276 | 16 ( 6%) | 8 ( 3%) |
| Extraglandular | 33 | 17 (52%) | 13 (39%) |
| | | P <0.0001 | P <0.0001 |

*From Rossi, R. L., Cady, B., Silverman, M. L., et al.: Current results of conservative surgery for differentiated thyroid carcinoma. World J. Surg., *10*:616, 1986, with permission.

**TABLE 14–6. Risk of Recurrence and Death by Age Decade, 1931–1970**

| SEX | AGE | TOTAL NO. | RECURRENCE | DEATH NO. | DEATH As Per Cent of Total | DEATH As Per Cent of Recurrence |
|---|---|---|---|---|---|---|
| Men* | <30 | 28 | 5 (18%) | 3 | 11% | 60% |
| | 31–40 | 34 | 4 (12%) | 2 | 6% | 50% |
| | 41–50 | 31 | 10 (32%) | 5 | 16% | 50% |
| | 51–60 | 25 | 8 (32%) | 6 | 24% | 75% |
| | >61 | 14 | 6 (43%) | 4 | 29% | 67% |
| Women† | <30 | 115 | 17 (15%) | 3 | 3% | 18% |
| | 31–40 | 122 | 11 ( 9%) | 5 | 4% | 46% |
| | 41–50 | 85 | 5 ( 6%) | 2 | 2% | 40% |
| | 51–60 | 80 | 23 (28%) | 21 | 24% | 86% |
| | >61 | 66 | 24 (36%) | 22 | 33% | 92% |
| Total | | 600 | 113 | 73 | | |

*Recurrence, P = 0.02; deaths, P = NS.
†Recurrence, P = 0.001; deaths, P = 0.001.

less than 20 years of age at diagnosis eventually died of disease compared with 5 per cent between the ages of 20 and 40 years and 8 per cent between the ages of 40 and 50 years. The mortality rate of patients more than 50 years of age at diagnosis was considerably increased, with 34 per cent of patients dying of disease. This high risk began in women after 50 years of age and in men after 40 years of age. In our first study, 75 per cent of all deaths in our series occurred in the 33 per cent of patients more than 50 years; 85 per cent of deaths occurred in the 50 per cent of patients more than 40 years of age. The risk of recurrence and death by age of patients treated between 1931 and 1960 is shown in Table 14–6.

On the basis of these data, Cady et al.[13] described three risk groups for dying of differentiated thyroid carcinoma. The high-risk group included patients with follicular carcinoma and consisted of men more than 40 years of age and women more than 50 years of age. These patients had a recurrence rate of 40 per cent and a mortality rate of 36 per cent. The intermediate-risk group included men more than 40 years of age and women more than 50 years of age with papillary carcinoma. These patients had a recurrence rate of 29 per cent and a mortality rate of 21 per cent. The low-risk group included men 40 years of age and younger and women 50 years of age and younger who had either follicular or papillary carcinoma. These patients had a recurrence rate of 11 per cent and a mortality rate of 4 per cent. The differences in recurrence rates between the high-risk and the intermediate-risk groups was not significant. Therefore, for simplicity, risk group definition was divided into two groups: the high-risk group for recurrent disease and death consisted of men more than 40 years of age and women more than 50 years of age, and the low-risk group consisted of all younger patients. The effect of the risk group as defined by sex and age was confirmed in our study[12, 34] of patients treated between 1961 and 1980 as shown in Table

**TABLE 14–7. Effect of Age-Based Risk Group on Outcome, 1961–1980***

| RISK GROUP | NO. | OUTCOME Recurred | OUTCOME Died of Disease |
|---|---|---|---|
| Low risk† | 192 | 10 ( 5%) | 2 ( 1%) |
| High risk‡ | 117 | 23 (20%) | 18 (15%) |
| | | P = 0.0001 | P <0.0001 |

*From Rossi, R. L., Cady, B., Silverman, M. L., et al.: Current results of conservative surgery for differentiated thyroid carcinoma. World J. Surg., *10*:616, 1986, with permission.
†Men less than 40 years of age and women less than 50 years of age.
‡Men more than 40 years of age and women more than 50 years of age.

**TABLE 14–8. Site of Recurrence and Outcome According to Age-Based Risk Group, 1961–1980***

| SITE OF RECURRENCE | LOW RISK No. | LOW RISK Patient Died of Disease | HIGH RISK No. | HIGH RISK Patient Died of Disease |
|---|---|---|---|---|
| Nodal | 5 | 0 | 6 | 3 |
| Local | 5 | 1 | 12 | 7 |
| Distant | 3 | 1 | 8 | 8 |

*From Rossi, R. L., Cady, B., Silverman, M. L., et al.: Current results of conservative surgery for differentiated thyroid carcinoma. World J. Surg., *10*:617, 1986, with permission.

**TABLE 14–9. Distant Metastasis in 17 Patients***

| AGE-BASED RISK GROUP | NO. OF PATIENTS | NO. (%) OF PATIENTS WHO DIED OF DISEASE | |
|---|---|---|---|
| Low risk | 5 | 2 ( 40%) | P = 0.055 |
| High risk | 12 | 11 ( 92%) | |
| Total | 17 | 13 ( 76%)† | |
| **SITE OF METASTASIS** | | | |
| Pulmonary | 10‡ | 6 ( 60%) | |
| Other | 7§ | 7 (100%) | |

*From Rossi, R. L., Cady, B., Silverman, M. L., et al.: Surgically incurable well-differentiated thyroid carcinoma: Prognostic factors and results of therapy. Arch. Surg., *123*:570, 1988, with permission.

†Median survival time, 6 months (range, 1 to 69 months).

‡Of five patients in the high-risk group, four died of disease; of five patients in the low-risk group, two died of disease.

§All patients were in the high-risk group.

14–7. Patients in the low-risk group had a recurrence rate of 5 per cent and a mortality rate of 1 per cent compared with patients in the high-risk group with recurrence and mortality rates of 20 and 15 per cent, respectively. This basic age-based risk group definition supersedes the prognostic effects of primary disease extension, pathologic type, and type of therapy. Of patients in the low-risk group treated between 1931 and 1960 and whose disease recurred, 36 per cent eventually died of disease. However, 74 per cent of patients in the intermediate-risk group with recurrent disease and 91 per cent of patients in the high-risk group with recurrent disease died of disease. The effect of the risk group and site of recurrence on the outcome of patients is shown in Table 14–8.

We[35] have reported on the effects of age on presentation in the outcome of patients with surgically incurable thyroid carcinoma defined as patients who present with distant metastatic disease, with unresectable neck disease, or who have residual tumor after operation. Of 17 patients who presented with metastatic disease, only 40 per cent of patients in the low-risk group but 92 per cent of patients in the high-risk group died of disease (Table 14–9).

Of 38 patients in the low-risk group with surgically incurable neck disease, only four patients (13 per cent) died of disease at 1 month, 3 years, 8 years, and 12 years, respectively. Of 42 patients in the high-risk group with locally incurable disease, 30 (71 per cent) died of disease at a median of 2 years (1 month to 14 years). This difference in survival was statistically significant ($P < 0.001$). Table 14–10 shows the effect of the risk group on the outcome of patients with surgically incurable neck disease. Of the 37 patients who had tracheal invasion on presentation, 79 per cent of patients in the high-risk group but only 11 per cent of patients in the low-risk group died of disease.[35]

A multiple regression analysis of variables affecting outcome in patients with papillary carcinoma at the Mayo Clinic[23, 28] identified four factors to be important in predicting death. They were *A*ge of the patient, *G*rade of tumor, *E*xtent of tumor (local invasion or distant metastases), and *S*ize of tumor (AGES). On the basis of the regression coefficients obtained from this analysis, a scoring system was devised (AGES score) that is capable of placing patients into risk groups with greatly different prognoses. We[11] have reported a simplified AMES clinical scoring system (*A*ge, distant *M*etastasis, *E*xtent, *S*ize) that separates 89 per cent of all patients at low risk of death (1.8 per cent) from the 11 per cent of patients at high risk of death (46 per cent death rate). The characteristics

**TABLE 14–10. Residual or Unresectable Local Neck Disease* in 80 Patients†**

| AGE-BASED RISK GROUP | NO. OF PATIENTS | NO. (%) OF PATIENTS WHO DIED OF DISEASE | MEDIAN SURVIVAL OF PATIENTS WHO DIED OF DISEASE, YEARS (RANGE) |
|---|---|---|---|
| Low risk | 38 | 5 (13%)‡ | 8 (1 mo–12 yrs) |
| High risk | 42 | 30 (71%)‡ | 2 (1 mo–14 yrs) |

*From Rossi, R. L., Cady, B., Silverman, M. L., et al.: Surgically incurable well-differentiated thyroid carcinoma: Prognostic factors and results of therapy. Arch. Surg., *123*:570, 1988.

†Of 37 patients with tracheal wall invasion, two (11%) of 18 patients in the low-risk group died of disease and 15 (79%) of 19 patients in the high-risk group died of disease.

‡$P < 0.001$.

**TABLE 14–11. Risk Group Definitions (1941–1980) Multifactorial System: AMES***

| |
|---|
| Low-risk group |
| All younger patients without distant metastases |
| Men less than 41 years |
| Women less than 51 years |
| All older patients with |
| Intrathyroidal papillary cancer or minor tumor capsular involvement follicular carcinoma and |
| Primary carcinoma less than 5 cm in diameter and |
| No distant metastases |
| High-risk group |
| All patients with distant metastases |
| All younger patients with follicular carcinoma with major capsular involvement |
| All older patients with |
| Extrathyroidal papillary carcinoma or major tumor capsular involvement follicular carcinoma and |
| Primary carcinoma 5 cm in diameter or larger regardless of extent of disease |

*From Cady, B., and Rossi, R.: An expanded view of risk-group definition in differentiated thyroid carcinoma. Surgery, *104*:948, 1988, with permission.

of the low-risk group and the high-risk group are listed in Table 14–11. The distribution of patients by the AMES and AGES scores is shown in Table 14–12. The vast majority of patients seen today with thyroid carcinoma in the United States have "minimal" risk of dying of the disease. A small group of patients with a higher risk of dying of carcinoma could be identified by the prognostic factors described by us (AMES) or by the Mayo group (AGES). These prognostic signs are available to the surgeon at the time of the operation and can help with the selection of the surgical procedure.

## DNA Ploidy

Studies are under way to improve and standardize the technology of DNA ploidy determinations,[3] to assess their prognostic and therapeutic implications, and to determine whether they add to the already available clinical and pathologic data to define the risk of dying of the disease. Bäckdahl et al.[4] have shown in retrospective studies that patients with papillary carcinoma who died of disease within 12 years had increased nuclear DNA values whereas patients who were alive at least 10 years after diagnosis had diploid DNA levels. Of patients with follicular carcinoma who died of disease, 89 per cent had increased or aneuploid nuclear DNA content whereas 95 per cent of patients with follicular carcinoma who survived and 96 per cent of patients with follicular adenoma had tumors with diploid DNA content. However, in the DNA measurements using flow cytometry techniques performed on archival tissues for follicular neoplasms at the Mayo Clinic,[8] the DNA ploidy did not differentiate well between the benign and malignant neoplasms, and although the aneuploidy was more common in follicular carcinoma, its presence did not correlate well with increased mortality, presenting an appreciable overlap between the different groups.

As the technique of DNA measurement improves and when performed in conjunction with fine needle aspiration[5] and established clinical and morphologic prognostic criteria, it may help to define more precisely the malignant potential of the lesion in each patient. Determination of nuclear DNA could thus add additional information to assist in therapeutic decisions in patients with thyroid carcinoma. Its exact place in the management of patients with these carcinomas will require further evaluation.

**TABLE 14–12. Comparison of Risk-Group Definitions***

| | TOTAL CASES | | DEAD OF DISEASE | | RATIO OF DEATH RATES |
|---|---|---|---|---|---|
| | No. | Incidence, per cent | No. | Death Rate, per cent | |
| | Mayo Clinic: Papillary Carcinoma | | | | |
| AGES (1946–1970) | | | | | |
| Low risk | 737 | 86 | — | 2 | 1:23 |
| High risk | 121 | 14 | — | 46 | — |
| | Lahey Clinic: Papillary and Follicular Carcinoma | | | | |
| AMES (1961–1980) | | | | | |
| Low risk | 277 | 89 | 5 | 1.8 | 1:26 |
| High risk | 33 | 11 | 15 | 46 | — |

*From Cady, B., and Rossi, R.: An expanded view of risk-group definition in differentiated thyroid carcinoma. Surgery, *104*:951, 1988, with permission.

## THERAPY

Surgery continues to be the basic treatment for patients with differentiated thyroid carcinoma. Other therapeutic modalities include the use of radioactive iodine, thyroid suppression, and external beam radiotherapy. The extent of surgery and the use of other therapeutic modalities remain controversial. Our therapeutic recommendations are strongly influenced by the risk group definition of the patient as defined by age and sex and the extent of disease (tumor size, presence or absence of capsular and extracapsular involvement, and presence initially of metastatic disease).

### *Thyroid Gland Surgery*

Patients in the low-risk age group (men less than 41 years of age and women less than 51 years of age), patients with small tumors (less than 2 cm), and patients without major capsular involvement of follicular carcinoma have an excellent prognosis. Patients in the low-risk AMES group seldom die of disease, even with limited resection of the thyroid. In this selected low-risk group of patients, we favor near total or total lobectomy on the side of the lesion. When subtotal lobectomy is performed for benign disease and an occult tumor is found days later on final pathologic analysis, no further operation is advised because the prognosis with such a lesion is 100 per cent cure. Of 57 selected patients treated with a unilateral lobectomy between 1961 and 1980, no patient had recurrent carcinoma or died of disease, and none of the 20 patients with occult carcinoma had recurrent disease. This suggests that conservative surgery can be adequate for limited disease in selected patients.[34] Radioactive iodine ablation is not necessary in young patients with a small intraglandular papillary carcinoma or in a patient in the low-risk AMES category. Thyroid suppression may be prescribed but is not essential.

When the primary carcinoma is at high risk by AMES criteria, total lobectomy on the side of the carcinoma and contralateral subtotal or near total lobectomy is our operation of choice. These patients will probably receive radioactive iodine ablation and thyroid suppression. A review of the Mayo Clinic[24] experience has shown that unilateral thyroid resection in this group of patients might produce a significantly higher incidence of local recurrent disease than in patients with some form of bilateral resection. However, the impact on survival of the more extensive operation was not different. No difference in local recurrence rates was observed when different types of bilateral resection (subtotal or total thyroidectomy) were compared.[20] Bilateral resection, but not necessarily total thyroidectomy, was therefore advocated by the Mayo Clinic group and appears to offer excellent results and lessen the possibility of persistent hypoparathyroidism or recurrent laryngeal nerve injury.

The review by Høie et al.[26] of the thyroid carcinoma experience in Norway failed to show any differences in local recurrent disease or survival comparing total thyroidectomy and hemithyroidectomy. They concluded that unless obvious malignant residual disease was left behind, the impact of the type of surgical procedure on the prognosis of patients with papillary thyroid carcinoma appeared to be minor. Although total thyroidectomy can remove a microfocus of tumor in the opposite lobe of the gland, it does not address micrometastasis to lymph nodes left behind in most patients with papillary thyroid carcinoma but no clinically involved lymph nodes.

Clark et al.[15, 16] demonstrated that total thyroidectomy in experienced hands can be performed with minimal morbidity. However, this does not appear to be true in the surgical community at large.[19, 22] Therefore, for patients in the low-risk group with a low likelihood of dying of disease, total thyroidectomy should not be used.

### *Lymph Node Surgery*

In the low-risk group of patients, node resection consists of limited or modified neck dissection. When nodes are palpable preoperatively, a modified node dissection is carried out after extending the collar incision to the mastoid process. The ipsilateral paratracheal nodes are excised down to the superior mediastinum. The spinal accessory nerve is always preserved. The submandibular space rarely requires dissection, and the jugular vein and sternocleidomastoid muscle are preserved if possible, although resection may be necessary to remove massive disease or nodes that directly invade these structures. When nodes are palpable only during operation, a limited lymph node dissection is performed through the collar incision. When node metastasis is not palpable intraoperatively, no deliberate node dissection is performed because no proof exists that prophylactic node dissection improves survival.

In the high-risk group, palpable lymph node metastases are encountered less often. However, when they are found preoperatively or at the time of operation, modified neck dissection should be considered. All palpable disease and all suspicious lymph nodes should be removed from the paratracheal region and tracheoesophageal groove and into the anterosuperior mediastinum. Postoperatively, the protocol should include a neck scan using radioactive iodine followed by thyroid ablation of any thyroid remnant. After thyroid ablation, a whole body scan is recommended to determine the presence of metastasis and the need for treatment. After successful surgical and radioactive iodine ablation, patients are given thyroid suppression and monitored by thyroid-stimulating hormone assay.

## *Special Therapeutic Situations*

Patients who have had irradiation to the head and neck during childhood more often have multifocal bilateral thyroid involvement. Therefore, some surgeons[37, 39] have advocated total thyroidectomy for such patients. However, their prognosis is identical to that of patients without a history of radiation in a similar risk group. Patients who have had radiation therapy are treated the same way as patients who have not had radiation therapy, that is, treatment is based on risk group definition. In most patients, a conservative approach to the treatment of small tumors with no associated risk of spread suffices.

## *Surgically Incurable Differentiated Thyroid Carcinoma*

This group includes patients who have extensive nonresectable local neck disease when first seen or who have residual carcinoma at the time of resection. Our results[35] suggest that when technically possible, patients with surgically incurable differentiated thyroid carcinoma should undergo resection of as much disease as possible, including thyroidectomy with excision of soft tissues and nodes when involved but without routine sacrifice of functioning recurrent laryngeal nerves or anything but minor portions of esophagus, trachea, or larynx. The overwhelming feature that controls outcome is the age of the patient. Less clear is the role of extensive surgical procedures, such as laryngectomy, tracheal resection, and resection of the esophagus. They should be reserved for recurrent disease in highly selected, usually younger, patients in whom all other therapy has been attempted. Intraluminal involvement of the larynx or trachea and impending obstruction of the airway are indications for tracheostomy and may be indications for laryngectomy or tracheal resection in patients with differentiated thyroid tumors, especially when disease is unresponsive to conservative therapy or is recurrent. Laryngectomy or segmental tracheal resection for disease invading the trachea without intraluminal involvement is controversial and should be used selectively. Grillo and Zannini[21] have reported on the use of resection and primary reconstruction of the trachea involved by carcinoma of the thyroid with good results in selected young patients. Total thyroidectomy may facilitate the use of radioactive iodine therapy but has no proved survival advantage over more conservative bilateral thyroidectomy. Any thyroid remnants may be ablated with radioactive iodine. Thereafter, patients with carcinoma that takes up radioactive iodine as seen on a diagnostic scan should be treated with radioactive iodine. External beam radiotherapy should be considered in patients with inoperable residual carcinoma that does not take up radioactive iodine and in patients with local recurrent disease not amenable to operation or therapy with radioactive iodine. Thyroid-stimulating hormone suppression should be used in all such patients. Patients in the low-risk group with incurable neck disease in our series seldom died of local (3 per cent) or metastatic (3 per cent) disease, but patients in the high-risk group frequently died of local or metastatic disease (26 and 31 per cent, respectively).

### *Distant Metastatic Disease*

For patients who have distant metastatic disease when first seen, bilateral thyroidectomy should be followed by radioactive iodine ablation of any residual normal thyroid tissue. The use of radioactive iodine for metastatic disease that takes up the isotope can be decided on only after complete ablation of normal thyroid tissue. Administration of thyroid hormone is necessary thereafter. In our series[35] of 17 patients with distant metastatic disease, 60 per cent of the patients in the low-risk group but 8 per cent of the patients in the high-risk group were long-term survivors. Patients with metastatic disease to the lung do better than patients with metastatic disease to bones or other organs largely because pulmonary metastases are more common in young patients. External beam radiotherapy can accomplish palliation in patients with metastatic disease to bone that does not take up radioactive iodine.

## FOLLOW-UP

After initial postoperative follow-up visits, the patient with differentiated thyroid carcinoma is usually seen at 6-month intervals for the first 2 years and then yearly. Thyroglobulin assays may be performed, especially in patients in the high-risk group or in patients with an increased risk of local or distant metastatic disease. Scanning with iodine 131 is usually not performed in the absence of symptoms.

## RECURRENT DISEASE

The likelihood of recurrent disease is determined by risk group definition (AMES). The prognosis after disease recurs depends primarily on the age of the patient at the time of the initial diagnosis of thyroid carcinoma, on the site of recurrent disease, and on the histology of the tumor.[13, 34] For example, nodal recurrent disease is seldom associated with death in patients in the low-risk group but in 67 per cent of patients in the high-risk group (Table 14–13). Local recurrent disease in the thyroid bed and soft tissues of the neck is more lethal than nodal recurrent disease and resulted in death in one third of patients in the low-risk group and in two thirds of patients in the high-risk group (Tables 14–7 and 14–13). Aggressive management of patients with recurrent disease is recommended with an attempt to remove all obvious disease surgically.

### *Surgery of Recurrent Disease*

Nodal recurrent disease in the low-risk group can be treated surgically, achieving cure in the vast majority of patients. Local recurrent disease in the thyroid bed is treated successfully in more than 70 per cent of patients with surgery, radioactive iodine, and thyroid suppression. In tumors that take up radioactive iodine, radioactive iodine should be used even when all tumor can be removed. Otherwise, external beam radiotherapy for residual disease and in tumors that do not take up radioactive iodine can be considered,

**TABLE 14–13. Survival Related to Risk Group, 1931-1960, in All Patients with Recurrent Disease**

| RISK GROUP | TOTAL NO. | LOCAL RECURRENCE* | NODAL METASTASES* | DISTANT METASTASES† |
|---|---|---|---|---|
| High risk | | | | |
| Recurrence | 33 | 3 ( 9%) | 3 ( 9%) | 27 (82%) |
| Deaths | | 2 (67%) | 2 (67%) | 26 (96%) |
| Intermediate risk | | | | |
| Recurrence | 38 | 12 (32%) | 12 (32%) | 14 (37%) |
| Deaths | | 9 (75%) | 6 (50%) | 13 (93%) |
| Low risk | | | | |
| Recurrence | 42 | 9 (21%) | 17 (41%) | 16 (38%) |
| Deaths | | 3 (33%) | 2 (12%) | 10 (63%) |
| Total | 113 | 24 (21%) | 32 (28%) | 57 (50%) |

*Not significant.
†P = 0.006.

**TABLE 14–14. Complications of Conservative Therapy, 1961–1980***

| COMPLICATION | NO. | PER CENT |
|---|---|---|
| Bleeding | 2 | 0.6 |
| Unilateral vocal cord paralysis | | |
| Permanent | 1 | 0.3 |
| Transient | 1 | 0.3 |
| Hypoparathyroidism | | |
| Permanent | 1 | 0.3 |
| Transient | 4 | 1.3 |
| Thoracic duct fistula | 1 | 0.3 |
| Unilateral superior laryngeal nerve paralysis | 1 | 0.3 |
| Postoperative pancreatitis | 1 | 0.3 |
| Operative death† | 1 | 0.3 |

*From Rossi, R. L., Cady, B., Silverman, M. L., et al.: Current results of conservative surgery for differentiated thyroid carcinoma. World J. Surg., *10*:618, 1986, with permission.

†Death of cardiovascular cause occurred 1 week after operation.

especially in patients in the high-risk group. All patients should receive thyroid hormone in doses sufficient to suppress thyroid-stimulating hormone.

## COMPLICATIONS

Table 14–14 summarizes the complications of surgical therapy at the Lahey Clinic in 309 patients operated on from 1961 to 1980 (see the chapter on surgical complications and their management). Our conservative management of thyroid carcinoma is associated with a low morbidity and mortality as shown in this table. Of these patients, 77 per cent were treated with bilateral subtotal thyroidectomy, 18 per cent with unilateral thyroidectomy, 3.6 per cent with excision of thyroid nodules, and 0.6 per cent with biopsy only. Nodal dissection was performed in 31 per cent of patients.

## SUMMARY

The extent of therapy for patients with differentiated thyroid carcinoma should be tailored to the biologic characteristics of the disease as defined by pathologic findings and risk group definition. Therapeutic decisions, therefore, should be based on an understanding of the pathophysiology of the disease, the available retrospective data of results of treatment, the technical expertise and experience of the surgeon, and principally on the clinically apparent likelihood of recurrence and death.

Total thyroidectomy is seldom necessary, and total lobectomy should be the standard operation for patients with carcinoma of the thyroid. Removal of portions of the contralateral thyroid lobe should be undertaken selectively after analysis of risks and benefits. One advantage of conservative thyroid operations in minimal disease is the opportunity to avoid lifetime medication with thyroid hormone, a bothersome necessity in patients in whom risk of death is not a factor who have overly aggressive surgery.

## REFERENCES


1. American Joint Committee on Cancer: Manual for Staging of Cancer. Philadelphia, J. B. Lippincott Co., 1977.
2. Attie, J. N., Khafif, R. A., and Steckler, R. M.: Elective neck dissection in papillary carcinoma of the thyroid. Am. J. Surg., *122*:464–471, 1971.
3. Bäckdahl, M., and Hamberger, B.: Ploidy in thyroid tumors. *In* van Heerden, J. A. (ed.): Common Problems in Endocrine Surgery. Chicago, Year Book Medical Publishers, Inc., 1989, pp. 49–53.
4. Bäckdahl, M., Carstensen, J., Auer, G., and Tallroth, E.: Statistical evaluation of the prognostic value of nuclear DNA content in papillary, follicular, and medullary thyroid tumors. World J. Surg., *10*:974–980, 1986.
5. Bäckdahl, M., Wallin, G., Löwhagen, T., et al.: Fine-needle biopsy cytology and DNA analysis: Their place in evaluation and treatment of patients with thyroid neoplasms. Surg. Clin. North Am., *67*:197–211, 1987.
6. Block, M. A.: Surgery of thyroid nodules and malignancy. Curr. Probl. Surg., *20*:133–203, 1983.
7. Bondeson, L., and Ljungberg, O.: Occult thyroid carcinoma at autopsy in Malmö, Sweden. Cancer, *47*:319–323, 1981.
8. Brennan, M. D.: Follicular cancer. *In* van Heerden, J. A. (ed.): Common Problems in Endocrine Surgery. Chicago, Year Book Medical Publishers, Inc., 1989, pp. 64–70.
9. Cady, B.: Surgery of thyroid cancer. World J. Surg., *5*:3–14, 1981.
10. Cady, B.: Cancer of the thyroid. *In* Nealon, T. F., Jr. (ed.): Management of the Patient with Cancer. Edition 3. Philadelphia, W. B. Saunders Co., 1986, pp. 160–168.
11. Cady, B., and Rossi, R.: An expanded view of risk-group definition in differentiated thyroid carcinoma. Surgery, *104*:947–953, 1988.
12. Cady, B., Rossi, R., Silverman, M., and Wool, M.:

Further evidence of the validity of risk group definition in differentiated thyroid carcinoma. Surgery, *98:*1171–1178, 1985.
13. Cady, B., Sedgwick, C. E., Meissner, W. A., et al.: Changing clinical, pathologic, therapeutic, and survival patterns in differentiated thyroid carcinoma. Ann. Surg., *184:*541–553, 1976.
14. Cady, B., Sedgwick, C. E., Meissner, W. A., et al.: Risk factor analysis in differentiated thyroid cancer. Cancer, *43:*810–820, 1979.
15. Clark, O. H.: Total thyroidectomy: The treatment of choice for patients with differentiated thyroid cancer. Ann. Surg., *196:*361–370, 1982.
16. Clark, O. H., Levin, K., Zeng, Q. H., et al.: Thyroid cancer: The case for total thyroidectomy. Eur. J. Cancer Clin. Oncol., *24:*305–313, 1988.
17. Doll, R.: The geographical distribution of cancer. Br. J. Cancer, *23:*1–8, 1969.
18. Favus, M. J., Schneider, A. B., Stachura, M. E., et al.: Thyroid cancer occurring as a late consequence of head-and-neck irradiation: Evaluation of 1056 patients. N. Engl. J. Med., *294:*1019–1025, 1976.
19. Foster, R. S., Jr.: Morbidity and mortality after thyroidectomy. Surg. Gynecol. Obstet., *146:*423–429, 1978.
20. Grant, C. S., and Hay, I. D.: Local recurrence of papillary thyroid carcinoma after unilateral or bilateral thyroidectomy. Wien. Klin. Wochenschr., *100:*342–346, 1988.
21. Grillo, H. C., and Zannini, P.: Resectional management of airway invasion by thyroid carcinoma. Ann. Thorac. Surg., *42:*287–298, 1986.
22. Harness, J. K., Fung, L., Thompson, N. W., et al.: Total thyroidectomy: Complications and technique. World J. Surg., *10:*781–786, 1986.
23. Hay, I. D., Taylor, W. F., and McConahey, W. M.: A prognostic score for predicting outcome in papillary thyroid carcinoma. Endocrinology, *119* (Suppl):T–15, 1986.
24. Hay, I. D., Grant, C. S., Taylor, W. F., and McConahey, W. M.: Ipsilateral lobectomy versus bilateral lobar resection in papillary thyroid carcinoma: A retrospective analysis of surgical outcome using a novel prognostic scoring system. Surgery, *102:*1088–1095, 1987.
25. Hedinger, C., and Sobin, L. H.: Histological Typing of Thyroid Tumours. International Histological Classification of Tumours. Number 11. Geneva, World Health Organization, 1974, pp. 17–24.
26. Høie, J., Stenwig, A. E., and Brennhovd, I. O.: Surgery in papillary thyroid carcinoma: A review of 730 patients. J. Surg. Oncol., *37:*147–151, 1988.
27. Lang, W., Borrusch, H., and Bauer, L.: Occult carcinomas of the thyroid: Evaluation of 1,020 sequential autopsies. Am. J. Clin. Pathol., *90:*72–76, 1988.
28. McConahey, W. M., Hay, I. D., Woolner, L. B., et al.: Papillary thyroid cancer treated at the Mayo Clinic, 1946 through 1970: Initial manifestations, pathologic findings, therapy, and outcome. Mayo Clin. Proc., *61:*978–996, 1986.
29. Meissner, W. A., and Warren, S.: Tumors of the thyroid gland. *In* Atlas of Tumor Pathology. Second series, fascicle 4. Washington, D.C., Armed Forces Institute of Pathology, 1969.
30. Noguchi, S., Noguchi, A., and Murakami, N.: Papillary carcinoma of the thyroid. I. Developing pattern of metastasis. Cancer, *26:*1053–1060, 1970.
31. Perkel, V. S., Gail, M. H., Lugin, J., et al.: Radiation-induced thyroid neoplasms: Evidence for familial susceptibility factors. J. Clin. Endocrinol. Metab., *66:*1316–1322, 1988.
32. Rossi, R. L.: Lymph node metastasis in thyroid carcinoma: Incidence, patterns of progression, and significance. Le Ganglion non envahi N-. Paris, France, Institut Gustave-Roussy, 1982, pp. 91–100.
33. Rossi, R. L., Nieroda, C., Cady, B., and Wool, M. S.: Malignancies of the thyroid gland: The Lahey Clinic experience. Surg. Clin. North Am., *65:*211–230, 1985.
34. Rossi, R. L., Cady, B., Silverman, M. L., et al.: Current results of conservative surgery for differentiated thyroid carcinoma. World J. Surg., *10:*612–622, 1986.
35. Rossi, R. L., Cady, B., Silverman, M. L., et al.: Surgically incurable well-differentiated thyroid carcinoma: Prognostic factors and results of therapy. Arch. Surg., *123:*569–574, 1988.
36. Rothman, K. J., and Boice, J. D., Jr.: Epidemiological Analysis with a Programmable Calculator. New edition. Boston, Epidemiology Resources, Inc., 1982.
37. Samaan, N. A., Schultz, P. N., Ordonez, N. G., et al.: A comparison of thyroid carcinoma in those who have and have not had head and neck irradiation in childhood. J. Clin. Endocrinol. Metab., *64:*219–223, 1987.
38. Sampson, R. J.: Prevalence and significance of occult thyroid cancer. *In* DeGroot, L. J., Frohman, L. A., Kaplan, E. L., et al. (eds.): Radiation-Associated Thyroid Carcinoma. New York, Grune & Stratton, Inc., 1977, pp. 137–153.
39. Schneider, A. B., Recant, W., Pinsky, S. M., et al.: Radiation-induced thyroid carcinoma: Clinical course and results of therapy in 296 patients. Ann. Intern. Med., *105:*405–412, 1986.
40. Silverberg, E.: Cancer statistics: 1982. CA, *32:*15–31, 1982.

# 15

# MEDULLARY THYROID CARCINOMA

*David I. Soybel, M.D., and Samuel A. Wells, Jr., M.D.*

In this chapter we review the pathology, natural history, clinical presentation, and management of patients with medullary thyroid carcinoma. Medullary carcinomas are derived from the C cells of the thyroid gland. These tumors are of great interest to biologists because they secrete many polypeptide hormones, but primarily calcitonin, which serves as an excellent plasma marker for medullary thyroid carcinoma. In addition to its sporadic occurrence, medullary thyroid carcinoma may develop in distinct subgroups of patients through autosomal dominant inheritance patterns. Also, the familial forms of medullary thyroid carcinoma may occur in association with neoplasia of other extrathyroidal tissues. These familial tumors may provide opportunities to characterize genes that regulate cellular proliferation, histogenesis, and differentiation. Medullary thyroid carcinoma represents a clinically important subgroup of thyroid carcinoma, and the life expectancy of patients with extrathyroidal spread of medullary thyroid carcinoma is less than that for patients with papillary carcinoma but much greater than that for patients with anaplastic carcinoma. The diagnosis and treatment of patients with early disease can improve the long-term prognosis and in many patients can result in cure.

## HISTORICAL ASPECTS

Although investigators had previously recognized that certain thyroid carcinomas were characterized by small clusters of cells and the extracellular deposition of amyloid,[33, 86] it was not until 1959 that Hazard et al.[29] established the distinctness of these tumors. In a review of 600 cases of thyroid carcinoma seen over a 31-year period at the Cleveland Clinic, they found 21 cases characterized by a nonfollicular sheetlike histologic pattern, the extracellular deposition of amyloid, and a high incidence of lymph node (48 per cent) and distant (38 per cent) metastases. Compared with highly malignant anaplastic carcinoma, however, the cells from medullary carcinoma were distinguished by less frequent mitoses, absence of bizarre nuclear forms, and absence of focal necrosis or polymorphonuclear cell infiltrates.

In 1961 Sipple[76] reported on a patient with bilateral pheochromocytomas and a thyroid tumor characterized as a "poorly differentiated follicular adenocarcinoma." In 1963, Manning and associates[47] described the case of a young woman with bilateral familial pheochromocytomas, multiple parathyroid adenomas, and a solid thyroid carcinoma with amyloid stroma. In 1965, Williams[101] reviewed two personal and 15 previously published cases in which thyroid carcinoma was associated with pheochromocytoma. His review suggested a high incidence of bilateral pheochromocytomas (11 cases), a high incidence of medullary thyroid carcinoma (at least 11 cases), and a high frequency of familial history of either tumor (at least seven cases). In 1968, Steiner and coworkers[82] proposed that the familial clinical syndrome characterized by medullary thyroid carcinoma, pheochromocytoma, and hyperparathyroidism with or without mucosal neuroma and marfanoid habitus be classified as multiple endocrine neoplasia (MEN) type II (MEN-II). This designation recognized the earlier description of familial syndromes characterized by the simultaneous occurrence of adenomas of the pituitary, parathyroids, and pancreatic islets[100] as MEN-I. Subsequently, two types of MEN-II syndromes became apparent. The MEN-IIa type defines patients with medullary thyroid carcinoma, pheochromocytoma, and hyperparathyroidism, and MEN-IIb or MEN-III is characterized by the concurrence of medullary thyroid carcinoma, pheochromocytoma, multiple mucosal neuromas, ganglioneuromatosis, and a typical phenotype.[15, 39] In this presentation, these syndromes are distinguished as MEN-IIa and MEN-IIb.

The chemistry and biologic properties of calcitonin were elucidated in an unrelated although parallel course with the clinical characterization of medullary thyroid carcinoma. Although Baber[3] had first described the C cells in 1876, it was not until 1962 that Copp and associates[17] demonstrated that arterial infusion of calcium salts into the thyroid-parathyroid complex of dogs initiated release of a humoral factor that lowered systemic blood calcium levels. In 1963, Hirsch and coworkers[32] extracted a substance inducing hypocalcemia from the thyroid gland, and in 1966, Bussolati and Pearse,[13] using immunofluorescence techniques, localized calcitonin to the C cells of the thyroid. Simultaneously in 1966, Williams[102] showed that spontaneous dog and rat medullary thyroid carcinomas were derived from the thyroid C cell. In 1970, Tashjian and coworkers[88] developed a radioimmunoassay for human calcitonin and demonstrated basal plasma levels in normal subjects and in patients with medullary thyroid carcinoma. Tashjian also demonstrated the different responses of normal subjects and patients with medullary thyroid carcinoma to the intravenous infusions of calcium and glucagon. DeLellis and associates[18] described the pathologic entity C cell hyperplasia, which occurs in patients with familial medullary thyroid carcinoma and represents the earliest stage of a C cell disorder and a premalignant stage of medullary thyroid carcinoma. At this time it was also becoming clear that C cells are derived embryologically from the neural crest, a site that may also give rise to cells of the adrenal medulla and other neuropeptide-secreting organs.[59] It remains a subject of active debate[85] whether all tumors expressed in the familial MEN syndromes can be embryologically traced to neural crest cells.

## INCIDENCE

Population-based surveys in the United States[61, 91] and Canada[75] indicate that medullary thyroid carcinoma constitutes 4 to 10 per cent of all thyroid carcinomas. These figures agree well with results reported in large institutional series.[7, 71] In children, the proportion of medullary thyroid carcinomas has been estimated at 2 to 3 per cent,[105] although Goepfert and associates[24] reported on eight cases (10.8 per cent) of medullary thyroid carcinoma among 74 cases of thyroid carcinoma in individuals less than 20 years of age seen from 1948 to 1978 at the M. D. Anderson Hospital.

In various series of patients with medullary thyroid carcinoma, the relative proportion of familial disease to nonfamilial (sporadic) disease may depend on referral patterns and screening practices. Between 80 and 90 per cent of patients reported in large institutional series[15, 64, 71] of medullary thyroid carcinoma have been classified as having nonfamilial disease based on history, clinical findings, and voluntary participation of family members in screening programs. Sizemore and associates[77] screened 219 primary relatives of 36 patients with histologically proved medullary thyroid carcinoma and no family history of thyroid tumor, hyperparathyroidism, or pheochromocytoma. In seven of the 36 patients, family screening identified 57 family members with elevated plasma calcitonin levels. Thus, in this report, 20 per cent of patients with presumed sporadic disease appeared to be index cases to kindreds with familial medullary thyroid carcinoma. In addition, Farndon and associates[21] described two large kindreds in which clinically evident medullary thyroid carcinoma was inherited in the absence of clinical, historical, or biochemical evidence of pheochromocytoma, hyperparathyroidism, or mucosal neuroma in any members of the affected families. This syndrome has been termed *familial nonMEN medullary thyroid carcinoma.* Thus, medullary carcinoma is not necessarily inherited as part of the MEN syndrome; however, the familial forms may constitute a greater proportion of medullary thyroid carcinomas than has previously been appreciated.

## INHERITANCE PATTERNS

Although indirect evidence exists that some medullary thyroid carcinomas may occur through an autosomal recessive inheritance pattern,[54] familial cases of this disease are most commonly inherited through an autosomal dominant pattern. When medullary thyroid carcinoma is transmitted as the sole lesion, it appears to have both a high degree of penetrance and expressivity. The genealogy of kindred O is shown in Figure 15–1 in a series of patients with familial nonMEN medullary thyroid carcinoma, which has previously been reported.[21] In older parts of this family tree, thyroid carcinoma is described as "suspected" when family members described surgery or symptoms compatible with the diagnosis and is described as "proved" only when supportive histologic evidence was available. From this genealogy, it would appear that the allele does not "skip" generations, that is, manifest itself in the children and grandparents' generation but not in the parents' generation. In addition, in this family, two consanguineous marriages involved individuals who both apparently carried the allele expressing medullary thyroid carcinoma. In both instances, a great majority of the offspring (greater than 75 per cent) manifested the tumor, as would be expected for the union of two heterozygous parents carrying the dominant gene. In no instance has clinical or biochemical evidence of pheochromocytoma or hyperparathyroidism been obtained in any member of this kindred.

The genealogy of a family with the MEN-IIa syndrome, which has been traced back eight generations to an affected member who was born in Virginia in 1845,[14] is shown in Figure 15–2. Again, expression of the syndrome has not skipped generations and conforms to an autosomal dominant pattern of transmission. The expression of the different components of the syndrome, however, has been variable. From a previously reported[14] series of patients, the data in Table 15–1 summarize some aspects of the variable expression. Medullary thyroid carcinoma or C cell hyperplasia has developed in 122 patients comprising 13 kindreds with MEN-IIa. Pheochromocytoma and parathyroid hyperplasia have each been diagnosed in about one third to one half of patients, often 5 to 10 years after the diagnosis of medullary thyroid carcinoma. In approximately 20 to 25 per cent of patients with MEN-IIa has the full syndrome of medullary thyroid carcinoma, pheochromocytoma, and parathyroid hyperplasia developed. In MEN-IIb, medullary thyroid carcinoma, the characteristic physical appearance, mucosal neuroma, and ganglioneuromatosis develop in virtually all patients. Pheochromocytomas develop in approximately 50 per cent of patients with MEN-IIb.[15, 39]

Although the diagnosis of pheochromocytoma may be made simultaneously or subsequent to the diagnosis of medullary thyroid carcinoma, this is not always the case. Jansson and associates[35] reviewed 64 consecutive patients treated surgically for pheochromocytoma. Ten persons (15.6 per cent) in this series were found to have C cell disease of whom seven had diagnosis simultaneously with pheochromocytoma and three had diagnosis in subsequent screening. Four of the patients were not members of previously recognized kindreds with MEN-IIa or MEN-IIb. These observations suggest that pheochromocytoma can be the presenting clinical abnormality in patients with MEN-IIa or MEN-IIb, particularly when no family history suggests that the patient should be screened for these syndromes. In addition, these find-

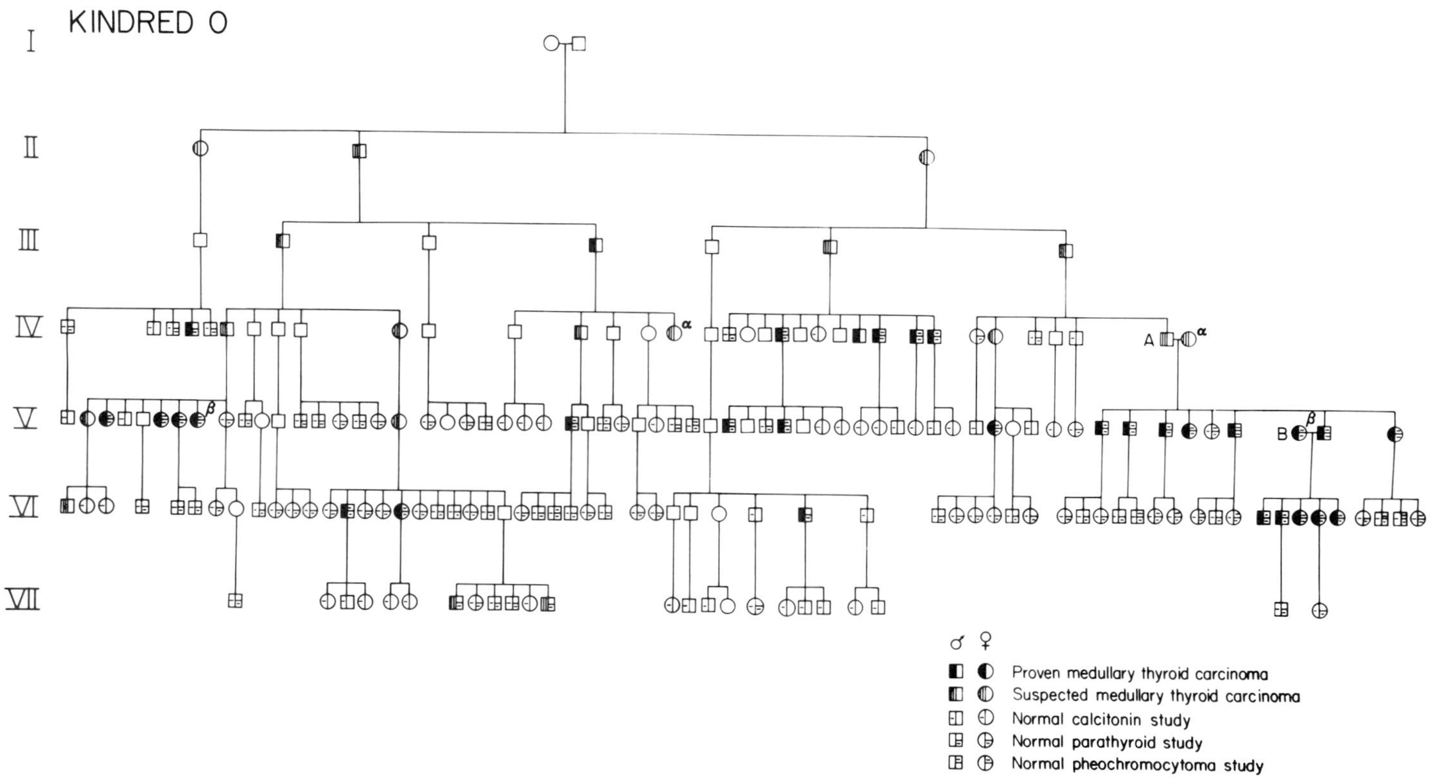


**FIGURE 15–1.** Kindred O, a genealogy of seven generations with transmission of medullary thyroid carcinoma in the absence of other endocrinopathy. Two individuals, designated by α and β, appear twice in the genealogy; they are wives involved in consanguineous marriages. (From Farndon, J. R., Leight, G. S., Dilley, W. G., et al.: Familial medullary thyroid carcinoma without associated endocrinopathies: A distinct clinical entity. Br. J. Surg., *73*:279, 1986, with permission.)

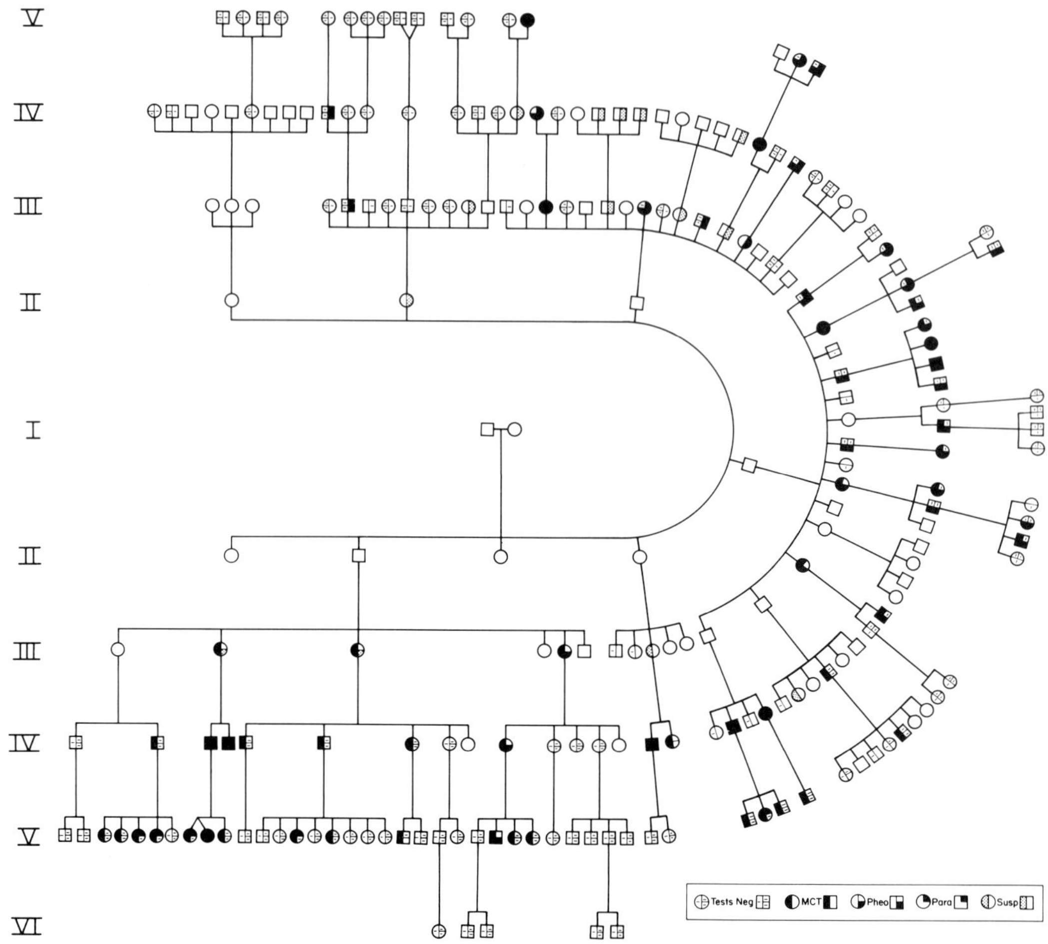


**FIGURE 15–2.** Kindred W, a genealogy with transmission of MEN-IIa (medullary carcinoma [MCT], pheochromocytoma [Pheo], hyperparathyroidism [Para]). Information is available only on descendants of the progenitor and his wife. O = Female; □ = Male; Susp = Suspected MTC. (Modified from Cance, W. G., and Wells, S. A., Jr.: Multiple endocrine neoplasia type IIa. Curr. Probl. Surg., *22*(5):18, 1985.)

**TABLE 15–1. Clinical Features of Patients with MEN-IIa**

| CLINICAL FEATURE | MEDULLARY THYROID CARCINOMA | PHEOCHROMO-CYTOMA | HYPERPARA-THYROIDISM |
|---|---|---|---|
| Patient numbers | 122 | 40 | 42 |
| Incidence, per cent | 100 | 33 | 34 |
| Average age at diagnosis, years | 27 ± 14 | 36 ± 13 | 31 ± 16 |
| Age range at diagnosis, years | 6–71 | 15–73 | 11–71 |
| Male to female ratio | 62:60 | 18:22 | 14:28 |

Reproduced with permission from Cance, W. G., and Wells, S. A., Jr.: Multiple endocrine neoplasia type IIa. Curr. Probl. Surg., *22*(5):18, 1985.

ings emphasize that family histories do not reliably exclude the diagnosis of MEN syndromes and that endocrinopathies may not all be apparent simultaneously. Any individual with medullary thyroid carcinoma or pheochromocytoma should undergo serial evaluation to exclude the presence of MEN-IIa or MEN-IIb. Immediate family members of affected persons should also be evaluated to exclude the presence of medullary thyroid carcinoma.

## ETIOLOGY

### *Cells of Origin*

The calcitonin-secreting cells or C cells cannot always be recognized in thyroid tissue using hematoxylin-eosin staining alone.[63] These cells are easily identified by using calcitonin antisera and immunoperoxidase staining.[28, 63] Under the light microscope, two cell variants have been described[63]: a small-bodied polygonal cell and a larger cell with streaming cytoplasm. Ultrastructurally, C cells contain numerous large mitochondria and electron-dense secretory granules that are argyrophilic and also stain positively with calcitonin antibodies.[28, 63]

In the normal adult, C cells occur singly and in clusters and are observed in both intrafollicular and parafollicular locations.[28] The cells are not distributed throughout the thyroid but tend to be concentrated along the central axes of the lateral lobes in the middle third and upper third of each lobe.[28] In the neonate, C cells morphologically resemble those of the adult. In the elderly individual, the density of C cells in tissue sections can be highly variable.[57] Reports[57, 79] have indicated that 15 to 20 per cent of thyroids in adults, especially in elderly patients, may harbor large aggregates of C cells. It is not yet certain whether such aggregates represent age-related hyperplasia, failure of cellular migration early in life, or perhaps latent neoplasms or premalignant lesions.

It is usually accepted that C cells, like the chromaffin cells of the adrenal medulla, are derivatives of embryonic neural crest cells and represent a larger class of cells designated by the acronym APUD. This acronym summarizes certain key cytochemical characteristics that include high *A*mine content, amine *P*recursor *U*ptake, amino acid *D*ecarboxylation, and other features, such as the presence of neuron-specific enolase,[34, 72] an enzyme not normally found outside of neuroectoderm-derived tissue.[72] It is no longer accepted that all cells with APUD characteristics (e.g., beta cells of pancreatic islets, anterior pituitary cells) necessarily derive from the neural crest.[85] Some cells in the parathyroid glands do stain for neuron-specific enolase.[93] Such cells probably reflect neuroendocrine elements other than parathyroid principal cells, which do not manifest APUD cytochemical characteristics. The embryologic relationships of neuroectodermal APUD cells, non-neuroectodermal APUD cells, and nonAPUD peptide-secreting cells remain unclear. Clinically, however, the concept of embryologically and functionally related APUD cells may be important in that it emphasizes the possibility that specific components of the multiple endocrine neoplasia syndromes may originate in a defect of differentiation of a common precursor cell or in a common defective response of such cells to stimuli of malignant transformation. In addition, the APUD concept indicates that such cells may share cytochemical properties for synthesizing a number of neuroendocrine substances (e.g., ACTH, somatostatin, serotonin), any one of which might be secreted by a malignant cell line that has undergone dedifferentiation.

### *Oncogenesis*

As already discussed, familial forms of medullary thyroid carcinoma are inherited in an autosomal dominant pattern. The exact genetic defects in these syndromes are not known. Some investigators[71] have demonstrated chromosomal deletions or high rates of spontaneous chromosomal instability in cultured peripheral lymphocytes of patients with the MEN syndromes, but other investigators[71, 107] have not been able to confirm these findings. Consistent constitutional chromosomal abnormalities are only now coming to light by use of newer techniques of molecular biology.

Despite the absence of information regarding initial steps in cell transformation, good evidence exists that familial medullary thyroid carcinoma arises through a sequence of proliferative changes in C cells. The earliest thyroid abnormality in this sequence involves C cell hyperplasia, which is characterized by multicentric patches of C cells in the lateral lobes.[106] These initial cell clusters do not exhibit nuclear atypic or vascular invasion but are a source of increased calcitonin secretion.[14] Ultrastructurally, the basal lamina surrounding hyperplastic cells may be duplicated in some areas and absent in others.[19] Such lesions progress variably to foci of carcinoma and ultimately grow to become clinically palpable. Baylin and associates[5] evaluated multifocal carcinoma in black female patients and found that each focus of carcinoma contained either type A or type B glucose-6-phosphate dehydrogenase. These findings suggested that the inherited defect leading to medullary thyroid carcinoma provides an initial mutation leading to multiple susceptible clones of C cells; each focus of carcinoma would then arise from a final mutation or selection of one cell in each clone. It seems likely that pheochromocytoma would develop against a background of diffuse or nodular adrenal medullary hyperplasia in a similar manner.[46]

The origin of diffuse parathyroid hyperplasia in the MEN-IIa syndrome is not resolved. It has been hypothesized[59] that these cells would proliferate and grow secondarily in response to the chronic hypocalcemic effects of increased circulatory levels of calcitonin. This hypothesis seems unlikely, however, because parathyroid hyperplasia is rare or virtually never occurs in patients with MEN-IIb, sporadic medullary thyroid carcinoma, or familial nonMEN medullary thyroid carcinoma.[14]

The cause of sporadic forms of medullary thyroid carcinoma also remains unknown. Various stimuli, such as hypervitaminosis A and D, irradiation, and experimentally induced hypercalcemia, have been associated with an increased incidence of medullary thyroid carcinoma in animals.[71] C cell hyperplasia[44] and rarely medullary thyroid carcinoma[43] have been described in association with parathyroid tumors. Most sporadic medullary thyroid carcinomas are not associated with hypercalcemia. Sporadic medullary thyroid carcinoma is much less frequently bilateral and less often associated with areas of C cell hyperplasia in contrast to the much higher incidence of bilaterality (greater than 90 per cent) and associated C cell hyperplasia in familial forms of the disease.[9, 14, 71, 90] These findings would argue that sporadic medullary thyroid carcinoma does not arise from the sequence of transforming events that give rise to familial forms of the disease.

## PATHOLOGY

### *Macroscopic Findings*

Medullary thyroid carcinoma is solid and gray-white or tan. The cut surface may dem-

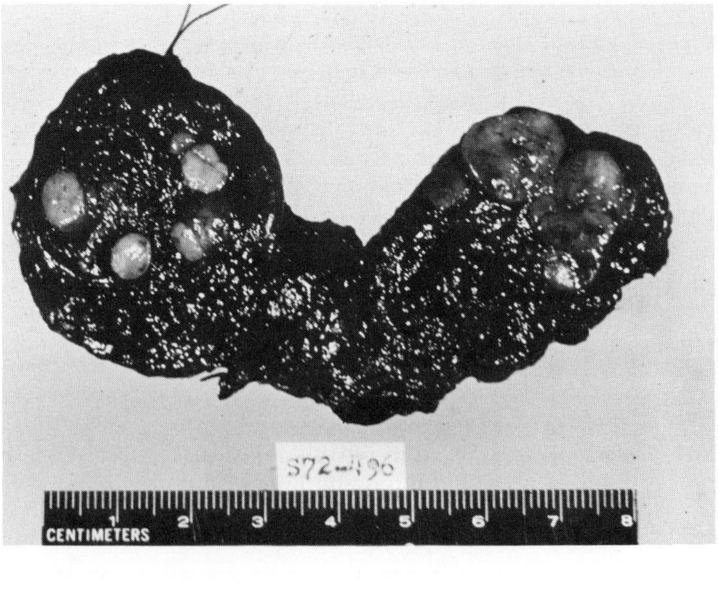


**FIGURE 15–3.** Primary medullary thyroid carcinoma in total thyroidectomy specimen. Tumor exhibits a solid growth pattern, is multicentric, and is situated laterally and superiorly in the thyroid lobes. (From Keiser, H. R., Beaven, M. A., Doppman, J., et al.: Sipple's syndrome: Medullary thyroid carcinoma, pheochromocytoma, and parathyroid disease. Ann. Intern. Med., *78:*571, 1973, with permission.)

onstrate areas of hemorrhage, necrosis, fibrosis, and calcification. In patients with familial disease, medullary thyroid carcinoma is virtually always present in both thyroid lobes, but the tumor may be multicentric, and foci vary greatly in size (Fig. 15–3). Characteristically, medullary thyroid carcinoma is located in the middle to upper portions of the thyroid lobe.[8, 9] In sporadic medullary thyroid carcinoma, the tumor is usually confined to one thyroid lobe. In some series,[67, 71] 30 per cent of patients with sporadic medullary thyroid carcinoma had bilateral or multicentric tumors; however, the proportion of patients with bilateral disease was under 5 per cent in other series.[9, 15]

## *Microscopic Findings*

Medullary thyroid carcinoma exhibits a variety of histologic patterns as seen in sections stained with hematoxylin-eosin or silver. At least three separate histologic classification systems have been used for describing these tumors. Keiser et al.[37] classified specimens from 23 patients with the MEN-IIa syndrome into cellular, intermediate, and fibrotic types (Fig. 15–4). Tumors of the cellular type, found in four patients, were composed of multiple nests of ovoid spindle shaped cells separated by delicate fibrovascular septae. Only small amyloid deposits were present in these specimens. The intermediate type of tumors, seen in nine patients, were divided by broad bands of fibrous tissue and contained extensive stromal amyloid deposits. In the ten patients exhibiting the fibrotic type, the central portion of the tumor was largely replaced by a cellular stroma that was frequently calcified and interspersed with amyloid deposits throughout. In this series, histologic type seemed to be related to the age of the patient and the spread of the tumor; all four patients with the cellular type were less than 27 years old and had no evidence of metastases to lymph nodes at operation. Of the 19 patients with the intermediate or fibrotic types, 16 were older than 29 years, were operated on 3 or more years after the detection of a thyroid mass, or had lymph node metastases. These patients also had larger tumors.

Subsequently, in a review of 72 patients with the MEN-IIa syndrome, Bigner and coworkers[8] divided tumors by size. In 22 patients (group 1) characterized as having tumors less than 0.7 cm in diameter (five patients had C cell hyperplasia alone), the histologic pattern was similar to the "cellular" type of Keiser et al.[37] (see earlier), and amyloid deposits were observed in 13 patients. Patients in group 1 were younger than the patients in other groups (mean 19.7 years) and had a lower prevalence of regional lymph node metastases (20 per cent) discovered at surgery. In 19 patients (group 2), the tumors were 0.7 to 1.5 cm in size, the mean age of the patients at diagnosis was 33.7 years, and the prevalence of nodal metastases was 30 per cent. Histologically, the tumors in patients in group 2 were characterized by increased amounts of amyloid, variable cell morphology, and rarely tumor necrosis. In 26 patients (group 3), the tumors were larger than 1.5 cm, the mean age of the patients at diagnosis was 32.7 years, and the prevalence of nodal metastases was 80 per cent. Histologically, the tumor margins were circumscribed, but true fibrous encapsulation was not observed. Stromal components were predominant in 20 patients, cell types were variable, amyloid was more abundant, and tumor necrosis was noted in specimens from three patients.

Saad and associates[71] and Zaatari and associates[108] distinguished at least five histologic patterns of medullary thyroid carcinoma. Incidences of nodal metastases in relation to these subtypes have not been evaluated.[71, 108] At present, the relationship between tumor size, histologic pattern, and clinical characteristics is still incompletely defined, especially for patients with the sporadic form of medullary carcinoma. Nevertheless, larger size, abundance of amyloid and stromal elements, and tumor necrosis seem to indicate a greater likelihood of extrathyroidal spread. Multicentricity, bilaterality, and the presence of C cell hyperplasia strongly suggest that the disease is familial,[9, 15, 71] while unilaterality and absence of C cell hyperplasia suggest sporadic disease.[9]

## *Cytochemical and Cytopathologic Features*

Medullary carcinoma secretes calcitonin, which can be localized in the secretory gran-

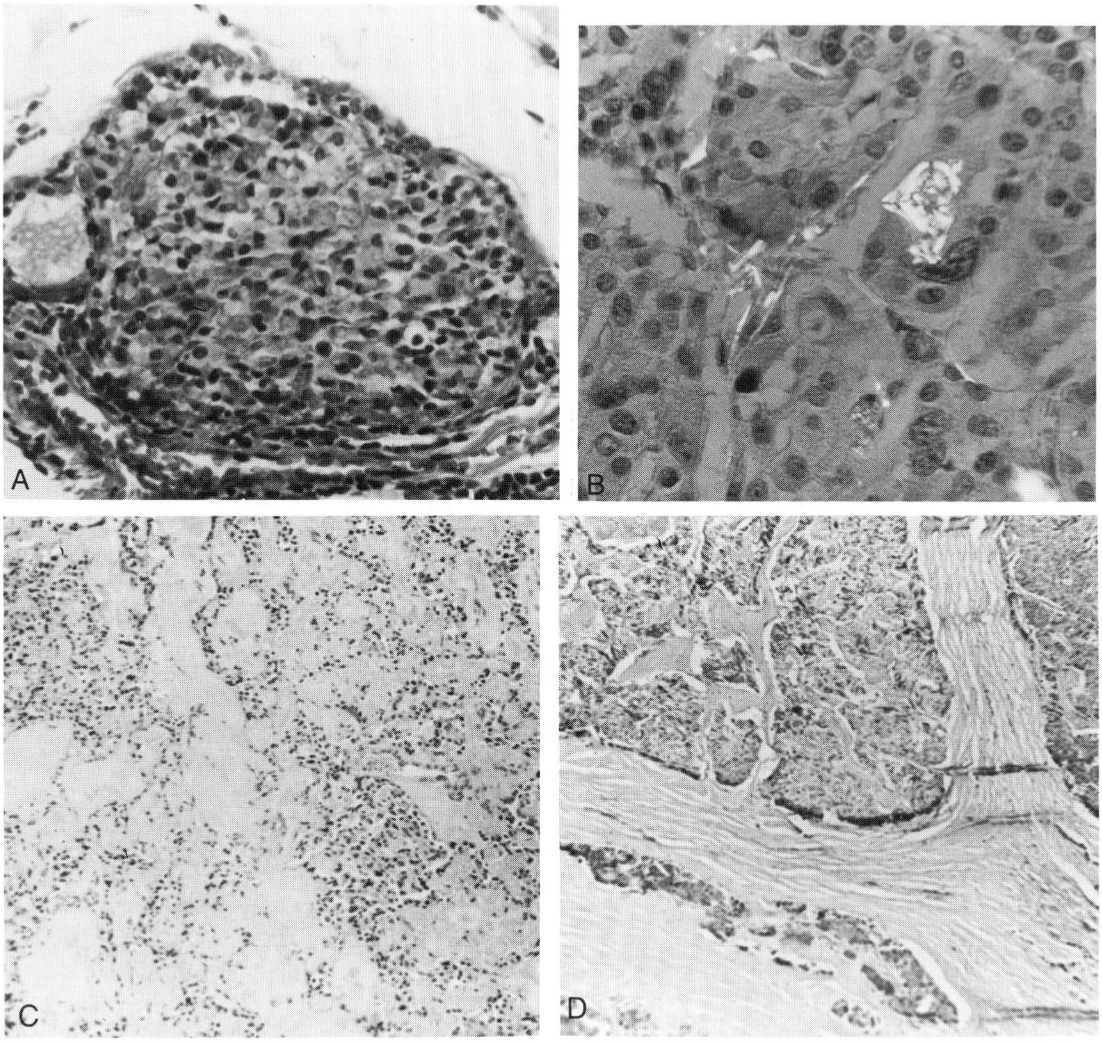

**FIGURE 15–4.** Histopathologic patterns of medullary carcinoma. *A,* C cell nodule without evidence of carcinoma. *B,* Cellular type of medullary carcinoma. Tumor nodules contain sheets and nests of ovoid cells with little connective tissue. *C,* Intermediate type of medullary carcinoma. Nests of tumor cells are separated by bands of amyloid-containing fibrous stroma. *D,* Fibrotic type of medullary carcinoma. Foci of tumor cells and amyloid deposits are scattered within dense fibrous stroma.

ules of normal and malignant C cells.[28, 63] A number of other peptides and amines have been identified in the secretory granules of sporadic and familial medullary thyroid carcinoma and these include gastrin, serotonin, adrenocorticotropin hormone (ACTH), bombesin, substance P, and others.[14, 74, 90] Other bioactive substances that medullary thyroid cells may synthesize in excess include prostaglandins,[14, 104] carcinoembryonic antigen,[14, 90] and mucin.[108]

The most important of these secretory products is calcitonin, a 3,500 dalton polypeptide that is composed of 32 amino acid residues. Tashjian and coworkers[88, 106] found that elevated plasma levels of this hormone, either in the basal state or after stimulation with certain calcitonin secretagogues, are highly sensitive and specific for the presence of a C cell disorder. Immunostaining of primary tumors using specific calcitonin antisera may also be useful in assessing the likelihood of extrathyroidal spread and the virulence of disease. Lippman and associates[41] found that homogeneous staining of C cells from resected medullary thyroid carcinoma predicted a low rate of tumor recurrence after thyroidectomy, whereas heterogeneous staining of cells from the primary tumor predicted high rates of regional and distant metastases and shortened survival. In 44 patients with medullary carcinoma, Saad and coworkers[70] also found that homogeneity of calcitonin staining correlated with survival and that homogeneity of staining in nodal metastases predicted higher long-term survival for the patient than did heterogeneous staining.

Other tissue staining characteristics that may prove useful in the diagnosis of medullary thyroid carcinoma and in the assessment of virulence of disease have been described as well. Immunochemical techniques have been used to demonstrate high levels of histaminase and L-dopa decarboxylase in medullary thyroid carcinoma. In particular, levels of histaminase per gram of tumor tissue appear to increase in the transition from C cell hyperplasia to microscopic carcinoma to palpable medullary thyroid carcinoma.[6] In one patient[70] it was possible to demonstrate, by immunocytochemical staining of medullary thyroid carcinoma, that the content of histaminase inversely correlated with the content of calcitonin. Tissue distribution of carcinoembryonic antigen, demonstrated by similar immunocytochemical techniques, may also correlate inversely with the distribution of calcitonin in medullary thyroid carcinoma cells,[49] and carcinoembryonic antigen levels in the circulation appear to correlate directly with recurrence of the tumor and metastasis.

One final cytopathologic procedure that may aid in identifying primary tumors with a high risk of occult metastasis and poor prognosis is the analysis of cellular DNA content. Bäckdahl and associates[4] retrospectively studied nuclear DNA distributions in paraffin specimens of 36 patients with medullary thyroid carcinoma, two of whom had familial disease and 34 of whom had no family history or endocrinopathy. Of patients who died less than 10 years after thyroidectomy for medullary thyroid carcinoma, 90 per cent had aneuploid tumors; 60 per cent who lived more than 10 years exhibited diploid tumors. Patients with diploid tumors in whom recurrent disease developed and who died of tumor had unresectable disease at the time of operation; of patients with aneuploid tumors who lived more than 10 years, almost all had resectable lesions and uninvolved regional lymph nodes. These findings suggest that nuclear DNA distribution may be used, in conjunction with assessment of extrathyroidal spread, as a means of determining prognosis. It is not known whether DNA distribution correlates with other cytochemical or histologic properties of these tumors.

## *Patterns of Extrathyroidal Spread*

Medullary thyroid carcinoma most commonly spreads to regional lymph nodes in the neck. In a 1969 review of 249 cases collected from six institutions, Fletcher[22] found that patients presenting with symptomatic medullary thyroid carcinoma had a 56 per cent incidence of unilateral cervical lymph node involvement and an 11 per cent incidence of bilateral lymph node involvement. These figures are similar to the 54 per cent overall incidence of lymph node involvement observed in the Mayo Clinic series[67] and the 52 per cent overall incidence in the M. D. Anderson series[71] for patients with sporadic medullary thyroid carcinoma. In patients with MEN-IIa or MEN-IIb, medullary thyroid carcinoma may be diagnosed while clinically occult by documenting increased plasma calcitonin levels. In these patients, the regional lymph nodes are infrequently involved. Russell and associates[67] found cervical node metastases in only two of 14 patients (14 per cent) whose medullary thyroid carcinoma was diagnosed by detection of elevations in basal plasma calcitonin levels. Wells and associates[99] had previously observed a similar incidence (18 per cent) of nodal involvement in 28 patients diagnosed biochemically compared with an incidence of 62 per cent in 24 patients in whom the carcinoma was palpable. These findings are consistent with those of Bigner and associates[8] who found that the incidence of cervical node metastasis is primarily related to tumor size, which also correlates importantly with preoperative plasma calcitonin levels.[99]

The incidence of metastasis to nodes in regions other than the neck is less well documented. Chong and coworkers[15] reported initial mediastinal involvement in 8 per cent of patients undergoing surgery for medullary thyroid carcinoma, and evidence of associated cervical adenopathy was present in each patient. After 128 resections for cure, recurrent disease subsequently developed in 44 patients. Of these 44, 18 per cent had recurrent disease in mediastinal nodes. Of patients with recurrent mediastinal disease, cervical node recurrent disease was found in 89 per cent and metastases to distant sites in 50 per cent. Similarly, Saad and coworkers[71] reported that the mediastinum was the sole site of recurrent disease in 1.3 per cent of patients undergoing curative thyroidectomy and was associated with recurrent disease in the neck or distant sites in 8.4 per cent. Thus, mediastinal involvement is unusual in the absence of cervical node involvement and strongly suggests the possibility of tumor in more distant locations.

The most common sites for distant metastases have included bone, 30 to 40 per cent; lung, 20 to 25 per cent; liver, 20 to 25 per cent; thoracic viscera, 2 to 4 per cent; and abdominal viscera, 2 to 5 per cent.[15, 25, 71] Metastases to distant sites may not always be associated with cervical node involvement. Chong and associates[15] found distant organs as the sole recurrence site in 8 of 44 patients in whom recurrent disease followed curative thyroidectomy, whereas distant disease was associated with simultaneous cervical or mediastinal recurrent disease in 10 patients. Saad and associates[71] found recurrent disease in distant sites, in the absence of simultaneous cervical node recurrent disease, in at least 7 per cent of patients who had previously undergone curative thyroidectomy. Chong and coworkers,[15] however, found that 84 per cent of patients with subsequent recurrent disease had nodal involvement at the initial operation. It is not clear whether the incidence of distant metastasis is related primarily to the characteristics of the primary tumor (e.g., size, histologic pattern, nuclear DNA distributions) and direct invasion of thyroid blood vessels or to an intermediate event of nodal metastasis.

## CLINICAL EXAMINATION AND PRESENTATION

An increasing proportion of patients with familial medullary thyroid carcinoma can be diagnosed while asymptomatic. Nevertheless, virtually all patients with sporadic medullary thyroid carcinoma and a high percentage of patients with familial disease present with clinical symptoms or signs. A patient who has a thyroid mass should be questioned closely regarding the onset of neck swelling and the presence of hoarseness, dysphagia, or respiratory difficulty. It is also important to seek evidence suggestive of pheochromocytoma or hyperparathyroidism. In addition, even in patients with apparently sporadic disease, a careful family history should be sought for evidence of multiple endocrine neoplasia. The physical examination should involve a detailed examination of the dimensions of the thyroid and the location and characteristics of any thyroid nodules and regional lymph nodes. Mucosal neuroma, a marfanoid habitus, café-au-lait spots, hypertrophied ocular nerves, and other features of the MEN-IIb syndrome should specifically be noted or excluded. Although the history and physical examination do not themselves provide a diagnosis of medullary thyroid carcinoma in a thyroid nodule, such information will be helpful in staging the carcinoma and in identifying whether family members are at risk of acquiring the disease.

Summarized in Tables 15–2, 15–3, and 15–

**TABLE 15–2. Clinical Presentation of Sporadic Medullary Carcinoma of the Thyroid**

| SERIES | NO. OF PATIENTS | AGE AT DIAGNOSIS, MEAN, YEARS | AGE AT DIAGNOSIS, RANGE, YEARS | RATIO OF MALES TO FEMALES |
|---|---|---|---|---|
| Gordon et al.[25] | 40 | 48 | 20–75 | 21:19 (1.1:1.0) |
| Block et al.[9] | 24 | 50 | 22–74 | 11:13 (1.0:1.2) |
| Rossi et al.[64] | 34 | 52, females; 61, males | 21–76 | 12:22 (1.0:1.8) |
| Russell et al.[64] | 50 | 50 | 27–73 | — |
| Saad et al.[71] | 125 | 46 | 15–80 | 62:63 (1.0:1.0) |

4 are some clinical characteristics of patients in whom medullary thyroid carcinoma has been diagnosed. Patients with apparently sporadic forms of the disease most commonly present in the fifth and sixth decades of life, although these forms may occur in individuals as young as 20 years of age (Table 15–2). Patients with MEN-IIa or MEN-IIb characteristically present first with a thyroid tumor (Table 15–3). The majority of patients summarized in this table were identified because of signs or symptoms, usually by the fourth decade in the MEN-IIa syndrome and by the second or third decade in the MEN-IIb syndrome. In patients with MEN-IIb, the appearance of a thyroid mass has been recorded in children 2 and 4 years of age,[11, 39, 56, 67] indicating that thyroid neoplasms in this group may be extremely virulent. In kindreds who display medullary thyroid carcinoma without associated endocrinopathy, the average age at diagnosis (43 years) is much closer to the age at which sporadic forms present. In contrast to the higher incidence of papillary and follicular carcinomas among women,[10] no clear evidence suggests that medullary thyroid carcinoma is more frequent among men or women.

Commonly, medullary thyroid carcinoma presents as a thyroid mass (Table 15–4). In 70 to 80 per cent of patients, sporadic medullary carcinoma is detected because of the finding of a painless palpable thyroid nodule. Up to 10 per cent of patients may have evidence of invasion of adjacent structures characterized by hoarseness, inspiratory difficulty, or dysphagia. From 25 to 50 per cent of patients may have palpable cervical adenopathy. In 6 to 10 per cent of patients with medullary thyroid carcinoma, adenopathy may be present in the absence of a thyroid mass.[15, 64]

Diarrhea may be the chief complaint in occasional patients,[15] but it may be associated with other signs or symptoms of disease in more than 25 per cent of patients with medullary thyroid carcinoma (Table 15–4). The diarrhea is usually loose, watery, and mild. More than half of the patients with these symptoms will complain of an excess of five stools per 24 hours, and one third may describe urgency. Steatorrhea or malabsorption is rare.[15, 84] Steinfeld and associates[84] found that almost 80 per cent of patients with medullary thyroid carcinoma and diarrhea had evidence of regional lymph node or distant metastases.

The pathogenesis of the diarrhea in association with medullary thyroid carcinoma remains incompletely understood. Clinical

**TABLE 15–3. Clinical Presentation of Medullary Carcinoma in Multiple Endocrine Neoplasias**

| SERIES | MEN TYPE | NO. OF PATIENTS | AGE AT DIAGNOSIS, MEAN, YEARS | AGE AT DIAGNOSIS, RANGE, YEARS | RATIO OF MALES TO FEMALES |
|---|---|---|---|---|---|
| Russell et al.[67] | II | 58 | 34 | 4–72 | — |
| Block et al.[9] | II | 58 | 36* | 20–67 | 22:36 (1.0:1.6) |
| Saad et al.[71] | II | 31 | 32 | 15–60 | 13:18 (1.0:1.4) |
| Cance and Wells[14] | II | 122 | 27 | 6–71 | 62:60 (1.0:1.0) |
| Khairi et al.[39] | III | 41† | 22 | 4–53 | 19:22 (1.0:1.2) |
| Russell et al.[67] | III | 15 | 20 | 2–51 | — |
| Brunt and Wells[11] | III | 10 | 16 | 4–36 | 4: 6 (1.5:1.0) |

*Includes four new cases and review of cases reported up until 1975.
†Includes only 20 cases diagnosed before availability of serum calcitonin assay for screening.

**TABLE 15–4. Symptomatic Presentation of Medullary Thyroid Carcinoma**

| SERIES | NO. OF PATIENTS | PER CENT DIAGNOSED THROUGH SCREENING PROGRAM | PER CENT PRESENTING WITH PALPABLE THYROID ENLARGEMENT OR NECK SWELLING | PER CENT WITH SYMPTOMS OF COMPRESSION (HOARSENESS, DYSPHAGIA) | PER CENT WITH DIARRHEA | PER CENT WITH PALPABLE CERVICAL ADENOPATHY |
|---|---|---|---|---|---|---|
| Williams et al.[104] | 67* | 0 | Most common | — | 21 | — |
| Gordon et al.[25] | 40† | 0 | 90 | 2 | 25 | — |
| Chong et al.[15] | 139‡ | 8 | 80 | 11 | 29 | — |
| Saad et al.[71] | 125§ | 0 | 94 | 13 | 29 | 52 |

*Unspecified number of patients (>5) may have had MEN syndromes.
†Includes three patients with possible MEN syndromes.
‡Includes 29 patients with MEN syndromes.
§Sporadic medullary carcinomas only; does not specify whether adenopathy was palpable in all instances.

investigations[18, 27] have suggested that high plasma calcitonin levels inhibit absorption and stimulate secretion of fluid and electrolytes in the jejunum and ileum. Calcitonin may elicit these effects locally, in the intestinal wall,[109] or perhaps through mechanisms mediated by the central nervous system.[62] Calcitonin infusions in humans have been shown to alter circulating levels of several gastrointestinal regulatory peptides, including gastrin, pancreatic glucagon, motilin, pancreatic polypeptide, and glucose-dependent insulinotropic peptide.[109] In addition, medullary carcinoma may secrete additional substances that can induce diarrhea, such as prostaglandins or serotonin.[9, 84] It is not clear whether circulating plasma calcitonin levels correlate significantly with the incidence of diarrhea, although patients with more advanced carcinoma (presumably those who secrete greater quantities of plasma calcitonin) have a higher incidence of diarrhea.

## DIAGNOSTIC MODALITIES AND STRATEGIES

At present, strategies for identifying and staging medullary thyroid carcinoma are required for two different groups of patients. The first group involves patients with symptoms or signs of thyroid carcinoma but a questionable or absent family history for familial disease or MEN. The second group is composed of patients who are first-degree or second-degree relatives of a patient with medullary thyroid carcinoma and who may harbor familial disease. In this section, we will discuss the diagnostic modalities used to detect and diagnose medullary thyroid carcinoma.

### *Diagnostic Modalities*

***Imaging.*** Several methods are available for imaging medullary thyroid carcinoma, some of which may specifically suggest the diagnosis. Plain films of the neck and thorax may demonstrate evidence of a thyroid mass[48, 92] and possibly compression of adjacent structures.[92] A characteristic feature that can be seen on a plain film involves irregular calcifications within the primary tumor or in metastatic deposits in cervical or mediastinal lymph nodes, lung, or liver. Such calcifications, which may be observed in 10 per cent of patients having symptoms,[92] are different from the faint homogeneous calcifications described with other thyroid tumors.[37, 48] Tumor masses that are large enough to calcify are usually associated with advanced disease.[92] Williams and coworkers,[103] however, suggested that such calcifications may be associated with an absence of mitotic activity in the tumor and do not necessarily imply poor long-term survival. Overall, plain films of the neck are not useful for detecting early lesions.

Thyroid scintigraphy using pertechnetate or radioactive iodine is not sensitive enough to identify early lesions. Medullary carcinoma does not concentrate $^{99m}$Tc or radioactive iodine and thus appears as hypofunctioning nodules on scintigraphy.[1] Anderson and associates[1] found that scintigraphy was not substantially more sensitive than palpation, and neither identified more than 31 per cent of familial medullary thyroid carcinomas, which were detectable through plasma calcitonin assay. Nevertheless, these authors noted that five of 35 patients with familial disease presented with bilateral symmetric hypofunctioning nodules coinciding with histologically verified multicentric medullary thyroid carcinoma. Thus, scintigraphy may not be recommended in routine diagnostic evaluation for suspected medullary thyroid carcinoma, but the finding of bilateral or multiple "cold" nodules may raise suspicion of familial disease.

Scintigraphic techniques are, perhaps, being more effectively applied to localize residual disease in patients who have undergone thyroidectomy for medullary thyroid carcinoma and who continue to have elevated plasma calcitonin levels postoperatively. Johnson and associates[36] used $^{99m}$Tc sulfur colloid to detect metastatic medullary thyroid carcinoma in 11 of 34 such patients. In eight patients with metastases demonstrated by $^{99m}$Tc phosphate, four had osseous metastases confirmed by skeletal films, two had osseous metastases not detected on bone films, and two had soft tissue lesions in cervical or mediastinal nodes. In nine patients with metastases demonstrated by $^{99m}$Tc sulfur colloid, eight had liver metastases, and one had splenic carcinoma. Recently, Arnstein and coworkers[2] used thallium 201 scanning to localize cervical or mediastinal metastases in two such patients, and in neither patient was recurrent disease detected clinically or by computed tomographic scan. Talpos and associates[87] used a subtraction technique with thallium 201 and $^{99m}$Tc pertechnetate to identify residual disease in five of ten patients evaluated. The number of patients undergoing these evaluations has been small, and it remains unclear how frequently these scintigraphic techniques will identify lesions not detectable clinically or through other imaging techniques.

Scintigraphy using radionuclide tracers that may be concentrated specifically in a medullary thyroid carcinoma or its metastases remains largely experimental. Miyauchi and coworkers[51] updated their experience with $^{99m}$Tc (V)-dimercaptosuccinic acid in ten patients with medullary thyroid carcinoma. This tracer was clearly concentrated in seven primary tumors, none of which was less than 2.5 cm in its smallest dimension. Lymph nodes as small as 0.8 by 1.2 cm were detected in one patient, but equally sized lymph nodes in another were not. In all of the patients with primary medullary thyroid carcinoma, plasma calcitonin levels were high (mean, 14,600 pg/ml; range, 1,700 to 30,000 pg/ml). Hilditch and associates[30] found poor visualization of documented primary or metastatic medullary thyroid carcinoma in five patients with plasma calcitonin levels ranging from 140 to 10,000 pg/ml. Their findings cast serious doubt on the usefulness of $^{99m}$Tc-dimercaptosuccinic acid to localize early metastases. Case reports[16, 20] also suggested that $^{131}$I-metaiodobenzylguanidine (MIBG) might be taken up by primary and metastatic medullary thyroid carcinoma. Other authors,[30, 60] however, have suggested that this uptake is also inconsistent and may be limited to large and advanced tumors. Further work to evaluate the usefulness of scintigraphic techniques for imaging medullary thyroid carcinoma and its metastases will require correlation with tumor size, plasma calcitonin levels, and comparisons with other imaging modalities.

One imaging technique that may prove useful in the diagnosis of primary medullary thyroid carcinoma and in the evaluation of spread is high-resolution ultrasonography.[26, 73] In one study[73] of six patients with sporadic medullary thyroid carcinoma and nine patients with familial medullary thyroid carcinoma, ultrasonography correctly detected 12 of 15 primary or recurrent lesions, many under 1 cm in diameter. Plasma calcitonin levels in patients with detected tumors ranged from 196 to more than 10,000 pg/ml, whereas primary or metastatic medullary thyroid carcinomas associated with basal plasma calcitonin levels below 140 pg/ml were not detected. Gorman and associates[26] noted that ultrasonography correctly identified cervical metastases in 12 patients, and in only four of these patients were lymph nodes palpable. A characteristic sonographic pattern was observed, which included bright echogenic foci corresponding to areas of amyloid deposition and calcification.[26, 73] An overall hypoechogenicity of the tumor compared with surrounding thyroid tissue was also noted.[73] This latter feature is not distinctive, however, because other thyroid carcinomas are also hypoechogenic.[26] Nevertheless, high-resolution sonography may prove to be useful in localizing primary medullary thyroid carcinoma and extrathyroidal cervical spread.

***Needle Aspiration for Cytologic Analysis.*** Tumors that are palpable or visualized sonographically can be aspirated using a 22-gauge needle. When stained either using the May-Grünwald-Giemsa[81] or Papanicolaou[23, 40] method, certain features are characteristic of medullary thyroid carcinoma including a spindle cell pattern or admixture of polygonal and spindle shaped cells, presence of cytoplasmic granules, and a background matrix containing amyloid. The May-Grünwald-Giemsa stain is said to enhance the appearance of cytoplasmic granules, which are identified by metachromatic red staining in 5 to 15 per cent of cells examined in the specimen.[81] Amyloid stains gray-blue or violet with May-Grünwald-Giemsa[81] and is lightly eosinophilic with the Papanicolaou stain.[23]

Routine processing of all thyroid nodule aspirates may correctly identify 60 to 85 per cent of medullary thyroid carcinomas.[40, 81] In one series[23] of 338 thyroid neoplasms removed surgically, the fine needle aspirate diagnosis of medullary thyroid carcinoma was made incorrectly (false positive) in nine patients, was omitted incorrectly (false negative) in six, and was made correctly in ten (true positive). Use of calcitonin antisera for immunocytochemical staining can clearly confirm cytologic analysis,[23, 40] but the high cost-to-benefit ratio of this methodology limits its usefulness.

***Plasma Calcitonin Assay.*** Radioimmunoassay of plasma calcitonin levels has proved invaluable in the diagnosis and follow-up of patients with medullary thyroid carcinoma. A number of sensitive and specific assays for plasma calcitonin are available. Although some can detect as little as 1 to 4 pg in a 0.2 ml sample,[58, 78, 88] assays with limits of detection as high as 15 to 20 pg (100 pg/ml) are useful in most clinical situations. Considerable variation, however, has been observed in reports of circulating calcitonin levels in normal subjects. The upper (95 per cent confidence) limits of circulating calcitonin levels in normal individuals has been reported as low as 75 pg/ml[58, 77] but often is reported in the range of 100 to 200 pg/ml.[78, 88] Interpretation of plasma calcitonin measurements can be complicated by the presence of high molecular weight components that cross-react in the assay but which are not functionally important. Interpretation can also be complicated by alterations in calcitonin secretion or metabolism, such as might occur in pregnancy, hypergastrinemia, or renal failure.[42, 80] Calcitonin may also be produced ectopically by tumors of the lung, breast, and gastrointestinal tract or by malignant lymphoma.[42] Patients harboring such tumors, however, have relatively modest increases in plasma calcitonin levels. Thus, interpretation of a specific calcitonin measurement requires an understanding of the assay sensitivity, specificity, individual upper and lower limits for control subjects, and other aspects of the health of the patient.

The calcitonin assay can be used in several ways. In patients with a thyroid mass and cytologic or histologic findings suggesting medullary thyroid carcinoma, the assay is used to confirm the diagnosis preoperatively and to evaluate the patient for residual disease or subsequent recurrence after the primary tumor has been excised. In their initial characterization of a radioimmunoassay for human calcitonin, Tashjian and coworkers[88] noted basal levels greater than 1,000 pg/ml in all 18 patients with clinically evident and histologically proved medullary thyroid carcinoma whereas plasma calcitonin levels ranged from 20 to 4,300 pg/ml in 12 patients who had been treated previously for medullary thyroid carcinoma but had no clinical evidence of recurrent disease. All 58 normal control subjects had basal plasma calcitonin levels of 400 pg/ml or less. Sizemore and associates[77] also found that virtually all patients with clinically detected sporadic forms will have clear elevations of basal plasma calcitonin levels. Similarly, Wells and associates[99] found elevations in basal plasma calcitonin levels in all 46 patients with MEN-IIa who had clinically apparent medullary thyroid carcinoma. Thus, in patients with clinically evident sporadic or familial medullary thyroid carcinoma, the basal plasma calcitonin level will almost always be elevated.

In patients with a family history of medullary thyroid carcinoma or of MEN-IIa or MEN-IIb, basal plasma calcitonin levels may not be elevated in the presence of C cell hyperplasia or early medullary thyroid carcinoma. Both Sizemore and coworkers[77] and Wells and associates[99] noted that between 25 and 35 per cent of such patients with histologically proved medullary thyroid carcinoma may not have basal elevations in plasma calcitonin. Therefore, these authors[77, 99] emphasized the importance of provocative testing to stimulate calcitonin secretion. Agents that provoke calcitonin secretion include intravenous infusions of calcium, glucagon, gastrin, or pentagastrin[58, 78, 88] and the oral ingestion of alcohol.[31] Use of these agents in provocative screening has been reviewed elsewhere.[14, 71] The method presently used in our laboratory evolved from a comparison of regimens using different combinations of intravenous infusions of calcium salts and pentagastrin.[97] In that study, each of 26 patients with previously resected or suspected medullary thyroid carcinoma underwent four studies: intravenous infusion of calcium gluconate, 2 mg/kg over 1 min; intravenous infusion of pentagastrin, 0.5 μg/kg over 5 sec; intravenous infusion of calcium chloride, 3 mg $Ca^{++}$/kg over 10 min; and sequential intravenous infusion of calcium gluconate, 2 mg/kg over 1 min followed by intravenous pentagastrin, 0.5 μg/kg over 5 sec. None of the patients had plasma calcitonin levels higher than 200 pg/ml; however, each exhibited a rise in plasma calcitonin levels (more than 300 pg/ml) within 1 to 5 min after at least one of the provocative tests. The combination of calcium gluconate and pentagastrin elicited higher peak plasma calcitonin levels than did calcium gluconate alone (22 of 24 patients tested [$p < 0.002$]), pentagastrin alone (25 of 26 patients tested [$p < 0.002$]), or calcium chloride alone (17 of 17 patients tested [$p < 0.002$]).

In another study[96] of 90 individuals in MEN-IIa kindreds, the relationship between stimulated plasma calcitonin levels and pathologic disease of thyroidectomy specimens was evaluated. In 61 patients with stimulated plasma calcitonin levels of 300 to 5,000 pg/ml, C cell hyperplasia or microinvasive medullary thyroid carcinoma was diagnosed in 56 per cent, although macroscopic medullary thyroid carcinoma was present in 44 per cent. Of these 61 patients, only one (1.6 per cent) had palpable disease, and only four (6.6 per cent) had regional lymph node metastases. In contrast, all 23 patients with stimulated plasma calcitonin levels greater than 10,000 pg/ml had extensive intrathyroidal disease, and 13 (57 per cent) had regional lymph node metastases. Despite the extent of disease seen intraoperatively, only 13 (57 per cent) of the patients had palpable thyroid nodules preoperatively. These observations confirm that regional lymph node metastases may occur well before a lesion is palpable clinically and that biochemical screening in high-risk patients can detect premalignant C cell hyperplasia or occult malignant disease that is in a curable stage.

In attempting to detect medullary thyroid carcinoma or C cell hyperplasia as early as possible, further investigations[98] were performed in 25 individuals from MEN-IIa kindreds who, at the time of screening, had normal basal plasma calcitonin levels (less than 250 pg/ml in our assay) that increased modestly (280 to 1,000 pg/ml) after provocative testing. During repeat provocative testing in these patients, blood samples were taken peripherally and also from the inferior thyroid vein (through a catheter that had been placed transfemorally). Among eight individuals who had demonstrated no increases in peripheral calcitonin levels after stimulation, one demonstrated a marked increase in inferior thyroid vein plasma calcitonin levels in response to stimulation, and this patient had microinvasive medullary thyroid carcinoma in the thyroidectomy specimen. Among 17 individuals with mild elevations in peripheral plasma calcitonin levels in response to stimulation, all demonstrated elevations of inferior thyroid vein plasma calcitonin levels above basal values. Six of these 17 patients had nonpalpable but visible medullary thyroid carcinoma at operation, four had microinvasive medullary thyroid carcinoma, and seven had C cell hyperplasia. One patient had cervical lymph node metastases, 13 had no evidence of nodal metastases, and in four patients, nodal metastases were not searched for. Again, these findings emphasize the usefulness of the plasma calcitonin assays to detect early carcinoma or premalignant lesions in individuals at high risk for medullary thyroid carcinoma.

The calcitonin assay may also be useful postoperatively in patients who have undergone total thyroidectomy for medullary thyroid carcinoma. In a follow-up study[94] of 200 patients with medullary thyroid carcinoma (123 with MEN-IIa, ten with MEN-IIb, 41 with familial nonMEN medullary thyroid carcinoma, and 26 with sporadic medullary thyroid carcinoma), it became clear that elevations in basal or stimulated plasma calcitonin levels postoperatively indicated residual disease. Illustrated in Figure 15–5 is how postoperative stimulated plasma calcitonin levels are related to the initial method of diagnosis and subsequent surgical therapy. Patients with familial medullary thyroid carcinoma diagnosed by provocative testing and selective venous catheterization have the lowest incidences of regional lymph node spread and evidence of residual medullary thyroid carcinoma after operation. Patients with sporadic disease or MEN-IIb who most frequently are identified only after development of symptoms or signs have the highest incidence of residual disease and poor survival. In an additional refinement in the interpretation of postoperative calcitonin levels, Miyauchi and associates[52] provided evidence that the doubling time of plasma calcitonin levels may correlate with prognosis. A doubling time of less than 6 months uniformly indicated recurrence of disease and postoperative survival of 3 years or less in five of five patients, a doubling time of 6 months to 1 year indicated recurrence of medullary thyroid carcinoma in four of five patients, and a doubling time of greater than 1 year indicated clinical recurrent disease in only three of 15 patients. Further work is necessary to determine whether the doubling time of plasma calcitonin levels would have usefulness in the planning of therapy for recurrent disease.

***Plasma Carcinoembryonic Antigen Determinations.*** Carcinoembryonic antigen is a plasma tumor marker for several carcinomas, including medullary thyroid carcinoma. As discussed earlier, immunostaining techniques indicate that carcinoembryonic antigen can be localized to medullary thyroid carcinoma cells, particularly in neoplasms that have a high risk of dissemination. Wells and associates[95] found an important positive correlation between basal plasma carcinoembryonic antigen levels and stimulated plasma calcitonin levels in patients before and after surgical excision of medullary thyroid carcinoma. They found plasma levels of both calcitonin and carcinoembryonic antigen to

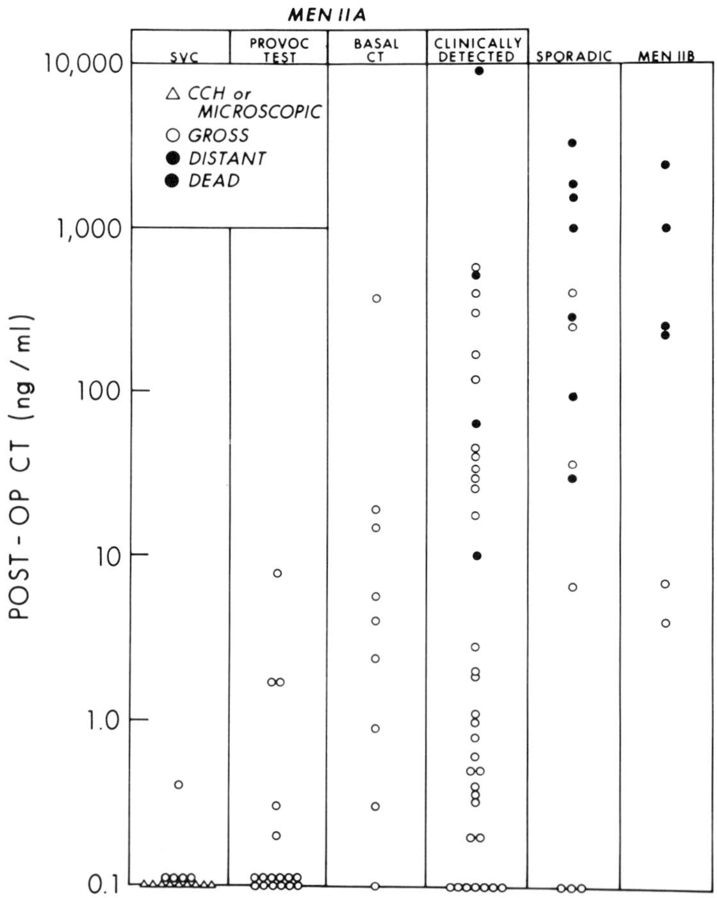


**FIGURE 15–5.** Stimulated plasma calcitonin levels in patients after total thyroidectomy for medullary thyroid carcinoma. Each column represents the method that was used preoperatively for diagnosis. SVC = Selective venous catheterization; CCH = C cell hyperplasia. (From Wells, S. A., Jr., Dilley, W. G., Farndon, J. A., et al.: Early diagnosis and treatment of medullary thyroid carcinoma. Arch. Intern. Med., *145:*1251, 1985, with permission.)

be increased in patients with disseminated disease but undetectable in patients with occult disease. After stimulation with calcium or pentagastrin, however, plasma calcitonin levels increase greatly, although plasma carcinoembryonic antigen levels do not change from basal values. Busnardo and coworkers[12] also described a general correlation of basal plasma carcinoembryonic antigen and calcitonin levels in 41 patients with medullary thyroid carcinoma but noted a few patients in whom carcinoembryonic antigen levels continue to rise after operation in the absence of parallel rises in calcitonin levels. Rougier and associates[65] and Saad and associates[68, 71] noted that postoperative plasma carcinoembryonic antigen levels, in contrast with plasma calcitonin levels, may correlate more closely with progression of residual disease. Saad et al.[68] found that four patients with plasma carcinoembryonic antigen doubling times of less than 13 months all died with disseminated disease, but those with a carcinoembryonic antigen doubling time greater than 24 months survived for longer periods of time, even in the presence of disseminated disease. Although plasma carcinoembryonic antigen is not a specific marker for medullary thyroid carcinoma, it may prove useful in identifying subgroups with a poor prognosis.

### *Evaluation of the Patient*

Patients with medullary thyroid carcinoma are identified because of signs and symptoms of thyroid carcinoma or because of an increased basal or stimulated plasma calcitonin level. The specific diagnosis of medullary thyroid carcinoma is usually made by fine needle aspiration cytology or after open biopsy or partial thyroidectomy for management of a cold nodule found by radionuclide scan. Although patients with proved medullary thyroid carcinoma may not report signs or symptoms of other endocrinopathies or of a family history of endocrine tumors, they should routinely have evaluation of urine excretion rates for epinephrine, norepinephrine, metanephrine, and vanillylmandelic acid. They should also have serum levels of calcium and parathormone determined.

Patients with a family history of MEN-IIa or MEN-IIb or evidence of familial transmission of medullary thyroid carcinoma are at high risk for the development of medullary thyroid carcinoma. Results of intensive screening efforts indicate that these tumors occur much earlier in life than does sporadic medullary thyroid carcinoma. It has previously been shown that patients with medullary thyroid carcinoma have a much better prognosis when their disease is diagnosed biochemically rather than by physical examination. Moreover, the diagnosis of other associated endocrine neoplasias may be delayed for several years unless sought for. We recommend, therefore, that individuals who are at risk for the development of familial medullary thyroid carcinoma undergo evaluation beginning at 5 years of age and annually thereafter until 40 years of age. Approximately 10 per cent of our patients with MEN-IIa initially had symptoms of pheochromocytoma; however, in none was hyperparathyroidism the first disease detected.[54] Because medullary thyroid carcinoma occurs in virtually all patients affected with MEN-IIa, MEN-IIb, and familial nonMEN medullary thyroid carcinoma and because it is the first endocrinopathy becoming manifested in patients with MEN-IIa and MEN-IIb, it is not necessary to screen for other endocrinopathies until a specific diagnosis of medullary thyroid carcinoma has been established.

When high-risk patients demonstrate elevations in basal or stimulated plasma calcitonin levels above 1,000 pg/ml, they are advised to have total thyroidectomy. When the stimulated levels are elevated but not above 1,000 pg/ml, patients should undergo selective thyroid venous catheterization with determination of stimulated plasma calcitonin levels or they should be retested in 6 months. Patients who have undergone thyroidectomy should have annual routine evaluation for the detection of persistent or recurrent medullary thyroid carcinoma and for the presence of pheochromocytoma and hyperparathyroidism.

## SURGICAL MANAGEMENT

In patients with the familial diseases, medullary thyroid carcinoma is almost always multicentric and bilateral. In patients with apparently sporadic forms of the disease, the incidence of bilaterality has ranged from less than 5 per cent[9, 15] to almost 30 per cent.[67, 71] The potential for bilaterality of disease, coupled with the difficulty of excluding familial disease in many patients, argues that all patients with medullary thyroid carcinoma should have total thyroidectomy. A transverse cervical incision (Fig. 15–6) is used, and all thyroid tissue is removed. Each of the parathyroid glands is identified (Fig. 15–7). In patients with MEN-IIa, total parathyroidectomy is performed with autotransplantation of parathyroid tissue to the forearm only when multiple glands are enlarged. When the glands are not enlarged, they are left in situ or transplanted to the sternocleidomastoid muscle when the blood supply appears inadequate. Even when distant metastases are apparent, lymph nodes in the central zone and obviously diseased areas of the neck are removed to diminish local recurrent disease. In patients with no obvious extrathyroidal disease or with only biochemically detected disease, the incidence of nodal metastases is 15 per cent or less[67, 99]; therefore, prophylactic dissection of lymph nodes in the central zone of the neck is recommended. The dissection encompasses lymph nodes located between the hyoid bone superiorly, the innominate vessels inferiorly, and the internal jugular veins laterally. When the lateral neck lymph nodes are enlarged, the patient should have modified neck dissection.

Two weeks after operation, basal and stimulated plasma calcitonin levels are measured to detect residual disease. When the calcitonin level is elevated, it may be beneficial to attempt to localize disease with radionuclide scans or even selective venous catheterization of the neck. Norton and associates[55] used selective venous catheterization and pentagastrin stimulation to localize residual disease to the neck or superior mediastinum in seven patients with persistently elevated peripheral calcitonin levels but no clinical or radiologic evidence of residual tumor. Surgical resection of this disease was possible in all patients, although in only one patient was the postoperative calcitonin level reduced to an undetectable level. In other patients, the stimulated plasma calcitonin level was reduced after operation, suggesting a mild to substantial decrease in tumor burden. Only one of the seven patients had clinically apparent recurrent disease in follow-up studies ranging from 6 months to 3 years.

Tisell and coworkers[89] performed reoperations in 11 patients whose stimulated plasma calcitonin levels were elevated after operation. The second operation was performed to eradicate tumor tissue in the neck and supe-

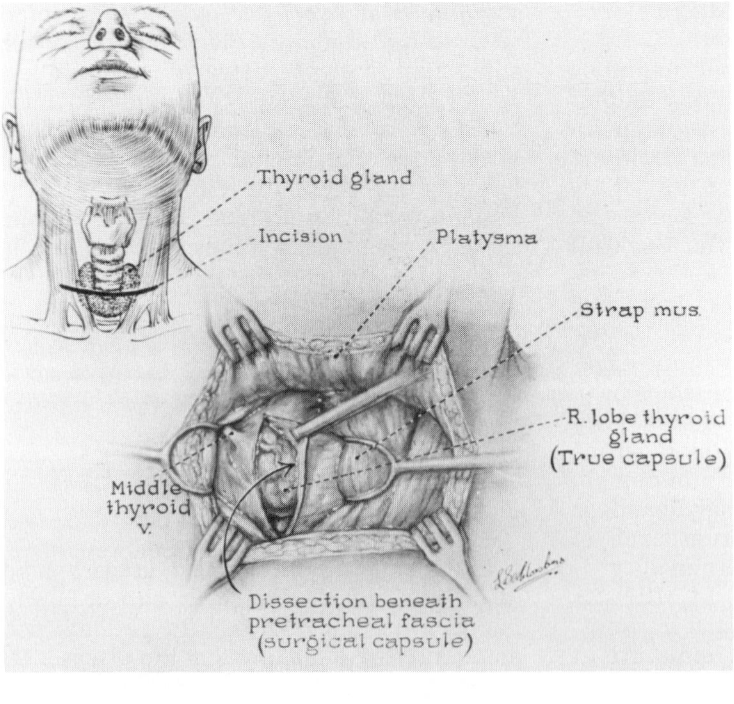


**FIGURE 15–6.** Standard operative approach to the thyroid gland through a transverse cervical incision. (From Cance, W. G., and Wells, S. A., Jr.: Multiple endocrine neoplasia type IIa. Curr. Probl. Surg., *22*(5):27, 1985, with permission.)

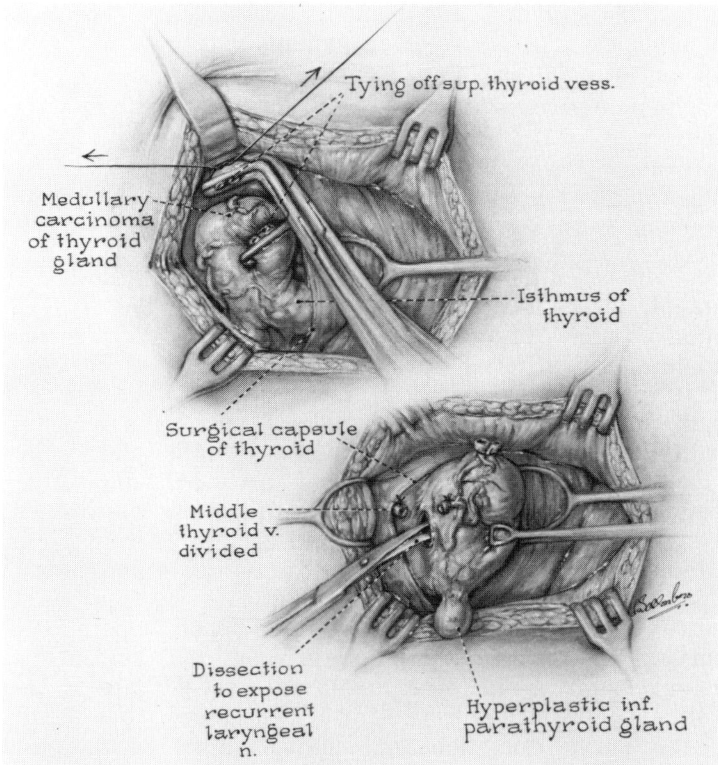


**FIGURE 15–7.** Total thyroidectomy for medullary thyroid carcinoma in a patient with MEN-IIa. The recurrent laryngeal nerves and all parathyroid glands are identified. (From Cance, W. G., and Wells, S. A., Jr.: Multiple endocrine neoplasia type IIa. Curr. Probl. Surg., *22*(5):28, 1985, with permission.)

rior mediastinum and involved a meticulous node-by-node dissection under a magnifying lens. Stimulated plasma calcitonin levels normalized after the second operation in four patients, suggesting that it might be possible to eradicate biochemically detected residual disease. Long-term follow-up on these four patients and another four with substantially reduced stimulated plasma calcitonin levels are not presently available. It seems reasonable to attempt to localize residual tumor when early postoperative plasma calcitonin levels are high and to perform meticulous removal of cervical and superior mediastinal nodes when the disease is confined to the neck. Further investigation is required to determine whether such aggressive therapy will improve patient survival.

## PROGNOSIS AFTER SURGICAL THERAPY

Assessment of the long-term outcome in patients with medullary thyroid carcinoma requires evaluation of the primary tumor characteristics and evidence of extrathyroidal spread to regional and distant sites. To compare recurrence rates and long-term survival between patients with medullary thyroid carcinoma and patients with other types of thyroid carcinoma, physicians have distinguished the following groups: patients with carcinoma confined to the thyroid gland, patients with carcinoma invading local structures, patients with cervical lymph node metastases, and patients with distant metastases. Russell and associates[67] found that of 67 patients with tumor confined to the thyroid, 45 (67 per cent) were clinically and biochemically free of disease with a mean follow-up period of 66 months. Of 49 patients with cervical node metastases at the time of operation, only four were free of disease with a mean follow-up period of 68 months. Patients with extrathyroidal tissue or distant metastases were too few to analyze with confidence, but both groups fared poorly. In analyzing survival, these authors[67] were careful to note that patients undergoing thyroidectomy for medullary thyroid carcinoma frequently die of other causes. Of the 67 patients with disease confined to the thyroid, two died of their disease and one died of other causes. Of the 49 patients with cervical metastases, nine died of medullary thyroid carcinoma and two died of other causes. Of the seven patients with local invasion or distant metastases, five died of their disease and none died of other causes.

Saad and coworkers[71] used a slightly different staging system to evaluate patient outcome (Fig. 15–8). In 67 patients with stage 1 disease (disease confined to the thyroid), 39 per cent eventually had clinical or radiographic evidence of recurrent disease, and approximately 90 per cent survived 5 years, while approximately 80 per cent were alive at 10 years (life table method). In 43 patients with stage 2 disease (intrathyroidal disease with involved but mobile regional nodes), 44 per cent had recurrent disease and survival patterns similar to those of patients with stage 1 disease. In 33 patients with stage 3 disease (invasion of local structures or fixation of diseased regional nodes), the cumulative recurrence rate was 61 per cent, with a 5-year survival rate of just under 60 per cent and a 10-year survival rate of 20 to 25 per cent. Patients with stage 4 disease (distant disease at the time of operation) had survival rates of 40 per cent at 5 years and 20 to 25 per cent at 10 years.

The time interval from thyroidectomy to clinical recurrence has not been analyzed closely by stage but clearly can be variable. In our recently updated series of patients with MEN-IIa,[54] nine of 93 patients (9.6 per cent) who had stimulated plasma levels of calcitonin less than 300 pg/ml in the immediate postoperative period eventually demonstrated elevated plasma calcitonin levels from 1 to 10 years after operation (mean, 4.4 years). Of these nine patients, clinical signs of recurrent disease eventually developed in eight, but all remained alive, a mean of 8.7 years after operation. Chong and associates,[15] in a follow-up study of 128 patients who underwent thyroidectomy for cure, found a cumulative rate of clinical recurrence of 34 per cent. Recurrent disease was documented from 2 months to 19 years after operation, and 90 per cent of patients who experienced recurrence did so by 8 years after the initial operation. Saad and coworkers[71] found recurrent disease as early as 1 month and as late as 25 years after operation and noted that recurrent disease was documented 10 years after operation in 8 per cent. These observations emphasize the importance of prolonged follow-up in these patients.

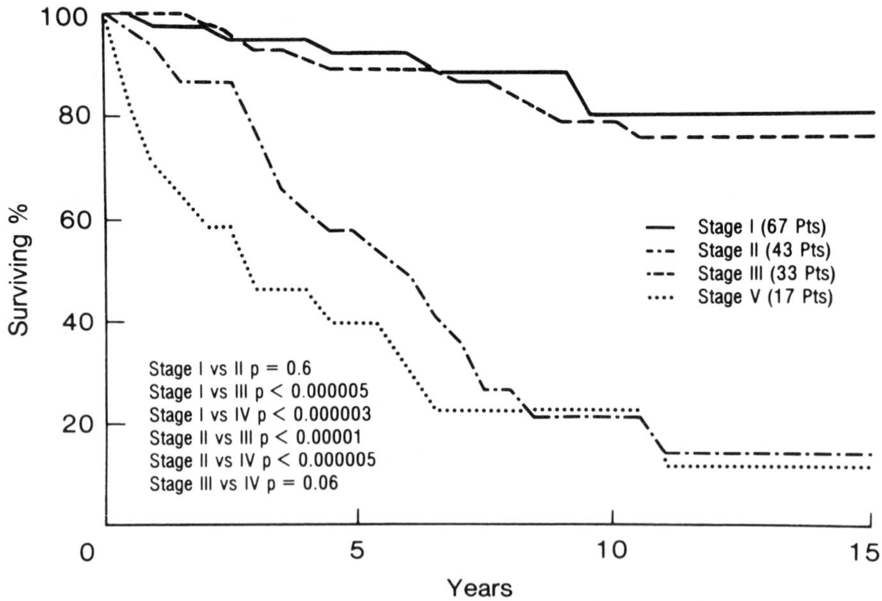


**FIGURE 15–8.** Survival curves for patients presenting with different stages of medullary thyroid carcinoma summarized by the life table method of Berkson-Gage. Stages are designated as in the text. Comparisons of survival curves were performed using the generalized Wilcoxon test. (From Saad, M. F., Ordonez, N. G., Guido, J. J., et al.: Medullary carcinoma of the thyroid: A study of the clinical features and prognostic factors in 161 patients. Medicine, *63*:326, 1984, with permission.)

Although clinicopathologic staging systems are useful in predicting recurrent disease and survival, they do not identify further subgroups who might be at high risk for recurrent disease, especially in patients with stages 1 and 2 disease. In this regard, it seems helpful to evaluate prognosis as a function of preoperative or immediate postoperative plasma calcitonin determinations as discussed earlier. In addition, a normal level of plasma calcitonin after operation is virtually always associated with an absence of clinical disease, whereas the presence of an elevated plasma calcitonin level after operation defines the group in whom residual medullary thyroid carcinoma can be expected. Finally, cytopathologic characteristics, such as cell nuclear DNA distribution or heterogeneous staining with antisera specific for calcitonin histaminase and L-dopa decarboxylase, may also prove to be independent factors in predicting progression of disease.

## ADJUVANT THERAPIES FOR UNRESECTABLE DISEASE

Adjuvant therapies, such as external beam radiation, radioactive iodine, and chemotherapy, have not proved consistently beneficial in patients with metastatic or residual medullary thyroid carcinoma. Steinfeld and associates[83] reported that combinations of large and small field doses of 4,000 to 5,000 cGy each achieved some measure of local control in four of five patients. Rougier and coworkers[66] also found that external beam therapy achieved some improvement in symptoms in five of eight patients with metastasis to bone and tumor regression of more than 50 per cent. Other authors[14, 71] have not observed any consistent benefits of radiation to areas of unresectable disease. Appropriate use of this therapy may remain undefined in the absence of a well-designed prospective randomized clinical trial.

Investigators have also attempted to evaluate the benefits of administration of iodine 131. Ljunberg and associates[45] used autoradiography to demonstrate that these tumors usually do not concentrate radioactive iodine. In one series[50] of patients with medullary thyroid carcinoma treated using iodine 131, only mild regression of metastases was observed when two doses of more than 100 mCi each were administered. Uptake of iodine 131 in a residual thyroid follicle might indirectly concentrate radiation in the neck and thus facilitate local control of disease. In patients who have undergone total thyroidectomy, however, no rationale for this therapy exists, and, accordingly, no substantial reduction in the size of the tumor or the plasma calcitonin level has been observed in such patients given iodine 131.[53, 69]

In general, chemotherapy, including doxorubicin, 5-fluorouracil, *cis*-platinum, bleomycin, and methotrexate, has not been found to diminish tumor burden or symptoms for long, if at all.[14, 66, 71] Kessinger and associates[38] suggested that DTIC (5-(3-3-dimethyl-1-triazino)-imidazole-4-carboxamide) may represent an agent effective in palliating unresectable disease in a variety of APUD cell-derived tumors. It is possible that other agents that localize in cells because of their APUD cytochemical properties (e.g., such toxins as streptozotocin or antibodies specific for calcitonin) might be used selectively to impair proliferation and growth of the tumor. Effectiveness of such agents in the treatment of a C cell-derived tumor remains to be established.

## SUMMARY

Medullary carcinoma of the thyroid is characterized by distinctive histologic properties and the production of an almost unique tumor marker, calcitonin. Such a tumor marker has made it possible to detect this carcinoma in its earliest stages before it has become invasive or spread to regional and distant sites. Medullary thyroid carcinoma may develop in 5 to 10 per cent of patients in the setting of a well-documented family history. In these individuals, cure or prevention is virtually certain when aggressive screening programs are used in all branches of the family known to transmit medullary thyroid carcinoma with or without associated endocrinopathy. The unique immunocytochemical staining properties of medullary thyroid carcinoma cells, in conjunction with long-term serial determinations of plasma calcitonin levels, have identified patients who may be at high risk for the development of extrathyroidal spread and early death after diagnosis. The mainstay of therapy for this disease, whether familial or sporadic, is surgery. Adjuvant treatments for unresectable metastasis or residual disease do not appear beneficial as of this writing. It remains a highly intriguing question whether the genomes transmitting the expression of medullary thyroid carcinoma MEN-IIa and MEN-IIb syndromes are unique to the APUD cell system or whether they represent a broader class of regulatory functions that render these cells susceptible to malignant transformation and dedifferentiation.

## REFERENCES


1. Anderson, R. J., Sizemore, G. W., Wahner, H. W., and Carney, J. A.: Thyroid scintigram in familial medullary carcinoma of the thyroid gland. Clin. Nucl. Med., *3:*147–151, 1978.
2. Arnstein, N. B., Juni, J. E., Sisson, J. C., et al.: Recurrent medullary carcinoma of the thyroid demonstrated by thallium-201 scintigraphy. J. Nucl. Med., *27:*1564–1568, 1986.
3. Baber, E. C.: Contributions to the minute anatomy of the thyroid gland of the dog. Proc. R. Soc. London (Biol.), *24:*240–241, 1876.
4. Bäckdahl, M., Tallroth, E., Auer, G., et al.: Prognostic value of nuclear DNA content in medullary thyroid carcinoma. World J. Surg., *9:*980–987, 1985.
5. Baylin, S. B., Hsu, S. H., Gann, D. S., et al.: Inherited medullary thyroid carcinoma: A final monoclonal mutation in one of multiple clones of susceptible cells. Science, *199:*429–431, 1978.
6. Baylin, S. B., Mendelsohn, G., Weisburger, W. R., et al.: Levels of histaminase and L-DOPA decarboxylase activity in the transition from C-cell hyperplasia to familial medullary thyroid carcinoma. Cancer, *44:*1315–1321, 1979.
7. Beaugié, J. M., Brown, C. L., Doniach, I., and Richardson, J. E.: Primary malignant tumours of the thyroid: The relationship between histological classification and clinical behaviour. Br. J. Surg., *63:*173–181, 1976.
8. Bigner, S. H., Cox, E. B., Mendelsohn, G., et al.: Medullary carcinoma of the thyroid in the multiple endocrine neoplasia IIA syndrome. Am. J. Surg. Pathol., *5:*459–472, 1981.
9. Block, M. A., Jackson, C. E., Greenawald, K. A., et al.: Clinical characteristics distinguishing hereditary from sporadic medullary thyroid carcinoma: Treatment implications. Arch. Surg., *115:*142–148, 1980.
10. Brennan, M. F., and Macdonald, J.: Cancer of the endocrine system. *In* DeVita, V. T., Jr., Hellman, S., and Rosenberg, S. A. (eds.): Cancer: Principles and Practice of Oncology. Philadelphia, J. B. Lippincott Co., 1985, pp. 1179–1192.
11. Brunt, L. M., and Wells, S. A., Jr.: Advances in the diagnosis and treatment of medullary thyroid carcinoma. Surg. Clin. North Am., *67:*263–279, 1987.
12. Busnardo, B., Girelli, M. E., Simioni, N., et al.: Nonparallel patterns of calcitonin and carcinoembryonic antigen levels in the follow-up of medullary thyroid carcinoma. Cancer, *53:*278–285, 1984.
13. Bussolati, G., and Pearse, A. G.: Immunofluorescent localization of calcitonin in the "C" cells of pig and dog thyroid. J. Endocrinol., *37:*205–209, 1967.
14. Cance, W. G., and Wells, S. A., Jr.: Multiple endocrine neoplasia type IIa. Curr. Probl. Surg., *22*(5):1–56, 1985.
15. Chong, G. C., Beahrs, O. H., Sizemore, G. W., and Woolner, L.: Medullary carcinoma of the thyroid gland. Cancer, *35:*695–704, 1975.
16. Connell, J. M., Hilditch, T. E., Elliott, A., and Semple, P. F.: $^{131}$I-MIBG and medullary carcinoma of the thyroid (Letter). Lancet, *2:*1273–1274, 1984.
17. Copp, D. H., Cameron, E. C., Cheney, B. A., et al.: Evidence for calcitonin—a new hormone from the parathyroid that lowers blood calcium. Endocrinology, *70:*638–649, 1962.
18. Cox, T. M., Fagan, E. A., Hillyard, C. J., et al.: Role of calcitonin in diarrhoea associated with medullary carcinoma of the thyroid. Gut, *20:*629–633, 1979.
19. DeLellis, R. A., Nunnemacher, G., and Wolfe, H. J.: C-cell hyperplasia: An ultrastructural analysis. Lab. Invest., *36:*237–248, 1977.
20. Endo, K., Shiomi, K., Kassi, K., et al.: Imaging of medullary thyroid cancer with 131I-MIBG (Letter). Lancet, *2:*233, 1984.
21. Farndon, J. R., Leight, G. S., Dilley, W. G., et al.: Familial medullary thyroid carcinoma without associated endocrinopathies: A distinct clinical entity. Br. J. Surg., *73:*278–281, 1986.
22. Fletcher, J. R.: Medullary (solid) carcinoma of the thyroid gland: A review of 249 cases. Arch. Surg., *100:*257–262, 1970.
23. Geddie, W. R., Bedard, Y. C., and Strawbridge, H. T.: Medullary carcinoma of the thyroid in fine-needle aspiration biopsies. Am. J. Clin. Pathol., *82:*552–558, 1984.
24. Goepfert, H., Dichtel, W. J., and Samaan, N. A.: Thyroid cancer in children and teenagers. Arch. Otolaryngol., *110:*72–75, 1984.
25. Gordon, P. R., Huvos, A. G., and Strong, E. W.: Medullary carcinoma of the thyroid gland: A clinicopathologic study of 40 cases. Cancer, *31:*915–924, 1973.
26. Gorman, B., Charboneau, J. W., James, E. M., et al.: Medullary thyroid carcinoma: Role of high-resolution US. Radiology, *162* (Pt 1):147–150, 1987.
27. Gray, T. K., Brannan, P., Juan, D., et al.: Ion transport changes during calcitonin-induced intestinal secretion in man. Gastroenterology, *71:*392–398, 1976.
28. Hazard, J. B.: The C cells (parafollicular cells) of the thyroid gland and medullary thyroid carcinoma: A review. Am. J. Pathol., *88:*213–250, 1977.
29. Hazard, J. B., Hawk, W. A., and Crile, G., Jr.:

Medullary (solid) carcinoma of the thyroid—A clinicopathologic entity. J. Clin. Endocrinol. Metab., *19:*152–161, 1959.
30. Hilditch, T. E., Connell, J. M., Elliot, A. T., et al.: Poor results with technetium-99m (V) DMS and iodine-131 MIBG in the imaging of medullary thyroid carcinoma. J. Nucl. Med., *27:*1150–1153, 1986.
31. Hillyard, C. J., Evans, I. M., Hill, P. A., and Taylor, S.: Familiar medullary thyroid carcinoma. Lancet, *1:*1009–1011, 1978.
32. Hirsch, P. F., Gauthier, G. F., and Munson, P. L.: Thyroid hypocalcemic principle and recurrent laryngeal nerve injury as factors affecting the response to parathyroidectomy in rats. Endocrinology, *73:*244–252, 1963.
33. Horn, R. C., Jr.: Carcinoma of the thyroid: Description of a distinctive morphological variant and report of 7 cases. Cancer, *4:*697–707, 1951.
34. Iwase, K., Nagasaka, A., Kato, K., et al.: Enolase subunits in patients with neuroendocrine tumors. J. Clin. Endocrinol. Metab., *63:*94–101, 1986.
35. Jansson, S., Hansson, G., Salander, H., et al.: Prevalence of C-cell hyperplasia and medullary thyroid carcinoma in a consecutive series of pheochromocytoma patients. World J. Surg., *8:*493–500, 1984.
36. Johnson, D. G., Coleman, R. E., McCook, T. A., et al.: Bone and liver images in medullary carcinoma of the thyroid gland: Concise communication. J. Nucl. Med., *25:*419–422, 1984.
37. Keiser, H. R., Beaven, M. A., Doppman, J., et al.: NIH Conference. Sipple's syndrome: Medullary thyroid carcinoma, pheochromocytoma, and parathyroid disease. Ann. Intern. Med., *78:*561–579, 1973.
38. Kessinger, A., Foley, J. F., and Lemon, H. M.: Therapy of malignant APUD cell tumors: Effectiveness of DTIC. Cancer, *51:*790–794, 1983.
39. Khairi, M. R., Dexter, R. N., Burzynski, N. J., and Johnston, C. C., Jr.: Mucosal neuroma, pheochromocytoma and medullary thyroid carcinoma: Multiple endocrine neoplasia type 3. Medicine, *54:*89–112, 1975.
40. Kini, S. R., Miller, J. M., Hamburger, J. I., and Smith, M. J.: Cytopathologic features of medullary carcinoma of the thyroid. Arch. Pathol. Lab. Med., *108:*156–159, 1984.
41. Lippman, S. M., Mendelsohn, G., Trump, D. L., et al.: The prognostic and biological significance of cellular heterogeneity in medullary thyroid carcinoma: A study of calcitonin, L-dopa decarboxylase, and histaminase. J. Clin. Endocrinol. Metab., *54:*233–240, 1982.
42. LiVolsi, V. A.: Calcitonin: The hormone and its significance. Prog. Surg. Pathol., *1:*71–103, 1980.
43. LiVolsi, V. A., and Feind, C. R.: Incidental medullary thyroid carcinoma in sporadic hyperparathyroidism: An expansion of the concept of C-cell hyperplasia. Am. J. Clin. Pathol., *71:*595–599, 1979.
44. LiVolsi, V. A., Feind, C. R., LoGerfo, P., and Tashjian, A. H., Jr.: Demonstration by immunoperoxidase staining of hyperplasia of parafollicular cells in the thyroid gland in hyperparathyroidism. J. Clin. Endocrinol. Metab., *37:*550–559, 1973.
45. Ljunberg, O.: Medullary carcinoma of the human thyroid gland: Autoradiographic localization of radioiodine. Acta Pathol. Microbiol. Scand., *68:*476–480, 1966.
46. Manger, W. M., and Gifford, R. W., Jr.: Pheochromocytoma. New York, Springer-Verlag, 1977, p. 42.
47. Manning, P. C., Jr., Molnar, G. D., Black, B. M., et al.: Pheochromocytoma, hyperparathyroidism and thyroid carcinoma occurring coincidentally: Report of a case. N. Engl. J. Med., *268:*68–72, 1963.
48. McCook, T. A., Putman, C. E., Dale, J. K., and Wells, S. A.: Review. Medullary carcinoma of the thyroid: Radiographic features of a unique tumor. A.J.R., *139:*149–155, 1982.
49. Mendelsohn, G., Wells, S. A., Jr., and Baylin, S. B.: Relationship of tissue carcinoembryonic antigen and calcitonin to tumor virulence in medullary thyroid carcinoma: An immunohistochemical study in early, localized, and virulent disseminated stages of disease. Cancer, *54:*657–662, 1982.
50. Michael, B. E., Forouhar, F. A., and Spencer, R. P.: Medullary thyroid carcinoma with radioiodide transport: Effects of iodine-131 therapy and lithium administration. Clin. Nucl. Med., *10:*274–279, 1985.
51. Miyauchi, A., Endo, K., Ohta, H., et al.: $^{99m}$Tc(V)-dimercaptosuccinic acid scintigraphy for medullary thyroid carcinoma. World J. Surg., *10:*640–645, 1986.
52. Miyauchi, A., Onishi, T., Morimoto, S., et al.: Relation of doubling time of plasma calcitonin levels to prognosis and recurrence of medullary thyroid carcinoma. Ann. Surg., *199:*461–466, 1984.
53. Nieuwenhuijzen Kruseman, A. C., Bussemaker, J. K., and Frölich, M.: Radioiodine in the treatment of hereditary medullary carcinoma of the thyroid. J. Clin. Endocrinol. Metab., *59:*491–494, 1984.
54. Normann, T.: Medullary thyroid carcinoma in Norway: Epidemiologic and genetic data. Acta Pathol. Microbiol. Scand., *85:*775–786, 1977.
55. Norton, J. A., Doppman, J. L., and Brennan, M. F.: Localization and resection of clinically inapparent medullary carcinoma of the thyroid. Surgery, *87:*616–622, 1980.
56. Norton, J. A., Froome, L. C., Farrell, R. E., and Wells, S. A., Jr.: Multiple endocrine neoplasia type IIb: The most aggressive form of medullary thyroid carcinoma. Surg. Clin. North Am., *59:*109–118, 1979.
57. O'Toole, K., Fenoglio-Preiser, C., and Pushparaj, N.: Endocrine changes associated with the human aging process. III. Effect of age on the number of calcitonin immunoreactive cells in the thyroid gland. Hum. Pathol., *16:*991–1000, 1985.
58. Parthemore, J. G., and Deftos, L. J.: Calcitonin secretion in normal human subjects. J. Clin. Endocrinol. Metab., *47:*184–188, 1978.
59. Pearse, A. G.: Common cytochemical and ultrastructural characteristics of cells producing polypeptide hormones (the APUD series) and their relevance to thyroid and ultimobranchial C cells and calcitonin. Proc. R. Soc. (Biol.), *170:*71–80, 1968.
60. Poston, G. J., Thomas, A. M., MacDonald, D.

W., et al.: $^{131}$I-MIBG uptake by medullary carcinoma of the thyroid (Letter). Lancet, *2*:560, 1985.

61. Pottern, L. M., Stone, B. J., Day, N. E., et al.: Thyroid cancer in Connecticut, 1935–1975: An analysis by cell type. Am. J. Epidemiol., *112*:764–774, 1980.
62. Primi, M. P., and Bueno, L.: Centrally mediated stimulation of jejunal water and electrolyte secretion by calcitonin in dogs. Am. J. Physiol., *250*(2 Pt 1):G172–G176, 1986.
63. Roediger, W. E. W.: The oxyphil and C cells of the human thyroid gland: A cytochemical and histopathologic review. Cancer, *36*:1758–1770, 1975.
64. Rossi, R. L., Cady, B., Meissner, W. A., et al.: Nonfamilial medullary thyroid carcinoma. Am. J. Surg., *139*:554–560, 1980.
65. Rougier, P., Calmettes, C., Laplanche, A., et al.: The values of calcitonin and carcinoembryonic antigen in the treatment and management of nonfamilial medullary thyroid carcinoma. Cancer, *51*:885–862, 1983.
66. Rougier, P., Parmentier, C., Laplanche, A., et al.: Medullary thyroid carcinoma: Prognostic factors and treatment. Int. J. Radiat. Oncol. Biol. Phys., *9*:161–169, 1983.
67. Russell, C. F., van Heerden, J. A., Sizemore, G.W., et al.: The surgical management of medullary thyroid carcinoma. Ann. Surg., *197*:42–48, 1983.
68. Saad, M. F., Fritsche, H. A., Jr., and Samaan, N.A.: Diagnostic and prognostic values of carcinoembryonic antigen in medullary carcinoma of the thyroid. J. Clin. Endocrinol. Metab., *58*:889–894, 1984.
69. Saad, M. F., Guido, J. J., and Samaan, N. A.: Radioactive iodine in the treatment of medullary carcinoma of the thyroid. J. Clin. Endocrinol. Metab., *57*:124–127, 1983.
70. Saad, M. F., Ordonez, N. G., Guido, J. J., and Samaan, N. A.: The prognostic value of calcitonin immunostaining in medullary carcinoma of the thyroid. J. Clin. Endocrinol. Metab., *59*:850–856, 1984.
71. Saad, M. F., Ordonez, N. G., Rashid, R. K., et al.: Medullary carcinoma of the thyroid: A study of the clinical features and prognostic factors in 161 patients. Medicine, *63*:319–342, 1984.
72. Schmechel, D., Marangos, P. J., and Brightman, M.: Nerone-specific enolase is a molecular marker for peripheral and central neuroendocrine cells. Nature, *276*:834–836, 1978.
73. Schwerk, W. B., Grün, R., and Wahl, R.: Ultrasound diagnosis of C-cell carcinoma of the thyroid. Cancer, *55*:624–630, 1985.
74. Sikri, K. L., Varndell, I. M., Hamid, Q. A., et al.: Medullary carcinoma of the thyroid: An immunocytochemical and histochemical study of 25 cases using eight separate markers. Cancer, *56*:2481–2491, 1985.
75. Simpson, W. J., and McKinney, S. E.: Canadian survey of thyroid cancer. Can. Med. Assoc. J., *132*:925–931, 1985.
76. Sipple, J. H.: The association of pheochromocytoma with carcinoma of the thyroid gland. Am. J. Med., *31*:163–166, 1961.
77. Sizemore, G. W., Carney, J. A., and Heath, H., 3d.: Epidemiology of medullary carcinoma of the thyroid gland: A five-year experience (1971–1976). Surg. Clin. North Am., *57*:633–645, 1977.
78. Sizemore, G. W., Go, V. L., Kaplan, E. L., et al.: Relations of calcitonin and gastrin in the Zollinger-Ellison syndrome and medullary carcinoma of the thyroid. N. Engl. J. Med., *288*:641–644, 1973.
79. Smith, L. H.: The APUD cell concept. J. Surg. Oncol., *8*:137–142, 1976.
80. Snider, R. H., Silva, O. L., Moore, C. F., and Becker, K.L.: Immunochemical heterogeneity of calcitonin in man: Effect on radioimmunoassay. Clin. Chim. Acta, *76*:1–14, 1977.
81. Söderstroöm, N., Telenius-Berg, M., and Akerman, M.: Diagnosis of medullary carcinoma of the thyroid by fine needle aspiration biopsy. Acta Med. Scand., *197*:71–76, 1975.
82. Steiner, A. L., Goodman, A. D., and Powers, S. R.: Study of a kindred with pheochromocytoma, medullary thyroid carcinoma, hyperparathyroidism and Cushing's disease: Multiple endocrine neoplasia, type 2. Medicine, *47*:371–409, 1968.
83. Steinfeld, A. D.: The role of radiation therapy in medullary carcinoma of the thyroid. Radiology, *123*:745–746, 1977.
84. Steinfeld, C. M., Moertel, C. G., and Woolner, L. B.: Diarrhea and medullary carcinoma of the thyroid. Cancer, *31*:1237–1239, 1973.
85. Stevens, R. E., and Moore, G. E.: Inadequacy of APUD concept in explaining production of peptide hormones by tumours. Lancet, *1*:118–119, 1983.
86. Stoffel, E.: Lokales amyloid der Schilddruse. Virchows Arch. (Pathol. Anat.), *201*:245, 1910.
87. Talpos, G. B., Jackson, C. E., Froelich, J. W., et al.: Localization of residual medullary thyroid cancer by thallium/technetium scintigraphy. Surgery, *98*:1189–1196, 1985.
88. Tashjian, A. H., Jr., Howland, B. G., Melvin, K. E. W., and Hill, C. S., Jr.: Immunoassay of human calcitonin: Clinical measurement, relation to serum calcium and studies in patients with medullary carcinoma. N. Engl. J. Med., *283*:890–895, 1970.
89. Tisell, L.-E., Hansson, G., Jansson, S., and Salander, H.: Reoperation in the treatment of asymptomatic metastasizing medullary thyroid carcinoma. Surgery, *99*:60–66, 1986.
90. Uribe, M., Fenoglio-Preiser, C. M., Grimes, M., and Feind, C.: Medullary carcinoma of the thyroid gland: Clinical, pathological, and immunohistochemical features with review of the literature. Am. J. Surg. Pathol., *9*:577–594, 1985.
91. Verby, J. E., Woolner, L. B., Nobrega, F. T., et al.: Thyroid cancer in Olmsted County 1935–1965. J. Natl. Cancer Inst., *43*:813–820, 1969.
92. Wallace, S., Hill, C. S., Paulus, D. D., Jr., et al.: The radiologic aspects of medullary (solid) thyroid carcinoma. Radiol. Clin. North Am., *8*:463–474, 1970.
93. Weber, C. J., Marangos, P. G., Richardson, S., et al.: Presence of neuron-specific enolase and somatostatin in human parathyroid tissues. Surgery, *98*:1008–1012, 1985.
94. Wells, S. A., Jr., Dilley, W. G., Farndon, J. A., et al.: Early diagnosis and treatment of medullary

thyroid carcinoma. Arch. Intern. Med., *145:*1248–1252, 1985.
95. Wells, S. A., Jr., Haagensen, D. E., Linehan, W. M., et al.: The detection of elevated plasma levels of carcinoembryonic antigen in patients with suspected or established medullary thyroid carcinoma. Cancer, *42:*1498–1503, 1978.
96. Wells, S. A., Jr., Baylin, S. B., Leight, G. S., et al.: The importance of early diagnosis in patients with hereditary medullary thyroid carcinoma. Ann. Surg., *195:*595–599, 1982.
97. Wells, S. A., Jr., Baylin, S. B., Linehan, W. M., et al.: Provocative agents and the diagnosis of medullary carcinoma of the thyroid. Ann. Surg., *188:*139–141, 1978.
98. Wells, S. A., Jr., Baylin, S. B., Johnsrude, I. S., et al.: Thyroid venous catheterization in the early diagnosis of familial medullary thyroid carcinoma. Ann. Surg., *196:*505–511, 1982.
99. Wells, S. A., Jr., Baylin, S. B., Gann, D. S., et al.: Medullary thyroid carcinoma: Relationship of method of diagnosis to pathologic staging. Ann. Surg., *188:*377–383, 1978.
100. Wermer, P.: Genetic aspects of adenomatosis of endocrine glands. Am. J. Med., *16:*363–371, 1954.
101. Williams, E. D.: A review of 17 cases of carcinoma of the thyroid and phaeochromocytoma. J. Clin. Pathol., *18:*288–292, 1965.
102. Williams, E. D.: Histogenesis of medullary carcinoma of the thyroid. J. Clin. Pathol., *19:*114–118, 1966.
103. Williams, E. D., Brown, C. L., and Doniach, I.: Pathological and clinical findings in a series of 67 cases of medullary carcinoma of the thyroid. J. Clin. Pathol., *19:*103–113, 1966.
104. Williams, E. D., Karim, S. M., and Sandler, M.: Prostaglandin secretion by medullary carcinoma of the thyroid: A possible cause of the associated diarrhoea. Lancet, *1:*22–23, 1968.
105. Winship, T., and Rosvoll, R. V.: Thyroid carcinoma in childhood: Final report on a 20 year study. Clin. Proc. Child. Hosp. Med. Ctr., *26:*327–348, 1970.
106. Wolfe, H. J., Melvin, K. E., Cervi-Skinner, S. J., et al.: C-cell hyperplasia preceding medullary thyroid carcinoma. N. Engl. J. Med., *289:*437–441, 1973.
107. Wurster-Hill, D. H., Noll, W. W., Bircher, L. Y., et al.: A cytogenetic study of familial medullary carcinoma of the thyroid. Cancer Res., *46*(4 Pt 2):2134–2138, 1986.
108. Zaatari, G. S., Saigo, P. E., and Huvos, A. G.: Mucin production in medullary carcinoma of the thyroid. Arch. Pathol. Lab. Med., *107:*70–74, 1983.
109. Ziegler, R., Deutschle, U., and Raue, F.: Calcitonin in human pathophysiology. Horm. Res., *20:*65–73, 1984.

# Commentary

*Blake Cady, M.D., and Ricardo L. Rossi, M.D.*

This superb chapter by leaders in the field of medullary thyroid carcinoma is a comprehensive overview. There is little to add. However, one aspect of management of patients with medullary carcinoma of the thyroid of the sporadic variety regards decisions after detection of a rising carcinoembryonic antigen or calcitonin level in the absence of clinical symptoms after curative regional surgical therapy. When patients have had adequate local and regional therapy by means of total thyroidectomy and appropriate neck dissection on the ipsilateral side and central compartment, the diagnostic pursuit of the location of other calcitonin-producing metastatic carcinoma is of little clinical use. Two features are important in understanding this recommendation: the clinical course of patients with medullary thyroid carcinoma is prolonged, even in patients whose distant dissemination of disease is widespread and who will eventually die of disease. Solitary metastatic lesions do not occur. In the absence of symptoms, even appreciably elevated calcitonin levels may be associated with a long-term, apparently disease-free state. Vigorous attempts to locate presumed metastatic disease detected by an elevated calcitonin level followed by therapy of asymptomatic lesions does not increase the cure rate or extend disease-free or total life. Therefore, for patients who do not have symptoms but who have an elevated calcitonin level, aggressive attempts at diagnosis and localization do not seem justified. One might even question the utility of obtaining frequent calcitonin values.

Familial medullary carcinoma of the thyroid is an ideal model for genetically related carcinomas in that a highly sensitive marker exists that, when elevated, can lead to curative treatment at a preclinical stage of C cell hyperplasia or microinvasive carcinoma. Thus, carcinoma usually associated with a poor prognosis can be treated at its earliest stage and produce a normal life expectancy.

Medullary carcinoma of the thyroid remains the only absolute indication for total thyroidectomy. However, even when a detailed pedigree is available before operation in a patient who is older than the norm and has a solitary focus of carcinoma, less than total thyroidectomy can be recommended because bilateral disease is extremely uncommon in sporadic carcinoma. The advantage of avoiding total thyroidectomy in such patients would be a reduction in parathyroid morbidity associated with that operation as well as elimination of the need for lifetime medication with thyroid hormone.

Despite extensive discovery of familial clusters of medullary thyroid carcinoma in the past two decades, family syndromes are still being encountered. This fact should be kept in mind by every surgeon who operates on the thyroid. Of all medullary carcinomas, 80 per cent are sporadic in occurrence, but the ability to cure a large pool of patients in familial clusters should stimulate us to seek these patients out. Patients whose family history is unknown should be treated by total thyroidectomy and ipsilateral neck dissection because they might be the index patient of such a familial group.

# 16

# UNDIFFERENTIATED CARCINOMA AND LYMPHOMA OF THYROID GLAND

*Ricardo L. Rossi, M.D., and Blake Cady, M.D.*

Undifferentiated thyroid carcinoma is uncommon and is associated with a poor prognosis. However, this carcinoma is of contemporary interest, and its treatment requires sound surgical and oncologic principles. In selected patients, reasonable palliation or occasionally cure can be achieved.

Undifferentiated thyroid carcinoma is decreasing in incidence for reasons that are not clear. A review[16] of 964 patients with thyroid carcinoma treated at the Lahey Clinic between 1931 and 1970 disclosed 126 patients with undifferentiated thyroid carcinoma. In consecutive decades, the proportion of undifferentiated thyroid carcinomas has steadily decreased from 19 to less than 5 per cent of all thyroid carcinomas seen at our institution currently. Thus, undifferentiated forms of thyroid carcinoma are much less frequent, and this shift is statistically significant although of unknown cause.

The histology of highly malignant undifferentiated carcinoma is often difficult to classify because these carcinomas may have little or no resemblance to the normal follicular cell of origin. As a result, terminology has been confusing. Classifications have been designed by the Armed Forces Institute of Pathology and the World Health Organization.[9] Basically, undifferentiated carcinoma is classified as small cell and large cell undifferentiated carcinoma. Small cell carcinoma constitutes a controversial group, and by strict diagnostic criteria, this carcinoma must be differentiated from lymphoma or anaplastic forms of medullary carcinoma.[16] Immunohistochemical studies and ultrastructural characteristics as defined by electron microscopy are essential in distinguishing these different malignant lesions.[6, 12, 15, 17] Even then, it may not be possible to differentiate all small cell neoplasms.[14]

Large cell undifferentiated carcinoma has been defined more specifically and consists of giant cell carcinoma, spindle cell carcinoma, anaplastic carcinoma, and carcinosarcoma.

The pathologic characteristics of these tumors are discussed in the chapter on pathology of the thyroid and parathyroid glands.

## GIANT AND SMALL CELL UNDIFFERENTIATED THYROID CARCINOMA

The median age of patients on presentation with these tumors is 60 years.[16] A history of long-standing goiter with recent sudden enlargement was reported in 33 per cent of our patients with giant cell carcinoma and in 21 per cent of all patients with undifferentiated carcinoma. The overall female to male ratio was 2.6 to 1, but it was 8 to 1 for patients with small cell diffuse carcinoma and 1.3 to 1 for patients with giant cell carcinoma. The most frequent carcinoma found in women was the small cell diffuse type; in men, the commonest carcinoma was the giant cell type.

The possibility of undifferentiated thyroid carcinoma originating from well-differentiated papillary thyroid carcinoma has been suggested. In one series[20] of 14 patients with anaplastic thyroid carcinoma, ten (71 per cent) followed or occurred simultaneously with a well-differentiated thyroid carcinoma, usually papillary carcinoma. Although this phenomenon does occur, in our review[16] of more than 600 patients with well-differentiated carcinoma and 94 total deaths, only four patients died with giant and spindle cell carcinoma. In one of these patients, only foci of anaplastic elements were discovered, and in another patient, foci of undifferentiated forms were present at the original resection for differentiated thyroid carcinoma. Thus, only two patients could truly be considered to have had a conversion from differentiated thyroid carcinoma to undifferentiated giant and spindle cell carcinoma with the attendant rapid growth of the carcinoma and prompt death of the patient. In addition, no recurrent disease or death occurred after 25 or 30 years, respectively, after primary therapy for differentiated carcinoma, suggesting that despite many presumed residual areas of papillary and mixed carcinoma in lymph nodes or contralateral thyroid lobes, late conversion to undifferentiated forms must be an exceedingly uncommon event.

A two-step process in the development of anaplastic carcinoma is suggested. Microscopic differentiated thyroid carcinoma is common. A distinct promoting factor may convert this innocuous stable occult focus of carcinoma to a clinically significant differentiated carcinoma and yet another promoting event convert such a focus to undifferentiated carcinoma. The relationship between radiation exposure either with radioactive iodine[2] or external beam radiotherapy and the later development of anaplastic thyroid carcinoma has been noted occasionally. In our series, only a few patients had received radiotherapy in childhood, and late conversion of presumed radiation-induced differentiated thyroid carcinoma was not present.

### *Clinical Presentation*

Hoarseness, dyspnea, and stridor are common presenting symptoms. The most frequent finding at presentation is a mass of recent onset or sudden enlargement of a previously known goiter. Approximately 10 per cent of patients had palpable lymph node metastasis, and 10 per cent had proved distant metastatic disease on presentation.

These carcinomas are aggressive and invade periglandular soft tissues early. In our series, only 20 per cent of patients had the primary carcinoma limited to the intraglandular location at operation. Extraglandular extension involved the trachea in 48 per cent of patients and the recurrent laryngeal nerves in 25 per cent of patients.

### *Diagnosis*

The clinical history and findings frequently suggest the presence of an undifferentiated thyroid carcinoma. Fine needle aspiration biopsy and cytology and core cutting biopsy can establish the diagnosis, can be used to avoid open biopsy, and can usually help distinguish between large cell undifferentiated thyroid carcinoma and benign conditions, such as hemorrhage or nontoxic nodular goiter. Small cell carcinoma, medullary carcinoma, and malignant lymphoma or thyroiditis can be difficult to differentiate, and often an open procedure is required for confirmation of the diagnosis. The serum calcitonin level can be helpful as a marker determining the presence of medullary carcinoma. In the treatment of patients with small cell undifferentiated carcinoma, immunohistochemical methods using immunoperoxidase techniques and monoclonal antibodies are important in differentiating this carcinoma from malignant lymphoma and medullary carcinoma because the treatment of patients with the latter two conditions is different.

When biopsy establishes the diagnosis, the extent of disease is assessed. Computed tomography of the neck and mediastinum can show the extent of disease and the degree of tracheal stenosis. The latter can also be assessed by plain frontal roentgenography of the neck with or without tomography. Indirect laryngoscopy can identify vocal cord paralysis. Laryngoscopy and esophagoscopy can be used selectively to demonstrate esophageal or tracheal involvement. Radiography of the chest can reveal pulmonary metastatic disease.

## *Treatment*

In the past, therapy consisted of surgery with an attempt to remove as much of the disease as was safely possible, short of esophagectomy and laryngectomy, and with liberal use of tracheostomy in selected patients. Surgical therapy was followed by external beam radiotherapy. The survival curve seen with this approach at our institution is depicted in Figure 16–1. The best 5-year survival rates were in patients with disease limited to the thyroid gland or in patients in whom all of the carcinoma could be removed surgically (Table 16–1). The 5-year survival rate for patients with giant cell carcinoma in whom all obvious tumor was removed was as high as 19 per cent. However, the overall 1-year survival rate for all patients with giant cell carcinoma was 14 per cent, and the 5-year survival rate was less than 10 per cent.

The median survival time for patients with giant cell carcinoma is about 6 months in most published reports, and the 5-year survival rate of less than 10 per cent has been a major incentive for the development of new treatment modalities. Recently, multimodality therapy—combining radiotherapy, chemotherapy, and surgery—has been used.[7, 11, 18, 21, 24] Although the increase in life expectancy with these therapies has not been well documented, local control of the carcinoma has sometimes been achieved, decreasing the number of patients who die of local compression and suffocation. Of 25 consecutive patients treated at the Karolinska Hospital[21] with hyperfractionated radiotherapy and bleomycin, cyclophosphamide, and 5-fluorouracil, tracheostomy was required in only three patients.

Regimens based on preoperative treatment with doxorubicin (Adriamycin), 20 mg/m$^2$/week, and hyperfractionated radiotherapy, 30 cGy, followed by neck exploration when the tumor is considered resectable and by postoperative treatment with doxorubicin, 20 mg/m$^2$/week, and radiotherapy, 16 cGy, have

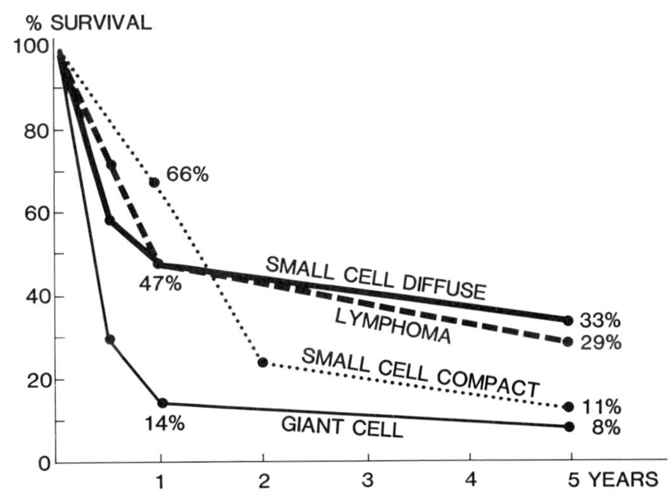


**FIGURE 16–1.** Survival curves of undifferentiated thyroid carcinoma and lymphoma. Note the similarity of small cell diffuse carcinoma and lymphoma. (From Rossi, R., Cady, B., Meissner, W. A., et al.: Prognosis of undifferentiated carcinoma and lymphoma of the thyroid. Am. J. Surg., *135*:591, 1978, with permission.)

**TABLE 16–1. Tumor Extent, Surgical Therapy, and Survival**

| | EXTENT AT SURGERY | | | | SURGICAL THERAPY | | | |
|---|---|---|---|---|---|---|---|---|
| | Intraglandular | | Extraglandular | | All Cancer Removed | | Gross Residual Cancer | |
| | *No.* | *Survived* | *No.* | *Survived* | *No.* | *Survived* | *No.* | *Survived* |
| Giant cell | 11 | 2 ( 18%) | 40 | 2 ( 5%) | 16 | 3 (19%) | 35 | 1 ( 3%) |
| Small cell diffuse | 7 | 4 ( 57%) | 29 | 8 (28%) | 12 | 6 (50%) | 24 | 6 (25%) |
| Lymphoma | 3 | 3 (100%) | 14 | 2 (14%) | 5 | 4 (80%) | 12 | 1 ( 8%) |
| Small cell compact | 3 | 1 ( 33%) | 6 | 0 | 2 | 1 (50%) | 7 | 0 |

From Rossi, R., Cady, B., Meissner, W. A., et al.: Prognosis of undifferentiated carcinoma and lymphoma of the thyroid. Am. J. Surg., *135*:591, 1978, with permission.

been reported by Farnebo and Wallin.[5] Other chemotherapeutic agents that have been used in the treatment of patients with undifferentiated carcinoma include actinomycin D and methotrexate.[10]

In surgical resection, an attempt should be made to remove all macroscopic tumor. An involved recurrent laryngeal nerve is likely to be sacrificed. Modified neck dissection is not performed routinely. When the tumor appears to be confined to the thyroid gland, total thyroidectomy to encompass the disease is the operation of choice. In most patients, however, only resection of the central gland is possible either to free the trachea or to place a tracheostomy. Laryngectomy and esophagectomy should be avoided, and tracheostomy is carried out selectively. For patients who are not candidates for surgery or who do not become candidates after initial radiotherapy and chemotherapy, further radiotherapy and other chemotherapeutic combinations (e.g., bleomycin, cyclophosphamide, and 5-fluorouracil) may be used selectively. Multimodality therapy is associated with severe side effects, some of which include spinal necrosis, pneumonitis, and bone marrow suppression, and therefore the efficacy of treatment must be weighed against the side effects. Despite aggressive therapy, the prognosis associated with these carcinomas remains poor. Patients should be given thyroid replacement hormone, primarily to avoid the hypothyroidism that can result from extensive involvement of the thyroid gland or the therapy used.

## LYMPHOMA

Lymphoma of the thyroid gland represented 2 per cent of all thyroid carcinomas treated at the Lahey Clinic between 1931 and 1970.[16] The median age of patients on presentation was 62 years; however, as reported by Compagno and Oertel,[4] a wide age range is found, and rarely patients in childhood are seen. A female to male predominance is apparent. The commonest form of presentation is a history of a rapidly enlarging painless mass in the thyroid. This sudden enlargement can occur in a patient with a long-standing goiter or in a patient who has a prior history of chronic lymphocytic thyroiditis. The association between chronic lymphocytic thyroiditis and the development of a lymphoma in the thyroid is well known. The possibility that a malignant thyroid lymphoma will develop in this context is increased by a factor of 67 in one report.[23]

Depending on the extent of the disease, signs and symptoms include hoarseness, tracheal compression with dyspnea or stridor or both, esophageal compression and dysphagia, or superior vena cava obstruction. Pain can be present. Hypothyroidism can be the result of the association of chronic lymphocytic thyroiditis with tumor involvement of the gland. The development of a dominant nodule in a patient taking thyroid suppression for chronic thyroiditis suggests the presence of a lymphoma of the thyroid.

### *Diagnosis*

Fine needle aspiration cytology of the thyroid is limited in its ability to differentiate a lymphoma of the thyroid from chronic lymphocytic thyroiditis and small cell carcinoma of the thyroid. The coexistence of chronic lymphocytic thyroiditis with lymphoma also adds to the difficulty in interpretation of the cytologic findings. Therefore, open biopsy will usually be required to obtain sufficient tissue to establish a sound differential diagnosis and to establish the pathologic classification of the lymphoma, although a core cutting biopsy may provide sufficient tissue for elaborate pathologic studies. Occasionally, a thyroid scan is helpful in identifying a nonfunctioning area in an asymptomatic goiter and in suggesting the site of biopsy. The diagnosis of specific lymphoma type can be assisted by electron microscopy, the study of cell surface markers, and tissue immunohistochemistry. The working formulation developed by the National Cancer Institute that separates tumors according to their grade appears to have significant prognostic implications.[1]

## Staging

When the diagnosis of thyroid lymphoma is suspected or proved, it is important to stage the disease and differentiate it from systemic lymphoma with secondary involvement of the thyroid gland. The presence of fever, unexplained sweating, pruritus, or weight loss suggests systemic disease. Node-bearing areas should be examined as should the liver and spleen. Laryngoscopy may be required to assess the function of the vocal cords or the presence of tracheal invasion. Esophagoscopy is required in selected patients. Patients should have roentgenography of the chest, computed tomography of the neck and chest, and abdominal computed tomography with oral and intravenously administered contrast material. In patients with high-grade lymphoma or when disease is suspected outside the neck, bone marrow biopsy may be required. An upper gastrointestinal series with small bowel follow-through is performed when symptoms suggest involvement. Laboratory studies should include a complete blood cell count and studies of liver function.

## Treatment

The role of surgery in the treatment of patients with thyroid lymphoma remains controversial. Reports from the Mayo Clinic[3] and our institution[16] suggest that thyroidectomy for lesions confined to the thyroid gland is associated with an excellent prognosis. In our series, all patients with only intraglandular disease were cured with thyroid lobectomy followed by external beam radiation. Of patients who had all obvious tumor removed, 80 per cent survived for a minimum of 5 years while patients with extraglandular disease or macroscopic residual cancer had a survival rate of only 14 and 8 per cent, respectively, despite receiving radiotherapy. In the review of the Mayo Clinic experience, Blair et al.[3] also noted that removal of obvious disease followed by radiotherapy of the neck and mediastinum was associated with a good prognosis. Therefore, when disease was resectable, they favored a surgical approach that included resection of the isthmus to ensure tracheal decompression and conservative bilateral subtotal thyroid lobectomy followed by external beam radiotherapy. When lobectomy has been performed for a thyroid neoplasm that later proves to be a lymphoma, subsequent irradiation is suggested. However, for disease confined to the neck, radiotherapy alone is highly effective and is advocated by others[13] as the primary modality of therapy.

The primary role of surgery is to establish an accurate diagnosis and to excise tumors limited to the thyroid gland. In patients with extensive involvement of the thyroid gland with extraglandular extension, extensive thyroidectomy is not indicated, and surgery is limited to an adequate biopsy. In the presence of tracheal compression, tracheal decompression should be attempted by resection of the isthmus. Tracheostomy is infrequently required.

The treatment of patients with lymphoma of the thyroid limited to the neck consists primarily of radiotherapy to the neck and superior mediastinum in doses of more than 4,000 cGy. In the presence of extensive disease, high-grade lymphoma, or disease outside the neck, multimodality therapy including chemotherapy should be used.[13, 22] Death occurs primarily from systemic disease. In the Mayo Clinic[3] experience with 38 patients, 12 patients had recurrent disease in the radiated field, but 18 patients had recurrent disease outside the radiated field. Radiotherapy failed to control the disease in most patients whose disease was present in multiple sites. For patients with recurrent disease, chemotherapy alone or in combination with radiotherapy should be employed.

### *Prognosis and Outcome*

The factors that affect outcome include histologic classification of the lymphoma and the extent of disease. As reported by Aozasa et al.,[1] low-grade and intermediate-grade lymphomas are associated with a 5-year survival rate of more than 75 per cent while high-grade lymphomas are associated with a survival rate of less than 20 per cent. The 5-year survival rate for patients with intraglandular disease is about 80 per cent; in patients with neck extension, the survival rate drops to 35 per cent. Patients with disseminated disease have a 5-year survival rate of less than 5 per cent. In our experience, before the current chemotherapeutic modalities were developed, the survival rate for patients with intraglandular disease was 100 per cent, and for patients with extraglandular disease, the survival rate was 14 per cent after surgery and radiotherapy. Nodal involvement was associated with a poor prognosis. The 5-year disease-free survival rate in the Mayo Clinic[3] study of 38 patients was 59 per cent, and the mean survival rate after a recurrence for patients receiving salvage therapy was 59 months compared with 2.9 months for patients not treated. Currently, the use of multidrug chemotherapy should strongly be considered in all but the earliest disease presentation.

## RARE TYPES OF THYROID CARCINOMA

A few rare types of thyroid carcinoma, such as epidermoid carcinoma, fibrosarcoma, unclassifiable carcinoma, or clear cell carcinoma, have been encountered. These lesions should be treated aggressively by surgical intervention because cures are possible. Nodal dissection should be performed when clinically detectable metastatic disease is present. Complete excision with postoperative radiotherapy may be curative, and even partial resection followed by external beam radiotherapy may provide short-term palliation. Two of four patients in our series[16] with fibrosarcoma survived 10 years after complete removal of intrathyroidal disease. The two patients whose disease could not be excised completely died within 1 year. In most patients with squamous cell carcinoma, disease is extensive on presentation.[19] Two patients with epidermoid carcinoma had extensive local disease that was resectable, but both patients died of disease. In one of the three patients with unclassified carcinoma, disease occurred in a completely excised intraglandular nodule, and the patient lived free of disease for 10 years. The other two patients had extraglandular extension and died of disease within 6 months. All six patients received radiotherapy. The patient with clear cell carcinoma had intraglandular disease that was completely excised and survived for 22 years. No radiotherapy was given. At autopsy, the kidneys were normal. The three patients with adenoacanthoma, adenosarcoma, and columnar cell carcinoma died of disease at 6, 8, and 64 months, respectively. All patients had undergone thyroidectomy and radiotherapy.

## METASTATIC CARCINOMA

Metastatic disease from melanoma, renal cell carcinoma, breast carcinoma, and other primary sites is not uncommon and must be considered in the differential diagnosis of unusual histology occurring in the thyroid gland.[8]

### REFERENCES


1. Aozasa, K., Inoue, A., Tajima, K., et al.: Malignant lymphomas of the thyroid gland: Analysis of 79 patients with emphasis on histologic prognostic factors. Cancer, *58:*100–104, 1986.
2. Baker, H. W.: Anaplastic thyroid cancer twelve years after radioiodine therapy. Cancer, *23:*885–890, 1969.
3. Blair, T. J., Evans, R. G., Buskirk, S. J., et al.: Radiotherapeutic management of primary thyroid lymphoma. Int. J. Radiat. Oncol. Biol. Phys., *11:*365–370, 1985.
4. Compagno, J., and Oertel, J. E.: Malignant lymphoma and other lymphoproliferative disorders of the thyroid gland: A clinicopathologic study of 245 cases. Am. J. Clin. Pathol., *74:*1–11, 1980.
5. Farnebo, L. O., and Wallin, G.: Anaplastic giant cell carcinoma of the thyroid. *In* Van Heerden, J. A. (ed.): Problems in Endocrine Surgery. Chicago, Year Book Medical Publishers, 1989, pp. 85–88.

6. Fauré, P., Chittal, S., Woodman-Mêmeteau, F., et al.: Diagnostic features of primary malignant lymphomas of the thyroid with monoclonal antibodies. Cancer, *61:*1852–1861, 1988.
7. Gottlieb, J. A., and Hill, C. S., Jr.: Chemotherapy of thyroid cancer with Adriamycin: Experience with 30 patients. N. Engl. J. Med., *290:*193–197, 1974.
8. Green, L. K., Ro, J. Y., MacKay, B., et al.: Renal cell carcinoma metastatic to the thyroid. Cancer, *63:*1810–1815, 1989.
9. International Histologic Classification of Tumors. Geneva, World Health Organization, 1967–1976 (15 numbers by various editors).
10. Jereb, B., Stjernswärd, J., and Löwhagen, T.: Anaplastic giant-cell carcinoma of the thyroid: A study of treatment and prognosis. Cancer, *35:*1293–1295, 1975.
11. Kim, J. H., and Leeper, R. D.: Treatment of anaplastic giant and spindle cell carcinoma of the thyroid gland with combination Adriamycin and radiation therapy: A new approach. Cancer, *52:*954–957, 1983.
12. Nambo, N. C., and Irwin, S. M.: Anaplastic small cell neoplasms of the thyroid: An immunoperoxidase study. Hum. Pathol., *15:*55–60, 1984.
13. Rasbach, D. A., Mondschein, M. S., Harris, N. L., et al.: Malignant lymphoma of the thyroid gland: A clinical and pathologic study of twenty cases. Surgery, *98:*1166–1170, 1985.
14. Rayfield, E. J., Nishiyama, R. H., and Sisson, J. C.: Small cell tumors of the thyroid: A clinicopathologic study. Cancer, *28:*1023–1030, 1971.
15. Rosai, J., and Carcangiu, M. L.: Pathology of thyroid tumors: Some recent and old questions. Hum. Pathol., *15:*1008–1012, 1984.
16. Rossi, R., Cady, B., Meissner, W. A., et al.: Prognosis of undifferentiated carcinoma and lymphoma of the thyroid. Am. J. Surg., *135:*589–595, 1978.
17. Shvero, J., Gal, R., Avidor, I., et al.: Anaplastic thyroid carcinoma: A clinical, histologic, and immunohistochemical study. Cancer, *62:*319–325, 1988.
18. Simpson, W. J.: Anaplastic thyroid carcinoma: A new approach. Can. J. Surg., *23:*25–27, 1980.
19. Simpson, W. J., and Carruthers, J.: Squamous cell carcinoma of the thyroid gland. Am. J. Surg., *156:*44–46, 1988.
20. Spires, J. R., Schwartz, M. R., and Miller, R. H.: Anaplastic thyroid carcinoma: Association with differentiated thyroid cancer. Arch. Otolaryngol. Head Neck Surg., *114:*40–44, 1988.
21. Tallroth, E., Wallin, G., Lundell, G., et al.: Multimodality treatment in anaplastic giant cell thyroid carcinoma. Cancer, *60:*1428–1431, 1987.
22. Tupchong, L., Hughes, F., and Harmer, C. L.: Primary lymphoma of the thyroid: Clinical features, prognostic factors, and results of treatment. Int. J. Radiat. Oncol. Biol. Phys., *12:*1813–1821, 1986.
23. Walfish, P. G.: Lymphoid: Malignant lymphomas of the thyroid. *In* Ingbar, S. H., and Braverman, L. E. (eds.): Werner's The Thyroid. Philadelphia, J. B. Lippincott Co., 1986, pp. 1368–1371.
24. Werner, B., Abele, J., Alveryd, A., et al.: Multimodality therapy in anaplastic giant cell thyroid carcinoma. World J. Surg., *8:*64–70, 1984.


# Commentary

*Chiu-an Wang, M.D.*

## UNDIFFERENTIATED CARCINOMA OF THYROID

Undifferentiated carcinomas of the thyroid are rare, and they cause death in the majority of patients. Rapid growth of a preexisting goiter in an elderly person is commonly the presenting clinical feature of this disease. When undifferentiated carcinoma of the thyroid is first diagnosed, the disease has often progressed beyond cure. Many patients have died within 6 months despite heroic measures of aggressive surgical treatment.

Clinically, undifferentiated thyroid carcinomas often appear diffusely enlarged, firm to stony hard, and are fixed to the adjacent structures of the neck. Local or distant metastatic disease is frequently present, and yet these patients are often euthyroid. Undifferentiated carcinoma of the thyroid may remain undiagnosed for a long time unless a tissue specimen is obtained for examination either by open biopsy or by percutaneous needle biopsy. We usually prefer large needle biopsy of the lesion.

Undifferentiated carcinoma of the thyroid may be classified into giant cell, spindle cell, or small cell carcinoma, and still others are mixed cell carcinomas. More than one cellular component may be present within an undifferentiated carcinoma, and a definitive diagnosis may not be easy to establish.

When the diagnosis of undifferentiated carcinoma of the thyroid is confirmed, the treatment is determined by the stage of the disease. Radical surgery is seldom performed, and then it is performed in only a few patients in whom the lesions are small enough to be resectable. We do not favor a radical surgical approach; rather, external beam radiation therapy is the preferred treatment in some patients. The size of the carcinoma may respond with transient subjective improvement, but ultimately many patients die of the disease. Partial excision of the tumor may be needed to institute temporary tracheostomy for the relief of respiratory compression.

## LYMPHOMAS AND OTHER RARE UNDIFFERENTIATED THYROID CARCINOMAS

Of the rare undifferentiated carcinomas of the thyroid, primary lymphoma poses a difficult diagnostic and therapeutic challenge because this lymphoma is clinically difficult to distinguish from small cell anaplastic carcinoma. A diagnosis by small needle biopsy may not be conclusive. Therefore, open biopsy is our preference when in doubt. The preferred treatment of patients with primary lymphoma of the thyroid is nonoperative. External beam radiation therapy and chemotherapy have been found effective in some patients. Although the result of treatment may look favorable initially, the ultimate outcome is often poor.

Other undifferentiated carcinomas are squamous cell carcinoma, mixed squamous cell carcinoma, and papillary carcinoma. These carcinomas are rare and exceedingly lethal. Surgery is rarely effective even in the early stages of the disease. With combined treatment of the disease with external beam radiation therapy and chemotherapy, a small percentage of patients may be salvaged. I endorse a conservative surgical approach to the treatment of patients with undifferentiated carcinoma of the thyroid.

# 17

# SURGERY OF THYROID GLAND

*Ricardo L. Rossi, M.D., and Blake Cady, M.D.*

The mortality rate of thyroidectomy approaches zero. This can be accomplished by a well-performed standardized technique. The morbidity rate should be less than 5 per cent. Morbidity consists of postoperative hemorrhage, wound infection, recurrent laryngeal nerve palsy, and postoperative hypoparathyroidism. A well-executed thyroidectomy will keep this morbidity to a minimum. The step-by-step technique of thyroidectomy as described in this chapter was originally designed and advocated by Dr. Lahey. Over the years, this technique has been modified by other surgeons of the Lahey Clinic and has stood the test of time (60 years) and numbers (more than 46,000 patients). It is particularly recommended for the surgeon who has not yet standardized a satisfactory procedure. For the thyroid surgeon who has mastered other techniques, it may be superfluous. The technique is easy to learn when special attention is paid to the details as outlined. It is the many details put together that make for a good result. At the Lahey Clinic, literally hundreds of surgical fellows and residents have learned this technique and may attest to its excellence.

Surgery plays only one part in the successful treatment of patients with thyroid disease. No matter how technically perfect thyroidectomy is performed, when the patient is brought into the operating suite in either a hypothyroid or hyperthyroid state, disaster may follow. When thyrocardiac disease is present, the services of a cardiologist are mandatory. When the patient is euthyroid but skilled anesthesiologists are not available, complications may occur. When an expert in diagnosing thyroid disease from a frozen section specimen is lacking, the wrong procedure may be elected. For the best results, treatment of the patient demands the services not only of the surgeon but also of the internist, the cardiologist, the anesthesiologist, and the pathologist—all experienced with thyroid disease.

## POSITION ON THE OPERATING TABLE

The proper position and draping of the patient on the operating room table are important for maximum exposure (Fig. 17–1). The patient should be in a semisitting position. A bar or rolled blanket or a firm pillow at least 4 or 5 inches thick is placed beneath the shoulders to permit maximum hyperex-

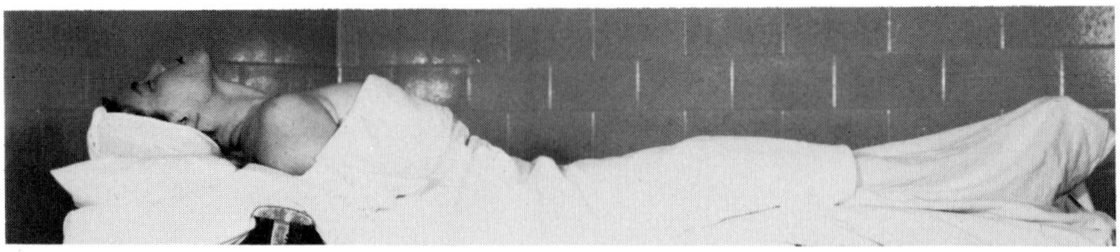

**FIGURE 17–1.** Position for patient. Note semisitting position with the neck flexed to bring the thyroid forward.

tension of the neck. Surgical drapes should be applied so that the entire anterior aspect of the neck from the chin to the suprasternal notch is exposed.

## TECHNIQUE OF THYROIDECTOMY

### *Anterior Exposure of Thyroid Gland*

#### The Incision

The thyroid scar may be the only lasting objective evidence to the patient who has recovered from thyroidectomy. A conspicuous scar as the result of a poorly planned and designed incision may be distressing. Long after recovery from the operation and the symptoms of thyroid disease, an ugly scar, because of its prominent location constantly exposed in the neck, may be a serious source of embarrassment to both patient and surgeon. Indeed, many patients are more concerned preoperatively about the resultant scar than the actual operation.

A proper incision should be well planned and well designed to provide as much concealment as possible and long enough so that the skin flap can be elevated for adequate exposure of the thyroid gland.

We prefer a low collar incision with a gentle curve upward performed in a freehand method about one fingerbreadth above the sternoclavicular joint (Fig. 17–2). It should be placed at a level at which a necklace will naturally rest to conceal the incision. When placed too high, it is constantly visible. It must not be straight but rather curved upward to disappear between the folds of the neck. One mistake that produces a more conspicuous scar is the horseshoe type of incision in which the lateral limbs run too high and can never be concealed. The incision must be symmetric, extending the same distance on each side from the midline; it must not be unbalanced, that is, with one side higher than the other, because this will make it more noticeable. Many times the incision must be planned according to the size and shape of the goiter. A unilateral enlargement of the thyroid requires that the limb of the incision over the enlarged lobe be at a higher level. After the enlarged lobe has been removed, the skin will slip downward to produce a balanced symmetric scar. Over a large and prominent goiter, the skin incision must be placed higher than normal. After the stretched skin has been relieved by removal of the goiter, it will descend to the proper level. Surgeons who give attention to these few simple details regarding the incision will be well rewarded many times over by the satisfaction of their patients.

#### Elevation of the Flap

The skin, subcutaneous fat, and platysma are elevated as one layer. The fascial plane between the posterior sheath of the platysma and the sheath of the sternohyoid muscle is relatively avascular and permits the flap to be raised with little, if any, bleeding. To find this plane for dissection requires attention to almost subtle details and is well worth the effort. In well-developed men, the platysma is prominent; in obese women, its fibers are not easily recognized in the subcutaneous fat. The platysmal fibers are more easily identified at the lateral portions of the incision. After the skin incision has been completed, the platysma muscle is identified laterally and its fibers divided, exposing the fascia of the sternocleidomastoid muscle and prethyroid muscles (the sternohyoid and the sternothyroid; Fig. 17–3). When the bared muscle fibers of the prethyroid muscle are exposed, the dissection has passed through the desired

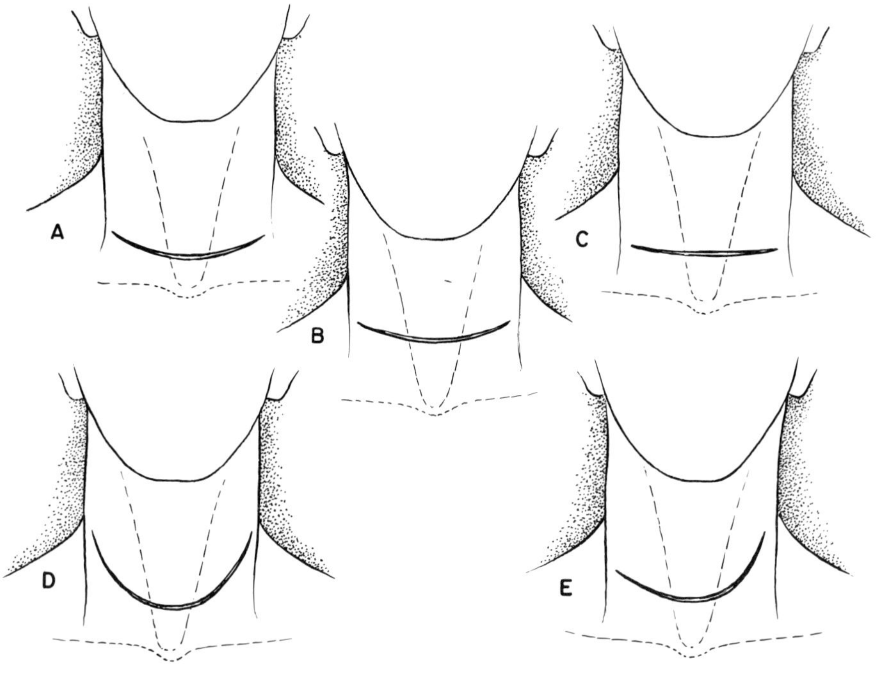


**FIGURE 17–2.** Skin incision for thyroidectomy. *A,* Proper—Symmetric curve at proper level. *B,* Too high—Cannot be concealed. *C,* Too straight with inadequate curve—Does not fall into folds of the neck. *D,* Too much of horseshoe type—Does not permit concealment. *E,* Asymmetric skin of right side has slipped down over front of chest. Had compensatory elevation of the incision been made (right side), it would have descended to the proper level.

fascial plane. As the surgeon approaches the midline, dividing the platysma, it will disappear. At this site, the subcutaneous fat is divided, exposing the fascia of the prethyroid muscles over which lie the superficial veins. The superficial veins are not elevated with the flap, and thus they act as a deep landmark to keep the proper fascial plane. Avoidance of injury to the superficial veins prevents unnecessary bleeding. The dissection is continued toward the opposite side, exposing and dividing the platysma. The flap with skin, platysma, and subcutaneous tissue is now ready for elevation by grasping with triple-hook clamps on the platysma and midline.

By application of strong upward traction, the flap is raised well above the thyroid notch by a combination of sharp and blunt dissection in a relatively avascular plane. At the upper aspect of this dissection, the flap appears to adhere securely to the underlying fascia. When the flap is first raised in the midline, then laterally, the plane is seen as a thin fibrous band beneath the platysma muscle. This fibrous tissue is sharply incised, permitting the flap to be pushed upward (Fig.

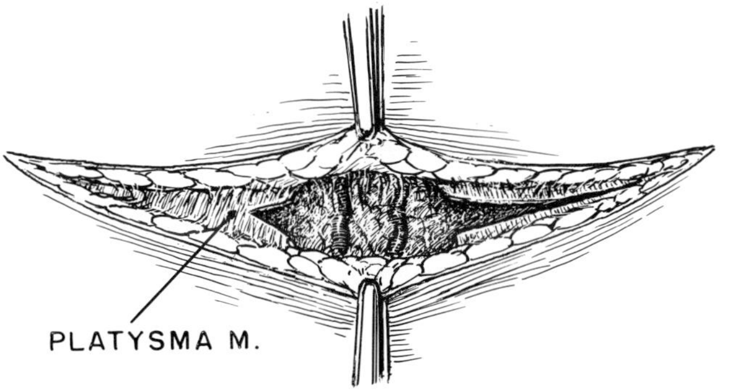


**FIGURE 17–3.** Division of platysma. Platysmal fibers well visualized laterally. Medially, fat has been elevated with flap. Superficial veins and fascia are seen over prethyroid muscles.

17–4). One of the most important technical steps in thyroidectomy is high elevation of the flap. The flap can be elevated satisfactorily only before the prethyroid muscles are divided. Failure to do so at this time will compromise the all-important feature of anatomic exposure. The lower flap is freed from the underlying fascia down to the level of the suprasternal notch in the plane beneath the platysma muscle.

### Division of Prethyroid Muscles (Sternohyoid and Sternothyroid)

Although this maneuver is not universally accepted, we divide the prethyroid muscles in all patients to obtain adequate exposure and to perform thyroidectomy safely. When the muscles are severed high, with their innervation preserved from the ascending branch of the ansa hypoglossal nerve (which enters the muscle low), and when they are later carefully sutured, no disability or disfigurement results. Disfiguring atrophy of the prethyroid muscles, with the sunken neck and prominent trachea, is the result of dividing the prethyroid muscles and their innervation too low in the neck.

The prethyroid muscles are mobilized for transection by freeing their lateral and medial fascial attachments (Fig. 17–4). The fascia of the lateral border of the sternohyoid is attached to the fascia of the medial anterior border of the sternocleidomastoid muscle. When this fascia between the two muscles is divided along the medial edge of the sternocleidomastoid muscle, the anterior jugular vein will be spared, and the communicating veins between the anterior jugular and external jugular veins can be visualized, ligated, and divided. The medial borders of the sternohyoid and sternothyroid muscles are best identified in the midline low in the neck. The midline of the trachea above the suprasternal notch should be determined by palpation and this area explored. Often a small amount of free fatty tissue is a clue to the midline (Fig. 17–5*A*). Before the midline fascia is divided, it is important to locate, ligate, and divide the communicating veins crossing the midline from the anterior jugular of one side to the anterior jugular of the other.

With the borders of the prethyroid muscle mobilized by sharp and blunt dissection, their posterior sheaths are separated from the underlying thyroid capsule. This procedure is accomplished better and bleeding is avoided when it is started over the lower section of the thyroid or the isthmus. A common error is to separate only the sternohyoid and leave the sternothyroid attached to the thyroid capsule. This is particularly true in hyperplastic glands, as found in Graves' disease. A pericapsular reaction seems to occur so that the sternothyroid adheres to the capsule of the thyroid gland. This may be avoided by first elevating the sternohyoid and then carefully looking for the medial border of the sternothyroid, which is more lateral and in an

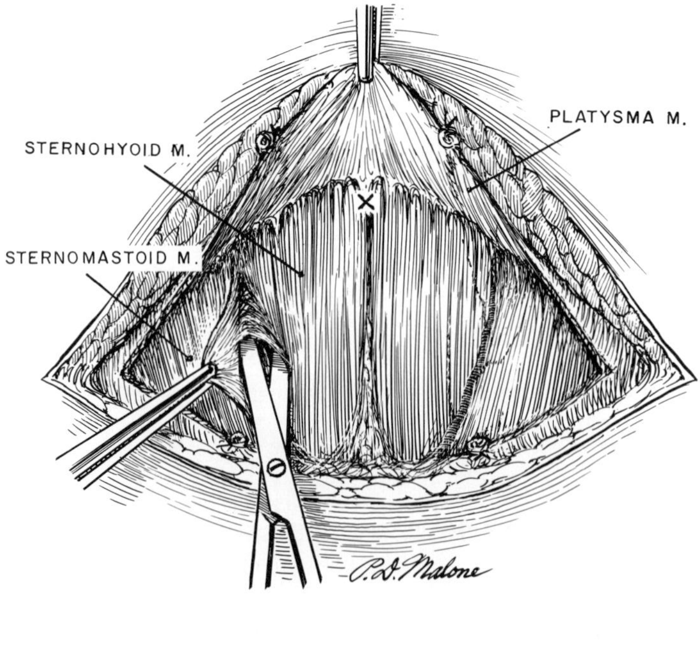


**FIGURE 17–4.** Elevation of flap, X, high to above thyroid notch. Fascia being divided between medial border of sternocleidomastoid muscle and lateral border of strap muscles (right side).

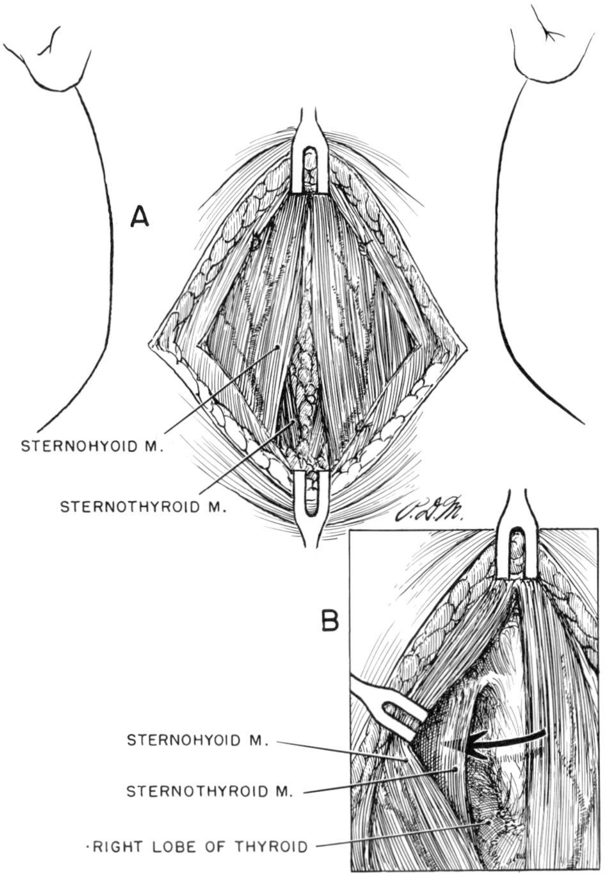


**FIGURE 17–5.** *A,* Dividing the pretracheal fascia in midline from below upward. Midline is best identified low in neck. Frequently a small amount of fat indicates the site of the midline. *B,* Freeing thyroid capsule from the sternothyroid muscle. Sternohyoid muscle is retracted laterally. Medial border of sternothyroid is identified, and muscle is separated from thyroid capsule. Arrow indicates plane between sternothyroid muscle and thyroid capsule.

enlarged gland may appear as the capsule of the thyroid itself (Fig. 17–5*B*). When the operator is aware of this situation, the sternothyroid muscle is identified and elevated from the capsule. Both prethyroid muscles are separated from the gland by blunt dissection. While the medial border of the sternocleidomastoid is retracted outward by the assistant, the surgeon applies Kocher clamps across the upper aspects of the prethyroid muscle from the median side toward the lateral side (Fig. 17–6). The prethyroid muscles are divided between the clamps. The lateral border of the strap muscles is divided superiorly and inferiorly (Fig. 17–7).

A Lahey triple-hook clamp is applied over the Kocher clamp for traction on the upper portion of the divided prethyroid muscles. Extreme gentleness is necessary to retract the upper portion of the divided prethyroid muscles to expose the upper pole and the superior thyroid vessels. This is aided by gentle downward traction on the gland. To permit better elevation of the prethyroid muscles and better exposure of the superior pole, fibers of the omohyoid joining the lateral border of the prethyroid muscles may be divided. As the area of the superior pole is unroofed, we have found it advantageous to incise the sternothyroid muscle below its attachment to the thyroid cartilage (Fig. 17–8). As the sternothyroid crosses the superior pole to the thyroid cartilage, it prevents further elevation of the sternohyoid and prevents access to the superior thyroid vessels. The plane between the sternohyoid and the sternothyroid is avascular. When this plane is entered, the sternothyroid may be divided. The sternohyoid is further elevated, and the superior thyroid vessels are well exposed in the operative field, although they are covered by a few fibers of the sternothyroid (Fig. 17–8). The lower divided prethyroid muscles are freed laterally and retracted downward. Both lobes are exposed in the same manner, and the anterior exposure of the thyroid is completed (Fig. 17–9).

When the anterior exposure has been per-

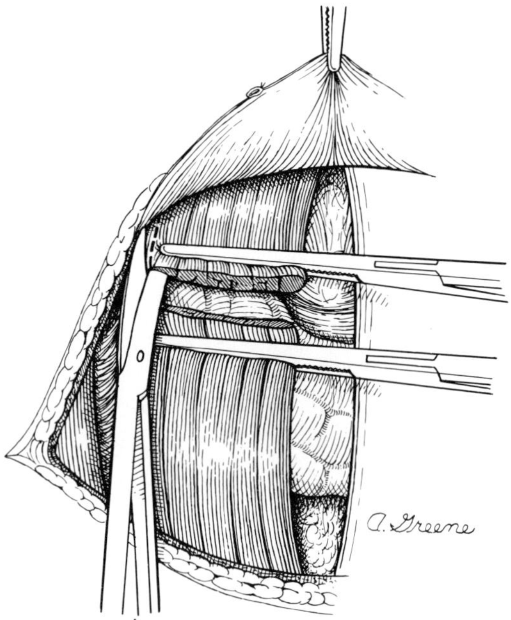


**FIGURE 17–6.** Cutting the prethyroid muscle high to avoid injury to the ansa hypoglossi, which descends lateral to the border of the muscle, entering the muscle low in the neck, and then ascends. (Reprinted with the permission of the Lahey Clinic.)

formed properly, the remainder of the operation should go smoothly. Difficulty encountered with mobilization, hemorrhage, and identification of the recurrent laryngeal nerves and the parathyroids is usually the result of poor anterior exposure.

## *Mobilization of Gland*

Mobilization of the thyroid gland involves division of the middle or lateral thyroid veins so that the internal jugular vein and carotid artery can be retracted laterally and the thyroid displaced up and out of its bed (Fig. 17–10). This gives access to the posterior aspect of the gland so that the inferior thyroid artery and the recurrent laryngeal nerve can be identified. The number of veins is variable. Usually one vein is seen at the upper pole, two or more veins drain the middle third of the gland, and frequently a plexus of veins is found in the region of the inferior pole.

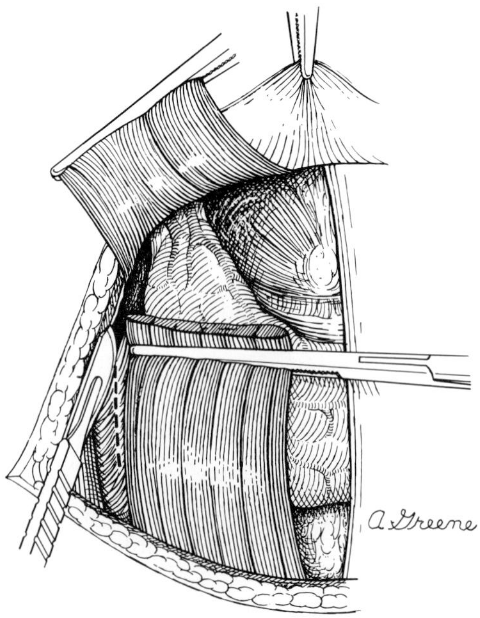


**FIGURE 17–7.** The lateral borders of the strap muscles are divided superiorly and inferiorly. (Reprinted with the permission of the Lahey Clinic.)

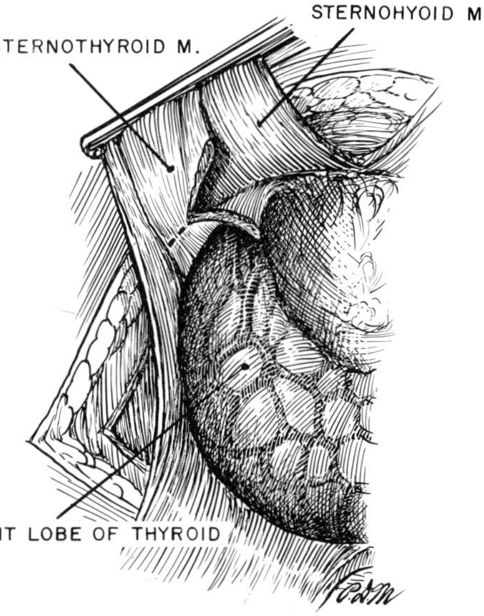


**FIGURE 17–8.** Exposure of the superior thyroid pole. The sternothyroid muscle inserts into the thyroid cartilage. The sternohyoid muscle inserts higher in the neck into the hyoid. The sternothyroid muscle fibers are divided, permitting the sternohyoid to be retracted more cephalad to expose the superior pole. The superior thyroid pole is exposed but covered with fibers of sternothyroid.

Gentle upward and medial traction on the gland places the lateral veins on the stretch so that by meticulous dissection they can be clamped and severed. As the lateral veins empty directly into the internal jugular vein, an inadvertent tear may flood the lateral compartment, making later identification of the inferior thyroid artery, recurrent laryngeal nerves, and parathyroid glands more difficult. As mentioned in the chapter on surgical anatomy, in large goiters that have expanded laterally, the cleavage plane between the capsule of the gland and the internal jugular vein may not be apparent immediately. The internal jugular vein may adhere tightly to the capsule, and the lateral veins may be pushed medially onto the capsule (Fig. 17–11). In large goiters, the lateral veins should be divided close to the capsule. When the gland is rotated anteriorly and medially, the cleavage plane will be apparent, the internal jugular vein is visualized and retracted laterally, and the remaining lateral veins are severed. Surgeons may misinterpret this situation and inadvertently excise the internal jugular vein and the lateral thyroid veins with the gland.

## *Isolation of Inferior Thyroid Artery*

The most vulnerable location for injury to the recurrent laryngeal nerve is the point at which the inferior thyroid artery approaches the lateral aspect of the thyroid. Before the thyroid gland is entered, the inferior thyroid artery may divide into two or more branches and be intimately associated with the recurrent laryngeal nerve and its branches (Fig. 17–12). (Readers not familiar with these all-important anatomic relationships are referred to the chapter on surgical anatomy.) The localization of the inferior thyroid artery is important because it plays an important part in identification of the recurrent laryngeal nerve.

The internal jugular vein and the carotid artery are retracted laterally, and the thyroid gland is retracted anteriorly and medially by placement of a triple-hook clamp deep into normal thyroid tissue and exposure of the entire posterolateral edge of the thyroid when the thyroid lobe is dislodged from its bed. For easy identification of the inferior thyroid artery and the recurrent laryngeal nerve, this compartment should be free of blood-stained tissue. By meticulous scissors dissection in this avascular field, the inferior thyroid artery will be visualized coming from beneath the carotid artery, in most instances at the level of the midportion of the thyroid gland. Occasionally, it appears as high as the superior pole, and in such instances, as it descends, it divides into two branches. This division may occur behind the carotid sheath and may present what appears to be a double inferior thyroid artery. Infrequently, it is found at the level of the inferior pole coming straight upward into the gland. As the inferior thyroid artery is followed to the capsule of the gland, attention is directed to the recurrent laryn-

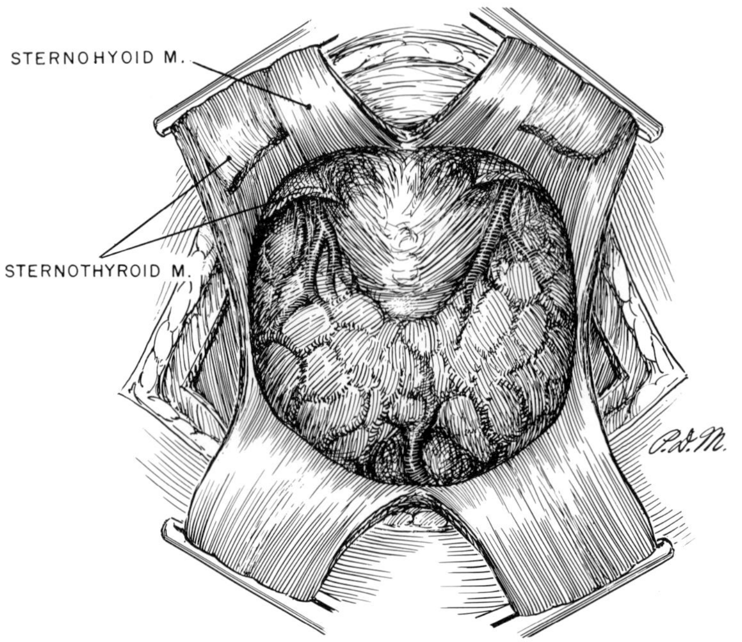


**FIGURE 17–9.** Completed anterior exposure.

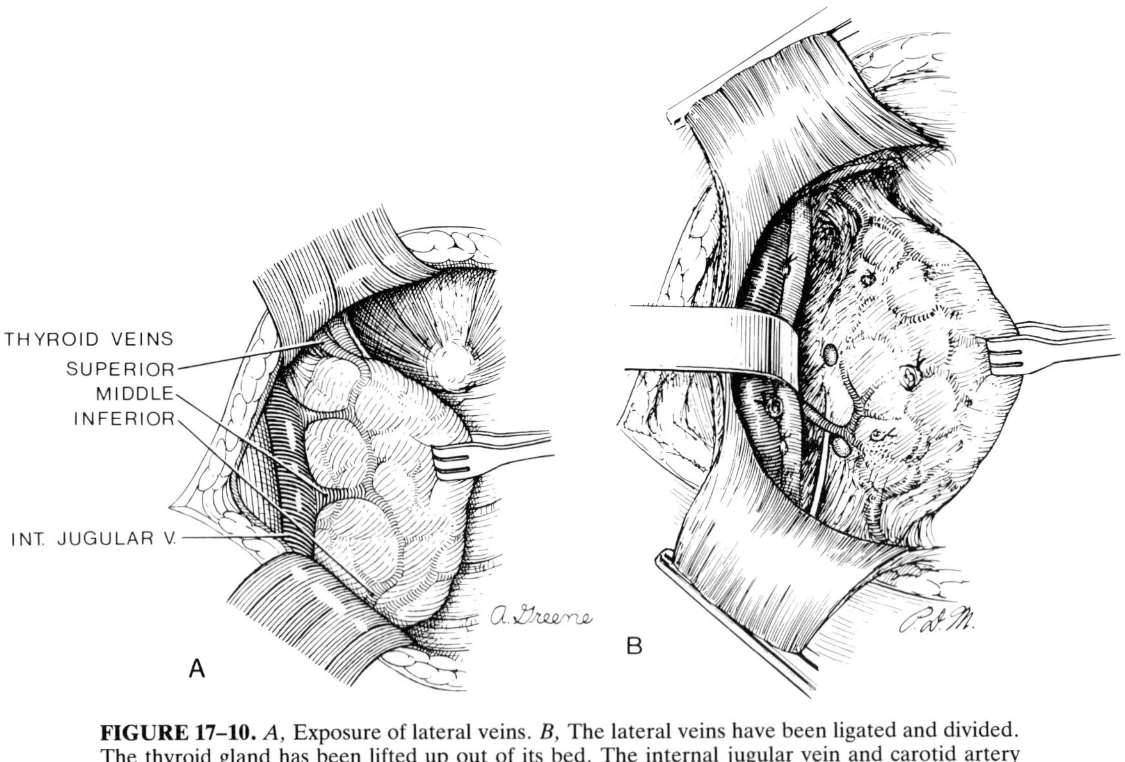


**FIGURE 17–10.** *A,* Exposure of lateral veins. *B,* The lateral veins have been ligated and divided. The thyroid gland has been lifted up out of its bed. The internal jugular vein and carotid artery are retracted laterally, and the lateral compartment is exposed for visualization of the recurrent laryngeal nerve and inferior thyroid artery. (Reprinted with the permission of the Lahey Clinic.)

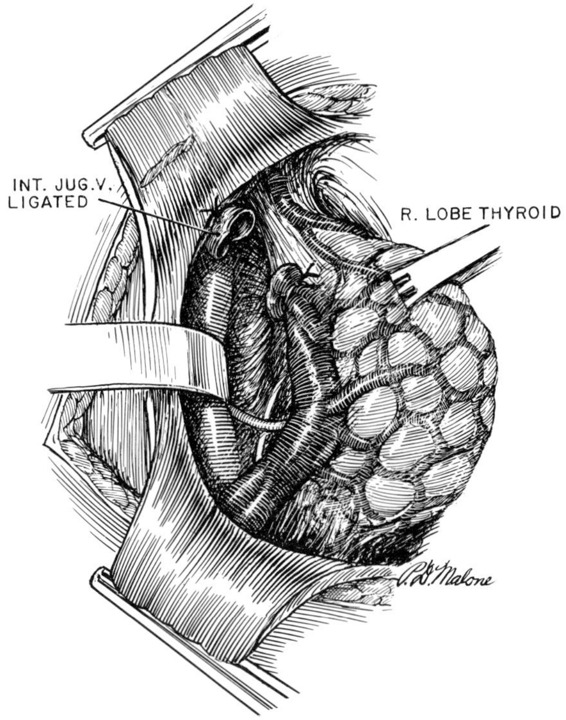


**FIGURE 17–11.** Large goiter with internal jugular vein and lateral inferior thyroid veins appearing clearly adherent to thyroid capsule. When these are not recognized, dissection may occur between the internal jugular vein and carotid artery with inadvertent excision of the internal jugular vein with the gland.

geal nerve; in most patients, this passes posterior to the artery, but it may be above or between the branches of the artery.

At the Lahey Clinic, it used to be routine to ligate the inferior thyroid artery laterally. Currently, this step has been replaced by separate and individual ligation of its branches at the level of the thyroid capsule when total or near total lobectomy is performed. The blood supply to the parathyroid glands is thus preserved.

Hemorrhage from a torn inferior thyroid artery is inexcusable. Obviously, it cannot be controlled with pressure on the carotid artery as is possible with a torn superior thyroid artery. When this catastrophe occurs, the carotid sheath must be retracted laterally and anteriorly and the proximal end of the artery clamped and ligated.

## *Isolation of Recurrent Laryngeal Nerve*

After the inferior thyroid artery has been identified, the recurrent laryngeal nerve must be demonstrated. Again, thorough knowledge of the anatomic relationships of the artery and nerve, adequate exposure, good light, and an avascular field are of paramount importance. Most often, the recurrent laryngeal nerve is identified at the time the inferior thyroid artery is isolated. If not, it is sought low in the neck in its usual location 1.0 to 1.5 cm lateral to the trachea as the nerve angles toward the larynx.

As it approaches the lower border of the thyroid, it may, as it ascends, be intimately associated with a plexus of delicate thyroid veins. Bleeding is avoided by meticulous scissors dissection; the scissors blades are always opened in the direction of the course of the nerve. The recurrent laryngeal nerve may have one or more extralaryngeal branches. Only one, however, contains the motor fibers supplying the laryngeal muscles. From a practical point of view, all branches must be considered as possible motor branches and spared injury. When identified, the nerve is followed to its junction with the inferior thyroid artery. The nerve can then be followed upward toward the larynx when total lobectomy is planned.

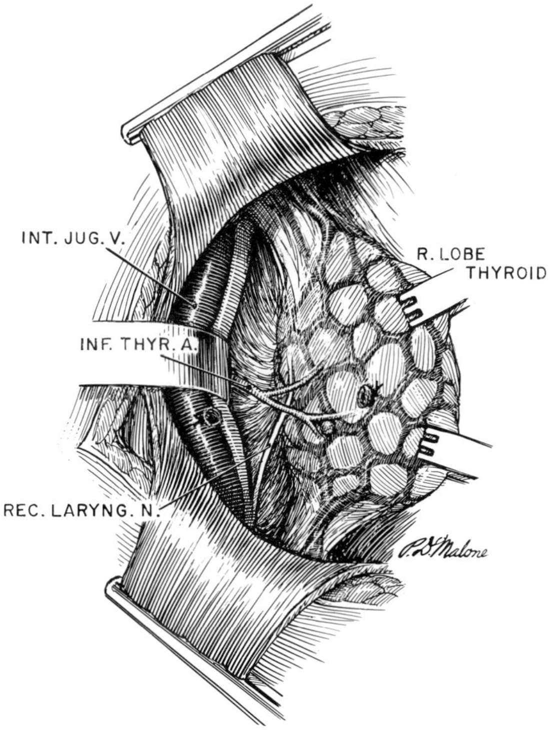


**FIGURE 17–12.** Relationship of inferior thyroid artery and recurrent laryngeal nerve.

## *Mobilization of Inferior Pole*

With the inferior thyroid artery and the recurrent laryngeal nerve visualized, the lower pole may be mobilized safely. The midline of the trachea is demonstrated below the isthmus (Fig. 17–13). The entire plexus of vessels below the isthmus and inferior poles (such as the lower thyroid or thyroidea ima vessels), may be cross-clamped (Fig. 17–14). During this maneuver, the recurrent laryngeal nerve must be constantly in view. The clamps are applied from the midline out. We prefer to use two hemostats below and one above and to divide between the upper one and the lower two. This is a safety measure and prevents any possibility of the vessels slipping from one clamp and escaping into the mediastinum where they may be difficult to retrieve. With the vessels divided, the lower pole is gently detached from the trachea and pulled upward and outward.

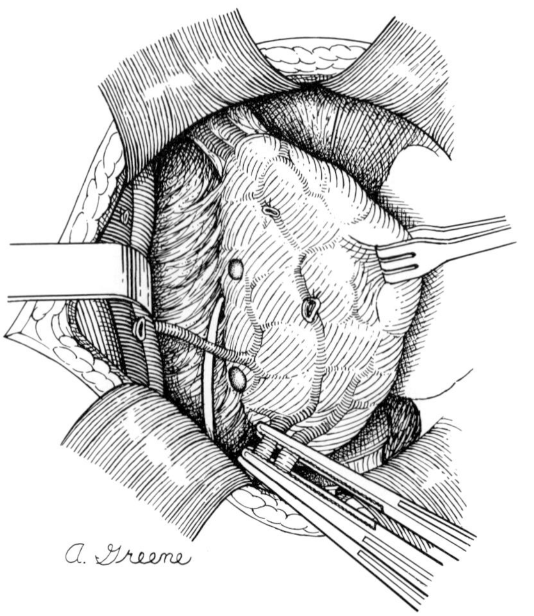


**FIGURE 17–14.** The inferior pole vessels are clamped after having identified the recurrent laryngeal nerve and the inferior parathyroid gland. (Reprinted with the permission of the Lahey Clinic.)

## *Division of Superior Thyroid Vessels and Mobilization of Upper Pole*

The superior thyroid vessels must be ligated under direct vision. With high elevation of the prethyroid muscle and downward and lateral traction of the superior pole, they can be separated from the inferior constrictor muscle. They may be hidden beneath a few fibers of the divided sternothyroid. It is safest to ligate the vessels with a ligature passing from inside out, that is, from medial to lateral to avoid the superior laryngeal nerve. The vessels are doubly ligated above and divided between the ligatures and a clamp placed below (Fig. 17–15). As previously described in the chapter on surgical anatomy, these vessels may approach the upper pole of the thyroid along its anterior and inner aspect. In hyperplastic glands, a lingula or tongue of thyroid tissue may ascend high, lateral to the entry of the vessels into the gland. In such instances, two mistakes may be made: a blind attempt may be made to pass a ligature around the vessels above the lingula or the lingula may be transected with the vessels, leaving remaining thyroid tissue intact—a difficult problem to remedy at a later date (Fig. 17–16). This may be avoided by isolating and dividing the superior thyroid vessels at a lower level; then, by excising the thyroid capsule, this extension of thyroid tissue exposed by outward and downward traction may be enucleated. Before complete enucleation, small posterior veins entering the gland should be clamped.

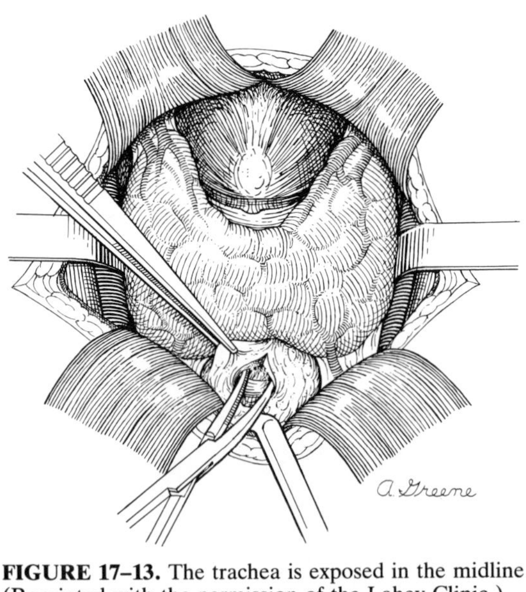


**FIGURE 17–13.** The trachea is exposed in the midline. (Reprinted with the permission of the Lahey Clinic.)

For decades at our institution, mass liga-

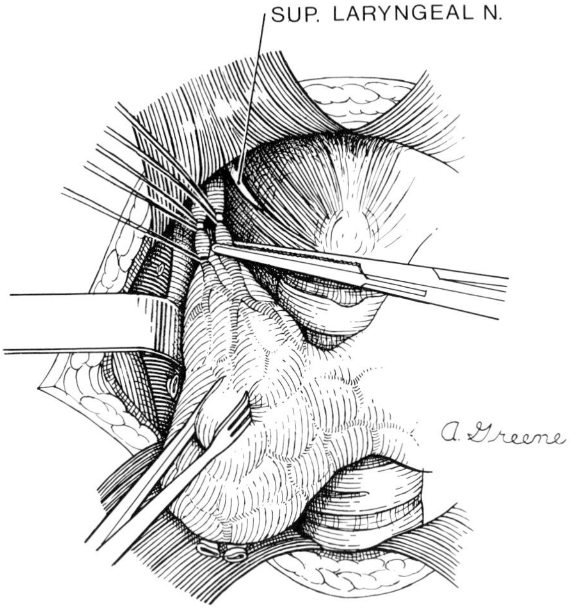


**FIGURE 17–15.** The superior thyroid vessels are ligated. (Reprinted with the permission of the Lahey Clinic.)

tion of upper pole vessels was performed by ligating low beside or on the pole or within the thyroid tissue to avoid injury to the superior laryngeal nerve. This technique has been modified to include isolation and individual ligation of upper pole vessels with identification of the superior laryngeal nerve. This technique is specifically indicated when performing total or near total lobectomy.

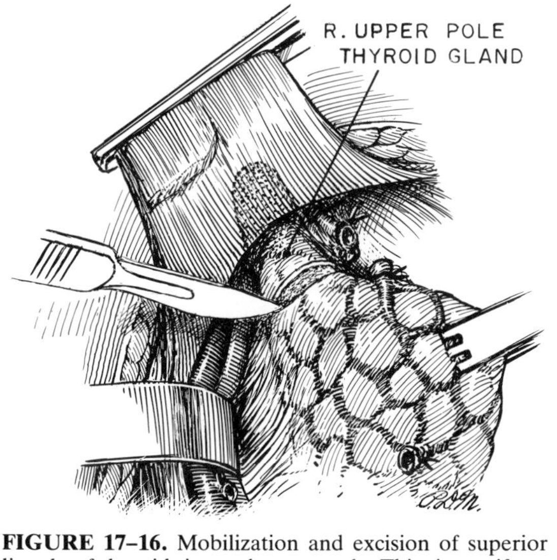


**FIGURE 17–16.** Mobilization and excision of superior lingula of thyroid tissue above vessels. This tissue, if not removed, is the most frequent cause of recurrent Graves' disease.

Meticulous attention must be paid to identification and preservation of the superior laryngeal nerve branches, which may intertwine branches of the superior thyroid artery.

## *Identification of Parathyroid Glands*

At this stage of thyroidectomy, with full exposure now obtained, the parathyroids should be identified. Every attempt is made to preserve at least one parathyroid on each side. With experience, they are easy to find. As familiarity is gained with their appearance—split pea–sized, lima bean–shaped, molded edges, tan to mahogany brown in color, appearing as distinct organs close to the thyroid capsule—they become more readily identified. Operative trauma or bruising of the parathyroids or adjacent lymph nodes may result in some capsule hemorrhage staining the tissues so that the thyroid, parathyroid fat, and lymphatic tissues cannot be clearly differentiated.

When the superior pole is rotated downward and inward, the superior parathyroid may usually be seen at about the junction of the upper and middle thirds of the thyroid gland along its lateral posterior aspect (Fig. 17–17). The inferior parathyroids are usually found just below the junction of the inferior thyroid artery and the recurrent laryngeal nerves. Frequently, a branch of the inferior thyroid artery leads to the inferior parathyroid gland. Clamps should be inserted into the thyroid capsule anterior to the parathyroids, and the capsule and the parathyroids should be dislodged gently from the thyroid gland so that they are not excised with the resected gland.

## *Division of Isthmus*

The isthmus is freed from its attachment to the trachea in the midline from below upward by blunt dissection and divided between a series of hemostats (Fig. 17–18). Care must be exercised in separating the isthmus from the underlying pretracheal fascia to avoid puncture of the trachea by the sharp points of this straight clamp. At the upper aspect of the isthmus, the suspensory

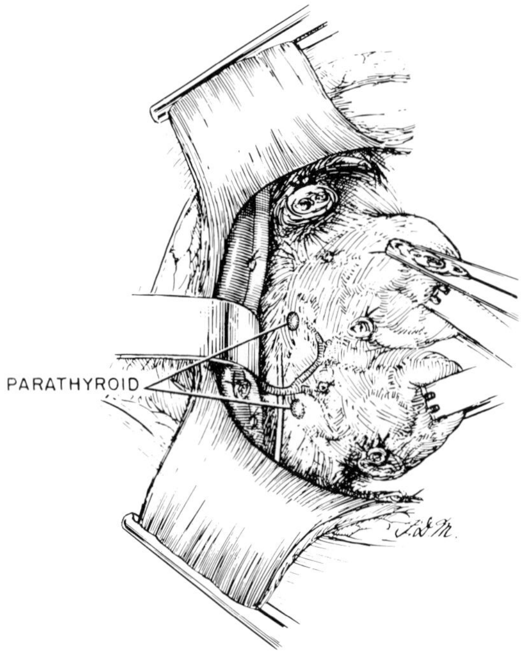


**FIGURE 17–17.** Identification of parathyroids. Superior, along the posterior capsule about the junction of the upper and middle thirds of the gland. Inferior, at the junction of the inferior thyroid artery and recurrent laryngeal nerve. (Reprinted with the permission of the Lahey Clinic.)

ligament is divided to complete mobilization of the gland.

## *Thyroidectomy*

At this moment in thyroidectomy, the amount of gland to resect or, conversely, the amount of gland to be left is determined by the pathologic condition for which thyroidectomy is being performed. In hyperthyroidism, it may depend on the severity of the thyrotoxicosis, the size of the gland, and the age of the patient. Usually about 90 per cent of the gland should be removed or 3 to 5 g left behind on each side. With a diffuse hyperplastic gland, such as that found in patients with Graves' disease, it is better to err on the side of more complete removal because surgically produced hypothyroidism is more easily controlled than recurrent hyperthyroidism. In toxic nodular goiter, the incidence of postoperative hyperthyroidism is almost zero, and the size of the remaining remnant is not so critical. In nontoxic nodular goiter, a larger remnant may be left so that the patient's postoperative thyroid requirements may be met without additional thyroid supplement, although usually suppressive therapy is given to prevent recurrence of the goiter. In chronic thyroiditis, removal of the isthmus is all that is usually necessary for relief of discomfort or pressure symptoms from the encircling arch of thyroid gland. The majority of patients with chronic thyroiditis have myxedema, which may develop regardless of the amount of gland removed. In benign tumors, less extensive subtotal lobectomy to remove the tumor completely will suffice. In malignant tumors, total thyroid lobectomy on one side may be indicated. Proficiency in judging the size of a remnant to be left comes with experience.

The line of division of the posterior thyroid capsule for subtotal thyroid lobectomy is illustrated in Figure 17–19. The recurrent laryngeal nerve and the parathyroids are again visualized to prevent injury. With the superior and inferior poles mobilized and the gland retracted medially, hemostats are applied to the lateral capsule outlining the amount of thyroid to be removed (Fig. 17–20). A row of capsular clamps is also placed medially after division of the isthmus to mark the medial posterior border. The capsule is incised above the line of hemostats. The thyroid tissue will appear to bulge out of the capsule. The incised lower edge of the capsule is pushed downward to help to preserve the parathyroids and their blood supply. A cuff of thyroid capsule and thyroid tissue is developed that will clearly establish the lateral border of the remnant and will later be sutured to the medial cuff to reconstruct the remnant.

The thyroid tissue between the lateral and medial lines of hemostats now outlines the boundaries of the thyroid to be excised. By the clamp and cut technique within the thyroid capsule, the gland is excised to free it from the remaining remnant (Fig. 17–20). All vessels and capsular hemostats are tied, and hemostasis is ensured (Fig. 17–21*A*). The remnant is reconstructed by suturing the lateral thyroid capsule to the medial capsule (Fig. 17–21*B*). When the medial capsule is not well defined, the sutures may be placed in the pretracheal fascia to buttress the cut edge of the gland against the trachea. To avoid injury to the recurrent laryngeal nerve and parathyroid glands, sutures should not

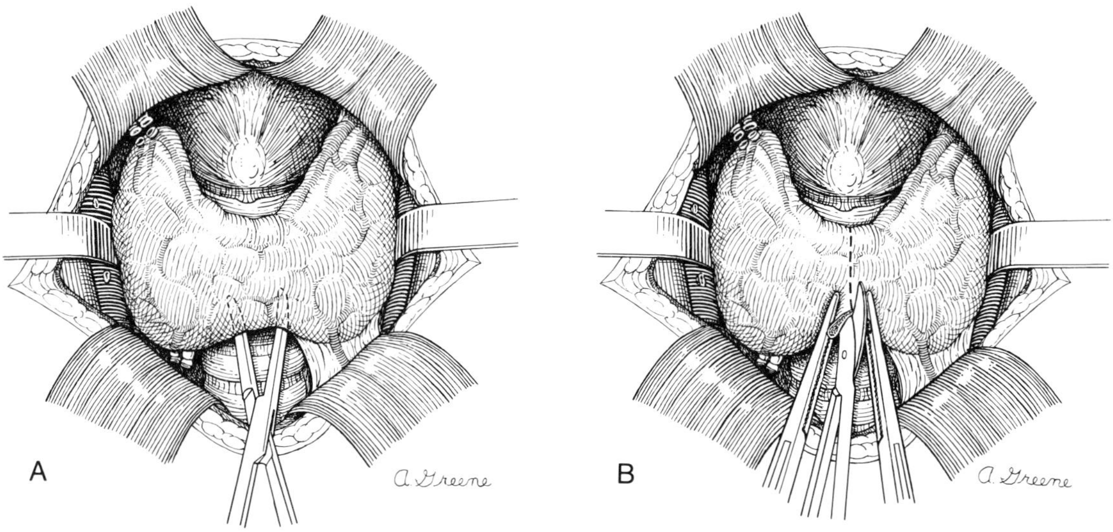


**FIGURE 17–18.** Division of the isthmus of the thyroid. *A,* Blunt dissection from trachea. *B,* Division between hemostats. (Reprinted with the permission of the Lahey Clinic.)

be placed deep in the tissue of the remnant (Fig. 17–22*A*).

Left subtotal hemithyroidectomy is performed in exactly the same manner. A pyramidal lobe, if present, is more common on the left; it may be small and consequently overlooked but should be excised. Recurrent hyperthyroidism after thyroidectomy for Graves' disease often develops secondary to thyroid tissue left either at the superior poles or as an overlooked pyramidal lobe. Although an overlooked pyramidal lobe may be small in a patient with Graves' disease, it may become hyperplastic after thyroidectomy, producing signs and symptoms of hyperplasia, and the patient will return with a sausagelike mass in the front of the neck. This can be avoided by excision of the pyramidal lobe completely up to the hyoid (Fig. 17–22*B*).

When total lobectomy is being performed, the recurrent laryngeal nerve is followed to

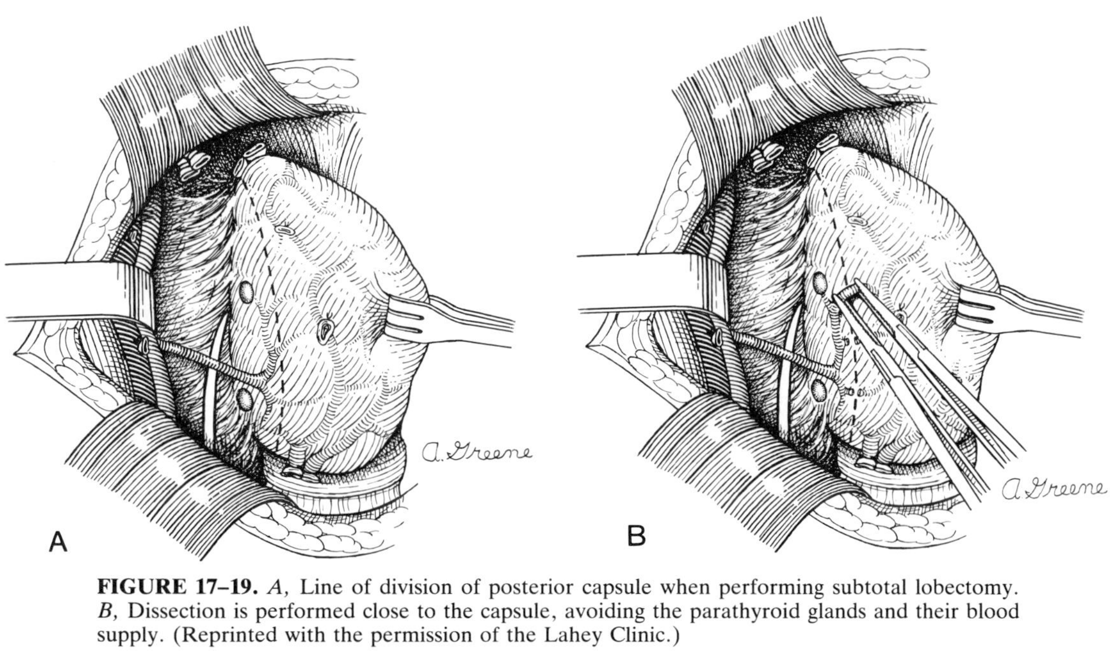


**FIGURE 17–19.** *A,* Line of division of posterior capsule when performing subtotal lobectomy. *B,* Dissection is performed close to the capsule, avoiding the parathyroid glands and their blood supply. (Reprinted with the permission of the Lahey Clinic.)

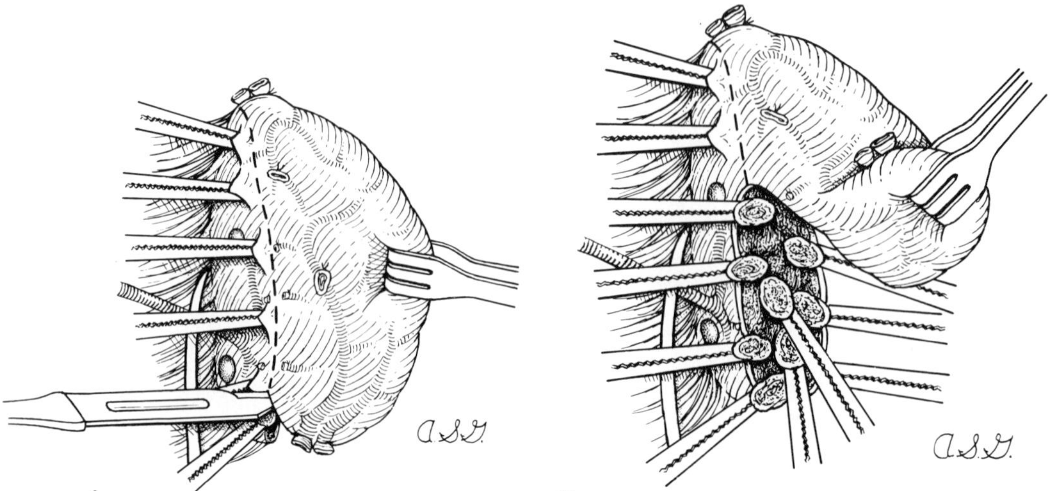


**FIGURE 17–20.** *A*, Hemostats are applied to the posterior capsule anterior to the parathyroid gland and recurrent laryngeal nerve. The capsule is incised. *B*, Intracapsular division of the thyroid gland. (Reprinted with the permission of the Lahey Clinic.)

its entrance into the larynx. The parathyroid glands are identified and preserved, and the inferior pole vessels and branches of the inferior thyroid artery are ligated individually at the level of the thyroid capsule. The superior pole vessels are also individually ligated after the superior laryngeal nerve is identified (Figs. 17–23 and 17–24).

## *Closure of Wound*

The head is slightly flexed, after removal of the rolled blanket that elevates the shoulders, to remove tension on the prethyroid muscles. The prethyroid muscles are approximated with mattress sutures (Fig. 17–22*C*). The anterior jugular veins may be ligated separately to prevent them from retracting from the mattress sutures approximating the prethyroid muscles and causing postoperative hemorrhage. We occasionally use interrupted sutures for the platysma, but this is optional. The skin edges are approximated with skin clips usually of the Michel type with protrusions for rapid removal (Fig. 17–22*D*). The excellence of the scar depends on careful approximation of the skin edges. Ordinarily, drains are not necessary. Drains of the Penrose type should not be used. When drains are required, they are of the Hemovac (Zimmer-Flynn Associates, Marshfield, Massachusetts) type and are brought out beyond the ends of the incision. Alternate clips are taken out on the second postoperative day and the remainder on the third postoperative day. Almost all patients can be discharged by the third postoperative day because diet and ambulation are almost always resumed on the first postoperative day and sometimes even late on the day of operation and because these operations are associated with little pain. Less than half of the patients require narcotics.

# THYROIDECTOMY COMBINED WITH NECK DISSECTION

The indicated surgical procedure for malignant disease of the thyroid is discussed elsewhere. The operative techniques involved are total or subtotal lobectomy on the side involved and frequently subtotal thyroidectomy on the opposite side or thyroidectomy combined with a modified or complete radical neck dissection. Total thyroidectomy is seldom necessary but is performed with few exceptions using the same technical steps described for total lobectomy. The need to define the lateral and medial borders of the remnant is eliminated. After the lateral aspects of the gland, the poles, and the isthmus

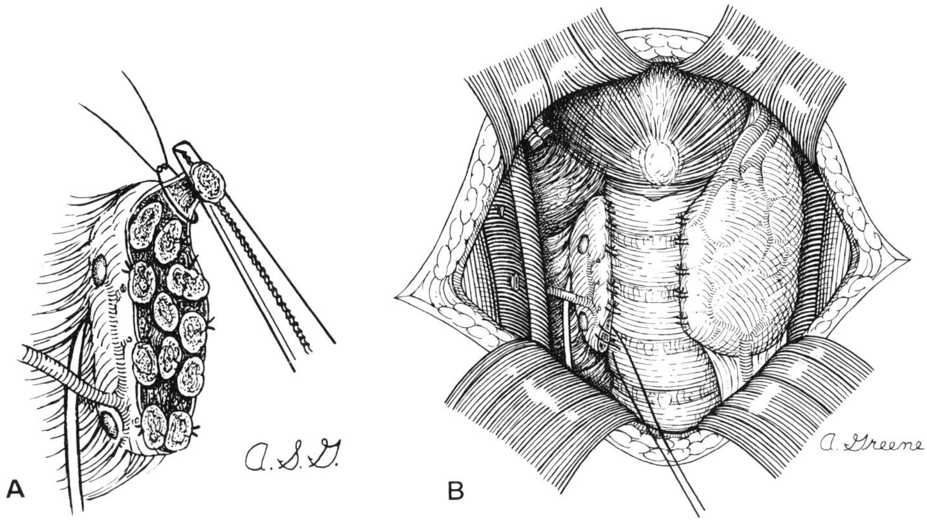


**FIGURE 17–21.** *A,* Hemostasis of transected thyroid. *B,* Reconstruction of the capsule. (Reprinted with the permission of the Lahey Clinic.)

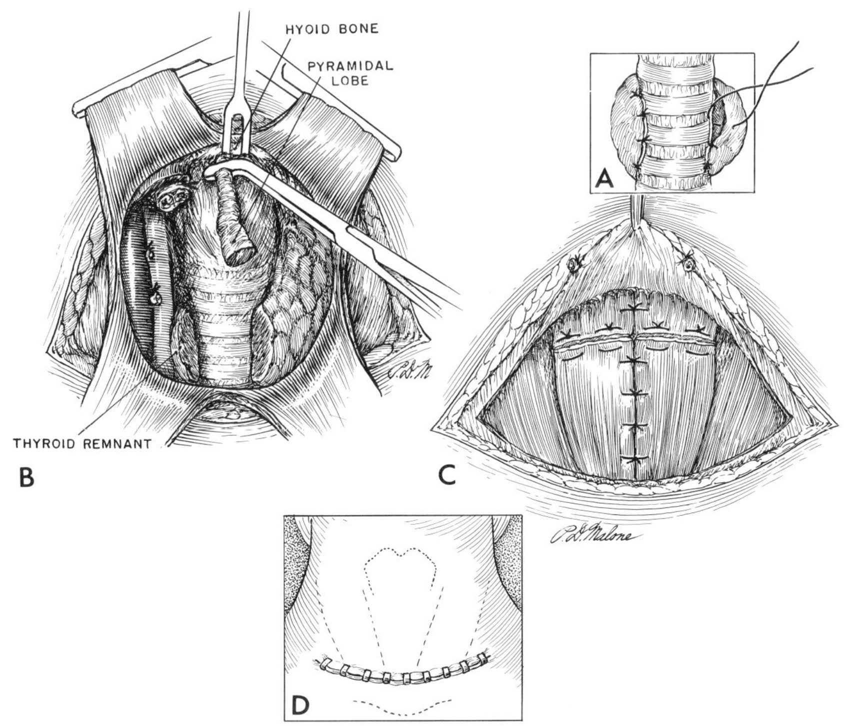


**FIGURE 17–22.** *A,* Reconstruction of thyroid remnant. The lateral thyroid capsule is sutured to the medial thyroid capsule or pretracheal fascia. *B,* Excision of pyramidal lobe. It usually arises from the left side and should be excised up to the hyoid. When not removed in hyperplastic glands, it may produce recurrent Graves' disease. *C,* Closure of muscles. *D,* Closure with skin clips.

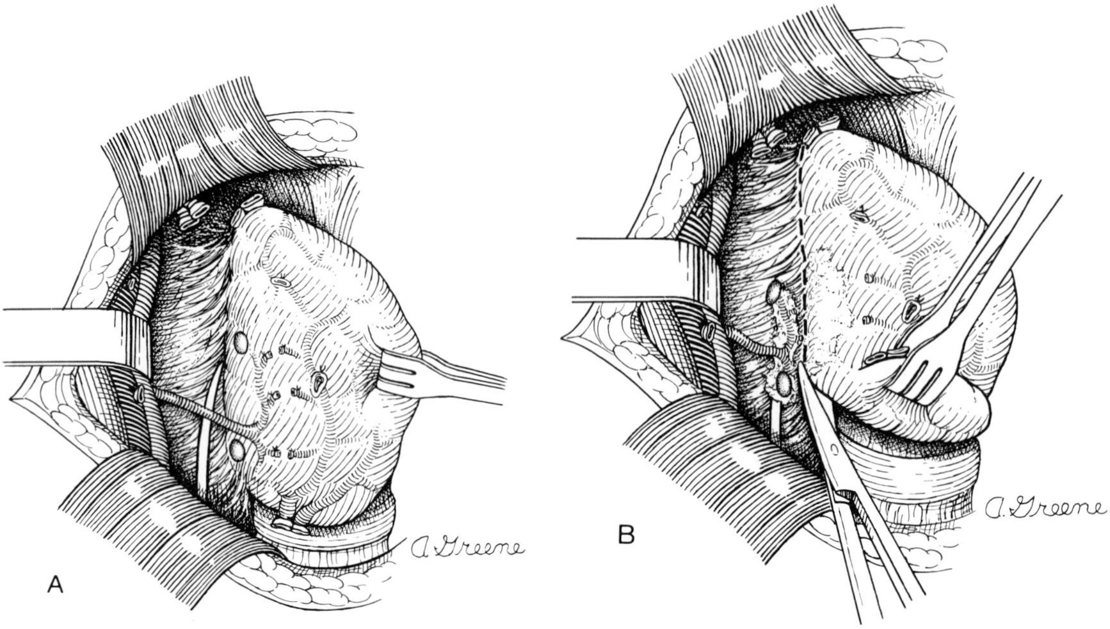


**FIGURE 17–23.** *A,* Incision of vessels at the level of the thyroid capsule with lateral displacement of the parathyroid glands. *B,* Division of attachments of the thyroid to the trachea with total extracapsular removal of the gland. (Reprinted with the permission of the Lahey Clinic.)

have been mobilized completely, the branches of the inferior thyroid artery are ligated close to the thyroid capsule, with care to preserve the parathyroid glands, and the recurrent laryngeal nerve is dissected free of all tissue to its entry into the larynx. The gland is excised completely from its bed, leaving the trachea bare of all thyroid tissue.

The diagnosis of malignant disease may be confirmed before neck dissection, preferably by needle cervical lymph node biopsy or needle thyroid biopsy, or the diagnosis may be made by frozen section at the time of thyroidectomy. The indications for and the types of neck dissection are discussed elsewhere. In most patients, particularly in a woman with a thin neck, the limb of the collar incision may be extended laterally and then upward, the skin flaps further elevated, and satisfactory exposure obtained (Fig. 17–25). In obese patients and patients with a lateral scar from previous biopsy of cervical nodes, the long incision is made to include the area of the biopsy incision if possible. Regardless of the type of incision, skin flaps must be raised to expose the superficial structures of the neck from the sternum and clavicle below, the area of the parotid and thyroid cartilage above, the entire thyroid lobe of the opposite side, and the anterior border of the trapezius behind the gland (Fig. 17–26). The sternothyroid, sternohyoid, and sternocleidomastoid muscles may be divided from their attachments to the sternum and clavicle.

The inferior thyroid veins (the thyroidea

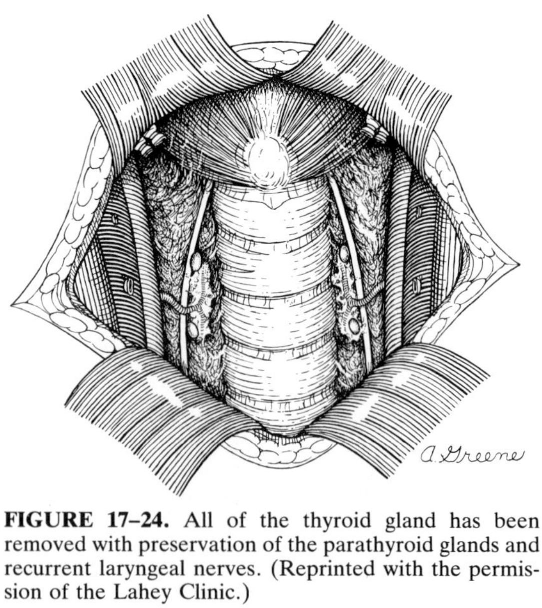


**FIGURE 17–24.** All of the thyroid gland has been removed with preservation of the parathyroid glands and recurrent laryngeal nerves. (Reprinted with the permission of the Lahey Clinic.)

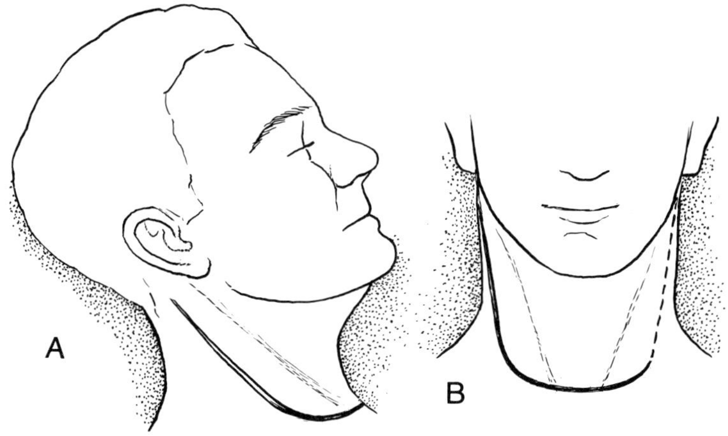


**FIGURE 17–25.** Skin incision for neck dissection that accompanies thyroidectomy for thyroid carcinoma. *A*, Lateral view. *B*, Incision possible for bilateral neck dissection.

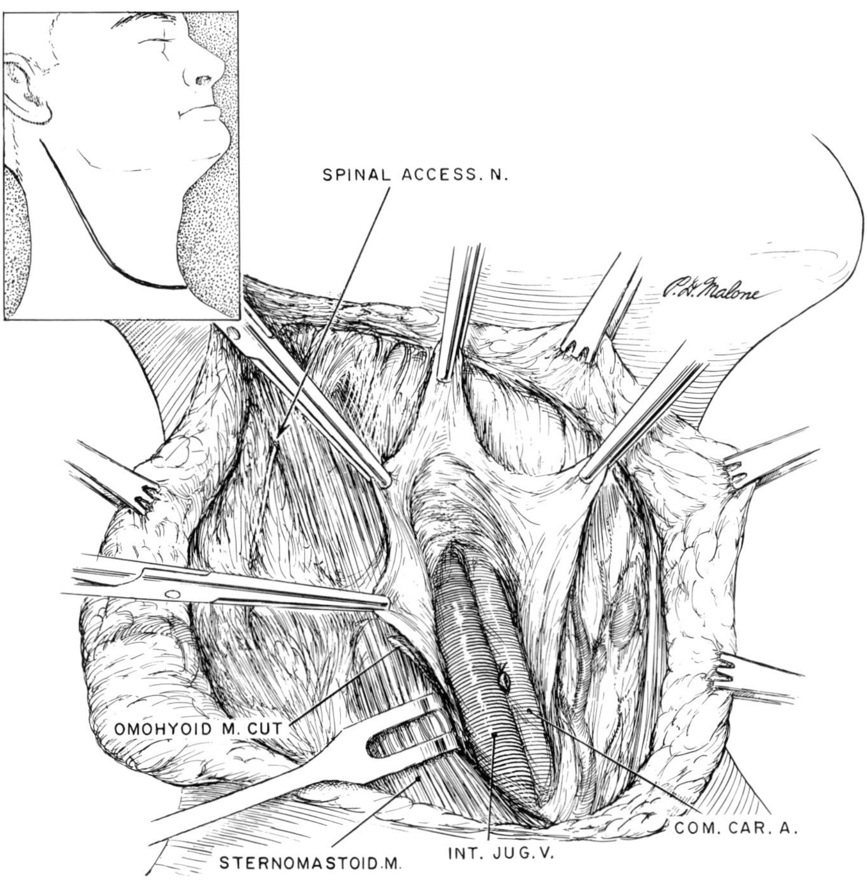


**FIGURE 17–26.** Anterior exposure for neck dissection. Wide exposure after dissection of skin flaps beneath platysma layer and vigorous retraction. Note the superficial location of the spinal accessory nerve overlying the region of the anterior border of the trapezius muscle. When this nerve is preserved in modified neck dissection, extreme caution must be exercised until the nerve is identified. The use of a nerve stimulator can be invaluable. Stripping of the lymphatic tissue about the internal jugular vein can be performed easily when preserving the vein.

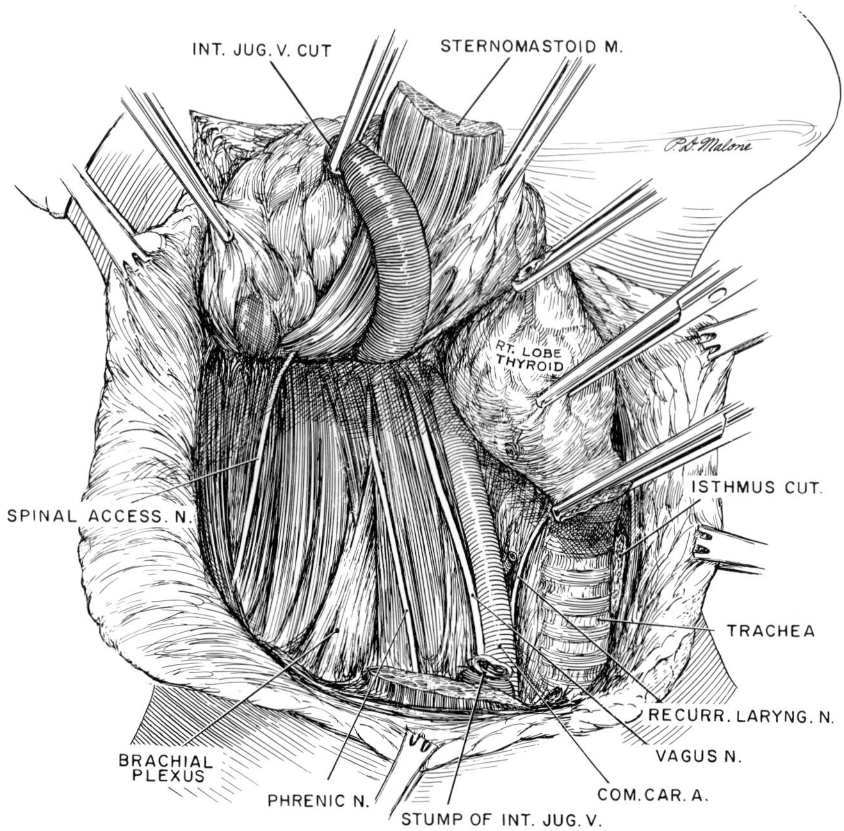


**FIGURE 17–27.** Radical neck dissection. The sternocleidomastoid muscle and internal jugular vein have been divided inferiorly and the dissection performed along the carotid sheath from below upward, exposing the underlying structures. The thyroid gland is dissected free from the trachea, sparing the recurrent laryngeal nerve. Of particular note is the course of the spinal accessory nerve, which runs through the substance of the sternocleidomastoid muscle. To preserve the nerve in modified dissections, the muscle and other tissue must be divided and cleared from around the nerve.

ima vessels when present) are divided in the midline. The internal jugular vein is isolated from its attachment to the carotid sheath. At this level, the vagus nerve is identified between the internal jugular vein and the carotid artery. The internal jugular vein is divided low in the neck, and the entire mass of lymphatics, muscles, and veins is retracted upward and dissected en bloc away from the underlying muscles and deeper structures, including the brachial plexus (Fig. 17–27). As the dissection proceeds upward in this avascular plane afforded by the carotid sheath, the phrenic and spinal accessory nerves are identified to avoid injury. The spinal accessory nerve will have to be dissected carefully out of the posterior neck contents. Medially, it runs through the substance of the sternocleidomastoid muscle, which will have to be divided over it or under it to enable the neck contents to be dissected free. When thyroid lobectomy has not been performed previously, as the dissection approaches the lower pole of the thyroid, the isthmus is freed, the inferior thyroid artery is ligated, the course of the recurrent laryngeal nerve is followed to the larynx, and the thyroid gland is excised from the trachea. The dissection is completed by excision of the insertion of the prethyroid muscles, high ligation of the internal jugular vein, and severance of the sternocleidomastoid muscle at the level of the parotid gland or mastoid process (Fig. 17–28).

The spinal accessory nerve is preserved in all instances because the major disability from neck dissection relates to shoulder dysfunction resulting from its sacrifice. No in-

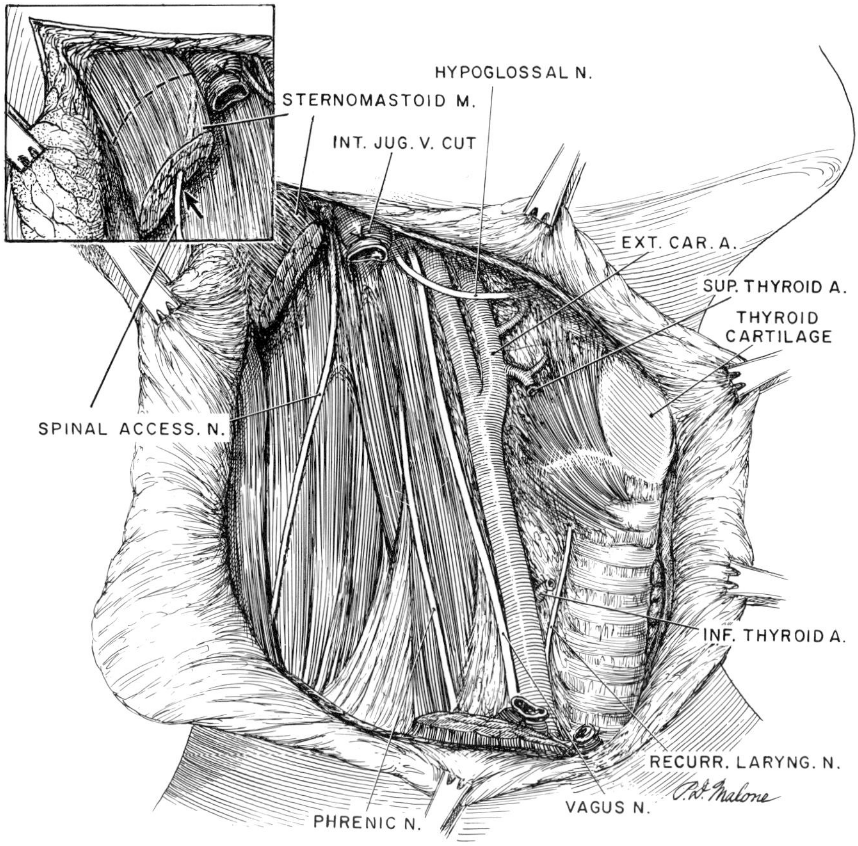


**FIGURE 17–28.** Radical neck dissection completed with preservation of the spinal accessory nerve. The internal jugular vein is ligated above and below. The vein can be preserved in modified neck dissection, as can the sternocleidomastoid muscle, when performing neck dissection for differentiated thyroid carcinoma. Note the course of the upper portion of the spinal accessory nerve through the substance of the sternocleidomastoid muscle, which has to be split over it to preserve the nerve.

creased incidence of recurrence within the neck area results from the preservation of this all-important structure. When the standard radical neck dissection is modified for patients with differentiated thyroid carcinoma, the structures preserved are, in order of descending cosmetic importance, the spinal accessory nerve, the submaxillary area, the jugular vein, and the sternocleidomastoid muscle. A more complete neck dissection should be performed for patients with medullary and undifferentiated thyroid carcinomas, however, because these patients are usually older or have a greater tendency for local recurrence. A more modest lymph node resection that preserves all these structures is acceptable in younger patients with papillary carcinoma because recurrent disease in the dissected neck is virtually unknown.

## FREEING SUBSTERNAL GOITERS

In our experience, almost all substernal goiters may be removed through the neck. On most occasions, venous hemorrhage before delivery of a substernal goiter into the neck may be serious and is more troublesome than arterial hemorrhage. The superficial and deep thyroid veins may be enlarged and dilated secondary to the tourniquet effect of the goiter pressing on the superior thoracic strait. Extreme care must be exercised to avoid tearing these veins. When serious venous bleeding occurs, the substernal goiter must be delivered rapidly from the superior mediastinum. The tourniquet effect is then

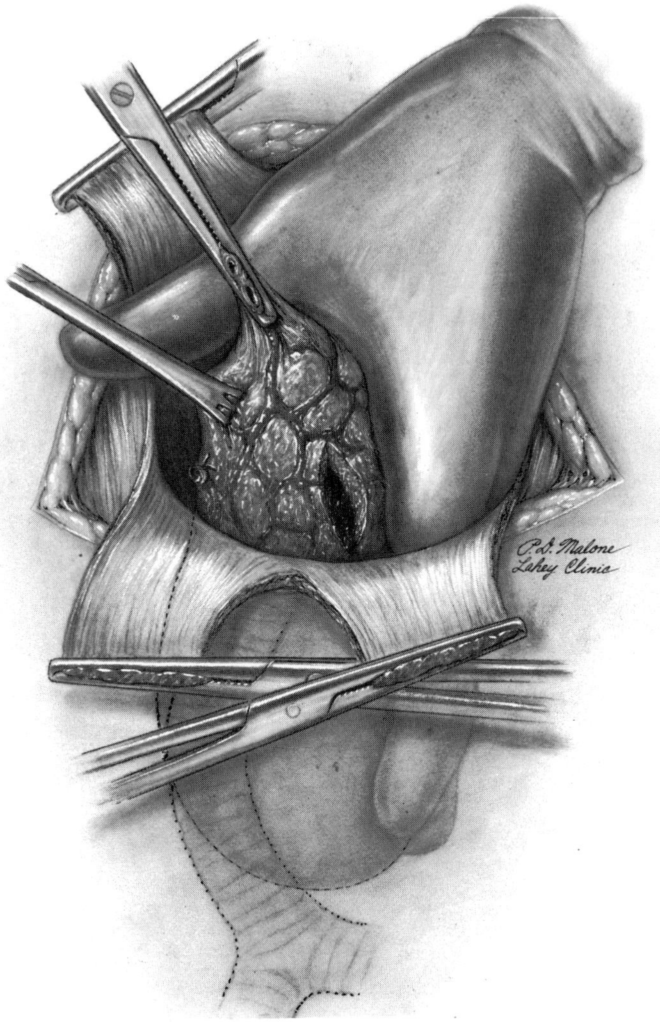


**FIGURE 17–29.** Finger dissection of substernal goiter. Note that the index finger is inserted into the mediastinum outside the thyroid capsule and is swept around until the gland is freed from the pleura and cellular tissue in the mediastinum. This may be the first step in removing intrathyroid goiter so as to release the tourniquet effect of the clavicles on the thyroid veins and to reduce hemorrhage. Occasionally, the substernal goiter cannot be made to pass out of the superior thoracic strait. In such instances, when venous hemorrhage from the tourniquet effect is encountered at the superior thoracic outlet, it may be necessary to enter the thyroid capsule and scoop out the contents, thus decreasing its diameter and reducing hemorrhage. Then, with gentle upward traction on the capsule, the gland is further separated with the index finger outside the capsule, freeing it from the pleura and surrounding structures.

released, the veins collapse, and the hemorrhage is controlled. The arterial supply to a substernal goiter arises in the neck and should be ligated, if possible, before attempting enucleation. After the inferior and superior thyroid arteries have been ligated, a cleavage plane is sought between the capsule of the thyroid and the surrounding tissue. The trachea may be compressed and pushed to one side. The best cleavage plane is usually lateral and posterior. By finger dissection, the goiter is freed from the pleura and the cellular tissue in the mediastinum and is delivered into the neck (Fig. 17–29). When the tumor is not carcinomatous and the substernal goiter cannot be freed by enucleation, the method described by Lahey may be useful (Fig. 17–29): The capsule of the goiter is opened, and its contents, which are usually seminecrotic or semicystic, are morcellated and scooped out, thus decreasing its diameter. Then, with gentle, gradual traction upward and with finger dissection outside the capsule to free it from the pleura, it may be delivered without further difficulty. Only rarely is a transsternal approach necessary for such goiters.

# Commentary

*Orlo H. Clark, M.D., and Allan E. Siperstein, M.D.*

Thyroid carcinomas represent a unique group of tumors with varying degrees of aggressiveness.[10] Most carcinomas (approximately 95 per cent) arise from the follicular cells of the thyroid gland (papillary, mixed papillary and follicular, follicular, Hürthle cell, and undifferentiated). Some carcinomas (approximately 5 per cent) arise from parafollicular C cells (medullary) and some from lymphoid tissue and stroma (lymphomas and sarcomas). Carcinomas may also metastasize to the thyroid, the most common being hypernephroma, carcinoma of the breast and lung, and melanoma.[31] Differentiated thyroid carcinomas of follicular cell origin are usually sporadic in origin, although 3 to 5 per cent are familial. The latter may be associated with Cowden's syndrome and Gardner's syndrome.[35, 56] Exposure to low-dose (600 to 2,000 cGy) therapeutic radiation, especially in childhood, dramatically increases the chance that carcinoma of the thyroid will develop.[18, 47, 64] Most papillary (70 per cent) and follicular (80 per cent) thyroid carcinomas take up radioactive iodine, and about 90 per cent make thyroglobulin.[52] Radioactive iodine scanning and thyroglobulin testing can be used to confirm the presence of residual thyroid carcinoma after thyroidectomy.

Medullary thyroid carcinoma may also be sporadic (approximately 60 per cent) or familial. The number of patients with familial disease appears to be increasing with more thorough screening of family members.[59] The familial type of medullary thyroid carcinoma occurs in association with multiple endocrine neoplasia syndrome type 2A (medullary thyroid carcinoma, pheochromocytoma, and hyperparathyroidism) or type 2B (medullary thyroid carcinoma, pheochromocytoma, marfanoid habitus, multiple neuromas, and ganglioneuromatosis). Medullary thyroid carcinoma may also be familial without other endocrinopathies (familial medullary thyroid carcinoma). Medullary thyroid carcinoma and premedullary thyroid carcinoma (C cell hyperplasia) can be detected by determining the calcitonin level in the basal state or after provocative testing with pentagastrin or calcium[24, 62] or both.[61]

At postmortem examination, the incidence of thyroid carcinoma is as high as 13 per cent in persons in Michigan and 28 per cent in persons of Japanese descent living in Hawaii.[22, 42] Most of these carcinomas are occult and are usually of follicular cell origin. Clinical thyroid carcinoma, although increasing slightly in frequency, occurs in about 40 persons per million and causes death in about six persons per million per year.[15] The natural history of patients with differentiated thyroid carcinoma of both follicular and papillary cell origin is highly variable. Fortunately, the commonest type of thyroid carcinoma is papillary (approximately 70 per cent), and most persons with papillary carcinoma do well. Factors suggesting a favorable prognosis for patients with differentiated thyroid carcinoma of follicular cell origin include young age (less than 40 years for men and 50 years for women),[6, 41] small tumor size (less than 1.5 cm),[6, 40, 41] absence of nodal invasion or distant metastatic disease,[5, 6, 27, 40, 41] female sex,[6, 40, 41] uptake of radioactive iodine,[13] well-differentiated histology,[50, 57] diploid DNA pattern,[2, 33] and response of adenylate cyclase to stimulation with thyroid-stimulating hormone.[55] Factors suggesting a favorable prognosis for patients with medullary thyroid carcinoma are similar and include young age, low tumor stage, small tumor size, and absence of nodal invasion or distant metastatic disease.[10]

Overall, about 50 per cent of patients with medullary thyroid carcinoma will die of disease within 5 years.[23] The prognosis is best for patients with familial medullary thyroid carcinoma without other manifestations of multiple endocrine neoplasia syndrome and worsens progressively for patients with multiple endocrine neoplasia syndrome type 2A, sporadic multiple endocrine neoplasia syndrome, and multiple endocrine neoplasia syndrome type 2B. Patients with a homogeneous distribution of calcitonin cells in the tumor as seen on immunohistochemical studies have a more favorable prognosis.[38, 49]

Carcinoma of the thyroid is fascinating because of the many factors associated with its natural behavior. Although most experts agree with the aforementioned comments, considerable confusion and controversy exist concerning the most effective treatment for patients with differentiated thyroid carcinoma.[9, 53] This is because most patients with carcinoma of the thyroid, especially the small (less than 1.5 cm) papillary tumors, do well regardless of treatment and because patients treated more aggressively have a higher rate of complications.

The real question, however, is, what is the best or preferred treatment for patients with thyroid carcinoma? Because no prospective studies concerning this subject have been carried out, no consensus exists. However, when it can be performed safely, total thyroidectomy is the preferred treatment for patients with differentiated thyroid carcinoma.[11] Why, then, do some experts in the field recommend lesser procedures? Most patients, especially patients younger than 40, with papillary thyroid carcinoma do well when treated by lobectomy with isthmectomy[6, 19, 60] and by near total thyroidectomy,[4] with survival rates that are similar to those for patients treated by more extensive operations. Almost all experts agree that a procedure less than lobectomy for any thyroid nodule that might be malignant is contraindicated except for small tumors (less than 1.5 cm) situated in the isthmus or on the anterior surface of the thyroid and leads to a higher complication rate when remnant tissue must be removed at a later date and a higher mortality rate.[4, 21] Most experts also agree that lobectomy with isthmectomy is the preferred treatment for patients with encapsulated or sclerosing papillary thyroid carcinoma confined to the thyroid gland that is less than 1.5 cm in size or for microinvasive follicular carcinoma. Lobectomy is also the preferred treatment for patients with thyroid carcinoma who are noncompliant and will not take thyroid hormone. Myxedema, which could be life threatening, will obviously develop in these patients when more extensive operations are performed and these patients fail to take thyroid hormone.

However, most patients with thyroid carcinoma have nodules greater than 1.5 cm in size and have at least microscopic involvement of regional ipsilateral lymph nodes.[43, 44] It would appear rational to treat these patients by total thyroidectomy when this can be accomplished safely. Total thyroidectomy is performed because with it all intrathyroidal tumor is removed, which occurs in up to 88.5 per cent of patients with papillary thyroid carcinoma.[48] It decreases the chance of recurrent disease in the central neck. It decreases the possibility of dedifferentiation from a differentiated to an undifferentiated or anaplastic carcinoma. This process has been reported to occur in about 1 per cent of patients with differentiated thyroid carcinoma.[14] It permits the use of thyroglobulin and calcitonin monitoring to detect the presence of persistent or recurrent disease. The major value of total thyroidectomy is that it also enables the use of radioactive iodine scanning to detect local or distant residual thyroid carcinoma and to ablate micrometastatic disease that is present in most patients.[39, 52]

Some surgeons[9] believe, however, that it is impossible to perform true total thyroidectomy because some thyroid tissue is almost always left in the thyroid bed. In our experience, all thyroid tissue was removed as assessed by no radioactive iodine uptake in 26 per cent of patients having total thyroidectomy, and in other patients, uptake was usually less than 1 per cent.[9] This residual uptake in most of these patients probably represents residual normal tissue in the thyroid bed, but in some patients it represents metastatic or recurrent disease. Lennquist et al.[37] recently developed a radioactive iodine probe for use during thyroidectomy to detect the presence of residual normal thyroid tissue or regional metastatic disease during operation. Dobyns[16] has previously recommended such an approach. When this method is used, more patients can have all diseased thyroid tissue removed, but a disadvantage is that patients cannot be receiving thyroid hormone because it will suppress the uptake of radioactive iodine by the thyroid tumor.

Obviously, a larger dose of radioactive iodine would be required to ablate a large thyroid remnant than would be the case for one composed of several milligrams of tissue. After all normal thyroid tissue has been removed, radioactive iodine therapy can be used to treat any remaining thyroid tumor. It is important not to use more radioactive iodine than necessary because when doses of radioactive iodine exceed 150 mCi, the incidence of leukemia[46] appears to be higher and the incidence of carcinoma in other organs that concentrate iodine (stomach and salivary glands) or eliminate radioactive iodine (bladder)[30] is possibly also higher. The dose of radioactive iodine received at different times is cumulative in its neoplastic potential.

Numerous retrospective studies, including those of Lennquist,[36] Massin,[39] Mazzaferri,[40] Samaan,[51] and Schlumberger[52] and their colleagues documented a lower recurrence rate and usually a better survival rate in patients with papillary and follicular thyroid carcinoma more than 2 cm in size who were treated by total thyroidectomy, postoperative radioactive iodine scanning, and ablative therapy when residual uptake of radioactive iodine was apparent followed by suppression therapy with thyroid-stimulating hormone.[8, 10, 40] Massin et al.[39] noted the lowest recurrence rate and best survival rate in patients treated initially by total thyroidectomy followed by radioactive iodine ablation. Lennquist[36] used a historic control and documented a marked decrease in the recurrence rate and mortality rate when patients were treated routinely by total thyroidectomy rather than by a variety of other procedures. Schlumberger et al.[52] reported that early recurrent thyroid carcinoma could be detected by monitoring serum thyroglobulin levels after total thyroidectomy. In patients with increasing serum thyroglobulin levels, regional and distant metastatic thyroid tumor was detected by scanning with radioactive iodine. In 33 patients with positive findings on scans and negative findings on radiography of the chest, complete remission (that is, no evidence of subsequent uptake of radioactive iodine and decrease in serum thyroglobulin levels to low levels) was possible in 64 per cent of patients, whereas in 186 patients with abnormal findings on radiography of the chest, only 8 per cent showed complete remission ($P < 0.001$).[52] This study clearly documented that it is easier to ablate micrometastatic disease than it is to ablate macrometastatic disease. A previous study by Wilson and Block[63] documented that radioactive iodine treatment is relatively ineffective for treating clinically evident nodal metastatic disease. These nodes should be removed surgically and the residual microscopic tumor ablated with a subsequent dose of 30 to 100 mCi of radioactive iodine.[10]

It is well known that more than 80 per cent of patients with papillary thyroid carcinoma have extrathyroidal disease at the time of initial treatment, and although in most patients this tumor does not grow or become clinically apparent, in some (approximately 15 to 20 per cent), it will eventually cause death.[4, 29, 43, 44, 54]

Studies documenting the benefits of total thyroidectomy and radioactive iodine ablation probably underestimate the benefits of this treatment because in many reported series[3, 40, 51] only patients with more aggressive tumors were treated in this fashion. Despite this fact, patients who receive this treatment do better in terms of having a lower recurrence rate and a better survival rate.

Why is treatment controversial? The controversy is based primarily on the higher complication rate in patients treated by more extensive thyroid operations. Foster[20] noted a higher complication rate associated with total thyroidectomy, and he suggested that the benefits of total thyroidectomy do not warrant the increased risks. Certainly, lobectomy is a safer operation than total thyroidectomy because only two parathyroid glands and one recurrent laryngeal nerve are at risk. Even when both parathyroid glands are removed or devascularized, parathyroid glands are almost always present on the contralateral side so that permanent hypoparathyroidism virtually never develops. Buckwalter and Thomas[4] advocated near total thyroidectomy, with all thyroid tissue removed on the side of the clinically evident tumor and a 2 to 3 g remnant left on the contralateral side to protect the parathyroid glands and recurrent laryngeal nerve. In some patients whose parathyroid glands are situated anteriorly, this procedure may be the treatment of choice because the risk of devascularizing the parathyroid glands is high when they are dissected off the thyroid gland on a long vascular pedicle. When a parathyroid gland does not have an adequate vascular supply after it is dissected from the thyroid gland, it should be removed. A biopsy is performed to confirm that it is a parathyroid gland, and the gland is autotransplanted into the contralateral sternocleidomastoid muscle. When the parathyroid glands are situated laterally to the thyroid gland, we see no advantage of near total thyroidectomy over total thyroidectomy, and the disadvantage of this procedure is that the remnant must be ablated with radioactive iodine before it can be scanned for residual tumor. When the recurrent laryngeal nerve or parathyroid glands are at risk, a small remnant of thyroid tissue should be left. When the recurrent laryngeal nerve is surrounded by tumor and the vocal cords are functioning normally, the tumor is dissected from the recurrent laryngeal nerve. Thyroid carcinoma does not behave like squamous cell carcinoma, and en bloc central neck dissection should be avoided because it will result in an unacceptable complication rate of 20 per cent or higher.[14]

The complication rate associated with total thyroidectomy as reported by Attie,[1] Clark,[9, 11] Harness,[25] Jacobs,[32] Karlan,[34] Lennquist,[36] and Perzik[45] and their colleagues is less than 2 per cent and is lower than the reported complication rate in many series[19, 20, 60] after less aggressive procedures. The low complication rate of hypothyroidism or recurrent laryngeal nerve injury that was reported in these studies usually occurred in patients with extensive bilateral carcinoma or highly invasive carcinoma with extensive nodal metastatic disease.[25] Our complication rate in 160 consecutive patients treated by total thyroidectomy is listed in Table 17–1. Only one of the permanent complications could have been avoided by a lesser procedure.[11] Other complications included seroma, bleeding, infection, injury to the external laryngeal nerve resulting in a performer's inability to sing high notes, and keloid formation. The incidence of these complications is no higher than in patients treated with lesser procedures than total thyroidectomy. Many surgeons who advocate total thyroidectomy are teaching senior or chief surgical residents how to perform these operations in university medical centers. The point is that total thyroidectomy is usually not a difficult procedure to perform, but physicians must train with a surgeon experienced in thyroid surgery to learn when and how to perform total thyroidectomy.

**TABLE 17–1. Complications of Total Thyroidectomy in 160 Consecutive Patients**

| COMPLICATION | NUMBER | PER CENT |
|---|---|---|
| Recurrent laryngeal nerve injury | | |
| Unintentional | | |
| Unilateral transient | 2 | 1.2 |
| Bilateral transient | 2 | 1.2 |
| Intentional | | |
| Unilateral permanent | 3 | 1.9 |
| Hypoparathyroidism* | 1 | 0.6 |
| Wound infection | 2 | 1.2 |

*Only one permanent complication could have been prevented by a lesser procedure.

## LYMPH NODE DISSECTION

Ipsilateral regional nodes contain metastatic papillary and medullary thyroid carcinoma in more than 50 per cent of patients.[10, 43, 44] About 80 to 90 per cent of patients less than 20 years of age with differentiated thyroid carcinoma have clinically palpable nodal metastatic disease whereas only 10 to 20 per cent of older patients have clinically palpable lymphadenopathy.[26, 27] Formerly, when prophylactic lymph node dissections were performed, metastatic disease was found in up to 80 per cent of patients even when disease was not clinically evident.[43, 44] Prophylactic node dissection is no longer advised because, despite the presence of micrometastatic disease in 80 per cent of patients, clinical evidence of involvement of these nodes only develops in 7 to 8 per cent of patients.[10, 27] It appears that the immune defense system in most patients can prevent the growth of these tumors for many years or for a lifetime.

Also controversial is the extent of nodal dissection required when nodes are clinically involved. Most surgeons experienced in endocrine surgery advise meticulous nodal dissection in the tracheoesophageal groove in the central neck on the side of the tumor. When bilateral thyroid carcinoma is present, bilateral central neck dissection is essential. This is especially true for patients with medullary thyroid carcinoma. The best and possibly only time to perform thorough dissection of this area is at the initial operation.[58] In patients with medullary thyroid carcinoma but not in patients with papillary thyroid carcinoma, the thymus is usually removed bilaterally through the cervical incision, all fibrofatty and lymphatic tissue is cleared out from the innominate vein inferiorly to the thyroid cartilage superiorly. This procedure obviously puts the parathyroid glands at increased risk because of devascularization and must be performed carefully. It is essential, however, for successful results in patients with medullary thyroid carcinoma.

For patients with papillary thyroid carcinoma with clinically palpable ipsilateral regional lymph nodes, we perform modified radical neck dissection. The rationale for a modified radical neck dissection rather than lumpectomy or "berry picking" is based on the excellent studies of Noguchi et al.,[43, 44] who documented that metastatic carcinoma to a lymph node of 3 mm or greater is always associated with papillary carcinoma in the smaller lymphatics. A modified neck dissection preserving the spinal accessory nerve, sternocleidomastoid muscle, and jugular vein (unless these structures are directly invaded or adherent to the tumor) is used for patients with papillary, follicular, and medullary thyroid carcinoma rather than a classic radical neck dissection because the surgical results are the same and the cosmetic results distinctly preferable.[63] A modified radical neck procedure is performed by extending the transverse Kocher incision laterally and dissecting to the level just below the mandible in a subplatysmal plane.[10] In most patients, a suprahyoid dissection is unnecessary unless the highest nodes, usually in the jugular chain, are involved in this area. Most patients with follicular thyroid carcinoma do not have regional node involvement, although nodal involvement in children with follicular thyroid carcinoma is common. Follicular carcinoma is unusual in children, but when it occurs, it usually behaves like papillary thyroid carcinoma.[12, 17, 27] Although studies[5, 7] suggest that the presence of lymph node metastasis does not influence survival, our studies[27] suggest a higher mortality rate in patients with clinically involved lymph nodes when patients are compared by age. Other studies[5, 40, 57] also suggest that node involvement is detrimental, especially when the nodes are matted together. When nodes are involved, however, the increased risk of dying of thyroid carcinoma is a minor rather than major factor and usually correlates with other prognostic factors except age.[5]

Patients with medullary thyroid carcinoma more than 2 cm in size or when regional cervical nodes in the central neck involved should have ipsilateral prophylactic node dissection. A therapeutic node dissection should almost always be carried out at the time of thyroidectomy for patients with medullary thyroid carcinoma. When no nodes are clinically palpable and the central nodes are free of tumor, ipsilateral neck dissection may be postponed. Serum calcitonin levels, both basally and after provocative tests (pentagastrin or calcium), should be reevaluated several weeks after total thyroidectomy in these patients. When the calcitonin level remains elevated, lateral neck dissection should be performed through the previous Kocher incision that is extended laterally. Occasionally, a parallel incision higher in the neck may be necessary for good exposure.[10]

Contralateral node involvement occurs in about 10 per cent of patients with unilateral thyroid carcinoma of follicular or parafollicular cell origin. The nodes most frequently involved are immediately adjacent to the lower pole of the thyroid gland.

## CONCLUSIONS

Although 80 per cent of patients do well with lesser procedures than total thyroidectomy for papillary and follicular thyroid carcinoma and about 5 per cent of patients die regardless of the extent of surgery, about 15 per cent of patients appear to benefit from total thyroidectomy because they have a lower recurrence rate and higher survival rate.[11] Hay et al.[28] noted improved survival in patients in the high-risk group treated by more aggressive operations, although the extent of thyroid resection in patients in the low-risk group made no difference in survival. It seems unfair, therefore, not to treat patients with thyroid carcinoma more than 1.5 cm in size by total thyroidectomy because this operation is associated with the lowest mortality rate. The complication rate associated with total thyroidectomy in patients with thyroid carcinoma can be minimal when these patients are treated by surgeons educated and trained in this technique. In the future, we may be able to treat patients selectively with more or less aggressive operations on the basis of DNA analysis or adenylate cyclase response to thyroid-stimulating hormone, but more studies are necessary before we accept this approach. A prospective study evaluating the effectiveness of the various forms of treatment for patients with thyroid carcinoma is recommended.

## REFERENCES


1. Attie, J. N., Moskowitz, G. S., Margouleff, D., and Levy, L. M.: Feasibility of total thyroidectomy in the treatment of thyroid carcinoma: Postoperative radioactive iodine evaluation of 140 cases. Am. J. Surg., *138:*555–560, 1979.
2. Bäckdahl, M., Auer, G., Forsslund, G., et al.: Prognostic value of nuclear DNA content in follicular thyroid tumors. Acta Chir. Scand., *152:*1–7, 1986.
3. Beierwaltes, W. H.: The treatment of thyroid carcinoma with radioactive iodine. Semin. Nucl. Med., *8:*79–94, 1978.
4. Buckwalter, J. A., and Thomas, C. G., Jr.: Selection of surgical treatment for well differentiated thyroid carcinomas. Ann. Surg., *176:*565–578, 1972.
5. Byar, D. P., Green, S. B., Dor, P., et al.: A prognostic index for thyroid carcinoma: A study of the E.O.R.T.C. Thyroid Cancer Cooperative Group. Eur. J. Cancer, *15:*1033–1041, 1979.
6. Cady, B., Rossi, R., Silverman, M., and Wool, M.: Further evidence of the validity of risk group definition in differentiated thyroid carcinoma. Surgery, *98:*1171–1178, 1985.
7. Cady, B., Sedgwick, C. E., Meissner, W. A., et al.: Changing clinical, pathologic, therapeutic, and survival patterns in differentiated thyroid carcinoma. Ann. Surg., *184:*541–553, 1976.
8. Clark, O. H.: TSH suppression in the management of thyroid nodules and thyroid cancer. World J. Surg., *5:*39–47, 1981.
9. Clark, O. H.: Total thyroidectomy: The treatment of choice for patients with differentiated thyroid cancer. Ann. Surg., *196:*361–370, 1982.
10. Clark, O. H. (ed.): Endocrine Surgery of the Thyroid and Parathyroid Glands. St. Louis, C. V. Mosby Co., 1985.
11. Clark, O. H., Levin, K., Zeng, O. H., et al.: Thyroid cancer: The case for total thyroidectomy. Eur. J. Cancer Clin. Oncol., *24:*305–313, 1988.
12. Crile, G., Jr., and Hazard, J. B.: Relationship of age of patient to natural history and prognosis of carcinoma of thyroid. Ann. Surg., *138:*33–38, 1953.
13. Crile, G., Jr., Antunez, A. R., Esselstyn, C. B., Jr., et al.: The advantages of subtotal thyroidectomy and suppression of TSH in the primary treatment of papillary carcinoma of the thyroid. Cancer, *55:*2691–2697, 1985.
14. Cohn, K., Bäckdahl, M., Forsslund, G., et al.: Prognostic value of DNA content in papillary thyroid carcinoma. World J. Surg., *8:*474–480, 1984.
15. Cutler, S. J., and Young, J. L. (eds.): Third National Cancer Survey Incidence Data. National Cancer Institute, Monograph No. 41. Washington, D.C., U.S. Department of Health, Education and Welfare, 1975.
16. Dobyns, B. M.: Extended total thyroidectomy with modified radical lymph node dissection for cancer. *In* Nyhus, L. M., and Baker, R. J. (eds.): Mastery of Surgery. Boston, Little, Brown & Co., 1984, p. 187.
17. Donohue, J. H., Goldfine, S. D., Miller, T. R., et al.: Do the prognoses of papillary and follicular thyroid carcinomas differ? Am. J. Surg., *148:*168–173, 1984.
18. Duffy, B. J., Jr., and Fitzgerald, P. J.: Thyroid cancer in childhood and adolescence: Report on 28 cases. J. Clin. Endocrinol. Metab., *10:*1296–1308, 1950.
19. Farrar, W. B., Cooperman, M., and James, A. G.: Surgical management of papillary and follicular carcinoma of the thyroid. Ann. Surg., *192:*701–704, 1980.
20. Foster, R. S., Jr.: Morbidity and mortality after thyroidectomy. Surg. Gynecol. Obstet., *146:*423–429, 1978.
21. France, C. J., Kouchy, C., Hergt, K., and Brines, O. A.: Relationship of histology to prognosis in thyroid carcinoma. Arch. Surg., *86:*588–592, 1963.
22. Fukunaga, F. H., and Yatani, R.: Geographic pathology of occult thyroid carcinomas. Cancer, *36:*1095–1099, 1975.
23. Gordon, P. R., Huvos, A. G., and Strong, E. W.: Medullary carcinoma of the thyroid gland: A clinicopathologic study of 40 cases. Cancer, *31:*915–924, 1973.
24. Greenspan, F. S.: Tumor markers in thyroid cancer. *In* Clark, O. H., and Roeher, H. D. (eds.): Thyroid Tumors. New York, S. Karger, 1988, pp. 54–77.
25. Harness, J. K., Fung, L., Thompson, N. W., et al.: Total thyroidectomy: Complications and technique. World J. Surg., *10:*781–786, 1986.
26. Harness, J. K., Thompson, N. W., and Nishiyama, R. H.: Childhood thyroid carcinoma. Arch. Surg., *102:*276–284, 1971.
27. Harwood, J., Clark, O. H., and Dunphy, J. E.: Significance of lymph node metastasis in differentiated thyroid cancer. Am. J. Surg., *136:*107–112, 1978.
28. Hay, I. D., Grant, C. S., Taylor, W. F., and McConahey, W. M.: Ipsilateral lobectomy versus bilateral lobar resection in papillary thyroid carcinoma: A retrospective analysis of surgical outcome using a novel prognostic scoring system. Surgery, *102:*1088–1095, 1987.
29. Hirabayashi, R. N., and Lindsay, S.: Carcinoma of the thyroid gland: A statistical study of 390 patients. J. Clin. Endocrinol. Metab., *21:*1596–1610, 1961.
30. Hoffman, D. A., McConahey, W. M., Fraumeni, J. F., Jr., and Kurland, L. T.: Cancer incidence

following treatment of hyperthyroidism. Int. J. Epidemiol., *11*:218–224, 1982.
31. Ivy, H. K.: Cancer metastatic to the thyroid: A diagnostic problem. Mayo Clin. Proc., *59*:856–859, 1984.
32. Jacobs, J. K., Aland, J. W., Jr., and Ballinger, J. F.: Total thyroidectomy: A review of 213 patients. Ann. Surg., *197*:542–549, 1983.
33. Joensuu, H., Klemi, P., Eerola, E., and Tuominen, J.: Influence of cellular DNA content on survival in differentiated thyroid cancer. Cancer, *58*:2462–2467, 1986.
34. Karlan, M. S., Catz, B., Dunkelman, D., et al.: A safe technique for thyroidectomy with complete nerve dissection and parathyroid preservation. Head Neck Surg., *6*:1014–1019, 1984.
35. Lee, F. I., and MacKinnon, M. D.: Papillary thyroid carcinoma associated with polyposis coli: A case of Gardner's syndrome. Am. J. Gastroenterol., *76*:128–140, 1981.
36. Lennquist, S.: Surgical strategy in thyroid carcinoma: A clinical review. Acta Chir. Scand., *152*:321–338, 1986.
37. Lennquist, S., Persliden, J., and Smeds, S.: Intraoperative scintigraphy in surgical treatment of thyroid carcinoma: Evaluation of a new technique. World J. Surg., *10*:711–717, 1986.
38. Lippman, S. M., Mendelsohn, G., Trump, D. L., et al.: The prognostic and biological significance of cellular heterogeneity in medullary thyroid carcinoma: A study of calcitonin, L-dopa, dicarboxylase and histaminase. J. Clin. Endocrinol. Metab., *54*:233–240, 1982.
39. Massin, J. P., Savoie, J. C., Garnier, H., et al.: Pulmonary metastasis in differentiated thyroid carcinoma: Study of 58 cases with implications for the primary tumor treatment. Cancer, *53*:982–992, 1984.
40. Mazzaferri, E. L., and Young, R. L.: Papillary thyroid carcinoma: A 10 year follow-up report of the impact of therapy in 576 patients. Am. J. Med., *70*:511–518, 1981.
41. McConahey, W. M., Hay, I. D., Woolner, L. B., et al.: Papillary thyroid cancer treated at the Mayo Clinic, 1946 through 1970: Initial manifestations, pathologic findings, therapy, and outcome. Mayo Clin. Proc., *61*:978–996, 1986.
42. Nishiyama, R. H., Ludwig, G. K., and Thompson, N. W.: The prevalence of small papillary thyroid carcinomas in 100 consecutive necropsies in an American population. *In* DeGroot, L. J. (ed.): Radiation-Associated Thyroid Carcinoma. New York, Grune & Stratton, 1976, pp. 123–135.
43. Noguchi, S., and Murakami, N.: The value of lymph-node dissection in patients with differentiated thyroid cancer. Surg. Clin. North Am., *67*:251–261, 1987.
44. Noguchi, S., Noguchi, A., and Murakami, N.: Papillary carcinoma of the thyroid: Value of prophylactic lymph node excision. Cancer, *26*:1061–1064, 1970.
45. Perzik, S.: The place of total thyroidectomy in the management of 909 patients with thyroid disease. Am. J. Surg., *132*:480–483, 1976.
46. Pochin, E. E., Myant, N. B., and Corbett, B. D.: Leukaemia following radioiodine treatment of hyperthyroidism. Br. J. Radiol., *29*:31–35, 1956.
47. Rosen, I. B., Simpson, J. A., Sutcliffe, S., and Gorenstein, L.: High-dose radiation and the emergence of thyroid nodular disease. Surgery, *96*:988–995.
48. Russell, W. O., Ibanez, M. L., Clark, R. L., and White, E. C.: Thyroid carcinoma: Classification, intraglandular dissemination, and clinicopathological study based upon whole organ sections of 80 glands. Cancer, *11*:1425–1460, 1963.
49. Saad, M. F., Ordonez, N. G., Guido, J. J., and Samaan, N. A.: The prognostic value of calcitonin immunostaining in medullary carcinoma of the thyroid. J. Clin. Endocrinol. Metab., *59*:850–856, 1984.
50. Sakamoto, A., Kasai, N., and Sugano, H.: Poorly differentiated carcinoma of the thyroid: A clinicopathologic entity for a high-risk group of papillary and follicular carcinomas. Cancer, *52*:1849–1855, 1983.
51. Samaan, N. A., Maheshwari, Y. K., Nader, S., et al.: Impact of therapy for differentiated carcinoma of the thyroid: An analysis of 706 cases. J. Clin. Endocrinol. Metab., *56*:1131–1138, 1983.
52. Schlumberger, M., Tubiana, M., De Vathaire, F., et al.: Long-term results of treatment of 283 patients with lung and bone metastases from differentiated thyroid carcinoma. J. Clin. Endocrinol. Metab., *63*:960–967, 1986.
53. Schroder, D. M., Chambors, A., and France, C. J.: Operative strategy for thyroid cancer. Is total thyroidectomy worth the price? Cancer, *58*:2320–2328, 1986.
54. Silliphant, W. M., Klinck, G. H., and Levitin, M. S.: Thyroid carcinoma and death: A clinicopathological study of 193 autopsies. Cancer, *17*:513–525, 1964.
55. Siperstein, A. E., Zeng, Q. H., Gum, E. T., et al.: Adenylate cyclase activity as a predictor of thyroid tumor aggressiveness. World J. Surg., *12*:528–533, 1988.
56. Sogol, P. B., Sugawara, M., Gordon, H. E., et al.: Cowden's disease: Familial goiter and skin hamartomas. A report of three cases. West. J. Med., *139*:324–328, 1983.
57. Tennvall, J., Biörklund, A., Möller, T., et al.: Is the EORTC prognostic index of thyroid cancer valid in differentiated thyroid carcinoma? Retrospective multivariate analysis of differentiated thyroid carcinoma with long follow-up. Cancer, *57*:1405–1414, 1986.
58. Tissell, L. E., Hansson, G., Jansson, S., and Salander, H.: Reoperation in the treatment of asymptomatic metastasizing medullary thyroid carcinoma. Surgery, *99*:60–66, 1986.
59. Wahl, R. A., and Roeher, H. D.: Surgery of C cell carcinoma of the thyroid. *In* Clark, O. H., and Roeher, H. D. (eds.): Thyroid Tumors. New York, S. Karger, 1988, pp. 100–112.
60. Wanebo, H. J., Andrews, W., and Kaiser, D. L.: Thyroid cancer: Some basic considerations. Am. J. Surg., *142*:474–479, 1981.

61. Wells, S. A., Jr., Baylin, S. B., Linehan, W. M., et al.: Provocative agents and the diagnosis of medullary carcinoma of the thyroid gland. Ann. Surg., *188:*139–141, 1978.
62. Wells, S. A., Jr., Cooper, C. W., and Ontjes, D. A.: Stimulation of thyrocalcitonin secretion by ethanol in patients with medullary thyroid carcinomas: An effect apparently not mediated by gastrin. Metabolism, *24:*1215–1219, 1975.
63. Wilson, S. M., and Block, G. E.: Carcinoma of the thyroid metastatic to lymph nodes of the neck. Arch. Surg., *102:*285–291, 1971.
64. Witt, T. R., Meng, R. L., Economou, S. G., and Southwick, H. W.: The approach to the irradiated thyroid. Surg. Clin. North Am., *59:*45–63, 1979.

# 18

# SURGICAL TREATMENT OF INTRATHORACIC GOITER

*David M. Shahian, M.D.*

Cervical goiters may extend into the thorax in 0.2 to 21 per cent[4, 6, 7, 14, 19, 21, 24, 26, 29, 30, 38, 42] of patients, although less than 1 per cent[10] of goiters are totally contained within the thoracic cavity. Intrathoracic goiters account for 2.6 to 6.9 per cent of all mediastinal tumors.[16, 27, 44]

The anatomic factors responsible for intrathoracic extension of a goiter have been described by Lahey and Swinton.[22–24] The thyroid is bounded superiorly by the hyoid and thyroid cartilages, posteriorly by the trachea and prevertebral fascia, and anteriorly by the sternocleidomastoid, omohyoid, sternohyoid, and sternothyroid muscles. With progressive enlargement of the gland, the path of least resistance is inferiorly into the thorax. The weight of the goiter and normal swallowing and respiratory motions with negative intrathoracic pressure contribute to mediastinal displacement.

In some patients, the connection to the cervical gland may become attenuated and be apparent only as a fatty or fibrous band or vascular pedicle. Such goiters, which are usually described as heterotopic or ectopic, are a source of continuing controversy. Lahey[23] stated that he had encountered none in more than 24,000 thyroidectomies, and Sweet[40] believed that a connection, albeit small, could always be found between the mediastinal thyroid and the cervical gland. Nonetheless, other surgeons[9, 11, 25, 31, 36, 37] have reported isolated mediastinal goiters with no obvious connection to the cervical gland. Whether such apparently disconnected goiters arise from isolated embryologic anlagen[5] or result from progressive attenuation of their cervical connections,[10] little doubt exists that they do occur. The designation isolated mediastinal goiter may be preferable to ectopic or heterotopic, either of which implies an etiologic mechanism that cannot be proved. The incidence of isolated mediastinal goiter in patients undergoing thyroidectomy is estimated to be 0.2 to 0.25 per cent.[9, 37]

## LOCATION

From 75 to 94 per cent of intrathoracic thyroid tumors are found in the anterior substernal compartment.[6, 8, 13, 14, 35, 39] Such substernal goiters are anterior to the recurrent laryngeal nerve and to the subclavian and innominate vessels. Posterior mediastinal goiters, which constitute 10 to 25 per cent of intrathoracic thyroid tissue, are thought by

Sweet[40] to arise from the posterolateral portion of the thyroid lobe rather than from the inferolateral aspect. Such posterior intrathoracic goiters descend behind the innominate vein, carotid sheath, innominate and subclavian arteries, recurrent laryngeal nerve, and inferior thyroid artery. They ultimately occupy a space bounded posteriorly by the vertebral column, laterally by the first rib, medially by the trachea and esophagus, and anteriorly by the carotid sheath and subclavian and innominate vessels.[40]

Posterior mediastinal goiters may occur in the hemithorax ipsilateral to the thyroid lobe of origin or even in the opposite hemithorax. Ipsilateral posterior mediastinal goiters are commonly found on the right side, presumably because the aortic arch obstructs descent of the goiter on the left side. Less commonly, a goiter may descend between the trachea and esophagus into the contralateral posterosuperior mediastinum.[6, 14, 28, 38] The rarest presentation is retroesophageal descent of a goiter into the contralateral posterosuperior mediastinum.[3, 6, 17, 43]

Isolated mediastinal goiters, without demonstrable connection to the cervical gland, occur most frequently in an anterior substernal location, although several such goiters have been described in the right posterior mediastinum.[11, 37]

A proposed anatomic classification of mediastinal goiters is presented in Table 18–1.

**TABLE 18–1. Classification of Mediastinal Goiter***

| TYPE | SUBTYPE | DESCRIPTION |
|---|---|---|
| I | | Anterior |
| | A | Isolated anterior mediastinal thyroid |
| | B | Substernal extension |
| II | | Posterior |
| | A | Isolated posterior mediastinal thyroid |
| | B | Ipsilateral posterior mediastinal extension |
| | C | Contralateral posterior mediastinal extension |
| | 1 | Retrotracheal |
| | 2 | Retroesophageal |

*All types except $IIC_{1,2}$ result in tracheal displacement away from the side of the mass seen on the chest radiograph. Types $IIC_{1,2}$ result in displacement of the trachea toward the side of the mass seen on the chest radiograph.

## CLINICAL PRESENTATION AND DIAGNOSIS

Although some patients with intrathoracic goiter may present with an asymptomatic mass seen on roentgenography of the chest, commonly they will complain of obstructive symptoms, including dyspnea, neck swelling, cough, dysphagia, stridor, pain, choking, hoarseness, or acute respiratory distress. Manifestations of superior vena cava syndrome may be present. Intrathoracic goiter must be considered in the differential diagnosis of any patient with an anterosuperior or posterosuperior mediastinal mass, particularly with a previous history of medical or surgical thyroid treatment.

McCort[29] described the roentgenographic findings of anterior mediastinal or ipsilateral posterior mediastinal goiter. These include contralateral displacement of the hyoid, trachea, and larynx; movement of the mass with swallowing; flecks of calcifications; and compression of the trachea or esophagus. However, contralateral extension of the thyroid gland into the opposite posterosuperior mediastinum produces deviation of the trachea and esophagus to the same side as the mass itself on roentgenography of the chest.[17] These plain roentgenographic and computed tomographic findings, together with the pattern of anterior or posterior compression of the esophagus observed on barium esophagography, usually permit the thyroid origin of a mediastinal mass to be suspected preoperatively. Radioactive scanning may be of some additional value, but such lesions often fail to concentrate the tracer preparation. Positive findings on radioactive scan corresponding to the location of the mass support a thyroid origin. Negative findings on radioactive scanning are of little discriminatory value.

## INDICATIONS FOR SURGERY

Most patients with a large intrathoracic goiter require surgery for symptomatic relief. Even in asymptomatic patients, removal of the intrathoracic goiter is indicated unless significant medical contraindications are present. Progressive enlargement of the gland usually occurs, and removal becomes more difficult with time. A small risk of unsuspected carcinoma has been reported[2, 20, 29, 30, 34] in patients with such intrathoracic goiters.

## SURGICAL TECHNIQUES

### *Anterior Substernal Goiter*

The typical substernal goiter can almost always be removed through a cervical incision. This cervical approach permits optimal control of the blood supply from the thyroid vessels, diminishes the chance of injury to the recurrent laryngeal nerve, permits identification of the parathyroid glands, and allows removal of a concomitant cervical goiter.[1, 10, 19, 20, 22–24, 32] Resection begins with cervical exploration and mobilization of the gland. The inferior thyroid and superior thyroid arteries are ligated, thus controlling the arterial blood supply to the substernal goiter. The surgeon's hand is introduced into the superior mediastinum, and a cleavage plane is developed between the capsule of the goiter and the surrounding mediastinal and pleural tissues. The gland is delivered carefully through the thoracic inlet into the cervical wound. Occasionally, this may result in appreciable venous bleeding, which can usually be controlled with a temporary pack. When a large goiter is removed in this fashion, a drainage catheter may be left in the resulting superior mediastinal cavity until obliteration occurs from compression by surrounding tissues.

For a large substernal goiter, the technique described by Lahey[22, 23] may be of value. The capsule of the goiter is entered, and the contents are scooped out manually or with a suction device (morcellation). After this maneuver, the extracapsular dissection is resumed, and the goiter is easily delivered.

For a large substernal goiter with mediastinal fixation, for goiters associated with severe superior vena cava syndrome, or for patients in whom carcinoma is suspected or confirmed preoperatively, a median sternotomy may be the most appropriate approach (Figs. 18–1 through 18–4). This need should arise infrequently. Although older publications suggested that the sternotomy be confined to the upper sternum with transverse division of the sternum at its midportion, this antedated the widespread use of complete sternotomy for open heart surgery. Complete sternal division is faster, simpler, and affords superior exposure. The goiter can usually be separated easily from surrounding mediastinal and pleural structures. One or two No. 28 French chest catheters are left in the mediastinal space. The sternum is closed with multiple interrupted stainless steel wires fol-

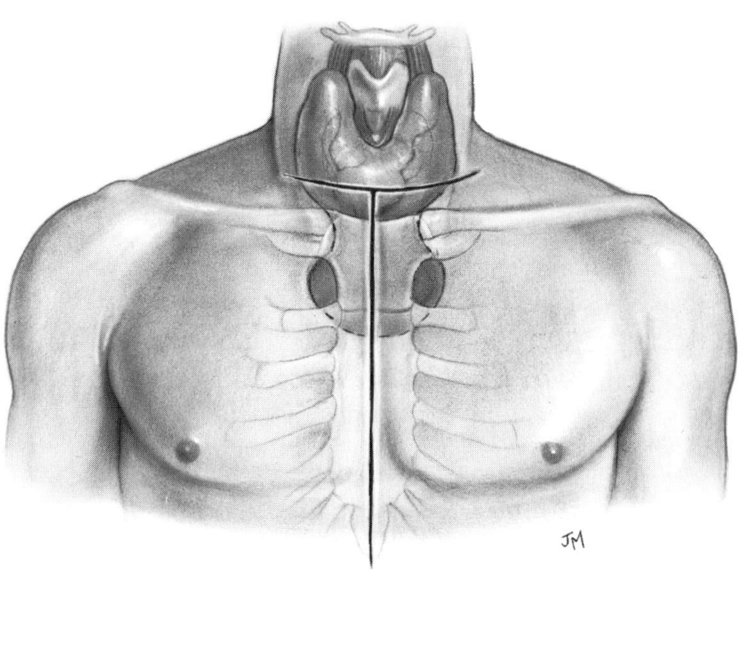

**FIGURE 18–1.** Transverse cervical incision combined with median sternotomy for excision of a large substernal goiter. (By permission of Lahey Clinic.)

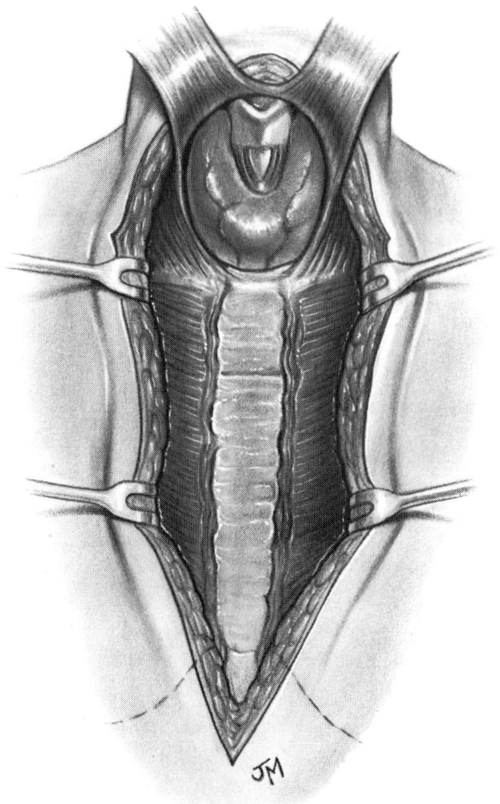


**FIGURE 18–2.** After preliminary cervical exploration, a midline incision is made over the sternum from the xiphoid process to the sternal notch. Partial division of only the upper sternum is preferred by some surgeons, but in general this results in inferior exposure and no advantage in wound healing. (By permission of Lahey Clinic.)

lowed by a running heavy polypropylene suture and standard skin closure.

Isolated substernal goiters derive most of their blood supply from mediastinal sources and have little or no connection to the cervical gland. Such isolated anterior mediastinal goiters are best removed through a sternotomy.

## *Posterior Mediastinal Goiter*

The correct surgical approach for removal of an ipsilateral posterosuperior mediastinal goiter remains controversial. On the one hand, substantial portions of the blood supply to the mediastinal gland may come from the inferior thyroid vessels, and inability to control this cervical blood supply from a thoracic approach may result in disastrous hemorrhage. Furthermore, the recurrent laryngeal nerve cannot be visualized adequately from the thoracic approach, and concomitant removal of the involved cervical portion of the gland may not be possible. On the other hand, serious hemorrhage may result from attempts to remove some posterior mediastinal goiters solely through a cervical approach.[12, 18, 33] This is particularly true of the occasional isolated posterior mediastinal goiter with little or no cervical component and in patients in whom prior cervical thyroidectomy has been performed. Although the original blood supply may have been from the inferior thyroid vessels, a collateral blood supply from the mediastinum often has developed in such situations. Furthermore, the typical right posterosuperior mediastinal goiter is intimately related both to the superior vena cava and the azygos vein and may cause substantial distortion of these vessels. Attempts to remove such goiters without direct visualization may result in severe hemorrhage. Although DeAndrade[6] described a large series of posterior mediastinal goiters removed solely though a cervical approach, most surgeons[10, 18, 19, 33, 40] favor an initial cervical approach with thoracotomy em-

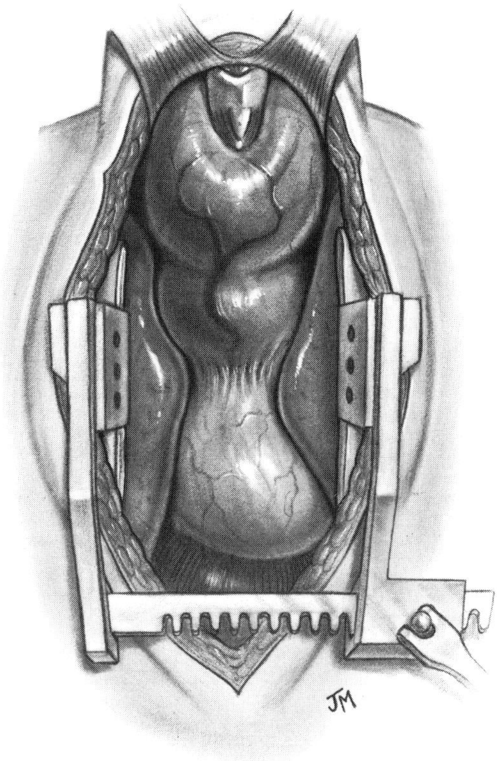


**FIGURE 18–3.** After sternotomy, the entire substernal extent of the goiter is apparent. Dissection of the goiter from surrounding structures is performed easily and precisely. (By permission of Lahey Clinic.)

ployed for larger lesions, especially when they are mainly intrathoracic and have little or no connection to the cervical gland.

For all posterior mediastinal goiters, we advocate initial cervical exploration and gentle attempt at extracapsular dissection of the gland from the surrounding tissues. However, we also have such patients positioned on the operating table for simultaneous thoracotomy, as described by Hart,[15] Hilton and Griffin,[17] and von der Lieth and Lester.[40] This approach combines the advantages of both the cervical and thoracic approaches, minimizes the disadvantages of a solely cervical or thoracic approach, and adds only the minimal additional risk of limited thoracotomy. Such a combined approach is especially useful in the rare instance of a contralateral retrotracheal posterior mediastinal goiter[28] or contralateral retroesophageal goiter (Figs. 18–5 and 18–6).[17, 43]

When a thoracotomy is anticipated for removal of a posterior mediastinal goiter, the patient should be placed in a 45 degree oblique position with the arm extended over the head with care to avoid stretch injury to the nerve. This approach permits simultaneous cervical and thoracic exploration, and the table may be rotated from side to side to facilitate whichever part of the dissection is occurring at a given time. Thoracotomy is performed through a fourth or fifth intercostal space incision, which may be either anterolateral or posterolateral depending on the surgeon's preference. The lung is retracted anteriorly, and the goiter is exposed easily. A double lumen endotracheal tube with deflation of the involved lung is unnecessary. The mass is found in the posterior mediastinum bounded anteriorly by the superior vena cava and inferiorly by the azygos vein, although occasionally more caudal extensions occur. The mediastinal pleura over the goiter is excised, and the capsule of the goiter is dissected free from the surrounding mediastinal structures. Its extension into the thoracic outlet is mobilized. A second surgeon working from the cervical approach can usually meet this thoracic dissection from above. With traction from above and pressure from below, the goiter is delivered into the cervical wound. Hemostasis is achieved in the chest,

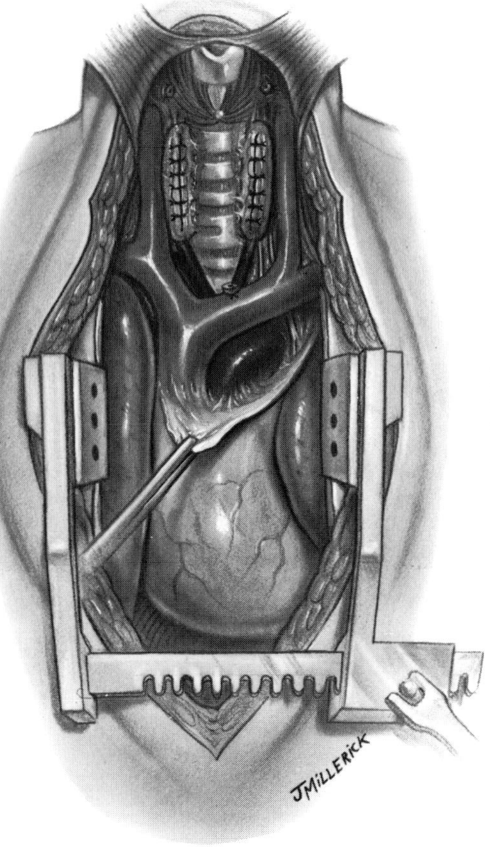


**FIGURE 18–4.** The trachea, thyroid remnants, and upper mediastinal structures are demonstrated after removal of the substernal goiter. (By permission of Lahey Clinic.)

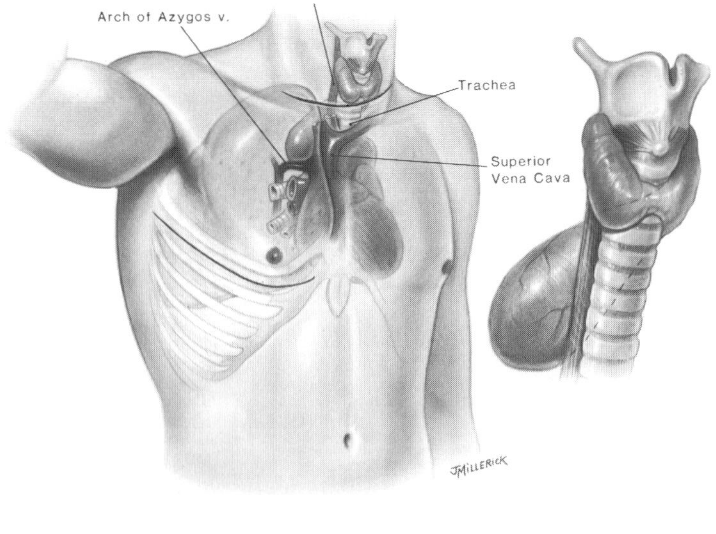


**FIGURE 18–5.** Incisions used for simultaneous cervical and right transthoracic exploration to remove a contralateral retroesophageal posterior mediastinal goiter. (By permission of Lahey Clinic.)

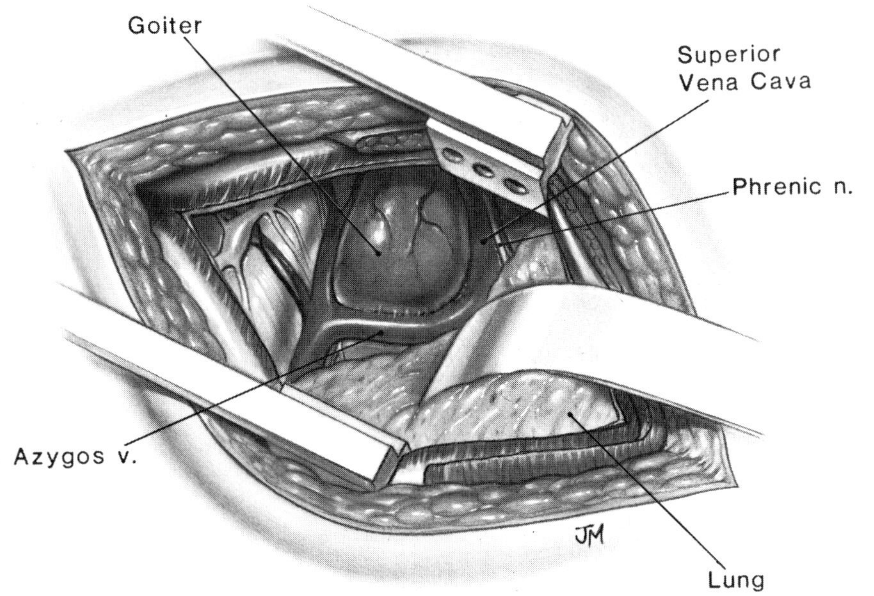


**FIGURE 18–6.** Operative view through the right thoracotomy shows the goiter bounded anteriorly by the superior vena cava and inferiorly by the azygos vein. (By permission of Lahey Clinic.)

the mediastinal pleura is left open to permit drainage of any resulting fluid or blood into the pleural cavity, and the pleural space is drained with two intercostal catheters.

In the rare instance of an isolated posterior mediastinal goiter, removal solely through the thoracic approach may be possible. The connection through the thoracic outlet may be a fibrofatty band, which may be divided, or no connection may be found.

## REFERENCES


1. Adams, H. D.: Transthoracic thyroidectomy. J. Thorac. Surg., *19:*741–754, 1950.
2. Allo, M. D., and Thompson, N. W.: Rationale for the operative management of substernal goiters. Surgery, *94:*969–977, 1983.
3. Cho, H. T., Cohen, J. P., and Som, M. L.: Management of substernal and intrathoracic goiters. Otolaryngol. Head Neck Surg., *94:*282–287, 1986.
4. Crile, G., Jr.: Intrathoracic goiter. Cleve. Clin. Q., *6:*313–322, 1939.
5. Crohn, N. N., and Kobak, M. W.: True posterior mediastinal goiter. Am. J. Surg., *82:*283–286, 1951.
6. DeAndrade, M. A.: A review of 128 cases of posterior mediastinal goiter. World J. Surg., *1:*789–797, 1977.
7. DeCourcy, J. L., and Price, C. A.: Intrathoracic goiter: Case report. Am. J. Surg., *64:*257–262, 1944.
8. deSouza, F. M., and Smith, P. E.: Retrosternal goiter. J. Otolaryngol., *12:*393–396, 1983.
9. Dundas, P.: Intrathoracic aberrant goiter. Acta Chir. Scand., *128:*729–736, 1964.
10. Ellis, F. H., Jr., Good, C. A., and Seybold, W. D.: Intrathoracic goiter. Ann. Surg., *135:*79–90, 1952.
11. Falor, W. H., Kelly, T. R., and Jackson, J. B.: Intrathoracic goiter. Surg. Gynecol. Obstet., *117:*604–610, 1963.
12. Falor, W. H., Kelly, T. R., and Krabill, W. S.: Intrathoracic goiter. Ann. Surg., *142:*238–247, 1955.
13. Georgiadis, N., Katsas, A., and Leoutsakos, B.: Substernal goiter. Int. Surg., *54:*116–121, 1970.
14. Gourin, A., Garzon, A. A., and Karlson, K. E.: The cervicomediastinal approach to intrathoracic goiter. Surgery, *69:*651–654, 1971.
15. Hart, D.: Discussion. *In* Adams, H.D.: Transthoracic thyroidectomy. J. Thorac. Surg., *19:*741–754, 1950.
16. Heimburger, I., Battersby, J. S., and Vellios, F.: Primary neoplasms of the mediastinum: A fifteen-year experience. Arch. Surg., *86:*978–984, 1963.
17. Hilton, H. D., and Griffin, W. T.: Posterior mediastinal goiter. Am. J. Surg., *116:*891–895, 1968.
18. Hurwitz, A., and Skorneck, A. B.: Intrathoracic goiters situated in the posterior aspect of the superior mediastinum. Surgery, *39:*991–996, 1956.
19. Johnston, J. H., Jr., and Twente, G. E.: Surgical approach to intrathoracic (mediastinal) goiter. Ann. Surg., *143:*572–579, 1956.
20. Judd, E. S., Beahrs, O. H., and Bowes, D. E.: A consideration of the proper surgical approach for substernal goiter. Surg. Gynecol. Obstet., *110:*90–98, 1960.
21. Katlic, M. R., Grillo, H. C., and Wang, C. A.: Substernal goiter: Analysis of 80 patients from

Massachusetts General Hospital. Am. J. Surg., *149:*283–287, 1985.
22. Lahey, F. H.: The surgical management of intrathoracic goiter. Surg. Gynecol. Obstet., *53:*346–354, 1931.
23. Lahey, F. H.: Intrathoracic goiters. Surg. Clin. North Am., *25:*609–618, 1945.
24. Lahey, F. H., and Swinton, N. W.: Intrathoracic goiter. Surg. Gynecol. Obstet., *59:*627–637, 1934.
25. Le Roux, B. T.: Heterotopic mediastinal thyroid. Thorax, *16:*192–196, 1961.
26. Lindskog, B. I., and Malm, A.: Diagnostic and surgical considerations on mediastinal (intrathoracic) goiter. Dis. Chest, *47:*201–207, 1965.
27. Lyons, H. A., Calvy, G. L., and Sammons, B. P.: The diagnosis and classification of mediastinal masses. I. A study of 782 cases. Ann. Intern. Med., *51:*897–932, 1959.
28. Maurer, E. R.: The surgical treatment of retrotracheal intrathoracic goiter. Arch. Surg., *71:*357–365, 1955.
29. McCort, J. J.: Intrathoracic goiter: Its incidence, symptomatology, and roentgen diagnosis. Radiology, *53:*227–236, 1949.
30. Nielsen, V. M., Løvgreen, N. A., and Elbrønd, O.: Intrathoracic goitre: Surgical treatment in an ENT department. J. Laryngol. Otol., *97:*1039–1045, 1983.
31. Nwafo, D. C.: Heterotopic mediastinal goitre. Br. J. Surg., *65:*505–506, 1978.
32. Pemberton, J. de J.: Surgery of substernal and intrathoracic goiters. Arch. Surg., *2:*1–20, 1921.
33. Pitt, L. P.: Aberrant posterior mediastinal goiter: A review of the literature and report of a case. Am. J. Surg., *103:*397–399, 1962.
34. Reeve, T. S., Rundle, F. F., Hales, I. B., et al.: The investigation and management of intrathoracic goiter. Surg. Gynecol. Obstet., *115:*222–229, 1962.
35. Rietz, K. A., and Werner, B.: Intrathoracic goiter. Acta Chir. Scand., *119:*379–388, 1960.
36. Rives, J. D.: Mediastinal aberrant goiter. Ann. Surg., *126:*797–810, 1947.
37. Salomon, J., and Levy, M. J.: Mediastinal aberrant goiter: Report of two cases. Dis. Chest, *52:*413–416, 1967.
38. Sand, M. E., Laws, H. L., McElvein, R. B.: Substernal and intrathoracic goiter: Reconsideration of surgical approach. Am. Surg., *49:*196–202, 1983.
39. Sherman, P. H., and Shahbahrami, F.: Mediastinal goiter: Review of ten cases. Am. Surg., *32:*137–142, 1966.
40. Sweet, R. H.: Intrathoracic goiter located in the posterior mediastinum. Surg. Gynecol. Obstet., *89:*57–66, 1949.
41. von der Lieth, W. C., and Lester, C. W.: Posterior mediastinal goiter: Use of a combined thoracocervical approach for excision. Am. J. Surg., *85:*811–814, 1953.
42. Wakeley, C. P. G., and Mulvany, J. H.: Intrathoracic goiter. Surg. Gynecol. Obstet., *70:*702–710, 1940.
43. Weissberg, D., and Thau, M.: Intrathoracic retroesophageal nodular goiter. Thorac. Cardiovasc. Surg., *29:*122–123, 1981.
44. Wychulis, A. R., Payne, W. S., Clagett, O. T., and Woolner, L. B.: Surgical treatment of mediastinal tumors: A 40-year experience. J. Thorac. Cardiovasc. Surg., *62:*379–392, 1971.

# Commentary

*Blake Cady, M.D., and Ricardo L. Rossi, M.D.*

This excellent exposition about intrathoracic goiter by Dr. Shahian is comprehensive. However, only a small fraction of the patients with substernal goiter will need open thoracotomy for removal of the goiter. The majority of these lesions can be extracted through the collar incision as has been described in other chapters in this book. One maneuver to keep in mind when trying to remove these goiters from the thyroidectomy incision is Dr. Lahey's description of the method of morcellation or internal scooping out of a lesion that might be in or below the thoracic inlet. This technique deflates the mass and takes enough pressure off the surrounding structures so that the residual intrathoracic or substernal goiter can then be extracted safely and relatively easily.

These lesions are discovered early because radiography of the chest is performed often, adenomatous goiter is an infrequent occurrence, and patients are operated on at earlier stages because a large goiter is cosmetically unacceptable to the patient. Transthoracic thyroidectomy will be an uncommon procedure in the future, but this operation needs to be part of every thyroid surgeon's armamentarium.

# 19

# ROLE OF THYROID-STIMULATING HORMONE SUPPRESSION AND RADIOACTIVE IODINE IN DIFFERENTIATED CARCINOMA OF THYROID GLAND

*Mary Beth Hodge, M.D.*

Several aspects of the treatment of patients with differentiated carcinoma of the thyroid are controversial. Physicians agree that thyroid carcinomas should be excised but disagree concerning the optimal surgical procedure. The use of radioactive iodine ablation—when to use it, the dose to be given, and determining its ultimate effectiveness—has generated much discussion. The beneficial effects of thyroid-stimulating hormone (TSH) suppression by thyroid hormone therapy have also been debated. This chapter clarifies the roles of TSH suppression and radioactive iodine ablation in the management of patients with differentiated carcinoma of the thyroid.

## THYROID-STIMULATING HORMONE AND CARCINOMA OF THE THYROID

Although patients with bilateral thyroidectomy require thyroid hormone therapy to obviate hypothyroidism, the need to give thyroid hormone is not always as clear in patients who have had hemithyroidectomy. It was first observed many years ago that thyroid extract given to patients with nontoxic goiter often caused regression and sometimes complete disappearance of the goiter. Dunhill[22] was the first researcher to show the beneficial effects of thyroid hormone and TSH suppression therapy in patients with carcinoma of the thyroid. He described the regression of papillary carcinoma of the thyroid in two children treated with thyroid hormone. In 1954, Balme[1] documented the regression of metastatic carcinoma of the thyroid in a patient treated with thyroid hormone. However, Crile,[17] Rawson and colleagues,[39] and Trunnell[54] showed that increasing serum levels of TSH by thyroidectomy or by thyroid ablation with radiation or goitrogens sometimes increased the growth rate of thyroid carcinomas. Crile[17, 18] also suggested that continued TSH stimulation of thyroid carcinoma could lead to transformation of differentiated slow-growing endocrine-dependent tumors to rapidly growing autonomously functioning metastasizing tumors.

Mazzaferri and coworkers[31] found that in 11 of 83 patients with thyroid nodules subsequently proved to be papillary carcinoma, the size of the lesion decreased with TSH suppressive therapy. In 1974, Hill and associates[25] showed that in two of 16 patients with papillary carcinoma and in two of six patients with follicular carcinoma, the size of the thyroid lesion decreased appreciably in response to thyroid hormone therapy, whereas in patients with medullary and undifferentiated carcinoma, the size of the thyroid lesion remained the same.

Mazzaferri and associates[31] also studied the effects of thyroid hormone therapy in preventing recurrence of differentiated carcinoma of the thyroid. In patients with papillary carcinoma treated with thyroid hormone, the cumulative recurrence rate was less than 20 per cent, but in patients with papillary carcinoma who were not treated with thyroid hormone, the recurrence rate was more than 40 per cent. Cady and colleagues[13] found no appreciable improvement in survival times of patients with operable differentiated carcinoma of the thyroid treated with adjuvant thyroid hormone when patients were categorized by risk group and type of tumor. They[13] concluded that age and sex risk factors outweighed the effects of adjuvant treatment with thyroid hormone. However, the study had some potential biases, that is, not all patients had TSH measured, patients seen before 1960 may have been treated with thyroid hormone to prevent myxedema rather than to suppress TSH, and some patients who received thyroid hormone may have had a large carcinoma and poor prognosis initially. Jesse[27] reported on 700 patients with carcinoma of the thyroid who were treated by total thyroidectomy and desiccated thyroid replacement, 3 grains daily. Jesse[27] did not mention whether measurements were taken to determine TSH suppression. In 34 per cent of Jesse's[27] patients, tumor recurred or the size of the metastatic tumor increased. Thus, the debate in the literature continues over the efficacy of thyroid hormone therapy in preventing recurrence of tumor and prolonging survival. However, treatment with thyroid hormone usually produces few side effects unless the dose is too high or the patient has underlying heart disease that could be unmasked by toxic levels of thyroid hormone. Until the problem regarding the efficacy of TSH suppression on tumor recurrence and patient survival is solved, thyroid hormone therapy should continue to be recommended after surgery for carcinoma of the thyroid.

## THYROID-STIMULATING HORMONE SUPPRESSION AND THYROID HORMONE

After the decision has been made to start thyroid hormone therapy to suppress TSH, the questions become what form of thyroid hormone should be given and how much should be prescribed. Several preparations of thyroid hormone are available. L-Thyroxine (Synthroid, Levothroid) is synthetic L-$T_4$. Liothyronine (Cytomel) is synthetic L-$T_3$. Desiccated thyroid (Thyroid, U.S.P.) is a mixture of L-$T_4$ and L-$T_3$ in their natural state and is derived from the thyroid glands of animals, usually cows. Because the content of animal hormone material is not uniform, various batches of the same dose tablet of desiccated thyroid lack biologic standardization.[40] For this reason, most physicians choose synthetic thyroid over desiccated thyroid. In general, levothyroxine (L-$T_4$) rather than liothyronine (L-$T_3$) is used for long-term suppression of TSH because L-$T_4$ has a longer half-life (approximately 1 week) than L-$T_3$ (approximately 1 day) and thus provides more sustained suppression of TSH. Because

L-$T_4$ is converted to L-$T_3$ in the periphery and in the pituitary gland,[26] it is not necessary to give both L-$T_4$ and L-$T_3$ (desiccated thyroid). Because L-$T_4$ is more stable than L-$T_3$, the dose is more precise.[15] Levothyroxine produces fewer side effects than L-$T_3$, which sometimes causes anxiety a few hours after the patient has ingested the medication. The fluctuating serum $T_3$ concentrations after oral ingestion of L-$T_3$ are less physiologic than the relatively constant $T_3$ concentration after oral ingestion of L-$T_4$. Also, compliance is better with L-$T_4$, which because of its longer half-life is taken only once daily, than with L-$T_3$, which is usually taken twice daily.

The dose of L-$T_4$ varies between 0.15 and 0.30 mg/d, and because the goal is to suppress TSH entirely, the dose required is usually greater than that normally required to achieve a euthyroid state in a patient with hypothyroidism. The adequacy of TSH suppression can be evaluated by obtaining a TSH level (the aim is to achieve an undetectable level of TSH) and adjusting the dose of L-$T_4$ accordingly. Conventional TSH assays have a normal range of 0 to 5 μU/ml, and therefore TSH should be suppressed to less than 1 μU/ml. New ultrasensitive TSH assays using monoclonal antibodies can detect levels of TSH of 0.1 μU/ml or less.[42] The normal range for TSH using the ultrasensitive assay is 0.5 to 5 μU/ml, but this will vary depending on the particular assay used. Hyperthyroid patients have a TSH value less than 0.08 μU/ml; the range should be less than 0.08 μU/ml when suppression of TSH is attempted. The ultrasensitive TSH assay eliminates the need for thyrotropin-releasing hormone (TRH) stimulation tests to determine the adequacy of TSH suppression.

Invariably, the doses of L-thyroxine recommended to suppress TSH can raise the serum total $T_4$ into the hyperthyroid range, but the clinical criteria are more important in determining whether to lower the dose of L-thyroxine. When a patient is tolerating a level of total $T_4$ of 13 or 14 μg/100 dl, the dose of L-$T_4$ does not need to be decreased. Usually, monitoring the level of total $T_4$ is not indicated unless the patient appears to have signs and symptoms of hyperthyroidism. However, one should try to use the least amount of L-$T_4$ necessary to suppress TSH because exogenous hyperthyroidism, even when asymptomatic, can cause osteopenia.

# ROLE OF RADIOACTIVE IODINE

Despite controversies regarding the management of patients with differentiated carcinoma of the thyroid, most physicians agree that operation is the most effective initial form of treatment available. The use of postoperative radioactive iodine ablative therapy of residual normal thyroid is controversial because it is uncertain whether it improves survival and decreases morbidity in patients with differentiated carcinoma of the thyroid. However, radioactive iodine may be effective in the treatment of patients with metastases, local tumor recurrence, and unresectable tumor.

Because the growth rate of differentiated carcinoma of the thyroid is slow, long-term follow-up is required to evaluate the effectiveness of any form of treatment.[55] In a large series of patients with differentiated carcinoma of the thyroid without evidence of disease after initial treatment, Gardet and coworkers[24] found relapse occurred in some patients as late as 25 years after initial treatment. Other problems in evaluating the effectiveness of radioactive iodine are the wide variability in the amount of thyroid tissue removed at operation,[50] the dose of radioactive iodine used to ablate remaining normal thyroid tissue,[20, 28, 33] and the scanning dose of radioactive iodine used to determine the completeness of ablation.[58] In consideration of the role of radioactive iodine in differentiated carcinoma of the thyroid, anticipatory radioactive iodine ablation of remaining normal thyroid tissue, radioactive iodine therapy for metastatic or recurrent disease, and radioactive iodine treatment of tumor after incomplete surgery must be differentiated from each other.

## *Postoperative Anticipatory Radioactive Iodine Ablation of Remaining Normal Thyroid Tissue*

Several authors[4, 31, 57, 59] have advocated postoperative administration of radioactive iodine to destroy remaining normal thyroid tissue and any neoplastic foci within the residual gland. One rationale for using radioactive iodine ablative therapy is to destroy all normal residual thyroid tissue in anticipation of giving subsequent radioactive iodine therapy. A second rationale is based on the presumption that thyroid carcinoma is a multifocal disease, and carcinoma may be found in the contralateral lobe. However, such carcinomas are unlikely to be troublesome clinically.

Sampson et al.[45] studied 3,000 autopsies of residents of Hiroshima and Nagasaki and found 536 thyroid carcinomas, 518 of which were occult papillary tumors. Although lymph node metastases were noted in 16 per cent of these occult tumors, the carcinoma was the cause of death in only one of the 518 patients.[45] Tollefson et al.[52] found that contralateral involvement developed in only 17 of 298 patients (5.7 per cent) with less than total thyroidectomy. Of these 17 patients, seven died of metastatic disease: three had clinically apparent contralateral involvement, and metastasis in the other four was discovered at biopsy or operation.[52]

Ablation of remaining normal thyroid tissue may enhance detection of recurrent tumor and metastases through subsequent radioactive iodine scans of the neck and body and through serum assays of thyroglobulin. The presence of normal residual thyroid tissue may make it difficult to determine whether a local recurrent tumor or metastasis can be treated with radioactive iodine or will require surgical excision. Unfortunately, not enough evidence is available to determine whether radioactive iodine ablation of remaining thyroid tissue is effective in prolonging survival or decreasing morbidity.

Part of the problem is lack of a good control group with which to compare survival and morbidity rates. Savoie and Garnier[47] administered radioactive iodine ablation after operation to 145 patients and observed local recurrence and metastases in 25 per cent of patients. However, without a control group, it was unclear whether treatment with radioactive iodine resulted in a decrease in the incidence of local recurrence and metastases. Varma and coworkers[57] compared the survival rate of 50 consecutive patients with differentiated carcinoma treated by surgery alone (1933 to 1947) with the survival rate of 263 consecutive patients treated by surgery followed by radioactive iodine ablation (1947 to 1964). The survival rates for patients less than 39 years of age in both groups were about equal, but in patients 40 years of age and older, the survival rate was appreciably higher in the group of 40 patients treated by the combination of surgery and radioactive iodine ablation.

In a retrospective study, Samaan and associates[44] collected data on 706 patients treated for differentiated carcinoma of the thyroid from 1951 to 1975 and followed up until 1981. Management and therapy were individualized according to the clinical findings and the experience of each attending physician. Of the total, 136 patients with no evidence of postoperative disease received radioactive iodine ablative therapy to the remaining normal thyroid tissue. When these 136 patients were compared with 390 patients with no evidence of postoperative disease who had not received radioactive iodine ablation regardless of the extent of disease, type of surgery, or histology, the frequency of recurrence was lower in patients treated with radioactive iodine ablation, but the survival rates of the two groups were not significantly different. When patients were subdivided according to histologic type of tumor, only the groups with follicular and mixed carcinoma had a significantly lower rate of recurrence ($P < 0.05$) when radioactive iodine ablation was administered. When patients were subdivided according to extent of surgery, those who had had total thyroidectomy plus radioactive iodine therapy had a significantly lower rate of recurrence ($P < 0.05$) and a higher rate of survival ($P < 0.05$) than patients who had had total thyroidectomy but no radioactive iodine treatment. This significance was lost when less than total thyroidectomy was performed.[44] Because the benefit of radioactive iodine ablation was apparent only in patients who underwent total thyroidectomy, these authors[44] postulated that the remaining normal thyroid tissue preferentially takes up iodine and little reaches any remaining malignant cells. Several other physicians[4, 31, 59] also found the recurrence rate was decreased with radioactive iodine ablative treatment after operation. Mazzaferri and associates[31] and Young and coworkers[59] have also shown that the use of thyroid hormone suppression resulted in a further decrease in the incidence of recurrent tumor in patients treated with surgery followed by radioactive iodine ablative therapy.

Snyder and colleagues[50] studied 69 patients with differentiated carcinoma of the thyroid who were treated surgically (the amount of thyroid tissue removed was variable) and were then given 30 mCi of radioactive iodine to ablate the remaining normal thyroid tissue. Thirteen patients required additional radioactive iodine for successful ablation. Of the 56 patients who underwent successful ablation with only 30 mCi of radioactive iodine, local recurrence developed in six patients within 5 to 37 months after ablation. Of these six patients, five had been considered to be free of disease after operation. Only one of the six patients had total thyroidectomy. These physicians[50] questioned whether a higher ablative dose might have prevented the recurrences, noting that one author[37] has proposed that higher doses of radiation may diminish the theoretical risk of exposing an initially "unseen" focus of carcinoma to a sublethal dose of radiation that might enhance its malignant potential and diminish its propensity to accumulate radioactive iodine.

As Snyder et al.[50] noted, many physicians[7, 16, 43] believe that remnants should be ablated because of the high incidence of multicentricity in patients with carcinoma of the thyroid. However, several large series[3, 7, 19, 41, 52] demonstrated recurrence rates varying from 2.6 to 17 per cent in patients who have had limited thyroid resection without postoperative radioactive iodine therapy. Thus, it is not clear whether postoperative ablation of remaining thyroid tissue with radioactive iodine is more effective than subtotal or near total thyroidectomy and adequate TSH suppression.[50] In a retrospective study of 859 patients with papillary carcinoma of the thyroid, McConahey and colleagues[32] showed that multicentricity was not a risk factor influencing survival. Of the 859 patients, 178 had two or more foci of carcinoma discovered at surgery. Other clinical and histologic features (that is, age and sex of the patient, size of tumor, and degree of invasiveness) are more predictive of the need for total thyroid ablation.[50] Until a prospective study is carried out to examine these issues, debate over the indications for ablation of thyroid remnants will continue. At the Lahey Clinic, we usually favor anticipatory ablation of thyroid remnants in patients with follicular or papillary carcinoma larger than 2.5 cm, in the presence of invasiveness beyond the tumor capsule (particularly for follicular carcinoma), in the presence of extensive local invasion beyond the thyroid capsule (follicular or papillary carcinoma), and in men over age 40 years and in women over age 50 at the time of diagnosis. The presence of cervical nodal involvement at the time of diagnosis in a patient in an otherwise low-risk group[10, 12] (men less than age 40 or women less than age 50) does not constitute an indication for anticipatory radioactive iodine ablation of thyroid remnants because the extent of cervical lymph node involvement has been shown to have no adverse effect on survival.[11]

The amount of radioactive iodine needed to achieve successful ablation of remaining normal thyroid tissue after operation is uncertain. The recommended dose of radioactive iodine varies from 30[19, 20, 24] to 150 mCi.[5, 34, 38, 57, 58]

Low-dose radioactive iodine (30 mCi) has the advantages of less radiation burden to the patient and it can be given on an outpatient basis, thus avoiding the cost of hospitalization. Determining the efficacy of low-dose radioactive iodine (30 mCi) over high-dose radioactive iodine (50 to 150 mCi) in ablating thyroid remnants after operation is difficult because patients have variable amounts of thyroid tissue remaining after operation, and investigators[5, 33, 38, 50] use diverse criteria for successful ablation and employ varying test doses (from 1 to 10 mCi) of radioactive iodine when performing scans of the neck and body after radioactive iodine therapy. The larger the scanning dose of radioactive iodine, the greater the chance of detecting a small focus of residual thyroid tissue.[58] In practice, however, the amount of the scanning dose is limited because of whole-body radiation incident to its use and diminishing benefits anticipated from display of tissue that is minute, may not be malignant, and may not accumulate sufficient radioactive iodine for effective treatment.[38, 50] Most centers use 1 or 2 mCi of radioactive iodine for a scanning dose because this amount usually displays thyroid tissue functioning at a level that could permit radioactive iodine ablative therapy.[50] A low iodine diet, diuretics to enhance excretion of iodine, and injection of TSH before the radioactive iodine scan are usually not necessary to enhance the uptake of radioactive iodine into any functioning residual thyroid tissue.

The success rate in ablating thyroid remnants with 30 mCi of radioactive iodine ranges from 11 to 83 per cent but seems to average about 60 per cent.[20, 33, 38, 50] The success rate in ablating thyroid remnants with 50 to 150 mCi of radioactive iodine ranges from 53 to 87 per cent.[5, 38] An ablative dose of 30 mCi of radioactive iodine may be chosen for patients who had a well-encapsulated carcinoma and who had undergone bilateral thyroidectomy with no evidence of persistent local or metastatic disease or for patients who refuse hospitalization for high-dose radioactive iodine therapy. However, some patients treated with 30 mCi of radioactive iodine may need additional treatment to achieve complete ablation of thyroid tissue, especially those with a substantial amount of thyroid tissue remaining in the neck.

Radioactive iodine ablation with 100 to 150 mCi should initially be given to patients who have evidence of invasive tumor, residual disease in the thyroid bed, or metastases (see later). Patients who had less than one lobe surgically removed for a malignant tumor larger than 2 cm may be candidates for additional surgery. When reoperation is not possible, these patients probably should be treated with 100 to 150 mCi of radioactive iodine because a large volume of thyroid tissue requires a large dose of radioactive iodine to achieve ablation.

The timing of radioactive iodine ablative treatment is important. At the Lahey Clinic Medical Center, patients who are to be treated with an ablative dose of radioactive iodine are withheld from thyroid hormone therapy until approximately 4 weeks after operation, at which time a radioactive iodine uptake and neck scan (using $^{123}I$) is obtained. When residual thyroid tissue and considerable uptake of radioactive iodine are seen, radioactive iodine ablation is given. Treatment with thyroid hormone (L-$T_3$) is started 1 week later in a split daily dose of 50 to 100 μg and is stopped approximately 3 or 4 months afterward. A repeat radioactive iodine scan (using 1 mCi of $^{131}I$) of the neck and body is obtained, and a serum thyroglobulin level is determined 2 weeks after discontinuing thyroid hormone (L-$T_3$). When no appreciable uptake (<1 per cent) or functioning tissue is seen, thyroid hormone (L-$T_4$) therapy is started.

Follow-up periodic examinations of the neck and determinations of the level of serum thyroglobulin are necessary. The level of TSH is also monitored to ensure the adequacy of thyroid hormone suppressive therapy. Radioactive iodine scans of the neck and body are repeated only when recurrent or metastatic disease is suspected, that is, elevated level of thyroglobulin, palpable neck mass, abnormal findings on radiography of the chest, or bone pain. The repeat scan should be obtained with 1 mCi of $^{131}I$ 4 weeks after L-$T_4$ is discontinued. When recurrent tumor or metastatic disease is radiosensitive, 100 to 150 mCi of radioactive iodine is given to destroy the tumor.

## *Use of Radioactive Iodine for Unresectable Tumor and Metastasis*

It is usually agreed that radioactive iodine therapy is indicated for patients with distant metastases, local recurrence, or residual tumor in the neck that concentrates radioactive iodine after operation. Based on a 25-year follow-up study of 103 patients with distant metastases from well-differentiated carcinoma of the thyroid, Beierwaltes and colleagues[5] found that patients whose metastases were treated successfully with radioactive iodine survived three times as long as patients whose metastatic disease was not treated successfully. Charbord and associates[14] studied 57 patients with local recurrence of differentiated carcinoma of the thyroid and found that the 15-year survival rate was 50 per cent in patients with a radiosensitive tumor compared with 30 per cent in patients whose recurrent tumor was not radiosensitive. Charbord and colleagues[14] noted that patients with radiosensitive tumor were younger than patients whose tumor did not take up radioactive iodine. Radioactive iodine treatment prolongs survival in patients with radiosensitive local recurrent tumor or pulmonary metastases. However, for many patients with radiosensitive bone metastases, such treatment is mainly palliative. Tubiana[55] thought that this may be because many patients with bone metastases are elderly, the proportion of moderately differentiated follicular carcinomas is high, and most distant bone metastases arise from hematogenous spread of tumor.

When residual tumor in the neck is radiosensitive, radioactive iodine therapy may improve survival. However, when the tumor does not take up radioactive iodine, the outlook is poor. In these situations, a trial of external beam radiotherapy may help in controlling local growth of the tumor,[49, 55] but the rate of tumor regression is often slow (2 to 34 months).[49]

When a patient has been free of disease since thyroidectomy and recurrent tumor or a metastasis develops in the neck and is not radiosensitive, consideration should be given to surgical removal of the tumor.

### *Complications of Radioactive Iodine Therapy*

In general, the majority of patients have no acute side effects with the oral administration of radioactive iodine. Some patients may complain of nausea and vomiting. Others may have discomfort in the area of the thyroid bed for several days, which is thought to represent radiation thyroiditis. Aspirin is usually helpful in this instance. Occasionally, transient submandibular or parotid sialadenitis may develop. Large doses of radioactive iodine may cause transient bone marrow suppression, especially in the presence of bone metastases.[37]

Potential long-term side effects of radioactive iodine include radiation pulmonary fibrosis and leukemia. Pulmonary fibrosis can develop several years after radioactive iodine has been given and is dependent on the presence of radiosensitive lung metastases and the cumulative dose of radioactive iodine. In a patient treated with radioactive iodine for lung metastases, the chance that pulmonary fibrosis will develop increases after a cumulative dose of 300 to 400 mCi of radioactive iodine has been given.[4, 23] In young patients, the rate of progression of lung metastases is often slow; when longer intervals elapse between treatments with radioactive iodine (for example, 1 year), the cumulative dose of radioactive iodine may be lessened.[9]

The possibility of leukemia developing also rises with an increasing cumulative dosage of radioactive iodine. In a review of five series of patients treated with radioactive iodine for carcinoma of the thyroid, Brincker and colleagues[8] found an incidence of leukemia of 2 per cent (10 cases of leukemia among 487 patients treated with radioactive iodine). However, the majority of patients in whom leukemia developed received a cumulative dosage of more than 400 mCi of radioactive iodine. Risks may be minimized further by spacing individual treatments at least 1 year apart. In 1984, Beierwaltes and associates[6] reported that leukemia did not develop in patients treated with ablative doses of 100 to 200 mCi of radioactive iodine. Because the development of leukemia is dose dependent, presumably this risk is remote for patients who receive only anticipatory ablative doses.

In general, the incidence of infertility, miscarriage, and major congenital anomalies is not increased in patients treated with radioactive iodine.[46] Patients should not be pregnant during treatment, and they are advised to wait 6 to 12 months after radioiodine treatment before becoming pregnant.

A mild increase in the incidence of bladder carcinoma may be apparent in patients treated with repetitive high doses of radioactive iodine.[23]

Although the long-term potential harmful effects of radioactive iodine should not be ignored, the beneficial effects of radioactive iodine in the treatment of unresectable tumor, recurrent tumor, and metastatic disease far outweigh potential risks associated with radioactive iodine. Anticipatory radioactive iodine ablation that involves no more than 100 mCi of $^{131}I$ is believed to be fairly safe and free of long-term harmful effects.

Pochin[36] reported that after radioactive iodine therapy, 2 to 3 per cent of well-differentiated thyroid carcinomas became anaplastic carcinomas. Although such conversions can occur spontaneously,[52] this iatrogenic effect cannot be ignored.

## USE OF SERUM THYROGLOBULIN IN MANAGEMENT OF PATIENTS WITH CARCINOMA OF THE THYROID

Thyroglobulin is a large glycoprotein that is synthesized by the thyroid follicular cell and secreted into the lumen of the follicular cell. It is found in the serum of most healthy adults. About 20 per cent of adults have antithyroglobulin antibodies that interfere with thyroglobulin measurement. The level of thyroglobulin increases with thyroidal stimulation by TSH or thyroid-stimulating immunoglobulins (TSI). Serum thyroglobulin is used as a tumor marker in differentiated thyroid carcinoma.

Although the level of serum thyroglobulin is often elevated in the presence of differentiated carcinoma of the thyroid,[56] it may also be elevated in other types of thyroid conditions, such as hyperthyroidism or goiter.[29, 53] Unfortunately, when any normal thyroid tissue remains in the neck after surgery for carcinoma of the thyroid, a detectable level of thyroglobulin may result. When all normal thyroid tissue has been removed either surgically or through radioactive iodine ablation and the level of thyroglobulin remains elevated, the presence of persistent carcinoma in the neck or metastatic carcinoma is implied.[21, 30, 51] Likewise, an undetectable level of thyroglobulin suggests but does not prove the absence of residual thyroid carcinoma.

Measurement of serum thyroglobulin is more meaningful when performed while the patient is not taking thyroid hormone (not taking L-$T_3$ for 2 weeks or not taking L-$T_4$ for 4 weeks) because thyroglobulin produced by either benign or malignant thyroid tissue may partially be suppressed by exogenous thyroid hormone. An elevated thyroglobulin level while the patient is taking thyroid hormone suggests the presence of residual or metastatic tumor. Thus, the serum thyroglobulin determination can be an important clinical tool in the evaluation of patients with mixed or pure follicular carcinoma of the thyroid provided all normal thyroid tissue has been excised or ablated. It is less useful in patients with pure papillary carcinoma.

Barsano and coworkers[2] believe the combination of a low level of serum thyroglobulin and negative findings on radioactive iodine scan of the neck and body substantially reduces the need for repetitive total body scanning during follow-up study of patients with carcinoma of the thyroid who have had successful ablation of thyroid remnants after thyroidectomy. Some investigators[2, 35, 48] reported that their patients had thyroidectomy and successful ablation of thyroid remnants but had elevated serum thyroglobulin levels and negative findings on radioactive iodine scans in the hypothyroid state. In a few of these patients, carcinoma recurred. Unfortunately, little information is available to help estimate the prognosis of patients with elevated levels of thyroglobulin and negative findings on scans taken after successful surgery and ablation of thyroid remnants. Barsano and associates[2] postulated that radioactive iodine therapy can impair the iodine concentrating capacity of thyroid or tumor tissue to a greater extent than its capacity to synthesize thyroglobulin. Thus, a patient with an elevated level of thyroglobulin in the absence of other clinical or scan abnormalities suggestive of recurrent tumor must be followed up closely with periodic radioactive iodine scans of the body to search for the development of a tumor. When carcinoma of the thyroid cannot be localized, no evidence is available to suggest that a patient with an elevated level of thyroglobulin and a negative finding on radioactive iodine scan requires treatment.[48]

After reviewing several studies to elicit the correlation between the level of thyroglobulin and radioactive iodine scans, Schneider and coworkers[48] reported that patients with recurrent or metastatic carcinoma of the thyroid rarely have a low level of serum thyroglobulin and that the level of serum thyroglobulin was sometimes more sensitive than the radioactive iodine scan in detecting functioning thyroid tissue. They showed that the use of both the thyroglobulin determination and the scan was superior to the use of either procedure alone when searching for metastases or recurrent tumor.[48] They further agreed with Barsano et al.[2] that a negative finding on scan and a low level of serum thyroglobulin suggest that all functioning thyroid carcinoma has probably been eliminated, and a plan of decreasing the frequency of follow-up scanning seems reasonable.[48]

Serum thyroglobulin and radioactive iodine scans cannot be expected to be useful in the management of medullary carcinoma or anaplastic carcinoma of the thyroid because these carcinomas have no ability to synthesize thyroglobulin and to concentrate iodine. Some differentiated carcinomas of the thyroid can become poorly differentiated and lose the ability to synthesize thyroglobulin and concentrate iodide. Because the frequency with which this occurs is not known, it is uncertain whether a low or undetectable level of serum thyroglobulin obviates the need for a scan.[48]

## SUMMARY

The roles of TSH suppression and radioactive iodine therapy in differentiated carcinoma of the thyroid have been discussed. Despite controversies, both of these therapeutic modalities may be important in the management of some patients with carcinoma of the thyroid. Adequate TSH suppression may decrease the rate of the development of recurrent tumor and may decrease the size of unresectable residual tumor or metastases. Radioactive iodine ablation of thyroid remnants will potentially facilitate treatment of radiosensitive recurrent tumors.

## REFERENCES

1. Balme, H. W.: Metastatic carcinoma of thyroid successfully treated with thyroxine. Lancet, *1*:812–813, 1954.
2. Barsano, C. P., Skosey, C., DeGroot, L. J., and Refetoff, S.: Serum thyroglobulin in the management of patients with thyroid cancer. Arch. Intern. Med., *142*:763–767, 1982.
3. Beaugié, J. M., Brown, C. L., Doniach, I., and Richardson, J. E.: Primary malignant tumours of the thyroid: The relationship between histological classification and clinical behaviour. Br. J. Surg., *63*:173–181, 1976.
4. Beierwaltes, W. H.: The treatment of thyroid carcinoma with radioactive iodine. Semin. Nucl. Med., *8*:79–94, 1978.
5. Beierwaltes, W. H., Nishiyama, R. H., Thompson, N. W., et al.: Survival time and "cure" in papillary and follicular thyroid carcinoma with distant metastases: Statistics following University of Michigan therapy. J. Nucl. Med., *23*:561–568, 1982.
6. Beierwaltes, W. H., Rabbani, R., Dmuchowski, C., et al.: An analysis of "ablation of thyroid remnants" with I-131 in 511 patients from 1947–1984: Experience at University of Michigan. J. Nucl. Med., *25*:1287–1293, 1984.
7. Black, B. M., Kirk, T. A., Jr., and Woolner, L. B.: Multicentricity of papillary adenocarcinoma of the thyroid: Influence on treatment. J. Clin. Endocrinol. Metab., *20*:130–135, 1960.
8. Brincker, H., Hansen, H. S., and Andersen, A. P.: Induction of leukaemia by $^{131}$I treatment of thyroid carcinoma. Br. J. Cancer, *28*:232–237, 1973.
9. Brown, A. P., Greening, W. P., McCready, V. R., et al.: Radioiodine treatment of metastatic thyroid carcinoma: The Royal Marsden Hospital experience. Br. J. Radiol., *57*:323–327, 1984.
10. Cady, B., Rossi, R., Silverman, M., and Wool, M.: Further evidence of the validity of risk group definition in differentiated thyroid carcinoma. Surgery, *98*:1171–1178, 1985.
11. Cady, B., Sedgwick, C. E., Meissner, W. A., et al.: Changing clinical, pathologic, therapeutic, and survival patterns in differentiated thyroid carcinoma. Ann. Surg. *184*:541–553, 1976.
12. Cady, B., Sedgwick, C. E., Meissner, W. A., et al.: Risk factor analysis in differentiated thyroid cancer. Cancer, *43*:810–820, 1979.
13. Cady, B., Cohn, K., Rossi, R. L., et al.: The effect of thyroid hormone administration upon survival in patients with differentiated thyroid carcinoma. Surgery, *94*:978–983, 1983.
14. Charbord, P., L'Heritier, C., Cukersztein, W., et al.: Radioiodine treatment in differentiated thyroid carcinomas: Treatment of first local recurrences and of bone and lung metastases. Ann. Radiol. (Paris), *20*:783–786, 1977.
15. Clark, O. H.: TSH suppression in the management of thyroid nodules and thyroid cancer. World J. Surg., *5*:39–47, 1981.
16. Clark, R. L., Jr., White, E. C., and Russell, W. O.: Total thyroidectomy for cancer of the thyroid: Significance of intraglandular dissemination. Ann. Surg., *149*:858–866, 1959.
17. Crile, G., Jr.: The endocrine dependency of certain thyroid cancers and the danger that hypothyroidism may stimulate their growth. Cancer, *10*:1119–1137, 1957.
18. Crile, G., Jr.: Endocrine dependency of papillary carcinomas of the thyroid. J.A.M.A., *195*:721–724, 1966.
19. Crile, G., Jr., McNamara, J. M., and Hazard, J. B.: Results of treatment of papillary carcinoma of the thyroid. Surg. Gynecol. Obstet., *109*:315–320, 1959.
20. DeGroot, L. J., and Reilly, M.: Comparison of 30- and 50-mCi doses of iodine-131 for thyroid ablation. Ann. Intern. Med., *96*:51–53, 1982.
21. Denney, J. D., Marty, R., Schor, R. A., and Van Herle, A. J.: Serum thyroglobulin as an indicator of metastatic well differentiated thyroid carcinoma. (Abstract.) J. Nucl. Med., *19*:678, 1978.
22. Dunhill, T. P.: The surgery of the thyroid gland: The Lettsomian Lectures. Trans. Med. Soc. Lond., *60*:234, 1937.
23. Edmonds, C. J., and Smith, T.: The long-term hazards of the treatment of thyroid cancer with radioiodine. Br. J. Radiol., *59*:45–51, 1986.
24. Gardet, P., Parmentier, C., Gerard-Marchant, R., et al.: Differentiated cancers of the thyroid: Course after treatment with special reference to frequency and chronology of the first relapse for 470 patients. Ann. Radiol. (Paris), *20*:831–840, 1977.
25. Hill, L. D., Beebe, H. G., Hipp, R., and Jones, H. W.: Thyroid suppression. Arch. Surg., *108*:403–405, 1974.
26. Ingbar, S, H., and Woeber, K. A.: The thyroid gland. *In* Williams, R. H. (ed.): Textbook of Endocrinology. Edition 6. Philadelphia, W. B. Saunders Co., 1981, pp. 117–247.
27. Jesse, R. H.: Discussion. *In* Harness, J. K., Thompson, N. W., Sisson, J. C., and Beierwaltes, W. H.: Differentiated thyroid carcinomas: Treatment of distant metastases. Arch. Surg., *108*:418, 1974.

28. Krishnamurthy, G. T., and Blahd, W. H.: Radioiodine I-131 therapy in the management of thyroid cancer: A prospective study. Cancer, *40*:195–202, 1977.
29. Lo Gerfo, P., Colacchio, T., Colacchio, D., and Feind, C.: Thyroglobulin in benign and malignant thyroid disease. J.A.M.A., *241*:923–925, 1979.
30. Lo Gerfo, P. L., Stillman, T., Colacchio, D., and Feind, C.: Serum thyroglobulin and recurrent thyroid cancer. Lancet, *1*:881–882, 1977.
31. Mazzaferri, E. L., Young, R. L., Oertel, J. E., et al.: Papillary thyroid carcinoma: The impact of therapy in 576 patients. Medicine, *56*:171–196, 1977.
32. McConahey, W. M., Hay, I. D., Woolner, L. B., et al.: Papillary thyroid cancer treated at the Mayo Clinic, 1946 through 1970: Initial manifestations, pathologic findings, therapy, and outcome. Mayo Clin. Proc., *61*:978–996, 1986.
33. McCowen, K. D., Adler, R. A., Ghaed, N., et al.: Low dose radioiodine thyroid ablation in postsurgical patients with thyroid cancer. Am. J. Med., *61*:52–58, 1976.
34. Nemec, J., Röhling, S., Zamrazil, V., and Pohunková, D.: Comparison of the distribution of diagnostic and thyroablative I-131 in the evaluation of differentiated thyroid cancers. J. Nucl. Med., *20*:92–97, 1979.
35. Pacini, F., Pinchera, A., Giani, C., et al: Serum thyroglobulin concentrations and $^{131}$I whole body scans in the diagnosis of metastases from differentiated thyroid carcinoma (after thyroidectomy). Clin. Endocrinol., *13*:107–110, 1980.
36. Pochin, E. E.: Prospects from the treatment of thyroid carcinoma with radioiodine. Clin. Radiol., *18*:113–125, 1967.
37. Pochin, E. E.: Radioiodine therapy of thyroid carcinoma. Semin. Nucl. Med., *1*:503–515, 1971.
38. Ramanna, L., Waxman, A. D., Brachman, M. B., et al.: Evaluation of low-dose radioactive iodine ablation therapy in postsurgical thyroid cancer patients. Clin. Nucl. Med., *10*:791–795, 1985.
39. Rawson, R. W., Rall, J. E., and Peacock, W.: Limitations and indications in the treatment of cancer of the thyroid with radioactive iodine. J. Clin. Endocrinol. Metab., *11*:1128–1142, 1951.
40. Rees-Jones, R. W., Rolla, A. R., and Larsen, P. R.: Hormonal content of thyroid replacement preparations. J.A.M.A., *243*:549–550, 1980.
41. Rose, R. G., Kelsey, M. P., Russell, W. O., et al.: Follow-up study of thyroid cancer treated by unilateral lobectomy. Am. J. Surg., *106*:494–500, 1963.
42. Ross, D. S.: New sensitive immunoradiometric assays for thyrotropin. Ann. Intern. Med., *104*:718–720, 1986.
43. Russell, W. O., Ibanez, M. L., Clark, R. L., and White, E. C.: Thyroid carcinoma: Classification, intraglandular dissemination, and clinicopathological study based upon whole organ sections of 80 glands. Cancer, *16*:1425–1460, 1963.
44. Samaan, N. A., Maheshwari, Y. K., Nader, S., et al.: Impact of therapy for differentiated carcinoma of the thyroid: An analysis of 706 cases. J. Clin. Endocrinol. Metab., *56*:1131–1138, 1983.
45. Sampson, R. J., Oka, H., Key, C. R., et al.: Metastases from occult thyroid carcinoma: An autopsy study from Hiroshima and Nagasaki, Japan. Cancer, *25*:803–811, 1970.
46. Sarkar, S. D., Beierwaltes, W. H., Gill, S. P., and Cowley, B. J.: Subsequent fertility and birth histories of children and adolescents treated with 131I for thyroid cancer. J. Nucl. Med., *17*:460–464, 1976.
47. Savoie, J. C., and Garnier, H.: A propos d'une série de 145 cas de cancers thyroïdien et du traitement par thyroïdectomie totale complétée par le radio-iode. Presse Med., *75*:2095–2100, 1967.
48. Schneider, A. B., Line, B. R., Goldman, J. M., and Robbins, J.: Sequential serum thyroglobulin determinations, $^{131}$I scans, and $^{131}$I uptakes after triiodothyronine withdrawal in patients with thyroid cancer. J. Clin. Endocrinol. Metab., *53*:1199–1206, 1981.
49. Simpson, W. J., and Carruthers, J. S.: The role of external radiation in the management of papillary and follicular thyroid cancer. Am. J. Surg., *136*:457–460, 1978.
50. Snyder, J., Gorman, C., and Scanlon, P.: Thyroid remnant ablation: Questionable pursuit of an ill-defined goal. J. Nucl. Med., *24*:659–665, 1983.
51. Tang Fui, S. C. N., Hoffenberg, R., Maisey, M. N., and Black, E. G.: Serum thyroglobulin concentrations and whole-body radioiodine scan in follow-up of differentiated thyroid cancer after thyroid ablation. Br. Med. J., *2*:298–300, 1979.
52. Tollefsen, H. R., Shah, J. P., and Huvos, A. G.: Papillary carcinoma of the thyroid: Recurrence in the thyroid gland after initial surgical treatment. Am. J. Surg., *124*:468–472, 1972.
53. Torrigiani, G., Doniach, D., and Roitt, I. M.: Serum thyroglobulin levels in healthy subjects and in patients with thyroid disease. J. Clin. Endocrinol. Metab., *29*:305–314, 1969.
54. Trunnell, J. B.: Iodine therapy in thyroid carcinoma. *In* Andrews, G. A., Brucer, M., and Anderson, E. H. (eds.): Radioisotopes in Medicine. A Course Given by the Oak Ridge Institute of Nuclear Studies, September 1953. Washington, D.C., U.S. Atomic Energy Commission, 1955, pp. 374–392.
55. Tubiana, M.: External radiotherapy and radioiodine in the treatment of thyroid cancer. World J. Surg., *5*:75–84, 1981.
56. Van Herle, A. J., and Uller, R. P.: Elevated serum thyroglobulin: A marker of metastases in differentiated thyroid carcinomas. J. Clin. Invest., *56*:272–277, 1975.
57. Varma, V. M., Beierwaltes, W. H., Nofal, M. M., et al.: Treatment of thyroid cancer: Death rates after surgery and after surgery followed by sodium iodide I 131. J.A.M.A., *214*:1437–1442, 1970.
58. Waxman, A., Ramanna, L., Chapman, N., et al.: The significance of I-131 scan dose in patients with thyroid cancer: Determination of ablation. Concise communication. J. Nucl. Med., *22*:861–865, 1981.
59. Young, R. L., Mazzaferri, E. L., Rahe, A. J., and Dorfman, S. G.: Pure follicular thyroid carcinoma: Impact of therapy in 214 patients. J. Nucl. Med., *21*:733–737, 1980.

# 20

# EXTERNAL BEAM RADIOTHERAPY IN CARCINOMA OF THYROID GLAND

*Ferdinand A. Salzman, M.D., and Charles F. Andrews, M.D.*

The precise role of external beam radiotherapy in each of the various histologic subtypes of carcinoma of the thyroid is difficult to assess. The low incidence of these tumors is a factor hindering controlled clinical trials that might give statistically valid answers to therapeutic queries. In its various histologic aspects, the disease seems either to grow and metastasize excessively slowly with relapses possible as long as 35 years after therapy (as in differentiated cell types)[35] or to progress so rapidly as to leave doubt in many cases as to the value of any treatment (as in anaplastic cell types). Furthermore, survival is higher for patients with differentiated thyroid carcinoma treated after 1960,[5, 16] but the precise reasons for this increased survival are unknown. Of perhaps most importance has been a failure of most reports to take into consideration the effect of age and sex on prognosis as has convincingly been pointed out in several reports from this institution[6–8, 23, 26] as well as from the E.O.R.T.C. thyroid tumor group,[3] which has constructed a prognostic index emphasizing age.

The modern era of radiotherapy dates to about 1955 to 1960 when most centers shifted from routine use of orthovoltage to megavoltage apparatus. Although it is doubtful whether any institution would have sufficient patients with the various subtypes of thyroid carcinoma treated by primary or adjuvant megavolt radiotherapy for statistically valid analysis, reports[13, 14, 20, 25, 27–29, 31, 34, 35] suggest the usefulness of radiotherapy in certain situations, particularly in inoperable or incompletely excised thyroid tumors.

## TECHNICAL ASPECTS

The radiotherapist has a wide choice of radiation energies. Linear accelerators that deliver photon (x-ray) energies from 4 to 6 Mev, telecobalt machines, and multimode accelerators delivering electron energies in the 12 to 30 Mev range are available and suitable for treatment of patients with thyroid carcinoma. Because the primary disease is mainly in the anterior aspect of the neck and anterior mediastinum, photon energies need not be more than 4 Mev. In this situation, opposed anterior and posterior fields are useful; the operator should bear in mind to apply spinal cord protection using posterior absorbers at the appropriate dose level. We prefer to exclude the cord from the primary beam at about 4,000 cGy. Alternatively, particularly in some well-differentiated carcinomas confined to the midline or thyroid bed, it may be possible to irradiate through opposing paired lateral fields so that the posterior margin does not extend to overlap the spinal cord and to use a compensator or wedge filter to modify the isodoses appropriately.

Electrons, preferably in the 20 to 30 Mev range, with their energy-dependent finite penetration are especially helpful and permit the use of a single anterior field with a central or midline absorber to reduce the high central dose at the level of the spinal cord to a safe level.

The problems of optimizing dose homogeneity and shielding sensitive structures, such as the esophagus and particularly the spinal cord, when photon radiation is used are solved with the 360-degree rotational technique.[40] A single shaped field that extends from the angle of the mandible down to include the anterosuperior mediastinum, if necessary, may be irradiated with the patient rotating through 360 degrees while in the sitting position. A 2-cm diameter lead rod, shaped to conform to the patient's cervical spinal curvature, rotates synchronously with the patient. The rod in effect "shadows" the spinal cord, thereby reducing the dose to it to an acceptable tolerance level. In the conventional fractionation regimens, a daily dose of 170 to 200 cGy is administered 4 to 5 days a week over 5 to 7 weeks.

Radiation doses are in the range of 5,000 to 6,000 cGy for the differentiated and medullary cell tumors, with boosts of 500 to 1,500 cGy to localized residue not uncommon. For the lymphomas, a minimum of 4,000 cGy with boost doses of 1,000 to 1,500 cGy to areas of disease suffice.

Dose recommendations for the anaplastic group of thyroid carcinomas are less dogmatic, and recent radiobiologic insights into altered fractionation regimens for more resistant tumors have some promise of improving the dismal results in this group.[29] These accelerated hyperfraction radiation schemes consist of giving smaller than conventional dose fractions two or three times a day.[38, 39] The radiobiologic aim is to increase radiation tolerance of the late responding normal tissues relative to early responding normal tissues for an acceptable long-term injury of the normal tissues while at the same time delivering higher than conventional daily doses to the tumor. The preferred scheme at present appears to be to administer a fraction size of 160 cGy twice a day with a minimum of 4 hours between fractions for a total dose of approximately 67 Gy.[38] This plan has resulted in acceptable late radiation effects in normal tissues and improved local control in many advanced epithelial carcinomas of the head and neck.

Radiation laryngitis, esophagitis, and tracheitis are expected concomitants of conventional treatment. Their severity will be related to the daily and total doses and in most instances can be ameliorated by advising a soft or liquid diet with appropriate dietary adjustment and the judicious use of analgesics and oral viscous lidocaine. On occasion, it is necessary to interrupt the treatments for 7 to 10 days. Appropriate hydration should be maintained.

Special laryngeal blocking devices are also useful, but care must be taken not to shield tumor. Skin tolerance to the conventional regimens is rarely a problem.

In accelerated fractionation techniques, such as twice daily treatment, all normal tissues react strongly early, and rest periods of 2 weeks or more are required after 2 to 2½ weeks of radiation therapy. A few patients may require hospitalization because of severe dehydration.

Damage to the spinal cord must be guarded against by careful attention to positioning of the treatment fields or by use of appropriate absorbers to block the spinal cord or both. Calculation, preferably computer assisted, of the resulting dose distribution in and around the vicinity of the spinal cord is mandatory.

## DIFFERENTIATED THYROID CARCINOMA: PAPILLARY, FOLLICULAR, AND MIXED PAPILLARY AND FOLLICULAR CARCINOMA

Routine prophylactic postoperative external beam radiotherapy is not recommended for patients with differentiated thyroid carcinoma because the results of surgery alone are excellent.[7, 23, 35] The available data do not justify this therapeutic approach, particularly in patients in the low-risk group as defined at our institution, that is, women 50 years of age and younger and men 40 years of age and younger.[8]

Our indications for adjuvant external beam radiotherapy are based on our studies[26] of the prognostic importance of the risk factors (age and sex) and a review of 940 patients treated between 1931 and 1980. Of the 940 patients with well-differentiated thyroid carcinoma initially seen at the Lahey Clinic Medical Center, a subset of 97 patients (10 per cent) was deemed to have surgically incurable disease, in 17 (1.8 per cent) because of distant metastatic disease. Of the 80 patients with locally incurable disease, 52 patients received external beam irradiation (Table 20–1). The risk category prognostic factor holds for radiotherapy response and for radioactive iodine and thyroid suppression as well. Only one of 21 patients in the low-risk group receiving adjuvant radiotherapy subsequently died of thyroid carcinoma, whereas 28 of 31 patients in the high-risk group eventually died of thyroid carcinoma.

Our indications for adjuvant external beam radiotherapy are, therefore, restricted to patients with inoperable or residual disease that does not take up radioactive iodine and particularly to patients in the high-risk category. In the older age group, radioactive iodine uptake is less frequent and less complete.[10, 18, 35] We also recommend the administration of thyroid hormone.

## Recurrent and Metastatic Disease

Surgery, external beam radiotherapy, and radioactive iodine all have a role in the treatment of patients with recurrent carcinoma. In differentiated thyroid carcinoma, local recurrent disease tends to evolve over an extended period, permitting sequential therapies. It is important to establish first whether surgery or radioactive iodine therapy is possible before external beam radiotherapy is begun. Not only small but large recurrent carcinomas are amenable to surgical intervention today. In the event of massive recurrent tumor, particularly inoperable invasion of the trachea or spread into the mediastinum, aggressive external beam radiation is indicated because salvage, if not cure, for long periods is possible. For localized tracheal invasion, supplemental iridium 192 seed endotracheal brachytherapy (endocurietherapy) is worthwhile in the absence of satisfactory radioactive iodine uptake. However, occasionally operation may be possible.[4]

Fortunately, pulmonary metastatic disease tends to be of the type that takes up radioactive iodine and is the first therapy considered for these patients. When uptake is demonstrated, long-term survival and even cure have been documented. External beam radiation is rarely necessary and is strictly limited to a lower than adequate total dose.

Osseous metastatic disease is seen in almost every bone but most commonly in the sternum, long bones, and the base of the skull. In the high-risk group, radioactive iodine uptake is poor, and aggressive external beam radiation should be administered after

**TABLE 20–1. Differentiated Thyroid Carcinoma: Adjuvant Therapy in 80 Patients with Surgically Incurable Neck Disease**

| | EXTERNAL BEAM RADIATION | | | | THYROID SUPPRESSION | | | | RADIOACTIVE IODINE | | | |
|---|---|---|---|---|---|---|---|---|---|---|---|---|
| | Treated | | Not Treated | | Treated | | Not Treated | | Treated | | Not Treated | |
| | No. | *No. (%) Dead of Disease* | No. | *No. (%) Dead of Disease* | No. | *No. (%) Dead of Disease* | No. | *No. (%) Dead of Disease* | No. | *No. (%) Dead of Disease* | No. | *No. (%) Dead of Disease* |
| High risk | 31 | 28 (90)* | 12 | 6 (50)* | 16 | 7 (44)† | 25 | 25 (100)† | 4 | 2 (50) | 33 | 25 (76) |
| Low risk | 21 | 1 (5) | 17 | 4 (24) | 25 | 2 (8) | 13 | 3 (23) | 8 | 2 (25) | 30 | 3 (10) |
| High vs low | P <0.001 | | P = 0.17 | | P = 0.01 | | P = 0.001 | | P = 0.47 | | P = 0.001 | |

From Rossi, R. L., Cady, B., Silverman, M. L., et al.: Surgically incurable well-differentiated thyroid carcinoma: Prognostic factors and results of therapy. Arch. Surg., *123*:572, 1988, with permission.
*Difference in number of patients dead of disease in high-risk group treated and not treated (P = 0.008).
†Difference in number of patients dead of disease in high-risk group treated and not treated (P <0.001).

attempts at stimulating uptake have failed. Even in the presence of radioactive iodine uptake, large osteolytic lesions may require supplementary external beam radiation to speed healing. A dose of at least 4,000 cGy may be needed to relieve pain and stimulate healing. Results are the poorest with follicular cell carcinoma. Again, we recommend administration of thyroid hormone for its suppressive effect.

## UNDIFFERENTIATED THYROID CARCINOMA: GIANT CELL, SPINDLE CELL, AND SMALL CELL

Undifferentiated thyroid carcinoma is rarely found in patients less than 40 years of age.[16, 24] As a group, these carcinomas are extremely aggressive and show poor radioresponse. Occasional excellent responses have been reported[30] in patients with the small cell compact type. Many of these radiosensitive small cell thyroid tumors have, on review and in light of recent ultrastructural and immunohistochemical studies, been reclassified as lymphomas. Other less radiosensitive small cell tumors may well be variants of anaplastic medullary or follicular carcinoma.[19, 21, 22]

Patients with the giant cell and spindle cell variety typically present with massive involvement of the thyroid by a hard mass with extension beyond the normal confines of the gland. Usually only biopsy is possible, and not infrequently tracheostomy is necessary. These tumors are among the most aggressive locally of any malignant neoplasms known, and they have not responded favorably to conventional radiotherapy. In our reported experience,[24] radiotherapy was administered to 89 per cent of 109 patients. Of the 109 patients, 51 had giant cell carcinoma, 36 had small cell diffuse carcinoma, 9 had small cell compact carcinoma, and in 13 patients, the tumor was unclassifiable. Doses usually exceeded 6,000 cGy using conventional fractionation. The 5-year disease-free survival was 8 per cent for patients with giant cell carcinoma, 33 per cent for patients with small cell diffuse carcinoma, and 11 per cent for patients with small cell compact carcinoma. All 5-year survivors had surgery and radiotherapy. Six of 24 patients with small cell diffuse carcinoma who had residual disease at completion of operation were cured. Patients cured of disease were younger than patients who died of disease.

A more promising radiotherapeutic approach has been reported by Simpson,[28] in which multiple daily fractions (100 cGy given four times a day) were administered to 11 patients with anaplastic thyroid carcinoma to a total dose of 3,600 cGy. Complete regression of tumor was possible in four patients, and three patients were alive and free of disease at 6½, 8, and 15 months. The fourth patient, although free of tumor, died of complications at 22 months. No further reports have appeared on the use of this accelerated hyperfractionation treatment in anaplastic thyroid carcinoma, although it is gaining in favor in other advanced head and neck carcinomas.[38] Wang (personal communication, 1988) stated that in the few patients with anaplastic thyroid carcinoma treated to date using two fractions daily, tumor shrinkage has been prompt and rapid, leading to good local control, but the patient is likely to die of metastatic disease. In his opinion, this is the most promising radiotherapeutic method of treating patients with anaplastic thyroid carcinoma.

### *Recurrent and Metastatic Disease*

In this group, survival after initial treatment is so low that recurrent carcinoma is rarely a clinical problem except possibly for the occasional patient with small cell carcinoma. In the unusual event that carcinoma recurs, the previous administration of high doses of radiotherapy, whether from conventional or hyperfractionation, precludes any further local irradiation. However, radiotherapy of metastatic disease may be necessary during the phase of primary neck therapy. As in any other progressing carcinoma, only palliation should be attempted. Depending on the site of the metastatic tumor, daily doses of 200 to 300 cGy carried to at least 3,000 cGy are administered. When relief of pain is not forthcoming by an accumulated dose of 4,500 cGy, therapy is discontinued, and narcotics are given. These patients are usually elderly, and they have poor tolerance for aggressive treatment, particularly when it is not palliative.

## MEDULLARY THYROID CARCINOMA

This unique tumor arising from the calcitonin-producing parafollicular C cells within the thyroid gland may occur sporadically or in familial groups. It constitutes approximately 5 per cent of all thyroid carcinomas. It has no avidity for radioactive iodine nor does it secrete thyroglobulin, but it does secrete calcitonin. The primary treatment is surgery. It is thought to be radioresistant, but this has not been the experience at our institution[25] or of some other workers.[29, 33] We have seen fewer patients for radiotherapy in recent years probably because earlier detection by calcitonin screening is making curative surgery more common. Patients with macroscopic tumor and patients with inoperable carcinoma fare well with aggressive radiotherapy. Tubiana[33] reported on 72 patients with medullary carcinoma of whom 29 patients received radiotherapy (15 prophylactically and 14 after incomplete excision) compared with 26 patients treated by surgery alone. The 20-year survival was higher in patients receiving radiation (50 per cent) than in patients receiving surgery only (25 per cent). Of eight patients with inoperable lesions, radiotherapy was effective in six patients. A smaller radiotherapy experience at our institution has not matched these results.[25]

Calcitonin is useful as a tumor marker, and an elevated level after operation may indicate persistence of clinically important disease. When the surgeon is satisfied that no local tumor persists, it does not seem justified to search aggressively for occult metastatic disease. After adequate surgery, calcitonin levels should return to normal levels slowly—as long as 12 years—despite the absence of clinical recurrence of tumor.[39]

### *Recurrent and Metastatic Disease*

When a patient has had previous definitive external beam radiation approaching or exceeding 5,000 cGy, further useful treatment is not possible. Additional exposure would exceed normal tissue tolerance in the neck and only add to and worsen the patient's discomfort. Soft tissue metastatic disease not previously irradiated requires doses approaching 5,000 cGy over a period of 5 weeks. Limited soft tissue disease should be pursued vigorously, and response and extent of residual tumor should be monitored with calcitonin assays. In this way, survival may be extended for years. Osseous metastatic disease is more ominous but does not necessarily imply a rapid demise. Relief of pain is the primary concern and can be achieved by appropriate external beam radiation.

Osteolytic lesions of the weight-bearing long bones are especially painful and in most patients carry the additional hazard of a pathologic fracture. In these circumstances, daily fractionated doses of 250 to 400 cGy of external beam radiation to a total dose of 2,500 to 4,000 cGy, depending on the size of the lesion, bring about a good response. When an osteolytic lesion in the femur, especially near the femoral neck, is 3 cm or larger and abuts a cortical surface, a pathologic fracture is considered imminent, and rod fixation is carried out before radiotherapy is started regardless of the histologic characteristics of the tumor.

## LYMPHOMA OF THYROID

Lymphomas of the thyroid constitute approximately 4 to 5 per cent of thyroid carcinomas.[12, 17, 32] The diagnosis is usually made after open biopsy or thyroidectomy for a rapidly enlarging thyroid mass. The most common histologic subtype is diffuse histiocytic lymphoma, which accounts for more than 75 per cent of thyroid lymphomas.[1, 2, 32, 36, 37] When the diagnosis has been made, postoperative evaluation and staging workup should be completed, which usually requires radiography of the chest, complete blood studies, bone marrow examination, and evaluation of abdominal lymph nodes with computed tomography, lymphangiography, or both.[1, 37] Although less applicable in non-Hodgkin's lymphomas, the Ann Arbor staging classification[9] should be used in evaluating these patients. In most patients, thyroid lymphoma is classified as either stage Iet or stage IIet. The "e" designates lymphoma arising in extranodal tissue, and the "t" designates the thyroid locus.

No clinical trials have compared different treatment modalities for patients with thyroid lymphomas, and guidelines must be formulated by examining results from multiple large referral centers. Surgery is the initial step and is usually needed for the diagnosis. However, some physicians[15] believe that as needle biopsy techniques improve, it may be possible to forego surgery.

Regardless of the type of surgery performed, postoperative irradiation is required for optimal control in patients with either stage Iet or stage IIet disease. Megavoltage equipment should be used, and the volume of treated tissue should include the neck bilaterally and the supraclavicular and mediastinal lymphatics.[1, 11, 32, 36, 37] The usual dose to these regions is at least 4,000 cGy with "boost" doses of 1,000 to 1,500 cGy to areas of residual disease. With doses greater than 4,000 cGy, local control rates approach 90 per cent.[36] A group from the M. D. Anderson Hospital[37] reported experience in 38 patients of whom 16 were treated by radiation alone with this volume and dose. Five-year rates of overall survival and disease-free survival for patients with stage Iet disease were 100 and 83 per cent, respectively, and for patients with stage IIet disease, rates were 88 and 75 per cent. In a review of 20 patients with thyroid lymphoma, the group from Princess Margaret Hospital[32] in Toronto found that all patients with stage Iet and nonmediastinal stage IIet disease treated with radiotherapy to the neck and mediastinum survived 5 years. No patient survived for 5 years with stage IIet mediastinal involvement or with stage Iet disease treated with irradiation only to the neck. Similarly, the Mayo Clinic experience[1] demonstrated fewer treatment failures among patients treated with irradiation to the neck and mediastinum than in patients who received treatment to the neck alone.

### *Recurrent and Metastatic Disease*

In patients with lymphoma of the thyroid, treatment failure is usually systemic, especially for patients in whom the initial presentation includes involvement of the mediastinum. Here, the principles governing treatment of lymphomas with chemotherapy, preferably multiagent, come into play. The patient's condition, extent of involvement, and lymphoma cell type are the important determinants of the drug to be administered and the aggressiveness of the treatment. In our experience, radiotherapy is not contraindicated for patients with tumor not previously irradiated and is useful for palliation. Doses in the range of 3,500 to 4,500 cGy help to relieve the pain of bone involvement.

## REFERENCES


1. Blair, T. J., Evans, R. G., Buskirk, S. J., et al.: Radiotherapeutic management of primary thyroid lymphoma. Int. J. Radiat. Oncol. Biol. Phys., *11*:365–370, 1985.
2. Burke, J. S., Butler, J. J., and Fuller, L. M.: Malignant lymphomas of the thyroid: A clinical pathologic study of 35 patients including ultrastructural considerations. Cancer, *39*:1587–1602, 1977.
3. Byar, D. P., Green, S. B., Dor, P., et al.: A prognostic index for thyroid carcinoma: A study of the E.O.R.T.C. thyroid cancer cooperative group. Eur. J. Cancer, *15*:1033–1041, 1979.
4. Cady, B.: Management of tracheal obstruction from thyroid diseases. World J. Surg., *6*:696–701, 1982.
5. Cady, B., and Wool, M. S.: Cancer of the thyroid. *In* Cady, B. (ed.): Cancer Manual. 7th Edition. Boston, American Cancer Society, Inc., Massachusetts Division, 1986, pp. 141–150.
6. Cady, B., Rossi, R. L, Silverman, M., and Wool, M. S.: Further evidence of the validity of risk group definition in differentiated thyroid carcinoma. Surgery, *98*:1171–1178, 1985.
7. Cady, B., Sedgwick, C. E., Meissner, W. A., et al.: Changing clinical, pathologic, therapeutic, and survival patterns in differentiated thyroid carcinoma. Ann. Surg., *184*:541–553, 1976.
8. Cady, B., Sedgwick, C. E., Meissner, W. A., et al.: Risk factor analysis in differentiated thyroid cancer. Cancer, *43*:810–820, 1979.
9. Carbone, P. P., Kaplan, H. S., Musshoff, K., et al.: Report of the committee on Hodgkin's disease staging classification. Cancer Res., *31*:1860–1861, 1971.
10. Charbord, P., L'Heritier, C., Cukersztein, W., et al.: Radioiodine treatment in differentiated thyroid carcinomas: Treatment of first local recurrences and of bone and lung metastases. Ann. Radiol., *20*:783–786, 1977.
11. Devine, R. M., Edis, A. J., and Banks, P. M.: Primary lymphoma of the thyroid: A review of the Mayo Clinic experience through 1978. World J. Surg., *5*:33–38, 1981.
12. Grimley, R. P., and Oates, G. D.: The natural

history of malignant lymphomas. Br. J. Surg., *67*:475–477, 1980.
13. Halnan, K. E.: Influence of age and sex on incidence and prognosis of thyroid cancer: Three hundred forty-four cases followed for ten years. Cancer, *19*:1534–1536, 1966.
14. Halnan, K. E.: The non-surgical treatment of thyroid cancer. Br. J. Surg., *62*:769–771, 1975.
15. Hamburger, J. I., Miller, J. M., and Kini, S. R.: Lymphoma of the thyroid. Ann. Intern. Med., *99*:685–693, 1983.
16. Heitz, P., Moser, H., and Staub, J.-J.: Thyroid cancer: A study of 573 thyroid tumors and 161 autopsy cases observed over a thirty-year period. Cancer, *37*:2329–2337, 1976.
17. Kapadia, S. B., Dekker, A., Cheng, V. S., et al.: Malignant lymphoma of the thyroid gland: A clinicopathologic study. Head Neck Surg., *4*:270–280, 1982.
18. Leeper, R. D.: The effect of $^{131}$I therapy on survival of patients with metastatic papillary or follicular thyroid carcinoma. J. Clin. Endocrinol. Metab., *36*:1143–1152, 1973.
19. Mambo, N. C., and Irwin, S. M.: Anaplastic small cell neoplasms of the thyroid: An immunoperoxidase study. Hum. Pathol., *15*:55–60, 1984.
20. McWhirter, R.: The value of clinical staging in thyroid cancer. *In* Hedinger, C. E. (ed.): Thyroid Cancer. U.I.C.C. Monograph series. Vol. 12, Berlin, Springer-Verlag, 1969, pp. 235–258.
21. Rayfield, E. J., Nishiyama, R. H., and Sisson, J. C.: Small cell tumors of the thyroid: A clinicopathologic study. Cancer, *28*:1023–1030, 1971.
22. Rosai, J., and Carcangiu, M. L.: Pathology of thyroid tumors: Some recent and old questions. Hum. Pathol., *15*:1008–1012, 1984.
23. Rossi, R. L, Nieroda, C., Cady, B., and Wool, M. S.: Malignancies of the thyroid gland: The Lahey Clinic experience. Surg. Clin. North Am., *65*:211–230, 1985.
24. Rossi, R. L., Cady, B., Meissner, W. A., et al.: Prognosis of undifferentiated carcinoma and lymphoma of the thyroid. Am. J. Surg., *135*:589–595, 1978.
25. Rossi, R. L., Cady, B., Meissner, W. A., et al.: Nonfamilial medullary thyroid carcinoma. Am. J. Surg., *139*:554–559, 1980.
26. Rossi, R. L., Cady, B., Silverman, M. L., et al.: Surgically incurable well-differentiated thyroid carcinoma: Prognostic factors and results of therapy. Arch. Surg., *123*:569–574, 1988.
27. Sheline, G. E., Galante, M., and Lindsay, S.: Radiation therapy in the control of persistent thyroid cancer. A.J.R., *97*:923–930, 1966.
28. Simpson, W. J.: Anaplastic thyroid carcinoma: A new approach. Can. J. Surg., *23*:25–27, 1980.
29. Simpson, W. J., and Carruthers, J. S.: The role of external radiation in the management of papillary and follicular thyroid cancer. Am. J. Surg., *136*:457–460, 1978.
30. Smedal, M. I., and Meissner, W. A.: The results of x-ray treatment in undifferentiated carcinoma of the thyroid. Radiology, *76*:927–935, 1961.
31. Smedal, M. I., Salzman, F. A., and Meissner, W. A.: The value of 2 mv. roentgen-ray therapy in differentiated thyroid carcinoma. A.J.R., *99*:352–364, 1967.
32. Souhami, L., Simpson, W. J., and Carruthers, J. S.: Malignant lymphoma of the thyroid gland. Int. J. Radiat. Oncol. Biol. Phys., *6*:1143–1147, 1980.
33. Tubiana, M.: External radiotherapy and radionuclide in the treatment of thyroid cancer. World J. Surg., *5*:75–84, 1981.
34. Tubiana, M., Lacour, J., Monnier, J. P., et al.: External radiotherapy and radioiodine in the treatment of 359 thyroid cancers. Br. J. Radiol., *48*:894–907, 1975.
35. Tubiana, M., Schlumberger, M., Rougier, P., et al.: Long-term results and prognostic factors in patients with differentiated thyroid carcinoma. Cancer, *55*:794–804, 1985.
36. Tupchong, L., Hughes, F., and Harmer, C. L.: Primary lymphoma of the thyroid: Clinical features, prognostic factors, and results of treatment. Int. J. Radiat. Oncol. Biol. Phys., *12*:1813–1821, 1986.
37. Vigliotti, A., Kong, J. S., Fuller, L. M., and Velasquez, W. S.: Thyroid lymphomas stages IE and IIE: Comparative results for radiotherapy only, combination chemotherapy only, and multimodality treatment. Int. J. Radiat. Oncol. Biol. Phys., *12*:1807–1812, 1986.
38. Wang, C. C., Blitzer, P. H., and Suit, H. D.: Twice-a-day radiation therapy for cancer of the head and neck. Cancer, *55*:2100–2104, 1985.
39. Withers, H. R.: Biologic basis for altered fractionation schemes. Cancer, *55*:2086–2095, 1985.
40. Wright, K. A., Proimos, B. S., Trump, J. G., et al.: Field shaping and selective protection in megavolt radiation therapy. Radiology, *72*:101, 1959.

# 21

# CHEMOTHERAPY FOR CARCINOMA OF THYROID GLAND

*John H. Wolff, M.D.*

Carcinoma of the thyroid gland is uncommon but when present is associated with a good prognosis. Surgery, radioactive iodine, hormone therapy, and occasionally external beam radiotherapy control the disease for most patients with differentiated carcinoma of the thyroid. Even for patients with distant metastases, these therapies can provide prolonged control of the disease. Only the few patients with differentiated thyroid carcinoma in whom multiple treatment modalities have failed and patients with undifferentiated tumors and lymphomas are referred for consideration for chemotherapy. As a consequence, data that define the role of cytotoxic drug therapy in carcinoma of the thyroid are scant.

The chemotherapeutic drug with the greatest reported experience in carcinoma of the thyroid is doxorubicin (Adriamycin). Gottlieb and Hill[1] reported on 30 patients treated with this agent. A wide variety of histologic types of tumor were represented, with responses seen in patients with all types of carcinoma (Table 21–1). The numbers of patients are too small to permit comparison of response rates by histologic factors. No patient had a complete response, but 11 patients had a partial response defined as at least a 50 per cent decrease in the product of the two largest perpendicular diameters of the marker lesions. The response rate in this series was 37 per cent, but subsequent experience has been considerably less positive. Other investigators[5] reported response rates of only 17 to 20 per cent.

**TABLE 21–1. Response to Adriamycin by Cell Type**

| CARCINOMA TYPE | NO. OF PATIENTS | PARTIAL RESPONSES |
|---|---|---|
| Differentiated | 10 | 3 |
| Spindle and giant cell | 9 | 2 |
| Medullary | 5 | 3 |
| Hürthle cell | 5 | 2 |
| Unclassified | 1 | 1 |

Data from Gottlieb, J. A., and Hill, C. S., Jr.: Chemotherapy of thyroid cancer with Adriamycin: Experience with 30 patients. N. Engl. J. Med., *290*:193–197, 1974.

Apart from doxorubicin, no good single-agent studies have been carried out. Activity for several agents has been suggested on the basis of small series of patients, often without adequate definition of response. Cisplatin

(Platinol) and bleomycin (Blenoxane) are among these drugs.[2]

Given the suggestion of activity for cisplatin, the Eastern Cooperative Oncology Group[6] performed a prospective randomized study comparing treatment with doxorubicin alone and treatment with a combination of doxorubicin and cisplatin. Evaluation of response was possible in 84 patients. The group treated with doxorubicin alone had a response rate of 17 per cent but no complete responses. Five complete responses plus six partial responses were seen in 43 patients treated with two drugs, and the rate for combined complete response plus partial response was 26 per cent. The difference in complete response rates was statistically significant whereas the difference in major (complete plus partial) response rates was not. Toxicity, as expected, was greater in the group treated with two drugs. In another study[8] of this combination of agents, admittedly smaller and not randomized, only a 9 per cent complete plus partial response rate was observed.

Throughout these studies, some of the responses have been prolonged. In some patients with differentiated tumors (invariably those who achieved complete response), disease has remained in remission for 3 to 5 years or more after cessation of therapy. Such lengthy remissions reflect the indolent nature of these tumors rather than their cure.

## ANAPLASTIC CARCINOMA

Anaplastic carcinoma of the thyroid is usually extremely aggressive, and death from uncontrolled local disease follows closely after the diagnosis is made. A combination of doxorubicin administered weekly and hyperfractionated (twice daily) radiation therapy was effective in controlling local disease in a series of nine patients.[3] One patient had all obvious disease resected before radiation therapy and chemotherapy. The other eight patients were treated after biopsy or partial resection. In seven of the eight patients, the tumor disappeared completely. Two of the seven patients experienced a subsequent relapse and died of local disease; in the other five patients, distant metastases developed. Median survival time was 10 months. In this treatment regimen, doxorubicin acts as a radiation sensitizer in addition to its direct cytotoxic effect. Sensitization occurs also in normal tissues, and the program causes moderate to severe mucositis. Despite the toxicity, this regimen represents a major improvement for patients with this rare tumor.

## LYMPHOMA

Treatment of patients with lymphoma of the thyroid, like that of lymphomas elsewhere, is complex and controversial. The pathologic process may be described in terms of one or more of a number of currently used classification schemes. Most thyroid lymphomas are high-grade lesions, such as diffuse histiocytic or undifferentiated (in the Rappaport classification). After the diagnosis has been made, staging must be designated carefully to permit detection of disease in extrathyroidal sites. Particular attention should be paid to the gastrointestinal tract because of the suggestion that a lymphoma of the thyroid may tend to involve this area more often than lymphoma of other sites.[7] Most lymphomas of the thyroid are localized to the gland at the time of diagnosis. Thyroid lymphoma is a rare disease, and published series involve small numbers of patients treated in many different ways. Guidelines for the treatment of this disease must be drawn from the general principles of lymphoma treatment. Therapy is determined by pathologic findings (grouped into high-grade and low-grade lesions) and stage.

Patients with localized high-grade lymphomas may be treated with radiation therapy with curative intent. Combination chemotherapy may also be curative. The relative worth of radiation and chemotherapy (as well as combined modality treatment) is currently a matter of heated controversy. Because many patients with this disease are elderly, it would be reasonable to treat them with radiation, withholding chemotherapy until relapse is evident. Young patients with this disease may be treated with combined modalities or with chemotherapy alone, although, again, the controversial nature of these treatments must be emphasized. Patients with disseminated high-grade lymphomas are treated with combination chemotherapy, and a portion of these patients are cured. The regimens used are complex aggressive multiagent protocols, such as combinations of methotrexate with leucovorin rescue, doxorubicin, cyclophosphamide, vincristine, prednisone, and bleomycin.[4]

When disease is localized, patients with low-grade lymphomas are treated with radiation therapy. Patients with disseminated low-grade lymphoma have incurable disease. For patients who are truly asymptomatic, careful observation without treatment is an appropriate approach; treatment is instituted whenever symptoms arise. When symptoms are localized, radiation to this region may be given in preference to systemic therapy. When chemotherapy is given, milder forms are used. The regimen may be as simple as a single oral alkylating agent.

## COMMENTS

Chemotherapy for patients with carcinoma of the thyroid is a potentially beneficial treatment with toxicity that is tolerable. When other modalities have failed or the disease is too widespread for local treatment, a trial of drug therapy is appropriate. When the performance status is good, the patient may benefit from aggressive combination therapy with doxorubicin and cisplatin. Prolonged responses are occasionally seen, and excellent palliation may be achieved. Lymphomas are, of course, sensitive to chemotherapy; these patients achieve excellent palliation and some cures with drug treatment.

## REFERENCES

1. Gottlieb, J. A., and Hill, C. S., Jr.: Chemotherapy of thyroid cancer with adriamycin: Experience with 30 patients. N. Engl. J. Med., *290*:193–197, 1974.
2. Harada, T., Nishikawa, Y., Suzuki, T., et al.: Bleomycin treatment for cancer of the thyroid. Am. J. Surg., *122*:53–57, 1971.
3. Kim, J. H., and Leeper, R. D.: Treatment of anaplastic giant and spindle cell carcinoma of the thyroid gland with combination adriamycin and radiation therapy: A new approach. Cancer, *52*:954–957, 1983.
4. Klimo, P., and Connors, J. M.: MACOP-B chemotherapy for the treatment of diffuse large-cell lymphoma. Ann. Intern. Med., *102*:596–602, 1985.
5. Leight, G. S., Farrell, R. E., Wells, S. A., and Falleta, J. M.: Effect of chemotherapy on calcitonin (CT) levels in patients with metastatic medullary thyroid carcinoma (MTC). Abstract 622. Proc. Am. Assoc. Cancer Res., *21*:155, 1980.
6. Shimaoka, K., Schoenfeld, D. A., DeWys, W. D., et al.: A randomized trial of doxorubicin *versus* doxorubicin plus cisplatin in patients with advanced thyroid carcinoma. Cancer, *56*:2155–2160, 1985.
7. Stone, C. W., Slease, R. B., Brubaker, D., et al.: Thyroid lymphoma with gastrointestinal involvement: Report of three cases. Am. J. Hematol., *21*:357–365, 1986.
8. Williams, S. D., Birch, R., and Einhorn, L. H.: Phase II evaluation of doxorubicin plus cisplatin in advanced thyroid cancer: A Southeastern Cancer Study Group Trial. Cancer Treat. Rep., *70*:405–407, 1986.

# 22

# HYPERPARATHYROIDISM

*Eugene P. Clerkin, M.D.*

Hyperparathyroidism may be caused by tumor or hyperplasia of the parathyroid glands resulting in excessive production of parathyroid hormone. The hormone acts directly on bone and kidney to exert a profound influence on mineral metabolism. Bone remodeling is increased, with release of calcium into the extracellular fluid. Production of 1,25-dihydroxyvitamin D by the kidney is also increased, thereby stimulating intestinal absorption of calcium. Parathormone also increases tubular reabsorption, although phosphorus and bicarbonate are decreased. The net effect is to increase movement of calcium into the extracellular fluid and to promote dissolution of bone mineral. This review presents the spectrum of the clinical manifestations resulting from these actions and the approach to therapy.

*Primary hyperparathyroidism* is usually a sporadic disease of unknown cause, although occasionally it results from genetic susceptibility (multiple endocrine neoplasia syndrome or familial hyperparathyroidism). Radiotherapy to the neck in childhood may increase the risk of the development of the disease in later years.[13] The disease is important for several reasons:

Primary hyperparathyroidism is relatively common. In patients older than 60 years of age, the annual incidence approaches 1:500 in women and 1:1000 in men.[12]

The clinical spectrum of the disease is so broad that it must be considered in the differential diagnosis of a number of common clinical problems.

The disease can be cured. Disabling symptoms can be prevented or even reversed when the patient is treated early enough.

## CLINICAL SPECTRUM

Renal calculi, once the hallmark of primary hyperparathyroidism, are now found in only a minority of patients, and the clinical course varies considerably. In some patients a single asymptomatic calculus may form, but in others multiple bilateral calculi are formed. Although the mechanism of formation of calculi is unclear, elevated circulating concentrations of 1,25-dihydroxyvitamin D and hypercalciuria are thought to be contributing factors.

Functional abnormalities of the kidney are even more common than the formation of calculi. Decreased renal tubular reabsorption of bicarbonate produces a tendency to hyperchloremic acidosis. A urine concentrating defect results from reduced responsiveness of the collecting ducts to vasopressin. The defect is usually mild, but occasionally the patient complains of polyuria and polydipsia. More important is a susceptibility to hypovolemia, particularly when complicating events, such as vigorous diuretic therapy, vomiting, and diarrhea, supervene. Although azotemia in the patient with hypercalcemia may be the result of interstitial nephritis, the possibility of prerenal failure caused by volume deficit must always be considered.

Osteitis fibrosa cystica, the classic skeletal lesion of patients with primary hyperparathyroidism, is characterized by bone pain, tenderness, and susceptibility to fracture. Serum alkaline phosphatase level is often mildly elevated, and radiography of the hands may show subperiosteal resorption of the phalanges or even resorption of the tufts of the distal phalanges. Fortunately, this complication is seldom seen today.

Peptic ulcer disease occurs with increased frequency in the presence of primary hyperparathyroidism, although the mechanism is unclear. Gastrinoma and milk-alkali syndrome should be excluded in the patient with peptic ulcer disease and hypercalcemia.

Several complications can be related to the systemic effects of hypercalcemia, but all are uncommon in patients with primary hyperparathyroidism. Hypercalcemic crisis may develop when the serum level of calcium approaches 15 mg/dl and is accompanied by anorexia, nausea, vomiting, fatigue, confusion, and eventually coma. This constitutes a medical emergency because it can progress to oliguric renal failure and tachyarrhythmia with the risk of sudden death.[11] Metastatic calcifications may appear at the corneal scleral junction (band keratopathy). Although unusual, band keratopathy can be important because it is the only clue for hypercalcemia that can be detected on physical examination. Calcifications may also occur in the lung, stomach, skin, pancreas, muscle, and, characteristically, in the renal parenchyma outside the caliceal system (nephrocalcinosis). Maternal hypercalcemia may induce functional atrophy of the fetal parathyroid glands with neonatal tetany. Occasionally, a patient has a debility syndrome characterized by weight loss, decreased appetite, anemia, and florid osteitis, all of which can be reversed by correction of the primary hyperparathyroidism.[5]

Psychiatric symptoms are usually subtle. Impaired concentration or mild depression can occasionally be recognized in retrospect but seldom cause the patient to seek medical attention.

Neuromuscular complications include a mild proximal muscle weakness, which occasionally becomes severe enough to be symptomatic despite normal levels of muscle enzymes.

Rheumatic complications include calcification of the articular cartilage (chondrocalcinosis) and episodes of painful effusion with deposition of calcium pyrophosphate crystals (pseudogout). Gout and calcific periarthritis also occur with increased frequency.

The role of primary hyperparathyroidism in osteoporosis is unclear. Although cortical bone density is appreciably reduced at the time of diagnosis compared with control subjects, trabecular bone is spared.[35] Moreover, the bone loss does not appear to be progressive,[27] and conflicting reports[15, 37] have appeared about the risk of vertebral fracture. The issue is especially important in older women who are at increased risk for the development of both primary hyperparathyroidism and osteoporosis.

Hypertension occurs with increased frequency in patients with primary hyperparathyroidism, but whether a causal relation is present is also unclear. Elevation of blood pressure is usually mild and is not related to the serum level of calcium or creatinine nor does it usually respond to successful treatment of the hyperparathyroidism.[28] When hypertension is found in a patient with primary hyperparathyroidism, pheochromocytoma related to multiple endocrine neoplasia syndrome type II must be considered. In one study,[25] a reduced survival time was reported in patients with untreated primary hyperparathyroidism caused by an increased risk of coronary artery disease. This finding needs confirmation.

Despite this foreboding symptom complex, the majority of patients with primary hyperparathyroidism appear to be asymptomatic at the time of diagnosis. The disease would never have been recognized were it not for the routine measurement of serum levels of calcium in hospital and office practice. Care must be taken, however, before a patient is declared to be asymptomatic because some complications are subtle or even asymptomatic and others are so common in the general population that it may be impossible to establish a causal relation to primary hyperparathyroidism. Moreover, no marker exists for predicting which patients will develop complications in later years.

## DIAGNOSIS

Measurement of total serum calcium is an inexpensive, reliable, and readily available screening test for primary hyperparathyroidism. Ionized calcium, which comprises about 50 per cent of the total serum calcium, is the biologically active portion of the total serum calcium and is tightly regulated by parathyroid hormone and vitamin D. Theoretically, measurement of ionized calcium would be the preferred way of assessing parathyroid function. Although the technology for performing this test is available,[4] it is not widely used, and its clinical advantage for routine testing has not been proved.

Until the early 1960s, the uneven quality of total serum calcium measurement by manual methods in hospital laboratories was a major problem in recognizing disorders of calcium metabolism. Today, the automated methods widely available offer a high degree of precision and accuracy. However, each laboratory must define the normal values for total serum calcium within the narrow range possible using present-day techniques. When doubt exists about the reliability of the result, serum calcium should be measured by atomic absorption spectroscopy.

The clinician must be alert to unexpected or intermittent hypercalcemia detected on routine chemistry profile testing. Although the tendency may be to view such a finding as a laboratory error or one that is not clinically significant, just the opposite is true. The laboratory is likely to be correct, and the patient may be at risk for all of the consequences of primary hyperparathyroidism.

Factitious hypercalcemia can occur when hemoconcentration increases serum levels of albumin as in severe hypovolemia or simply leaving a tourniquet on for too long at the time of phlebotomy. Rarely, massive increases in total globulin level or a myeloma paraprotein increase the total serum level of calcium.

Confusion also arises when an abnormality unrelated to parathyroid disease lowers the total serum calcium level, thereby setting the stage for masked hypercalcemia. The most common example is hypoalbuminemia, which lowers bound calcium and may obscure a rise in ionized calcium. Measurement of ionized calcium can be helpful when this is suspected.

Other events can mask hypercalcemia by reducing the ionized calcium. Chronic renal failure, for example, reduces renal synthesis of 1,25-dihydroxyvitamin D and induces hyperphosphatemia, both of which lower ionized calcium. Serum albumin may also be reduced, thereby lowering bound calcium. When renal insufficiency develops in a patient with primary hyperparathyroidism, the patient may present with a total serum level of calcium that is "normal" or slightly depressed but inappropriate for the degree of renal failure. Establishing the sequence of events may be virtually impossible unless laboratory data are available before the onset of renal failure.

The ionized calcium level may also be lowered in the tumor lysis syndrome because of hyperphosphatemia, vitamin D deficiency states, severe hypomagnesemia, acute pancreatitis, and occasionally primary hypothyroidism. Clearly, the clinician must be alert to the various determinants that can modify the total serum calcium level to interpret this test result properly.

## DIFFERENTIAL DIAGNOSIS OF HYPERCALCEMIA

The differential diagnosis of hypercalcemia is one of the classic problems in medicine and has been discussed in a recent review[3] (Table 22–1). Despite the array of laboratory tests now available for the evaluation of hypercalcemia, the comprehensive physical examination of the patient is a critical step in management. Not only will this examination provide information necessary for the differential diagnosis of hypercalcemia but it will serve as the basis for deciding the appropriate treatment.

Primary hyperparathyroidism is the most common cause of hypercalcemia. Although familiarity with the spectrum of the disease can be useful in suggesting the diagnosis, most patients are asymptomatic and are identified by the detection of hypercalcemia as part of a routine chemistry profile. In fact, the presence of normal findings on history and physical examination in a patient with

**TABLE 22–1. Etiology of Hypercalcemia**

| |
|---|
| **PRIMARY HYPERPARATHYROIDISM** |
| Malignancy |
| Granulomatous disease |
| Medications |
| Vitamin D toxicity |
| Lithium |
| Milk-alkali syndrome |
| Thiazides |
| Hormonal treatment of carcinoma of breast |
| Familial hypocalciuric hypercalcemia |
| Other endocrine disorders |
| Thyrotoxicosis |
| Adrenal crisis |
| Pheochromocytoma |
| Renal failure |
| Post-transplantation/dialysis |
| Aluminum intoxication |
| Diuretic phase of acute renal failure |
| Immobilization |
| Rare causes |

hypercalcemia strengthens the likelihood of this diagnosis.

Malignancy is the second most common cause of hypercalcemia and is usually associated with symptoms related to the tumor: loss of appetite, loss of weight, and fatigue. Furthermore, the symptoms of hypercalcemia tend to occur at a concentration of serum calcium that seems to be well tolerated in other hypercalcemic states. These include nausea, vomiting, lethargy, and confusion. Mistaking these symptoms for symptoms associated with terminal disease or the effects of chemotherapy or radiation therapy can be an unfortunate oversight because correction of the hypercalcemia may provide complete relief of symptoms.

Most of the malignancies associated with hypercalcemia are solid tumors with extensive skeletal metastatic disease (for example, carcinoma of breast or lung). Diagnosis is seldom a problem because of the size of the tumor burden. Intuitively, we may attribute the hypercalcemia to carcinoma cells destroying bone with release of calcium. This may be true to some extent, but some tumors with extensive skeletal metastases (such as prostate and small cell carcinoma of the lung) seldom cause hypercalcemia. It seems likely that certain metastatic tumors produce local factors that promote bone resorption and cause hypercalcemia.[36]

Other malignancies may be associated with hypercalcemia with minimal or no skeletal metastatic disease (for example, squamous cell carcinoma of the lung, esophagus, head, and neck and carcinoma of the kidney, ovary, or urinary bladder).[8] These tumors can be diagnostic problems because the tumor burden can be small. Hypercalcemia is believed to result from one or several substances secreted by the tumor (humoral hypercalcemia of malignancy). One of these substances appears to be a parathyroid hormone–related peptide that can bind to parathyroid hormone receptors and thereby mimic some of the actions of parathyroid hormone: increased osteoclastic bone resorption and decreased tubular resorption of phosphorus. However, unlike native parathyroid hormone, renal production of 1,25-dihydroxyvitamin D is not affected nor is osteoblastic bone formation increased.[14]

About 15 per cent of patients with hypercalcemia associated with malignancy have hematologic tumors. Multiple myeloma is the most common of these tumors, but occasionally lymphoma or leukemia is responsible. Local bone resorbing factors account for extensive osteolytic bone destruction, and hypercalcemia is usually aggravated by renal insufficiency. Increased production of 1,25-dihydroxyvitamin D has been reported in a few patients with Hodgkin's disease and non-Hodgkin's lymphoma.[23]

Overall survival of patients with hypercalcemia and malignancy is poor, although some patients with carcinoma of the breast and myeloma survive for years after an episode of hypercalcemia.

Other causes for hypercalcemia are much less common and can usually be recognized after a comprehensive history and physical examination. Sarcoidosis is usually recognized by the typical clinical findings together with abnormal findings on roentgenography of the chest. Hypercalcemia in this disorder has been related to increased production of 1,25-dihydroxyvitamin D.[29] Other granulomatous diseases occasionally associated with hypercalcemia include tuberculosis, disseminated candidiasis, histoplasmosis, berylliosis, eosinophilic granuloma, and silicone implants. Why hypercalcemia develops in some patients with these disorders and does not develop in others is unclear.

Several medications cause hypercalcemia. Vitamin D intoxication may occur after 2 or 3 months of daily doses of 100,000 units, an amount used in treating patients with hypoparathyroidism or vitamin D-resistant states. Occasionally, toxicity will develop with much lower doses, especially in the elderly. Vitamin A in doses exceeding 75,000 units a day may potentiate the action of vitamin D and contribute to hypercalcemia.

Hypercalcemia develops in about 10 per cent of patients treated with lithium on a long-term basis. Because the serum level of parathyroid hormone may also be elevated, distinguishing this cause from primary hyperparathyroidism may be possible only by the demonstration of hypercalcemia before starting lithium or persistence of hypercalcemia for more than 4 weeks after administration of lithium has been stopped.[20]

Milk-alkali syndrome was originally described in patients taking absorbable antacids and milk treatment for peptic ulcer disease. This treatment is no longer used, but the widespread use of calcium carbonate in the treatment of patients with osteoporosis may result in a similar clinical picture when excessive doses are used.

Thiazides increase total serum levels of calcium 0.5 to 1.0 mg/dl. About half of the increase can be explained by hemoconcentration increasing serum albumin and bound calcium, but the ionized calcium level is also increased, apparently because of increased bone resorption and renal tubular reabsorption of calcium. In the normal person, the effect usually subsides after several weeks, even with continued administration of the drug. However, when a preexistent high bone turnover state is present, hypercalcemia may appear and persist for as long as the drug is continued. Hormonal treatment of patients with metastatic carcinoma of the breast with estrogen, androgen, or tamoxifen may also cause prompt elevation of the serum level of calcium.

Familial hypocalciuric hypercalcemia is an autosomal dominant disorder with high penetrance that is found in less than 1 per cent of patients with hypercalcemia.[17] It is characterized by lifelong moderate hypercalcemia, apparently resulting from a cellular defect causing increased renal tubular reabsorption of calcium. The urine level of calcium is less than 100 mg/24 hours in 75 per cent of patients, and the ratio of calcium clearance to creatinine clearance is less than 0.01. The serum level of parathyroid hormone is normal to slightly elevated. The condition is almost always benign, but rare instances of neonatal hyperparathyroidism may develop in certain kindreds with the disease. The major complication comes from needless parathyroid surgery; when this is carried out, hypercalcemia either persists or is replaced by hypoparathyroidism. The presence of hypercalcemia in two generations of a family suggests the possibility of this diagnosis, especially when one member has had unsuccessful parathyroid surgery. When the diagnosis is made, all first-degree relatives should be examined. Multiple endocrine neoplasia syndrome and familial hyperparathyroidism must be excluded.

Other endocrine diseases may also cause hypercalcemia. Approximately 5 per cent of patients with thyrotoxicosis have hypercalcemia often associated with increased serum levels of phosphorus. The disease resolves when the euthyroid state is restored. Rarely, primary hypothyroidism may lead to hypercalcemia with hypocalciuria.[39] Hypercalcemia may be a transient finding in adrenal crisis or during withdrawal from steroid therapy, probably related to hemoconcentration. The affinity of albumin for calcium may also be increased in this setting. Pheochromocytoma has caused hypercalcemia, which is corrected by excision of the adrenal tumor. Nonbeta islet cell tumor of the pancreas associated with secretion of vasoactive intestinal peptide has also been associated with hypercalcemia.

Chronic renal failure may be associated with hypercalcemia after transplantation or during dialysis,[26] presumably because of a disequilibrium state resulting from the inability to reduce the massive parathyroid hyperplasia induced by the hypocalcemia of chronic renal failure. Excessive supplements with calcium or vitamin D may be a contributing factor. Aluminum intoxication, probably related to the ingestion of aluminum antacids and decreased renal excretion of aluminum, may also develop in patients undergoing renal dialysis. A low turnover osteomalacia and, in some instances, hypercalcemia may occur because of failure of the bone to take up calcium from the extracellular fluid.[33] Transient hypercalcemia may also appear during the diuretic phase of acute renal failure in patients with rhabdomyolysis.

Immobilization for 1 to 4 months may cause hypercalcemia, especially in children and occasionally in adults with high bone turnover (for example, patients with extensive Paget's disease or skeletal metastatic disease).

Other disorders that have occasionally been associated with hypercalcemia include acquired immunodeficiency syndrome, neuroleptic malignant syndrome, William's syndrome (infants with supravalvular aortic stenosis, mental retardation, elfin facies, and abnormal sensitivity to vitamin D), benign dysplastic breast disease, and prolonged total parenteral nutrition. Rarely, no explanation for the hypercalcemia can be found.[34]

The clinician must consider each of these causes for hypercalcemia in a systematic way and estimate the probability of each disease in an individual patient. The most difficult problems arise in the diagnosis of primary hyperparathyroidism, occult malignancy, familial hypocalciuric hypercalcemia, and sarcoid.

The possibility that the patient may have two diseases that potentially cause hypercalcemia must not be overlooked. Hypercalcemia may be caused by the synergistic effect of both diseases or the impugned disorder may not affect calcium metabolism at all. The most common example is coexistent malignant disease and primary hyperparathyroidism. Treatment of the latter may add considerably to the quality of life for the patient with malignancy who has prolonged survival.

## LABORATORY EVALUATION OF HYPERCALCEMIA

Although no single laboratory test establishes the diagnosis of primary hyperparathyroidism with certainty, combining several tests with a careful clinical evaluation permits a diagnosis to be made with reasonable certainty in almost all instances. A positive diagnosis cannot be made until it has been demonstrated that the abnormal parathyroid tissue has been removed and the hypercalcemia has been corrected.

The serum level of calcium should be measured on at least three occasions. Hypercalcemia is found in virtually all patients with primary hyperparathyroidism, but mild hypercalcemia (<11.5 mg/dl) is the rule rather than the exception. Intermittent and masked hypercalcemia are occasional confounding issues. It is also important to determine the duration of the hypercalcemia, when possible. When the duration exceeds 1 year and the results of the clinical examination are normal, primary hyperparathyroidism is likely, although familial hypocalciuric hypercalcemia must be considered. When the hypercalcemia can be shown to have developed within the past year, especially when the patient is symptomatic, malignancy must be suspected.

Clinical application of an assay for parathyroid hormone lagged behind that for other polypeptide hormones. Several reasons were responsible for this delay: low concentration of circulating parathyroid hormone, difficulty obtaining antibodies to react with human parathyroid hormone, and immunologic heterogeneity of circulating parathyroid hormone fragments. The procedure is technically difficult and costs several times that of the radioimmunoassay for growth hormone and insulin. Because no reference preparation is available, results vary among laboratories.

Measurement of intact parathyroid hormone by an immunoradiometric assay is now the procedure of choice for measuring parathyroid hormone. The test uses two antisera; one is directed to the N terminal fragment of the hormone, and the second has midmolecular specificity.[24] The test should be ordered only when hypercalcemia has been demonstrated or masked hypercalcemia is suspected. A definite elevation of the serum level of parathyroid hormone in the presence of hypercalcemia and normal renal function serves as solid evidence for primary hyperparathyroidism. C terminal assays are unreliable in the presence of renal failure because of retention of inactive parathyroid hormone fragments, and occasionally carcinoma and primary hyperparathyroidism overlap. N terminal parathyroid hormone assays measure biologically active hormone but have not proved clearly beneficial for the diagnosis of primary hyperparathyroidism.[19]

An increased serum level of parathyroid hormone with a normal serum level of calcium can be found in a number of physiologic and pathologic situations: vitamin D deficiency (usually resulting from malabsorption); therapy with anticonvulsants, corticosteroids, or cholestyramine; laxative abuse; vitamin D-resistant rickets; pseudohypoparathyroidism; hypomagnesemia; chronic renal failure; pregnancy; aging; and idiopathic hypercalciuria.

The urine level of calcium is greater than 200 mg/24 hours in the majority of patients with primary hyperparathyroidism who are following a regular diet (600 to 1,000 mg of calcium daily). Values less than 100 mg/24 hours may be helpful in identifying the rare situation of a patient with familial hypocalciuric hypercalcemia, but a low urine level of calcium is more often explained by an incomplete urine collection, failure to acidify the urine during collection, decreased renal function, or use of thiazides.

Other tests are routinely performed to aid in proper interpretation of the serum calcium and to alert the clinician to other possible causes of hypercalcemia. Creatinine, albumin, and phosphorus must always be measured concurrently with calcium because any abnormalities can modify the total serum calcium by mechanisms already described. Moreover, the presence of hypoalbuminemia, anemia, an elevated sedimentation rate, or hyperglobulinemia favors a diagnosis of malignant disease; serum chloride levels more than 103 mEq/L and, to a lesser extent, a fasting serum phosphorus level less than 3.0 mg/dl favor a diagnosis of primary hyperparathyroidism.[6] Thyroid function studies should also be performed because of the potential impact of thyroid disease on serum levels of calcium.

Roentgenography of the chest must be performed routinely to search for underlying malignant or granulomatous disease. Excretory urography or a plain film of the abdomen will help to establish the presence of asymptomatic renal calculi.

Additional tests are reserved for diagnostic problems and are determined by the clinical setting. Serum ionized calcium measurement may be helpful in the presence of hypoalbuminemia. Serum and urine protein electrophoresis and bone marrow examination may be helpful when multiple myeloma, leukemia, or lymphoma is being considered. Serum levels of magnesium should be measured in any clinical setting that can lead to magnesium depletion, such as malabsorption or chronic alcoholism. Angiotensin-converting enzyme is useful in identifying a patient suspected of having active sarcoidosis, but it is not specific for this disorder.[18] A corticosteroid suppression test may be helpful when sarcoidosis, myeloma, lymphoma, or vitamin D intoxication is suspected. Prednisone, 10 mg three times a day for 10 days, will usually normalize serum levels of calcium in these conditions but not in primary hyperparathyroidism or in most malignant diseases. However, false-positive and false-negative results may occur. Elevation of the level of 1,25-dihydroxyvitamin D is characteristic of sarcoidosis, but comparable levels are seen in patients with other granulomatous diseases as well as in patients with primary hyperparathyroidism and in an occasional patient with lymphoma. Elevation of the 25-hydroxyvitamin D can be helpful in establishing the diagnosis of vitamin D intoxication.

Because of the possible association with pheochromocytoma in multiple endocrine neoplasia syndrome type II, the urinary level of metanephrines should be measured in the hypertensive patient with primary hyperparathyroidism. Serum prolactin and gastrin are useful screening tests for multiple endocrine neoplasia syndrome type I in patients with symptoms or a family history to suggest this possibility. Mild elevations of gastrin may occur with primary hyperparathyroidism and are corrected by surgery.[40]

Localization techniques are being developed to identify the site of a parathyroid adenoma.[38] These techniques can be helpful for planning the surgical approach but should not be used to establish the diagnosis.

In patients with no prior surgery, noninvasive techniques can be considered. High-resolution real-time ultrasonography has a reasonable chance of success in expert hands for localizing eutopic tumors weighing more than 200 mg. Scintigraphic scanning of the parathyroid glands using thallium 201 and scanning of the thyroid gland using technetium 99m with computer subtraction techniques offer comparable reliability. Neither technique, however, surpasses the ability of the experienced surgeon to localize the adenoma, and both studies are associated with an appreciable risk of false-positive results because of thyroid nodules.

Invasive techniques, such as nonselective digital subtraction angiography and parathyroid venous sampling for parathyroid hormone, are reserved for the patient who has had previous parathyroid surgery. Computed tomography has proved useful in detecting ectopic parathyroid tumors.

## TREATMENT

The only effective treatment for patients with primary hyperparathyroidism is surgery. Parathyroid hormone antagonists are potentially useful for selected patients but are still in the developmental stage.[31] Assuming the patient's general medical status offers no contraindication to surgery, the decision for surgery is based on an estimate of the likelihood of future complications, the likelihood of cure with surgery, and, of course, the wishes of the patient.[16]

The risk for future complications is best determined by assessing the impact of the disease up to the time of diagnosis and the tempo with which these complications have developed. When renal calculi have formed within the past several years, when osteitis fibrosa is already evident, or when renal function is impaired, surgical intervention is strongly favored. These patients are not likely to improve spontaneously and must be considered at high risk for the development of serious complications in the future.

On the other hand, if the history of renal calculi or peptic ulcer disease is remote and both conditions have been inactive for years, the argument for surgery is less convincing. In my opinion, the result of a single bone densitometric reading or the presence of hypertension is not a valid indication for surgical treatment.

The age of the patient should also be considered. Surgery is a more attractive option for patients less than 60 years of age because these persons have a longer exposure to the disease and therefore a higher risk of complications. The inconvenience and cost of follow-up testing present an added burden for these patients.

The level of the serum calcium must also be considered. Mild hypercalcemia, variously defined as 11.0 to 11.5 mg/dl, in an asymptomatic individual appears to predict a lower risk of complications.

The next question to consider is the likelihood of cure with surgery. The experience of the surgeon is a major factor in determining a successful outcome. The role of noninvasive localization studies remains to be established.

The cure rate will also be influenced by the underlying pathologic condition. A single adenoma will be found in 90 per cent of patients with primary hyperparathyroidism. The success rate for surgery in these patients exceeds 90 per cent and is determined by the size and location of the adenoma.

About 5 to 10 per cent of patients have chief cell hyperplasia. All four glands are usually affected, although enlargement is often asymmetric. Most patients with multiple endocrine neoplasia syndrome and familial hyperparathyroidism will be in this category. Surgery for these patients is less likely to be successful because of the difficulty in predicting the amount of parathyroid tissue to remove.[7] Cure rate is decidedly reduced,[30] and efforts to improve response to surgery by autotransplantation or cryopreservation have not met with uniform success.

Rarely will a patient with primary hyperparathyroidism have parathyroid carcinoma. This will usually be suggested by a serum level of calcium of more than 14 mg/dl and a greatly increased parathyroid hormone level. Osteitis fibrosa cystica and a palpable neck mass are additional clues that can be helpful. Successful initial surgery is the key to therapy. Although the natural history is one of slow progression, only 50 per cent of patients survive to 5 years beyond the time of diagnosis.[32] Recurrent hypercalcemia after parathyroid surgery should always lead to review of the original pathologic specimen to exclude parathyroid carcinoma.

Patients who have had prior exploration for hyperparathyroidism will have a lower likelihood of cure with the second operation. Assuming the initial operation had been adequate, success will be compromised by a higher frequency of smaller or ectopic tumors as well as the complicating fibrosis of the previous operation. Localization techniques may be helpful in these patients, especially the invasive methods already mentioned. Complications from surgery, such as vocal cord paralysis and postoperative hypoparathyroidism, also occur with greater frequency in this group.

Finally, the options for surgery or medical observation must be explained to the patient so that he or she can make an informed decision. As is true in most medical decisions, the plan for treatment is based on probabilities rather than certainties and must be applied to the unique needs of the individual patient.

In general, I recommend operation for

patients with primary hyperparathyroidism when active complications of the disease are evident or when the mean serum level of calcium exceeds 11.5 mg/dl. Even milder hypercalcemia might justify surgery in persons less than 50 years of age.

A period of observation can be considered when no complications of primary hyperparathyroidism are present and the serum level of calcium is <11.5 mg/dl. This option is especially attractive when the patient is more than 60 years old but can also be considered in patients less than this age whose previous parathyroid exploration revealed negative findings or when parathyroid hyperplasia is suspected.

Treatment with estrogen appears to inhibit parathyroid hormone-mediated bone resorption and has been used for treating postmenopausal women suspected of having primary hyperparathyroidism with a serum level of calcium of <11.5 mg/dl. Serum and urine levels of calcium are usually normalized, but parathyroid hormone levels are unchanged, and the long-term effect on bone remains uncertain.[22] Although a risk-to-benefit analysis of lifelong estrogen treatment in patients with primary hyperparathyroidism has not been completed, conjugated estrogen, 1.25 mg daily, offers an option for the postmenopausal woman.

When surgery for primary hyperparathyroidism is not elected, prudent follow-up studies should include monitoring serum calcium and creatinine clearance every 6 to 12 months or more often when the patient is immobilized or hypovolemia develops. A plain film of the abdomen should be obtained periodically to monitor for asymptomatic renal calculi. The role of bone densitometry in identifying the patient in whom severe osteopenia might develop has not been established, but it offers another objective measure for assessing progress. Medications previously noted to cause hypercalcemia should be avoided. Patients are usually advised to follow a diet that provides approximately 600 mg of calcium a day.

*Secondary hyperparathyroidism* is a homeostatic response to hypocalcemia in an effort to normalize the serum level of calcium by promoting the release of calcium from bone and indirectly by increasing intestinal absorption of calcium. This attempt to maintain a normal calcium balance, however, exposes the person to progressive bone dissolution because of the action of parathyroid hormone on bone.

In chronic renal failure, hypocalcemia develops because of phosphate retention and reduced renal synthesis of 1,25-dihydroxyvitamin D. Secondary hyperparathyroidism results in osteitis fibrosa and is usually complicated by osteomalacia and osteoporosis. The most advanced form of renal osteodystrophy is seen in patients who require long-term treatment with dialysis and is characterized by bone pain and susceptibility to fracture.[9] The skeletal lesion can be minimized by early treatment with vitamin D and phosphate binders, although intermittent intravenous infusion of 1,25-dihydroxyvitamin D may also be helpful.[2] Subtotal parathyroidectomy can be considered in the patient undergoing dialysis who has disabling osteodystrophy and is not a candidate for renal transplantation. However, before this step is considered, osteitis must be identified as the predominant skeletal lesion and optimal medical treatment provided.[10] Roentgenography of the hands showing subperiosteal resorption and increased circulating levels of intact parathyroid hormone are consistent with osteitis. A serum level of calcium that is elevated or at the upper limit of normal suggests that medical measures to reduce parathyroid hormone secretion have been pushed to the limit. However, bone biopsy with histomorphometry should also be carried out to confirm that osteitis is the predominant lesion and to exclude extensive accumulation of aluminum.

A resistant form of osteomalacia may appear in renal osteodystrophy and has been accompanied by hypercalcemia, bone pain, fractures, and radiographic evidence of subperiosteal resorption. The condition resembles hyperparathyroidism, but the serum level of parathyroid hormone is actually lower than would be expected for end-stage renal disease. The pathogenesis is not clear, but it may be caused by accumulation of aluminum in bone, which blocks calcium uptake, thereby leading to hypercalcemia. Calcium supplements and vitamin D may accentuate the hypercalcemia.[33] Parathyroidectomy may accentuate the skeletal deformity and lead to enhanced aluminum deposition on bone.[1] Proper management requires elimination of exogenous aluminum to the extent possible and probably chelation therapy with deferoxamine to eliminate aluminum and reverse the bone changes associated with it.[21]

Subtotal parathyroidectomy is seldom required for the treatment of hypercalcemia in a patient in chronic renal failure. This complication is usually transient and can be managed by reducing exogenous sources of vitamin D and calcium.[26] All of the other causes of hypercalcemia should also be considered.

The response to parathyroid surgery for patients with secondary hyperparathyroidism can be compromised by ectopic or supernumerary parathyroid glands just as with surgery for primary hyperparathyroidism. Postoperative hypocalcemia and the later development of a skeletal mineralization defect have been problems seen in patients with renal osteodystrophy.

## REFERENCES


1. Andress, D. L., Ott, S. M., Maloney, N. A., and Sherrard, D. J.: Effect of parathyroidectomy on bone aluminum accumulation in chronic renal failure. N. Engl. J. Med., *312*:468–473, 1985.
2. Andress, D. L., Norris, K. C., Coburn, J. W., et al.: Intravenous calcitriol in the treatment of refractory osteitis fibrosa of chronic renal failure. N. Engl. J. Med., *321*:274–279, 1989.
3. Bilezikian, J. P.: Hypercalcemia. Dis Mon *34*:737–799, 1988.
4. Bowers, G. N., Jr., Brassard, C., and Sena, S. F.: Measurement of ionized calcium in serum with ion-selective electrodes: A mature technology that can meet the daily service needs. Clin. Chem., *32*:1437–1447, 1986.
5. Boxer, M., Ellman, L., Geller, R., and Wang, C. A.: Anemia in primary hyperparathyroidism. Arch. Intern. Med., *137*:588–590, 1977.
6. Boyd, J. C., and Ladenson, J. H.: Value of laboratory tests in the differential diagnosis of hypercalcemia. Am. J. Med., *77*:863–872, 1984.
7. Bruining, H. A., Birkenhäger, J. C., Ong, G. L., and Lamberts, S. W.: Causes of failure in operations for hyperparathyroidism. Surgery, *101*:562–565, 1987.
8. Burtis, W. J., Wu, T. L., Insogna, K. L., and Stewart, A. F.: Humoral hypercalcemia of malignancy. Ann. Intern. Med., *108*:454–457, 1988.
9. Cushner, H. M., and Adams, N. D.: Review: Renal osteodystrophy—pathogenesis and treatment. Am. J. Med. Sci., *290*:234–245, 1986.
10. Dawborn, J. K., Brown, D. J., Douglas, M. C., et al.: Parathyroidectomy in chronic renal failure. Nephron, *33*:100–105, 1983.
11. Fitzpatrick, L. A., and Bilezikian, J. P.: Acute primary hyperparathyroidism. Am. J. Med., *82*:275–282, 1987.
12. Heath, H., III, Hodgson, S. F., and Kennedy, M. A.: Primary hyperparathyroidism: Incidence, morbidity, and potential economic impact in a community. N. Engl. J. Med., *302*:189–193, 1980.
13. Katz, A., and Braunstein, G. D.: Clinical, biochemical and pathologic features of radiation-associated hyperparathyroidism. Arch. Intern. Med., *143*: 79–82, 1983.
14. Klee, G. G., Kao, P. C., Heath, H., 3d.: Hypercalcemia. Endocrinol. Metab. Clin. North Am., *17*:573–600, 1988.
15. Kochersberger, G., Buckley, N. J., Leight, G. S., et al.: What is the clinical significance of bone loss in primary hyperparathyroidism? Arch. Intern. Med., *147*:1951–1953, 1987.
16. Lafferty, F. W., and Hubay, C. A.: Primary hyperparathyroidism: A review of the long-term surgical and nonsurgical morbidities as a basis for a rational approach to treatment. Arch. Intern. Med., *149*:789–796, 1989.
17. Law, W. M., Jr., and Heath, H., III: Familial benign hypercalcemia (hypocalciuric hypercalcemia): Clinical and pathogenetic studies in 21 families. Ann. Intern. Med., *102*:511–519, 1985.
18. Lufkin, E. G., DeRemee, R. A., and Rohrbach, M. S.: The predictive value of serum angiotensin-converting enzyme activity in the differential diagnosis of hypercalcemia. Mayo Clin. Proc., *58*:447–451, 1983.
19. Lufkin, E. G., Kao, P. C., and Heath, H., III: Parathyroid hormone radioimmunoassays in the differential diagnosis of hypercalcemia due to primary hyperthyroidism or malignancy. Ann. Intern. Med., *106*:559–560, 1987.
20. Mallette, L. E., and Eichhorn, E.: Effects of lithium carbonate on human calcium metabolism. Arch. Intern. Med., *146*:770–776, 1986.
21. Malluche, H. H., Smith, A. J., Abreo, K., and Faugere, M. C.: The use of deferoxamine in the management of aluminum accumulation in bone in patients with renal failure. N. Engl. J. Med., *311*:140–144, 1984.
22. Marcus, R., Madvig, P., Crim, M., et al.: Conjugated estrogens in the treatment of postmenopausal women with hyperparathyroidism. Ann. Intern. Med., *100*:633–640, 1984.
23. Mundy, G. R.: Hypercalcemia of malignancy revisited. J. Clin. Invest., *82*:1–6, 1988.
24. Nussbaum, S. R., Zahradnik, R. J., Lavigne, J. R., et al.: Highly sensitive two-site immunoradiometric assay of parathyrin, and its clinical utility in evaluating patients with hypercalcemia. Clin. Chem., *33*:1364–1367, 1987.
25. Palmér, M., Adami, H. O., Bergström, R., et al.: Mortality after surgery for primary hyperparathyroidism: A follow-up of 441 patients operated on from 1956–1979. Surgery, *102*:1–7, 1987.
26. Piraino, B. M., Rault, R., Greenberg, A., et al.: Spontaneous hypercalcemia in patients undergoing dialysis: Etiologic and therapeutic considerations. Am. J. Med., *80*:607–615, 1986.
27. Rao, D. S., Wilson, R. J., Kleerekoper, M., and Parfitt, A. M.: Lack of biochemical progression or continuation of accelerated bone loss in mild asymptomatic primary hyperparathyroidism: Evidence for biphasic disease course. J. Clin. Endocrinol. Metab., *67*:1294–1298, 1988.
28. Rapado, A.: Arterial hypertension and primary hyperparathyroidism: Incidence and follow-up after parathyroidectomy. Am. J. Nephrol., *6*(Suppl. 1):49–50, 1986.

29. Reichel, H., Koeffler, H. P., and Norman, A. W.: The role of the vitamin D endocrine system in health and disease. N. Engl. J. Med., *320*:980–991, 1989.
30. Rizzoli, R., Green, J., 3d, and Marx, S. J.: Primary hyperparathyroidism in familial multiple endocrine neoplasia type I: Long-term follow-up of serum calcium levels after parathyroidectomy. Am. J. Med., *78*:467–474, 1985.
31. Rosenblatt, M.: Peptide hormone antagonists that are effective in vivo: Lessons from parathyroid hormone. N. Engl. J. Med., *315*:1004–1013, 1986.
32. Shane, E., and Bilezikian, J. P.: Parathyroid carcinoma: A review of 62 patients. Endocr. Rev., *3*:218–226, 1982.
33. Sherrard, D. J., Ott, S. M., and Andress, D. L.: Pseudohyperparathyroidism: Syndrome associated with aluminum intoxication in patients with renal failure. Am. J. Med., *79*:127–130, 1985.
34. Silver, J., and Popovtzer, M. M.: Hypercalcemia with elevated dihydroxycholecalciferol levels and hypercalciuria: A parathyroid concentration-independent mechanism. Arch. Intern. Med., *144*:162–163, 1984.
35. Silverberg, S. J., Shane, E., de la Cruz, L., et al.: Skeletal disease in primary hyperparathyroidism. J. Bone Miner. Res., *4*:283–291, 1989.
36. Strewler, G. J., and Nissenson, R. A.: Nonparathyroid hypercalcemia. Adv. Intern. Med., *32*:235–258, 1987.
37. Wilson, R. J., Rao, D. S., Ellis, B., et al.: Mild asymptomatic primary hyperparathyroidism is not a risk factor for vertebral fractures. Ann. Intern. Med., *109*:959–962, 1988.
38. Winzelberg, G. G.: Parathyroid imaging. Ann. Intern. Med., *107*:64–70, 1987.
39. Zaloga, G. P., Eil, C., and O'Brian, J. T.: Reversible hypocalciuric hypercalcemia associated with hypothyroidism. Am. J. Med., *77*:1101–1104, 1984.
40. Zaniewski, M., Jordan, P. H., Jr., Yip, B., et al.: Serum gastrin level is increased by chronic hypercalcemia of parathyroid or nonparathyroid origin. Arch. Intern. Med., *146*:478–482, 1986.

# 23

# FAMILIAL HYPERPARATHYROIDISM AND HYPERPARATHYROIDISM ASSOCIATED WITH MULTIPLE ENDOCRINE NEOPLASIA SYNDROMES

*Melvin A. Block, M.D.*

The familial and hereditary occurrence of endocrine neoplasms involving a single endocrine gland or multiple endocrine glands produces certain unique clinical manifestations of diagnostic and therapeutic importance. Parathyroid tumors, usually manifesting as primary hyperparathyroidism, have been a common component of these syndromes. Distinctive features of these associations of hyperparathyroidism along with treatment will be considered in this discussion.

Although hyperparathyroidism alone or associated with other endocrine neoplasms can occur sporadically or without an obvious pattern in families (familial), frequently this entity has a genetic basis (hereditary) whenever it involves more than one member of a family. Thus, the possibility of an occurrence in other family members should be considered for each patient for whom the diagnosis of hyperparathyroidism is made. The frequency of primary hyperparathyroidism in familial or hereditary patterns varies on the basis of the type of patient population in reported series but, in general, appears to approximate 5 to 10 per cent of patients. External radiation therapy, although an etiologic factor in producing primary hyperparathyroidism, does not appear to endanger later generations.

Hyperparathyroidism of genetic origin does not usually become manifested in early childhood. Hyperparathyroidism may appear in late adolescence in the multiple endocrine adenoma or neoplasia (MEN) syndromes. Thus, factors other than a purely genetic one may be involved.[29] In adult life, the clinical appearance of neoplasms of a genetic origin occurs earlier than that of the sporadic forms of the same neoplasm and may be evident earlier in life in succeeding generations of some families.[14]

For the multiple endocrine syndromes under consideration, both adenoma and neoplasia have been used to complete the designated terms. Because some of the neoplasms can be malignant in these multiple endocrine syndromes, we have considered neoplasia to be more descriptive.

## CLASSIFICATION

Hyperparathyroidism occurring in families or as a component of multiple endocrine neoplasia syndromes can be categorized as shown in Table 23–1.

**TABLE 23–1. Classification of Familial and Hereditary Hyperparathyroidism**

- Familial hyperparathyroidism
  - Producing complications of hypercalcemia
    - Dominant inheritance: All parathyroid glands usually hyperplastic for each family member involved
    - Recessive inheritance: Only one parathyroid gland may be hyperplastic for each family member involved
    - Familial cystic parathyroid adenomatosis with jaw fibromas
  - Familial benign hypocalciuric hypercalcemia: Does not produce complications from hypercalcemia in adults
- Multiple endocrine neoplasia (MEN) syndromes
  - Dominant inheritance
    - MEN-I: All parathyroid glands always hyperplastic
    - MEN-IIa: All parathyroid glands usually hyperplastic
- Miscellaneous endocrine syndromes (including hyperparathyroidism, which may be familial)
  - Hyperparathyroidism associated with foregut carcinoid tumors (occasionally other endocrine neoplasms present)
  - Familial hypophosphatemic rickets with secondary hyperparathyroidism
- Familial parathyroid carcinoma with hyperparathyroidism

## GENERAL CONSIDERATIONS

The severity of hyperparathyroidism in familial or hereditary forms, from the standpoints of degree of hypercalcemia and frequency and magnitude of complications, varies much from patient to patient. However, the severity of hypercalcemia and the incidence of complications appear less in patients with the MEN-IIa syndrome than in those with the MEN-I syndrome. Also, benign familial hypocalciuric hypercalcemia does not appear to produce complications in adult life.

Hyperparathyroidism may be the first clinical manifestation of the MEN-I or MEN-IIa syndrome or may become evident many years after other endocrine neoplasms are symptomatic or otherwise apparent. Thus, it is necessary to recognize the potential for the occurrence of clinical hyperparathyroidism in a given patient and to monitor appropriately for its occurrence. Provocative testing for subclinical hyperparathyroidism has not been found necessary to date. Simple monitoring of serum calcium levels has been considered cost effective in recognizing hyperparathyroidism in members of families at risk for the development of this condition. Unless other clues suggest the possibility of a familial or MEN syndrome, routine examination of all patients with primary hyperparathyroidism for elevated levels of serum gastrin and calcitonin is not cost effective.[25]

Important features of hyperparathyroidism are compared in Table 23–2 for the various familial and MEN syndromes. To be emphasized is that the dominant endocrine neoplasm for MEN-I and MEN-IIa syndromes occurs in both sporadic and inherited forms. Thus, gastrinomas occur both in the sporadic (Zollinger-Ellison syndrome) and in the MEN-I syndrome categories, and medullary thyroid carcinoma occurs sporadically as well as in the MEN-IIa syndrome.[14, 35] However, hyperparathyroidism is present only in the inherited forms of MEN syndromes. In the treatment of patients with hyperparathyroidism of the MEN syndromes, priorities must be established, with the relative risks of the other endocrine components of the syndromes taken into consideration.

In our experience, a precise clinical separation or correlation does not exist for the

**TABLE 23–2. Comparison of Features of Hyperparathyroidism in Familial and MEN Syndromes**

| FEATURE | MEN-I | MEN-IIA | FAMILIAL HYPER-PARATHYROIDISM | MISCELLANEOUS MEN SYNDROMES |
|---|---|---|---|---|
| Incidence of hyperparathyroidism | Syndrome occurs in autosomal dominant inheritance<br>Hyperparathyroidism always present in involved family member | Syndrome occurs in autosomal dominant inheritance<br>Hyperparathyroidism present only in some families<br>When it involves a family, only some MEN-IIa have hyperparathyroidism | Occurs in autosomal dominant (more frequent) and recessive inheritance | Sporadic involvement of members of a family usually on basis of information to date |
| Number of parathyroid glands involved when hyperparathyroidism present | All parathyroid glands hyperplastic<br>Hyperplasia of supernumerary parathyroids a significant occurrence | All parathyroid glands hyperplastic when hyperparathyroidism present in family member | For autosomal dominant inheritance, all parathyroid glands usually hyperplastic<br>For recessive inheritance, only one parathyroid gland usually hyperplastic | All parathyroid glands hyperplastic usually |
| Dominant endocrine neoplasm | Gastrinoma, frequently malignant | Medullary carcinoma of thyroid | Usually no other endocrine neoplasm | Foregut carcinoid tumors for one syndrome |
| Severity of hyperparathyroidism | Usually severe, requires operation | Hypercalcemia often not present despite hyperplasia of parathyroid glands<br>Severe in a few family members | Surgical correction usually required | Surgical correction required |
| Operative procedure indicated | Subtotal parathyroidectomy vs total parathyroidectomy with autotransplantation | Subtotal parathyroidectomy when hypercalcemic<br>Emphasize preservation of parathyroid function<br>Remove incidental enlarged parathyroid glands in patient not hypercalcemic | For hyperplasia of multiple parathyroid glands: subtotal parathyroidectomy vs total parathyroidectomy with autotransplantation<br>For single gland enlargement, remove this gland only | Usually subtotal parathyroidectomy |

pathologic entities of parathyroid adenomas, usually involving a single parathyroid gland, and chief cell hyperplasia, either diffuse or nodular, involving multiple parathyroid glands.[12, 27] Both histologic patterns can be present in a patient with multiple parathyroid gland enlargement producing primary hyperparathyroidism. The finding of an adenoma of one parathyroid gland does not rule out a second parathyroid adenoma or diffuse hyperplasia of other parathyroid glands.

Experience has suggested the occurrence, in some hereditary forms of hyperparathyroidism, of an increased risk for the development of neoplasms other than those characteristically constituting the syndrome. This fact has appeared particularly relevant for the MEN-IIa syndrome.[14]

The stimulus for hyperparathyroidism may continue indefinitely for the familial and hereditary forms. Thus, after surgical correction of the hyperparathyroidism, it is necessary to conduct periodic evaluations throughout the patient's lifetime.

The degree of enlargement of individual parathyroid glands varies widely even though all glands are microscopically hyperplastic in the familial and hereditary forms of primary hyperparathyroidism.[10, 12] Only one or several parathyroid glands may be huge and the other parathyroid glands only slightly enlarged. Rarely, although all parathyroid glands are only slightly enlarged, all are hyperplastic on microscopic study.[13]

It is of clinical importance to recognize that hyperparathyroidism does not occur in the sporadic Zollinger-Ellison syndrome (it consists only of gastrinoma and complications from this neoplasm) or in medullary thyroid carcinoma (it is unilateral in the thyroid gland). These sporadic forms also are not hereditary. The MEN-I and MEN-II syndromes imply a hereditary occurrence as well as the presence of multiple endocrine neoplasms, which may include hyperparathyroidism. (Hyperparathyroidism is present in all patients with MEN-I syndrome and in some families of MEN-IIa syndrome.)

## FAMILIAL HYPERPARATHYROIDISM

Familial hyperparathyroidism usually occurs in an autosomal dominant inheritance, with all parathyroid glands being hyperplastic (Fig. 23–1). The severity of hypercalcemia and the frequency of complications from hypercalcemia usually justify operation, either subtotal parathyroidectomy or total parathyroidectomy with autotransplantation of parathyroid tissue.

Rarely, hyperparathyroidism occurs sporadically in members of a family or in an apparent recessive inheritance.[33] In these patients, hyperplasia of a single parathyroid gland appears to be a common finding, with its surgical removal correcting the problem. In some families, solitary parathyroid adenomas occur with a dominant inheritance.[3]

Another rare form of familial hyperparathyroidism has been described as familial cystic parathyroid adenomatosis.[37] Hyperparathyroidism occurs at an early age and is corrected by removal of a single cystic parathyroid adenoma. However, the other normal parathyroid glands are also cystic, and hyperparathyroidism tends to recur after a 6- to 10-year interval of normocalcemia as a result of enlargement and hyperfunction of a second cystic parathyroid gland. In one family reported, the inheritance appeared to be dominant. Because the adenoma predominantly involved the inferior parathyroid glands, both inferior parathyroid glands should be removed when these patients undergo operation. Fibrous tumors of the jaw appear to be a common associated lesion. The jaw fibromas may appear and enlarge after correction of hypercalcemia. Other endocrine tumors were not evident in the family reported. That hereditary factors are complex is indicated by the presence of hypocalciuric hypercalcemia in some members of this family.

For patients with evidence of familial hyperparathyroidism, a search should be conducted for other endocrine neoplasms, especially those comprising the MEN-I and MEN-IIa syndromes. Also, benign hypocalciuric hypocalcemia should be ruled out.

## BENIGN FAMILIAL HYPOCALCIURIC HYPERCALCEMIA

Benign familial hypocalciuric hypercalcemia occurs with an autosomal dominant inheritance, appears in patients at an early age, and is sufficiently frequent to require its exclusion for patients with evidence of primary hyperparathyroidism, especially those without clinical manifestations of complications from hypercalcemia.[32] This entity can simulate primary hyperparathyroidism in terms of persistent mild hypercalcemia and elevated levels of serum parathyroid hormone in the absence of other causes for these laboratory findings. At operation, varying degrees of mild macroscopic and microscopic hyperplasia of parathyroid glands are found. However, subtotal parathyroidectomy does not correct hypercalcemia in this entity, and experience has shown that complications from hypercalcemia do not occur in adult patients even though the condition is present for a lifetime. Thus, operation is not justified for these patients. A report[39] indicated that neonates born of parents with benign hypocalciuric hypercalcemia may have severe hy-

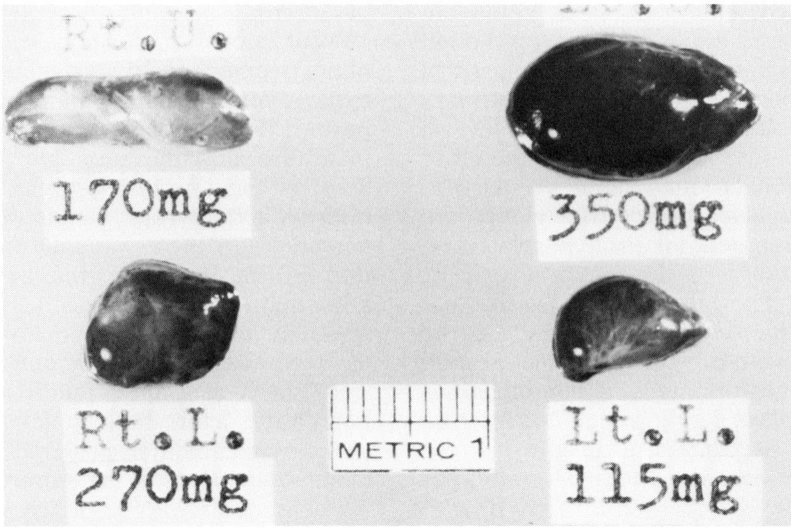


**FIGURE 23–1.** Parathyroid glands removed during subtotal parathyroidectomy for patient with familial hyperparathyroidism. All four parathyroid glands are enlarged. Part of the left lower parathyroid gland was preserved.

perparathyroidism producing hypotonia and skeletal undermineralization with skeletal complications that require total parathyroidectomy for control. Clear cell hyperplasia of parathyroid glands has been found in these infants.

The diagnosis of benign familial hypocalciuric hypercalcemia is best made by demonstrating urine calcium levels below 100 mg per 24 hours and a urine calcium to creatinine clearance ratio of less than 0.01 (about a 15 per cent overlap). Serum levels of magnesium in this condition are elevated or at upper limits of normal instead of the below normal or low levels in the presence of hyperparathyroidism. A high renal tubular absorption of filtered calcium characterizes this entity. No evidence of an association with other endocrine disease is known.

In view of the complexity of hypocalciuric hypercalcemia and evolving evidence that hyperparathyroidism of a standard variety and with complications occurs in some familial cases, members of families affected by benign hypocalciuric hypercalcemia require individual assessment relative to the characteristics of hypercalcemia and the risk for the development of complications. (Attention is called to earlier comments concerning familial cystic parathyroid adenomatosis.) Hypothyroidism can also influence parathyroid function and aggravate diagnostic difficulties.

## HYPERPARATHYROIDISM AND MEN-I SYNDROME

The MEN-I syndrome comprises gastrinomas (usually in the pancreas but occasionally in the duodenum or other ectopic locations), hyperparathyroidism, and pituitary adenomas. The variants of the syndrome include the presence of insulinomas instead of gastrinomas.[42] In a few patients, additional abnormalities are present, including thymoma, lipoma, and Cushing's syndrome. Pituitary adenomas are characteristically prolactinomas.

Hyperparathyroidism is a constant component of the MEN-I syndrome.[35] The age of the patient at the time of clinical appearance and the temporal relationship of occurrence relative to other components of the syndrome vary considerably among patients. Experience suggests that hyperparathyroidism is frequently the first manifestation of the MEN-I syndrome that can readily be identified and appears after the patient reaches the age of 18 years.[4] Surgical correction of hyperparathyroidism associated with the MEN-I syndrome is usually justified because of the degree of severity of hypercalcemia, complications resulting from hypercalcemia, and evidence that gastric hyperacidity is ameliorated by elimination of hypercalcemia. Mild hypercalcemia without complications poses questions of the advisability of operative correction similar to those for primary hyperparathyroidism in general. For most patients, however, a bias for operative correction has been followed. The gastric hyperacidity often can be controlled medically now but is aided by alleviation of hypercalcemia.[34] Before the availability of effective agents to control gastric acid hypersecretion, however, correction of hypercalcemia alone was usually not adequate for this purpose.[7]

All parathyroid glands are hyperplastic in the MEN-I syndrome (Fig. 23–2). A continuous stimulation of all parathyroid tissue seemingly is present in this syndrome.[16] Thus, bits of accessory or supernumerary parathyroid tissue also become hyperplastic, increasing technical difficulties in performing an adequate subtotal parathyroidectomy or total parathyroidectomy.[2] Furthermore, late recurrence of hyperparathyroidism may result, in part, from increasing hyperplasia of these small embryologic fragments (accessory or supernumerary) of parathyroid tissue.

A high recurrence rate of hyperparathyroidism in the MEN-I syndrome after either subtotal parathyroidectomy or total parathyroidectomy and autotransplantation has been experienced.[8, 11, 38, 43] Long-term studies have shown recurrence rates approaching 50 per cent after subtotal parathyroidectomy, with one report[36] of even a higher recurrence rate after total parathyroidectomy and autotransplantation. Technical considerations relative to these two procedures will be considered in greater detail later. Because of the high frequency of recurrence and the relative ease of reoperation to remove a portion of autotransplanted parathyroid tissue from the forearm contrasted with reoperation in the neck after subtotal parathyroidectomy, a bias to total parathyroidectomy and autotransplantation is considered justified for patients with MEN-I. In my experience, total parathyroidectomy and autotransplantation of parathyroid tissue is particularly indicated for patients in whom all parathyroid glands are large. In such patients, it is technically difficult to preserve a viable fragment of 30 to 100 mg of parathyroid tissue by subtotal parathyroidectomy, and the likelihood of overlooked hyperplastic supernumerary parathyroid tissue appears significant. When the capability for freezing parathyroid tissue exists, autotransplantation can be delayed until the need is established after operation and the presence of hyperplastic supernumerary parathyroid tissue sufficient to maintain normal serum calcium levels is ruled out. In patients with the MEN-I syndrome in whom one parathyroid gland is only slightly enlarged, subtotal parathyroidectomy is technically easy. Subtotal parathyroidectomy is considered justified in this situation by an experience demonstrating long-term control of hypercalcemia for most patients and the avoidance of at least a temporary period of hypoparathyroidism after operation, which occurs with total parathyroidectomy and autotransplantation.

The need for indefinite monitoring of serum calcium levels of patients with the MEN-I syndrome is well established.

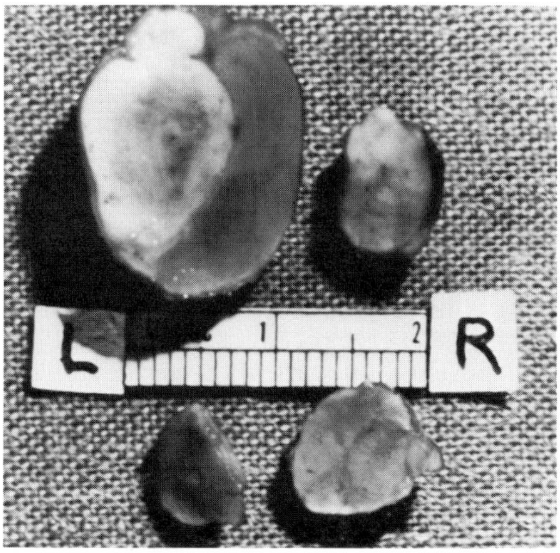


**FIGURE 23–2.** Cross-section of parathyroid glands from a patient with MEN-I syndrome showing nodular hyperplasia involving all glands. Great enlargement of all parathyroid glands can make preservation of 30 to 100 mg of viable parathyroid tissue (subtotal parathyroidectomy) technically difficult.

## HYPERPARATHYROIDISM IN MEN-IIa SYNDROME

The MEN-II syndrome comprises bilateral medullary thyroid carcinoma in all patients. Members of some families with the MEN-IIa syndrome also demonstrate hyperparathyroidism.[14] The MEN-IIa syndrome also includes pheochromocytomas, also usually bilateral in adrenal glands of some members of some affected families. The MEN-IIb syndrome is distinguished by the presence of mucosal neuromas producing a characteristic facies that can be recognized in infancy; this syndrome is also characterized by an appearance early in life. However, hyperparathyroidism is not a component of the MEN-IIb syndrome.[9]

The hazards of pheochromocytoma make a search for this lesion advisable for patients with MEN-II, with priority given for treatment of this adrenal neoplasm when present. Also, precedence is usually given next to the surgical treatment of medullary thyroid carcinoma because of the life-endangering features of this carcinoma in the MEN-IIa syndrome.

An identifiable chromosomal abnormality has been demonstrated for patients with the MEN-II syndrome[20] (see addendum preceding references). However, at this time the finding of elevated levels of serum calcitonin serves as the clinical marker for evidence of the MEN-II syndrome in family members by documenting the presence of the basic lesion, medullary thyroid carcinoma or C cell hyperplasia or both, in each lobe of the thyroid gland.

Hyperparathyroidism is seen infrequently in the MEN-IIa syndrome and is usually mild when present. Although the tendency for hyperparathyroidism to be mild might be explained by the effect of elevated levels of serum calcitonin to suppress hypercalcemia, this seems unlikely, especially in that correction of hypercalcitoninemia by elimination of thyroid medullary carcinoma does not result in the flare-up of an underlying hyperparathyroidism.

One or more enlarged hyperplastic parathyroid glands are frequently found at the time of total thyroidectomy for hereditary medullary thyroid carcinoma, yet hypercalcemia or other evidence of hyperparathyroidism is not evident at any time before or after operation after removal of all medullary thyroid carcinoma[9] (Fig. 23–3). In such patients, removal of the enlarged parathyroid gland or glands is justified, but an effort is made to preserve other parathyroid glands to prevent permanent hypoparathyroidism. Identified normal-appearing parathyroid glands can be marked by placing a colored permanent suture nearby to be used in the event hyperparathyroidism later requires reoperation; however, this action is rarely required.

Another observation of interest has been the occasional finding of hyperplasia, either diffuse or nodular, in normal-sized parathyroid glands removed necessarily or incidentally during total thyroidectomy for the MEN-IIa syndrome.[9, 20] This may represent early or indolent hyperparathyroidism in such patients.

The infrequent occurrence of clinical hyperparathyroidism in patients with the MEN-IIa syndrome and the greater risk of permanent hypoparathyroidism because of the necessity for total thyroidectomy for patients with the MEN-IIa syndrome have stimulated efforts to preserve normal-sized parathyroid glands for patients with this syndrome. Deliberate parathyroid surgery has been needed only for patients with overt hyperparathyroidism.

Subtotal parathyroidectomy has appeared adequate to control hyperparathyroidism for the majority of patients with the MEN-IIa syndrome. When all parathyroid glands are greatly enlarged and levels of serum calcium are high or other manifestations of hyperparathyroidism are apparent, total parathyroidectomy with autotransplantation of parathyroid tissue is justified. Rarely, this situation evolves over a period of years after total thyroidectomy for medullary thyroid carcinoma in the MEN-IIa syndrome and produces an increase in technical problems in reoperative surgery for parathyroid hyperplasia. In general, however, the effects of hyperparathyroidism have been less serious in the MEN-IIa syndrome than in the MEN-I syndrome. Cance and Wells[20] preferred total parathyroidectomy with autotransplantation for patients with the MEN-IIa syndrome with evidence of clinical hyperparathyroidism. This procedure is preferred also when possible for patients who require surgery for hyperparathyroidism after total thyroidectomy to minimize technical problems related to reoperation and to maximize the control of hyperparathyroidism. Patients with the MEN-IIa syndrome should be monitored by periodic serum calcium determinations; the frequency of testing should be individualized on the basis of serum calcium levels, occurrence of hyperparathyroidism in other family members, and accompanying medical problems.

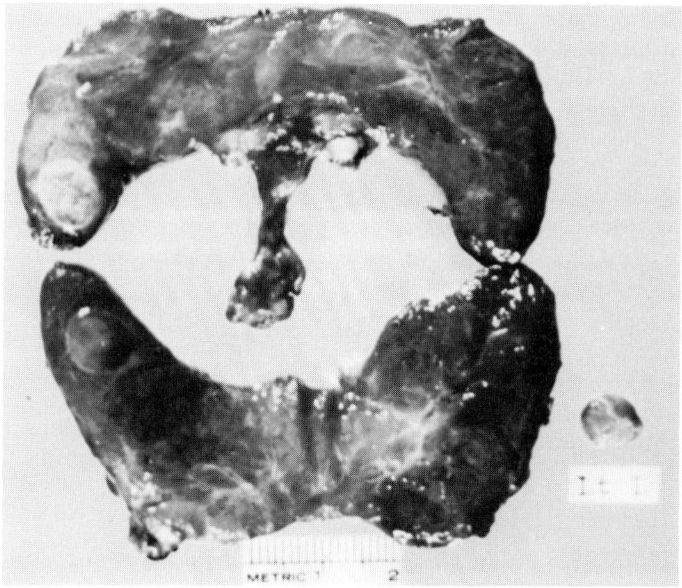

**FIGURE 23–3.** Cross-section of thyroid gland and incidental enlarged parathyroid gland (80 mg) removed at left lower position for patient with MEN-IIa syndrome. Patient had no clinical evidence of hyperparathyroidism. Nodule seen in thyroid tissue at left was an incidental benign nodule; only C cell hyperplasia was present microscopically in the thyroid lobes bilaterally. This finding indicates that asymptomatic parathyroid hyperplasia can occur in the MEN-IIa syndrome before overt medullary thyroid carcinoma.

## HYPERPARATHYROIDISM ASSOCIATED WITH FOREGUT CARCINOIDS

Carcinoid tumors, especially of the foregut, may be associated with hyperparathyroidism, and this condition may be familial.[22] Genetic relationships do not appear to have been well identified. Patients with foregut carcinoids should be screened for hyperparathyroidism, and, when these tumors or hyperparathyroidism is found, other members of the family should be examined for this entity. The carcinoid tumors produce a variety of hormones, resulting in a broad spectrum of clinical manifestations, the dominant hormone produced determining features of the clinical picture. Histochemical findings in studies of carcinoid tumors correlate with hormone production. The carcinoids should be distinguished from gastrinomas.

In the majority of patients, all parathyroid glands are hyperplastic in this syndrome of associated foregut carcinoid tumors and primary hyperparathyroidism. Thus, subtotal parathyroidectomy or, when appropriate, total parathyroidectomy with autotransplantation of parathyroid tissue is indicated.

## SPORADIC ASSOCIATION OF HYPERPARATHYROIDISM WITH OTHER ENDOCRINE NEOPLASMS

The sporadic association of hyperparathyroidism with virtually all other known endocrine neoplasms has been reported[47, 49] and may involve single or multiple occurrences. Carotid body tumors, which may be bilateral, have been present in a number of patients reported.[47] In sporadic associations, hyperparathyroidism is the result of enlargement of a single parathyroid gland in nearly all instances. When hyperplasia of multiple parathyroid glands is found, it is especially important to screen other family members for endocrine neoplasms, including hyperparathyroidism.

Other endocrine neoplasms can ectopically produce parathormonelike substances and simulate an associated hyperparathyroidism.[49] Thus, it is wise to suspect such an association and to manage the other endocrine neoplasm first and only later to explore parathyroid glands when evidence of hyperparathyroidism persists and operative correction is justified.

Other endocrine neoplasms can conceivably serve as a stimulus for later hyperparathyroidism. Thus, hypocalcemia induced by primary aldosteronism might serve to produce parathyroid autonomy.

## FAMILIAL HYPOPHOSPHATEMIC RICKETS WITH SECONDARY HYPERPARATHYROIDISM

Hereditary hypophosphatemic rickets is a congenital disease involving a proximal renal tubular phosphate transport abnormality that results in renal phosphate leak and hypophosphatemia. Hypercalciuria and stimulation of parathyroid hormone release evidently also occur with bone demineralization and abnormalities in skeletal growth. Autonomously functioning hyperplastic parathyroid tumors result with secondary hyperparathyroidism.[48] In such patients, severe bone disease may require total parathyroidectomy and autotransplantation.[31] These patients are also at risk for the development of graft-dependent recurrent hyperparathyroidism and later may require resection of grafted parathyroid tissue. These considerations apply to other familial renal disease, such as congenital cystic disease of the kidney, which can, by causing renal insufficiency, induce secondary hyperparathyroidism.

Of interest is the occurrence of familial isolated hyperparathyroidism.[1] Furthermore, features of pseudohypoparathyroidism and pseudopseudohypoparathyroidism can occur in different members of the same family.

## FAMILIAL PARATHYROID CARCINOMA

Parathyroid carcinoma has been reported[21] in members of families with hereditary hyperparathyroidism. The diagnosis of parathyroid carcinoma requires documentation of direct invasion of adjacent tissue or metastatic disease. Diffuse calcifications, especially in the lungs and in the skin of the extremities with ulcer formation, may be a complication. Parathyroid carcinomas are usually functioning, and hypercalcemia becomes difficult to control; thus it, rather than other effects of the malignant lesion, usually causes death. Acute pancreatitis with acute hypercalcemic crisis can also be the terminal event.

Wide excision of a parathyroid carcinoma usually requires at least partial thyroidectomy and removal of structures, including muscle, invaded by the carcinoma. On occasion, removal of a large distant metastatic lesion provides significant palliation. Methods of palliation also include use of medical measures, such as etidronate, mithramycin, and calcitonin, in an attempt to control hypercalcemia.

## OPERATIVE CONSIDERATIONS

### *Preoperative Steps*

The patient and appropriate family members should be aware of the implications of hyperparathyroidism in a familial occurrence or as a component of a MEN syndrome. Usually a final decision as to the precise operative procedure is best made at the time of operation, but either subtotal parathyroidectomy or total parathyroidectomy with autotransplantation of parathyroid tissue is anticipated.

Preoperative localization techniques are not sufficiently precise to identify all parathyroid glands in most instances of multiple gland enlargement, which is characteristic of most patients with familial or hereditary forms of hyperparathyroidism. At least one parathyroid gland in these patients may be too small for recognition by localization studies now available. It is the least enlarged or slightly enlarged, as well as ectopically located, parathyroid glands that present difficulties for the surgeon at operation. The cost effectiveness of routine preoperative localization studies for all patients has not yet been resolved, but no good evidence is available to mandate such testing. At this time, ultrasonography appears to be the most cost effective. The use of technetium 99m pertechnetate-thallium 201 techniques can be valuable in locating ectopic large parathyroid glands. Magnetic resonance imaging may provide improvement in accuracy of localization of parathyroid glands but is expensive. Most techniques have individual limitations and fail to provide dependable localization in approximately 20 to 40 per cent of patients with hyperparathyroidism. These studies are indicated for patients requiring reoperation for persistent or recurrent hyperparathyroidism and in patients in the high-risk group undergoing primary operation. In the latter group, it is important to minimize operative time and the possibility of overlooking ectopically located hyperplastic parathyroid glands.

## *Principles of Operative Techniques*

The objective in operation for hyperparathyroidism of familial or MEN types is to identify all parathyroid tissue and provide an appropriate removal of the hyperplastic parathyroid glands. The significant frequency of supernumerary glands requires a search for ectopically located parathyroid glands, especially high in the neck (for undescended parathyroid glands), in the thyroid gland, in the superior mediastinum, in the posterior mediastinum, and along the carotid sheaths.[23] It is usually advisable to mobilize and remove as much thymic tissue as possible through the cervical incision to ensure excision of abnormal parathyroid glands in this location.

When all parathyroid tissue has been identified, a decision is made as to the extent of removal and is individualized.[5, 6] From a technical standpoint, at least the volume of a viable normal parathyroid gland should be preserved in subtotal parathyroidectomy. The procedure should involve preservation of approximately 30 to 50 mg of normal parathyroid tissue. Because of the likelihood of injury in dividing an enlarged parathyroid gland to preserve a portion sufficient to provide normal serum calcium levels, sometimes it is necessary to err in preserving an amount of parathyroid tissue somewhat greater in size—up to an estimated 100 mg of tissue.

Initially in subtotal parathyroidectomy, it is best to perform subtotal removal of a parathyroid gland to ensure preservation of a viable fragment of 30 to 100 mg. When division of the parathyroid gland fails technically to preserve the desired amount of parathyroid tissue, the procedure is carried out on a second parathyroid gland. It usually is technically easier to perform partial removal of a parathyroid gland using the smallest of the parathyroid glands. After subtotal removal of parathyroid tissue from one parathyroid gland has been completed, the other enlarged and hyperplastic parathyroid glands can be removed. In some patients, one of the parathyroid glands, which may be normal in size or only slightly enlarged, may deserve preservation intact. No removal of a part of this parathyroid gland is performed except for a biopsy to confirm that it is a parathyroid gland.

The term 3½ gland parathyroidectomy often is inaccurate in describing subtotal parathyroidectomy inasmuch as removal of one half of a fourth parathyroid gland may not preserve sufficient parathyroid tissue. It is helpful to mark the preserved parathyroid fragment by a permanent colored suture to use in identifying the parathyroid tissue should reoperation ever be necessary.

For total parathyroidectomy, all parathyroid tissue is removed. The parathyroid tissue to be autotransplanted or frozen for possible later autotransplantation should be confirmed by microscopic study at the time of operation. The parathyroid tissue for autotransplantation or freezing is cut into fine slices. A high success rate of autotransplantation requires 60 to 70 mg of tissue.[38, 44] Many sites are satisfactory for placing the parathyroid tissue for autotransplantation. The forearm muscle is used frequently to permit ease of assessment of function by determination of levels of parathyroid hormone in blood from veins draining the site of parathyroid autotransplantation. Success is reduced when the parathyroid tissue is frozen and later used for autotransplantation when the need is verified.[46] Because supernumerary parathyroid tissue may not have been removed during total parathyroidectomy, some surgeons prefer to delay autotransplantation of parathyroid tissue until this question is resolved after operation.[17]

The presence of accessory parathyroid tissue as tiny fragments, not as identifiable glands, probably occurs more often than appreciated in the past. These residual or embryologic rests are often in close proximity to a normal or standard parathyroid gland.[2, 26]

This finding has been observed in the form of microscopic clumps of parathyroid tissue in fat surrounding a parathyroid gland or may form a tiny visible clump of parathyroid tissue at an independent location or in proximity to a normal parathyroid gland (Figs. 23–4 and 23–5). Such fragments of residual parathyroid tissue may, over an extended period of stimulation, become hyperplastic and enlarge enough to be of clinical importance. Hyperplasia of such accessory parathyroid tissue may contribute to recurrent hyperparathyroidism, particularly in the multiple endocrine syndromes or chronic uremia,[26, 36] and has introduced the question of whether total parathyroidectomy is often incomplete in a strict sense.

As indicated in the paragraphs concerning the MEN-I syndrome, the high recurrence rate of hyperparathyroidism in this syndrome has led some surgeons to prefer total parathyroidectomy with autotransplantation for this entity even though recurrence is often delayed for many years. Total parathyroidectomy with autotransplantation is performed when all parathyroid glands are huge and preservation of 30 to 100 mg of viable parathyroid tissue is technically difficult. When

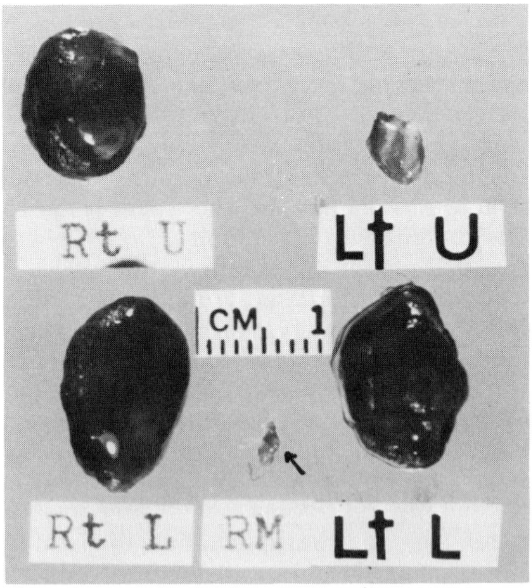


**FIGURE 23–4.** Parathyroid tissue removed in subtotal parathyroidectomy for familial hyperparathyroidism with removal also of a small remnant of accessory or supernumerary (fifth) parathyroid tissues (between the lower parathyroid glands at the arrow). These tiny fragments of supernumerary parathyroid tissue can enlarge and contribute to persistent or recurrent hyperparathyroidism.

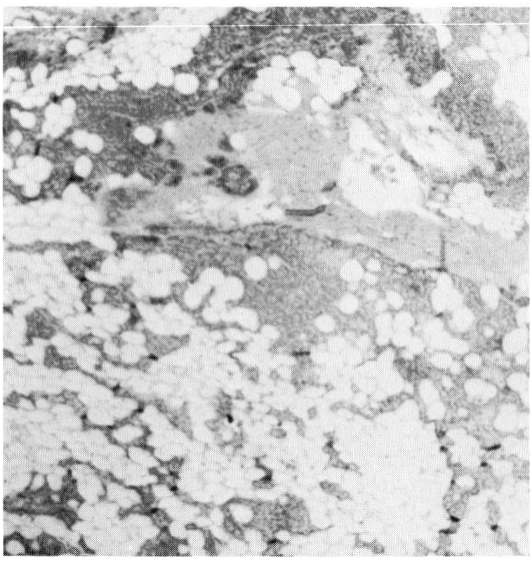

**FIGURE 23–5.** Photomicrograph of fragments of parathyroid tissue in fat surrounding a parathyroid adenoma. This accessory parathyroid tissue can enlarge in familial and hereditary hyperparathyroidism and contribute to persistent or recurrent hyperparathyroidism.

subtotal parathyroidectomy is technically possible, this operation has provided results that can justify its use in the MEN-I syndrome. When reoperation is needed for recurrent hyperparathyroidism, total parathyroidectomy with autotransplantation of parathyroid tissue is given preference. These policies are also followed in other situations in which all parathyroid tissue is hyperplastic. In facilities lacking equipment needed for proper freezing of parathyroid tissue, immediate autotransplantation of parathyroid tissue is considered justified when total parathyroidectomy is performed. When recurrent hyperparathyroidism is sufficient to require removal of a part of autotransplanted parathyroid tissue later, this procedure is performed.

A number of technical refinements are available for parathyroid surgery. Intraoperative ultrasonography can be used to locate elusive parathyroid tumors.[41] Fine needle aspiration biopsy under ultrasound or computed tomography guidance can be used to confirm parathyroid tissue localized by these or other techniques before operation in problem cases. Invasive localizing techniques, including arteriography and venous sampling for elevated parathyroid hormone levels, are available for difficult situations.

## RESULTS OF OPERATION

Control of hypercalcemia for patients with hyperparathyroidism of a familial or multiple endocrine neoplasia variety is not as high as for patients with sporadic hyperparathyroidism. Persistent or recurrent (6 months or more after operation but within a few years) hyperparathyroidism caused by an overlooked hyperplastic parathyroid gland or hyperplasia of a preserved parathyroid remnant occurs in approximately 8 to 10 per cent of patients (Tables 23–3 and 23–4).[15, 24, 50–52] Reoperation is reaching 90 per cent success now.[18, 28] However, for the MEN-I syndrome, long-term studies[2, 8, 38, 43] show recurrence of hyperparathyroidism to approximate 40 to 50 per cent after subtotal parathyroidectomy. In one of my patients with the MEN-I syndrome, evidence of recurrent hyperparathyroidism developed 17 years after subtotal parathyroidectomy. The recurrence of hyperparathyroidism in patients with MEN-I appears to be as great after total parathyroidectomy with autotransplantation as after subtotal parathyroidectomy.[36] However, correction is easier by removal of a part of hyperplastic autotransplanted parathyroid tissue from the forearm or similar location than by reexploration of the neck. Thallium 201 scanning can identify the hyperplastic parathyroid tissue producing graft-dependent recurrent hyperparathyroidism after autotransplantation.[40] Serum parathyroid hormone levels do not appear decisive in follow-up studies of patients after surgical correction of hyperparathyroidism, but further experience is needed.

In a review of 862 patients undergoing operation for primary hyperparathyroidism between 1955 and 1986 under diverse circumstances, Bruining and associates[19] reported that primary hyperparathyroidism was not confirmed in 67 patients or 8 per cent. Of the remaining 795 patients, operation failed in 89 patients or 11 per cent. In 48 patients, the surgeon failed to find and remove a single enlarged parathyroid gland; in the remaining 41 patients, the surgeon failed to remove adequate amounts of parathyroid disease in multiple parathyroid gland involvement. Of the 41 failures in multiple parathyroid gland involvement (28 per cent of the total series),

**TABLE 23–3. Management of Parathyroid Hyperplasia by Subtotal Parathyroidectomy: Reported Results for Primary Hyperparathyroidism**

| REPORT | OPERATIVE CRITERIA | NUMBER OF CASES | HYPERCALCEMIA CONTROLLED | PERMANENT HYPOCALCEMIA | FOLLOW-UP PERIOD |
|---|---|---|---|---|---|
| Block et al.,[8] 1978 | Preserve 50–100 mg | 2 Glands involved, 7 | 100% } 94% | 14% } 8% | 1–17 yrs; average, 4.4 yrs |
| | | 3 Glands involved, 9 | 89% | 0 | |
| | | All glands involved, 20 | 85% | 10% | |
| Block et al.,[11] 1979 | Preserve 50–100 mg | 3 Glands involved, 19 | 92% } 86% | | 1–19 yrs; average, 4.9 yrs |
| | | All glands involved, 25 | 79% | | |
| | | Nonfamilial, non-MEN, nonrenal insufficiency, 30 | 93% | 4.5% | |
| Edis et al.,[24] 1979 | Preserve 30–100 mg | 55 | 87% | 5% | 1–17 yrs; average, 3.9 yrs |
| | | MEN, 9; familial, 5 | All failures = 5% persistence | | |
| Wang et al.,[50] 1982 | Preserve 30–50 mg | Clear cell, 9 | 78% | 0 | 2–12 yrs |
| | | Chief cell, <4 glands involved, 24; | 100% | | |
| | | 4 glands involved, 21 | 95% | 5% | 1 mo–8 yrs |
| Bondeson et al.,[15] 1985 | Remove 2–3 glands, 26 patients | 39 Total (nonfamilial) I | 85% } 90% | 15% | 1–17 yrs; average, 3.9 yrs |
| | Remove 2–3 glands; partial removal 1–2 glands, 13 patients | II | 100% | | |
| Wells et al.,[51] 1985 | Remove all glands more than 50 mg | 76 (<4 glands involved) | 89.5% | 4% | 1–11 yrs |

**TABLE 23–4. Surgical Management of Parathyroid Hyperplasia Causing Primary Hyperparathyroidism: Comparison of Subtotal Parathyroidectomy with Total Parathyroidectomy and Autotransplantation**

| PRODEDURE | HYPERCALCEMIA CONTROLLED | PERMANENT HYPOCALCEMIA |
|---|---|---|
| Subtotal parathyroidectomy (summary reported cases) | | |
| For <4 gland involvement (approximately 200 cases; see Table 23–3) | 90% | 5% (0–15%) |
| Four-gland involvement (approximately 59 cases) | 87% | 5+% (5%–15%) |
| Total parathyroidectomy, autotransplantation Wells et al.[52] 1980 | | |
| Four-gland involvement (36 cases including 16 familial, 4 familial hypocalciuric hypercalcemic hyperparathyroidism) | 92% immediate<br>70% long-term | 5.6% |

approximately one half were the result of persistent disease and one half were the result of recurrent hyperparathyroidism recognized 6 months to 17 years later.

In a review of 416 patients undergoing operation for primary hyperparathyroidism from 1956 through 1979 (339 or 77 per cent adenomas and 77 or 23 per cent hyperplasia), Rudberg and associates[45] found that 33 patients or 8 per cent had persistent hypercalcemia after operation. Of these 33 patients, 15 underwent reoperation of which 11 were successful (missed adenoma in six patients, inadequate parathyroidectomy for hyperplasia in five); for 18 patients, reoperation was not considered necessary. Of the 22 (5 per cent) recurrences (hypercalcemia evident 6 months or later after operation), 12 patients with parathyroid hyperplasia evidenced recurrence up to 19 years, and 10 patients with adenoma experienced recurrence after 9 to 17 years. Of the patients with adenoma, in six patients or 2 per cent the lesion was not found at the initial operation, with 10 patients or 3 per cent having recurrence 9 to 17 years after operation. Of patients with parathyroid hyperplasia, five or 7 per cent showed persistent hypercalcemia, and 12 or 16 per cent evidenced recurrence as long as 19 years after operation. Of the latter group, a number of patients had the MEN-I syndrome.

Complications specific to subtotal parathyroidectomy relate primarily to permanent hypoparathyroidism. This complication has been reported at frequencies varying from 0 to 15 per cent, with an average of approximately 5 per cent (Tables 23–3 and 23–4). With greater use of autotransplantation of parathyroid tissue, the incidence of this complication may lessen. Permanent loss of function of a recurrent laryngeal nerve should be less than 1 per cent. No reliable data are available for the incidence of permanent loss of function of the external branch of the superior laryngeal nerve. Complications that can occur after any surgical operation, including wound hematomas or infection or both, pneumonia, thrombophlebitis and pulmonary embolism, myocardial infarction, and arrhythmias, can occur after subtotal parathyroidectomy or total parathyroidectomy with autotransplantation but should be unusual.

For patients with recurrent hyperparathyroidism of a mild degree, medical measures may suffice to provide reasonable control of hypercalcemia. Medical measures include the use of phosphate supplements and restriction of dairy products, a large fluid intake, and estrogens and progesterone in combination or separately. Nonoperative techniques, such as transarterial catheter ablation, can be of help in certain problem situations. Also, for patients at high risk in reoperation, ultrasonically guided percutaneous inactivation of parathyroid tumors using alcohol is reported[30] to control hypercalcemia for at least a period of months. The diagnosis of a parathyroid tumor is first confirmed by fine needle aspiration cytology in these patients. However, this treatment is not possible for patients with parathyroid gland hyperplasia because of difficulties in identifying and treating multiple parathyroid tumors.

Experience has demonstrated the need for periodic evaluations indefinitely of patients having hyperparathyroidism of the familial or multiple endocrine neoplasia varieties.

**Addendum.** Progress has been made recently in identifying the gene for the MEN-II syndrome to chromosome 10. The clinical role for this information in genetic screening is yet to be determined. (Ponder, B.: Multiple endocrine neoplasia type 2: The search for the gene continues. Br. Med. J., *300*:484–485, 1990.)

## REFERENCES


1. Ahn, T. G., Antonarakis, S. E., Kronenberg, H. M., et al.: Familial isolated hypoparathyroidism: A molecular genetic analysis of 8 families with 23 affected persons. Medicine, *65:*73–81, 1986.
2. Åkerström, G., Malmaeus, J., and Bergström, R.: Surgical anatomy of human parathyroid glands. Surgery, *95:*14–21, 1984.
3. Allo, M., and Thompson, N. W.: Familial hyperparathyroidism caused by solitary adenomas. Surgery, *92:*486–490, 1982.
4. Benson, L., Ljunghall, S., Åkerström, G., and Öberg, K.: Hyperparathyroidism presenting as the first lesion in multiple endocrine neoplasia type 1. Am. J. Med., *82:*731–737, 1987.
5. Block, M. A.: Exploration of parathyroid glands and subtotal resection for hyperplasia. *In* Nyhus, L. M., and Baker, R. J. (eds.): Mastery of Surgery. Boston, Little, Brown and Company, 1984, pp. 205–212.
6. Block, M. A., and Cerny, J. C.: The endocrine system. *In* Beahrs, O. H., and Beart, R. W., Jr. (eds.): General Surgery—Therapy Update Service. Media, PA, Harwal Medical Publications, 1987, pp. 1–45.
7. Block, M. A., Frame, B., and Fox, T. A., Jr.: The clinical course of duodenal ulcer associated with hyperparathyroidism. Henry Ford Hosp. Med. J., *19:*21–26, 1971.
8. Block, M. A., Frame, B., and Jackson, C. E.: The efficacy of subtotal parathyroidectomy for primary hyperparathyroidism due to multiple gland involvement. Surg. Gynecol. Obstet., *147:*1–5, 1978.
9. Block, M. A., Jackson, C. E., and Tashjian, A. H., Jr.: Management of parathyroid glands in surgery for medullary thyroid carcinoma. Arch. Surg., *110:*617–624, 1975.
10. Block, M. A., Frame, B., Jackson, C. E., and Horn, R. C., Jr.: The extent of operation for primary hyperparathyroidism. Arch. Surg., *109:*798–801, 1974.
11. Block, M. A., Frame, B., Kleerekoper, M., and Rao, D. S.: Surgical management of persistence or recurrence after subtotal parathyroidectomy for primary hyperparathyroidism. Am. J. Surg., *138:*561–566, 1979.
12. Block, M. A., Greenawald, K., Horn, R. C., Jr., and Frame, B.: Involvement of multiple parathyroids in hyperparathyroidism. Am. J. Surg., *114:*530–537, 1967.
13. Block, M. A., Frame, B., Jackson, C. E., et al.: Primary diffuse microscopical hyperplasia of the parathyroid glands: Surgical importance. Arch. Surg., *111:*348–354, 1976.
14. Block, M. A., Jackson, C. E., Greenawald, K. A., et al.: Clinical characteristics distinguishing hereditary from sporadic medullary thyroid carcinoma: Treatment implications. Arch. Surg., *115:*142–148, 1980.
15. Bondeson, A.-G., Bondeson, L., Ljungberg, O., and Tibblin, S.: Surgical strategy in nonfamilial primary parathyroid hyperplasia: Long-term follow-up of thirty-nine cases. Surgery, *97:*569–573, 1985.
16. Brandi, M. L., Aurbach, G. D., Fitzpatrick, L. A., et al.: Parathyroid mitogenic activity in plasma from patients with familial multiple endocrine neoplasia type 1. N. Engl. J. Med., *314:*1287–1293, 1986.
17. Brennan, M. F., and Brown, E. M.: Prediction of in vivo function of human parathyroid tissue autografts by in vitro testing. World J. Surg., *4:*747–751, 1980.
18. Brennan, M. F., and Norton, J. A.: Reoperation for persistent and recurrent hyperparathyroidism. Ann. Surg., *201:*40–44, 1985.
19. Bruining, H. A., Birkenhäger, J. C., Ong, G. L., and Lamberts, S. W. J.: Causes of failure in operations for hyperparathyroidism. Surgery, *101:*562–565, 1987.
20. Cance, W. G., and Wells, S. A., Jr.: Multiple endocrine neoplasia: Type IIa. Curr. Probl. Surg., *22:*1–56, 1985.
21. Dinnen, J. S., Greenwood, R. H., Jones, J. H., et al.: Parathyroid carcinoma in familial hyperparathyroidism. J. Clin. Pathol., *30:*966–975, 1977.
22. Duh, Q.-Y., Hybarger, C. P., Geist, R., et al.: Carcinoids associated with multiple endocrine neoplasia syndromes. Am. J. Surg., *154:*142–148, 1987.
23. Edis, A. J., and Levitt, M. D.: Supernumerary parathyroid glands: Implications for the surgical treatment of secondary hyperparathyroidism. World J. Surg., *11:*398–401, 1987.
24. Edis, A. J., van Heerden, J. A., and Scholz, D. A.: Results of subtotal parathyroidectomy for primary chief cell hyperplasia. Surgery, *86:*462–469, 1979.
25. Farndon, J. R., Geraghty, J. M., Dilley, W. G., et al.: Serum gastrin, calcitonin, and prolactin as markers of multiple endocrine neoplasia syndromes in patients with primary hyperparathyroidism. World J. Surg., *11:*252–257, 1987.
26. Farrington, K., Varghese, Z., Chan, M. K., et al.: How complete is a total parathyroidectomy in uraemia? Br. Med. J. (Clin. Res.), *294:*743, 1987.
27. Fialkow, P. J., Jackson, C. E., Block, M. A., and Greenawald, K. A.: Multicellular origin of parathyroid "adenomas." N. Engl. J. Med., *297:*696–698, 1977.
28. Grant, C. S., van Heerden, J. A., Charboneau, J. W., et al.: Clinical management of persistent and/or recurrent primary hyperparathyroidism. World J. Surg., *10:*555–565, 1986.
29. Jackson, C. E., Block, M. A., Greenawald, K. A., and Tashjian, A. H., Jr.: The two-mutational-event theory in medullary thyroid cancer. Am. J. Hum. Genet., *31:*704–710, 1979.
30. Karstrup, S., Holm, H. H., Torp-Pedersen, S., and Hegedüs, L.: Ultrasonically guided percutaneous inactivation of parathyroid tumours. Br. J. Radiol., *60:*667–670, 1987.

31. Kinder, B. K., and Rasmussen, H.: New applications of total parathyroidectomy and autotransplantation: Use in proximal renal tubular dysfunction. World J. Surg., *9:*156–164, 1985.
32. Law, W. M., Jr., and Heath, H., III: Familial benign hypercalcemia (hypocalciuric hypercalcemia): Clinical and pathogenetic studies in 21 families. Ann. Intern. Med., *102:*511–519, 1985.
33. Law, W. M., Jr., Hodgson, S. F., and Heath, H., III: Autosomal recessive inheritance of familial hyperparathyroidism. N. Engl. J. Med., *309:*650–653, 1983.
34. Macleod, A. F., Ayers, B., Young, A. E., et al.: Resolution of hypergastrinaemia after parathyroidectomy in multiple endocrine neoplasia syndrome type I (MEN type I). Clin. Endocrinol. (Oxf.), *26:*693–698, 1987.
35. Majewski, J. T., and Wilson, S. D.: The MEA-I syndrome: An all or none phenomenon? Surgery, *86:*475–484, 1979.
36. Mallette, L. E., Blevins, T., Jordan, P. H., and Noon, G. P.: Autogenous parathyroid grafts for generalized primary parathyroid hyperplasia: Contrasting outcome in sporadic hyperplasia versus multiple endocrine neoplasia type I. Surgery, *101:*738–745, 1987.
37. Mallette, L. E., Malini, S., Rappaport, M. P., and Kirkland, J. L.: Familial cystic parathyroid adenomatosis. Ann. Intern. Med., *107:*54–60, 1987.
38. Malmaeus, J., Benson, L., Johansson, H., et al.: Parathyroid surgery in the multiple endocrine neoplasia type I syndrome: Choice of surgical procedure. World J. Surg., *10:*668–672, 1986.
39. Marx, S. J., Attie, M. F., Spiegel, A. M., et al.: An association between neonatal severe primary hyperparathyroidism and familial hypocalciuric hypercalcemia in three kindreds. N. Engl. J. Med., *306:*257–264, 1982.
40. McCall, A. R., Calandra, D., Lawrence, A. M., et al.: Parathyroid autotransplantation in forty-four patients with primary hyperparathyroidism: The role of thallium scanning. Surgery, *100:*614–620, 1986.
41. Norton, J. A., Shawker, T. H., Jones, B. L., et al.: Intraoperative ultrasound and reoperative parathyroid surgery: An initial evaluation. World J. Surg., *10:*631–639, 1986.
42. Rasbach, D. A., van Heerden, J. A., Telander, R. L., et al.: Surgical management of hyperinsulinism in the multiple endocrine neoplasia, type 1 syndrome. Arch. Surg., *120:*584–589, 1985.
43. Rizzoli, R., Green, J., III, and Marx, S. J.: Primary hyperparathyroidism in familial multiple endocrine neoplasia type I: Long-term follow-up of serum calcium levels after parathyroidectomy. Am. J. Med., *78:*467–474, 1985.
44. Rothmund, M., and Wagner, P. K.: Assessment of parathyroid graft function after autotransplantation of fresh and cryopreserved tissue. World J. Surg., *8:*527–533, 1984.
45. Rudberg, C., Åkerström, G., Palmér, M., et al.: Late results of operation for primary hyperparathyroidism in 441 patients. Surgery, *99:*643–651, 1986.
46. Saxe, A.: Parathyroid transplantation: A review. Surgery, *95:*507–526, 1984.
47. Steely, W. M., Davies, R. S., and Brigham, R. A.: Carotid body tumor and hyperparathyroidism: A case report and review of the literature. Am. Surg., *53:*337–338, 1987.
48. Tieder, M., Modai, D., Shaked, U., et al.: "Idiopathic" hypercalciuria and hereditary hypophosphatemic rickets: Two phenotypical expressions of a common genetic defect. N. Engl. J. Med., *316:*125–129, 1987.
49. Vair, D. B., Boudreau, S. F., and Reid, E. L.: Pancreatic islet-cell neoplasia, with secretion of a parathormone-like substance and hypercalcemia. Can. J. Surg., *30:*108–110, 1987.
50. Wang, C.-A., Castleman, B., and Cope, O.: Surgical management of hyperparathyroidism due to primary hyperplasia. Ann. Surg., *195:*384–392, 1982.
51. Wells, S. A., Jr., Leight, G. S., Hensley, M., and Dilley, W. G.: Hyperparathyroidism associated with the enlargement of two or three parathyroid glands. Ann. Surg., *202:*533–538, 1985.
52. Wells, S. A., Jr., Farndon, J. R., Dale, J. K., et al.: Long-term evaluation of patients with primary parathyroid hyperplasia managed by total parathyroidectomy and heterotopic autotransplantation. Ann. Surg., *192:*451–458, 1980.

# 24

# IMAGING OF PARATHYROID GLANDS WITH RADIONUCLIDES

*Peter F. Winter, M.D.*

The combined use of $^{99m}Tc$ pertechnetate and Tl-201 chloride with appropriate subtraction technique has evolved as the radionuclide imaging method of choice for evaluation of the parathyroid glands.[8] The study is noninvasive and can be performed in about 45 minutes in a nuclear medicine department equipped with a computer for image processing.

Subtraction scintigraphy using $^{99m}Tc$/Tl-201 is based on the observation that the thyroid gland accumulates both $^{99m}Tc$ pertechnetate and Tl-201 chloride and the parathyroid gland accumulates only Tl-201 chloride. Thus, after injection of Tl-201 chloride alone, a composite image of the thyroid gland and the parathyroid gland is produced. Additional visualization of the thyroid gland with $^{99m}Tc$ pertechnetate permits subtraction of the thyroid image from the combined image, with the parathyroid image remaining (Fig. 24–1).

Normal parathyroid glands are too small to be seen on such a subtracted parathyroid image, but enlarged parathyroid glands, such as found in patients with hyperplasia and adenomas, can be visualized (Fig. 24–2). Ectopic parathyroid adenomas in the mediastinum should be apparent on the Tl-201 image alone.

## TECHNICAL CONSIDERATIONS

The technical aspects, such as the sequence of the injection of the radiotracers and their relative administered dose levels, remain under discussion and reflect different approaches to eliminate the mutual interference of the emitted unscattered and scattered photons on the image formation. $^{99m}Tc$ emits photons with an energy of 140 keV whereas the Tl-201 emits photons at various energy levels with 90 per cent of the photons in the 69 keV to 83 keV range, which are used for imaging, and the remaining 10 per cent at 135 keV and 169 keV. The scattered photons of the $^{99m}Tc$ photons fall into the energy window of the lower energy Tl-201 photons, causing degradation of the Tl-201 image, while the Tl-201 photons at 135 keV and 169 keV fall into the energy window of $^{99m}Tc$, degrading the $^{99m}Tc$ image.

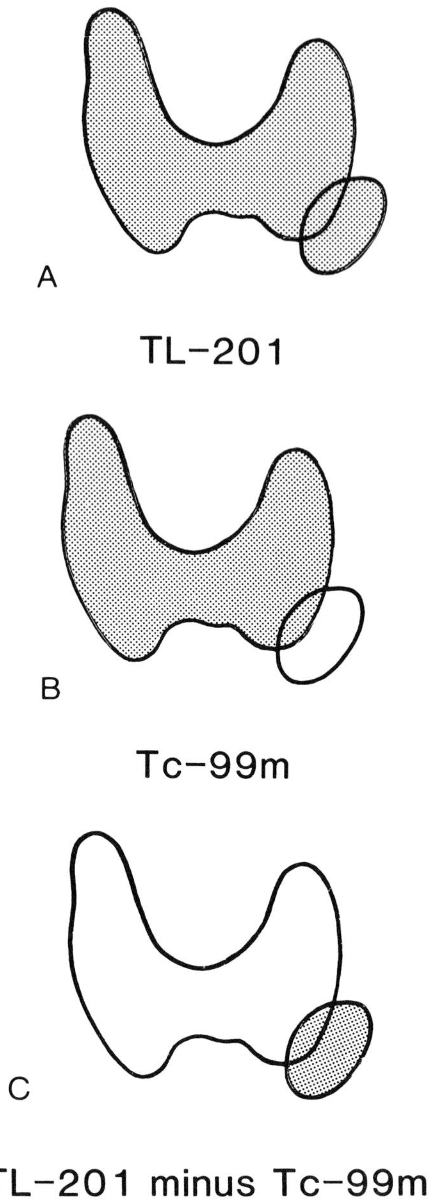


**FIGURE 24–1.** Diagram of principle of subtraction image formation. *A,* The thallium-201 image visualizes thyroid gland and parathyroid adenoma, which cannot be distinguished from each other. *B,* The $^{99m}$Tc image visualizes the thyroid gland only. *C,* The computer-generated subtraction view delineates the parathyroid adenoma.

An acceptable protocol is as follows: injection of 2 mCi of Tl-201 chloride and imaging of neck and chest at 10 minutes, injection of 1 mCi of $^{99m}$Tc pertechnetate and repeat imaging of the neck without having the patient moved after the initial images, and computer subtraction of the digitally stored images with manual adjustment of intensity differences for optimal display.

## CLINICAL CONSIDERATIONS

The sensitivity for accurate localization of parathyroid adenomas in patients with clinical and biochemical evidence of hyperparathyroidism approaches 90 per cent.[1, 6, 7, 12] The reported[8] sensitivity for the detection of hyperplastic glands is lower than that for adenomas. This difference in sensitivity is believed to reflect the discrepant glandular size found in these conditions, with adenomas usually being larger than glandular hyperplasia.

The specificity of this technique is adversely affected by Tl-201 uptake in thyroid abnormalities.[9, 10] For this reason, patients with known multinodular goiter are not well suited for $^{99m}$Tc/Tl-201 imaging. The possibility of a false-positive study can be reduced by correlating the scan with the clinical findings. Because thyroid nodules are easier to palpate than are parathyroid adenomas, a palpable finding in the area of Tl-201 uptake more likely represents a thyroid nodule rather than a parathyroid adenoma. A primary carcinoma in the neck, metastatic cervical lymph nodes, lymphoma, and sarcoidosis are other causes of false-positive results and affect the specificity.[9, 10]

Previous neck surgery lowers the sensitivity of detecting parathyroid hyperplasia or adenomas, impeding the localizing information when it is needed the most before contemplated reexploration.[5, 11] The reported sensitivity for localizing parathyroid adenoma in these patients ranges from 27 to 64 per cent.[5] The wide variance probably reflects the particular technique employed and the different patient groups studied in these reports.[5, 11]

## OTHER RADIONUCLIDE TECHNIQUES

The mechanism of the localization of thallium-201 in parathyroid tissue is nonspecific and appears to be related to cellularity and vascularity. In the past, Se-75 selenomethionine, a metabolic tracer following the incor-

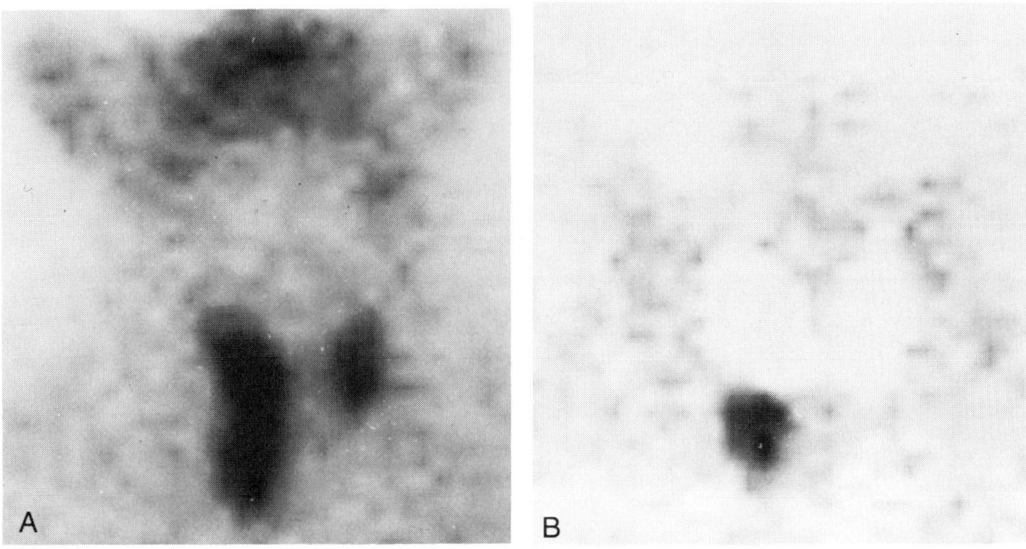


**FIGURE 24–2.** Parathyroid adenoma. *A,* The composite image shows a normal distribution of tracer in the thyroid gland. *B,* The subtraction image shows a focus of activity, which was a parathyroid adenoma.

poration of amino acids into protein, has been employed to localize parathyroid tissue. It has been abandoned because of the poor imaging characteristics of Se-75 and resultant low detection rate of parathyroid adenomas.

Occasionally, other radionuclide tracers, such as gallium-67 citrate and $^{131}$I metaiodobenzylguanidine (MBG), can visualize pathologic processes in the parathyroid glands. Gallium-67 citrate is a tracer with the propensity of accumulating in neoplastic or inflammatory processes. Anecdotal reports of a parathyroid adenoma[4] and a parathyroid carcinoma[3] visualized by gallium-67 scintigraphy have been published. The $^{131}$I MBG tracer has an affinity for neuroectodermally derived tumors and can localize in a parathyroid adenoma.[2]

## REFERENCES

1. Ferlin, G., Borsato, N., Camerani, M., et al.: New perspectives in localizing enlarged parathyroids by technetium-thallium subtraction scan. J. Nucl. Med., *24:*438–441, 1983.
2. Hayward, R. S., Bowering, C. K., and Warshawski, R. S.: I-131 metaiodobenzylguanidine uptake in a parathyroid adenoma. Clin. Nucl. Med., *13:*632–634, 1988.
3. Iwase, M., Shimuzi, Y., Kitahara, H., et al.: Parathyroid carcinoma visualized by gallium-67 citrate scintigraphy. J. Nucl. Med., *27:*63–65, 1986.
4. Katagiri, M., Harada, T., Kawano, R., et al.: Parathyroid adenoma imaged by gallium 67-citrate: A case report. Clin. Nucl. Med., *12:*788–790, 1987.
5. Miller, D. L., Doppman, J. L., Shawker, T. H., et al.: Localization of parathyroid adenomas in patients who have undergone surgery. Part 1. Noninvasive imaging methods. Radiology, *162* (1 Pt 1):133–137, 1987.
6. Peck, W. W., Higgin, C. B., Fisher, M. R., et al: Hyperparathyroidism: Comparison of MR imaging with radionuclide scanning. Radiology, *163:*415–420, 1987.
7. Percival, R. C., Blake, G. M., Urwin, G. H., et al.: Assessment of thallium-pertechnetate subtraction scintigraphy in hyperparathyroidism. Br. J. Radiol., *58:*131–135, 1985.
8. Winzelberg, G. G.: Parathyroid imaging. Ann. Intern. Med., *107:*64–70, 1987.
9. Winzelberg, G. G.: Thallium 201/99mTc parathyroid subtraction scintigraphy of the neck: Single area of increased thallium uptake. Semin. Nucl. Med., *17:*273–275, 1987.
10. Winzelberg, G. G.: Thallium 201/99mTc parathyroid subtraction scintigraphy of the neck: Multiple areas of increased thallium uptake. Semin. Nucl. Med., *17:*276–277, 1987.
11. Winzelberg, G. G., and Hydovitz, J. D.: Localization of parathyroid adenomas in patients who have undergone surgery (Letter). Radiology, *163:*828, 1987.
12. Winzelberg, G. G., Hydovitz, J. D., O'Hara, K. R., et al.: Parathyroid adenomas evaluated by Tl-201/Tc-99m pertechnetate subtraction scintigraphy and high-resolution ultrasonography. Radiology, *155:*231–235, 1985.

# 25

# CROSS-SECTIONAL IMAGING OF PARATHYROID GLANDS

*Carl R. Larsen, M.D.*

Several noninvasive imaging procedures are available for the accurate localization of parathyroid disease. Why any of these localization procedures are necessary is questioned because of the estimated surgical cure rate of 90 to 95 per cent in experienced hands without any preoperative localization studies.[1, 20, 25] Preoperative localization studies can direct the initial exploration to one side of the neck rather than bilaterally. The cost effectiveness of preoperative screening in promoting efficient use of operating room time remains controversial. It may be essential, however, for patients who have had previous parathyroid surgery. Postoperative changes within the soft tissues of the neck make reexploration difficult, with a higher incidence of complications.[1, 20] The reported surgical cure rate in patients undergoing reoperation is 30 to 40 per cent less than that for patients undergoing primary exploration.[9, 17] Less experienced surgeons frequently achieve less favorable results on initial exploration when a preoperative localization procedure has not been carried out.[25]

## ULTRASONOGRAPHY

High-resolution real-time ultrasonography is the procedure of choice for preoperative localization of parathyroid tumors. A reliable modality for imaging pathologic changes, its accuracy ranges from 76 to 92 per cent.[10, 20, 25] Ultrasonography, unlike other cross-sectional imaging modalities, is operator dependent, and accuracy rates in some clinical practices are somewhat lower. Simeone and associates[19] reported an overall sensitivity of 88 per cent, specificity of 96 per cent, and a positive predictive value of 90 per cent in their evaluation of 45 patients. Scintigraphy using combined technetium 99m (a thyroid imaging agent) and thallium 201 with a computer subtraction technique has a sensitivity of between 80 and 85 per cent and a specificity of 90 per cent.[25] Scintigraphy using this technique and high-resolution real-time ultrasonography are the initial screening tests, depending on which method is available at an institution. The roles of computed tomog-

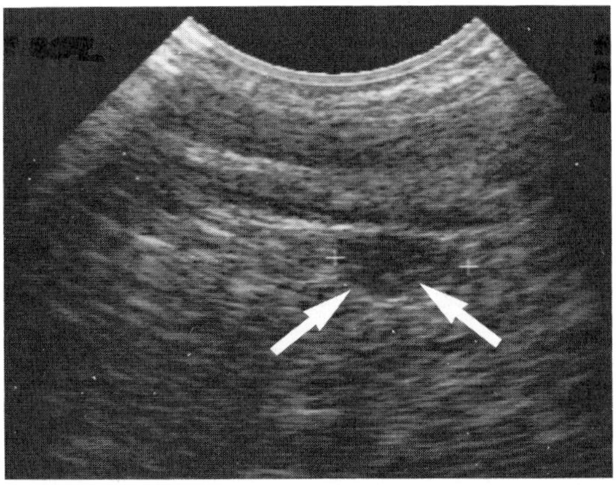

**FIGURE 25–1.** Ultrasonographic study of a parathyroid adenoma (*arrows*) measuring 1 cm and having decreased echogenicity.

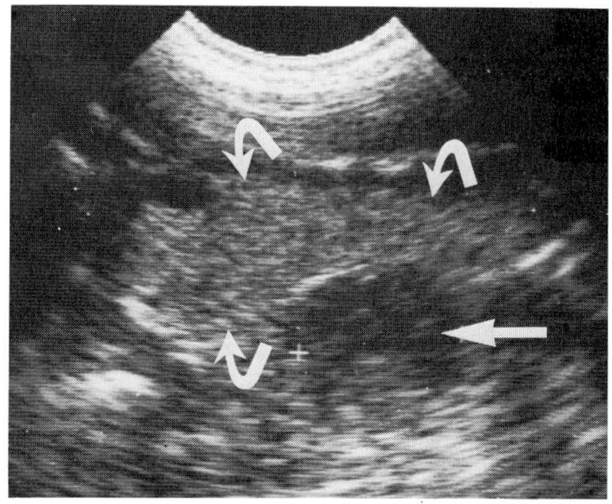

**FIGURE 25–3.** Relatively hypoechoic parathyroid adenoma (*straight arrow*) adjacent to homogeneous echo pattern of the thyroid (*curved arrows*).

raphy and magnetic resonance imaging will be discussed later. Several other noninvasive localization techniques are available but are of lesser value and are only of historic interest.

In the majority of patients, ultrasonography will not demonstrate the normal parathyroid gland.[1–3, 18] Parathyroid adenomas (Fig. 25–1) appear as discrete sharply marginated soft tissue masses with echogenicity usually lower than the adjacent thyroid tissue.[20, 25] The shape, echogenicity, size, and location are variable (Figs. 25–2 and 25–3). Adenomas may also be hyperechoic, cystic,[14] or mixed in echographic appearance (Figs. 25–4 and 25–5). Hyperplastic glands have been described as being less echogenic than adenomas; however, with the variable appearance of adenomas, this evaluation may be subjective and of little value for use in differentiation.[17, 24] Hyperplasia will usually involve more than one gland, which aids in clarification. Sometimes the only useful diagnostic suggestion of the presence of an enlarged parathyroid gland is a prominent neurovascular bundle, which is normally not distinguishable from the longus colli muscle. Hypertrophy of the inferior thyroid artery, which supplies the enlarged gland, will make it apparent, suggesting parathyroid disease.[19] Parathyroid carcinoma usually presents as a

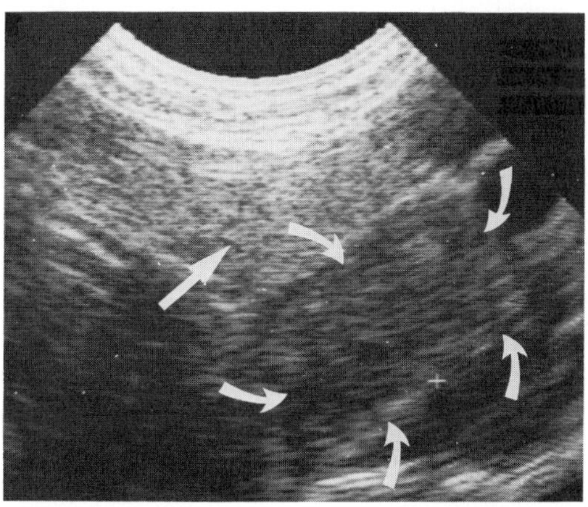

**FIGURE 25–2.** Ultrasonographic examination of parathyroid adenoma (*curved arrows*) showing less echogenicity compared with thyroid gland (*straight arrow*).

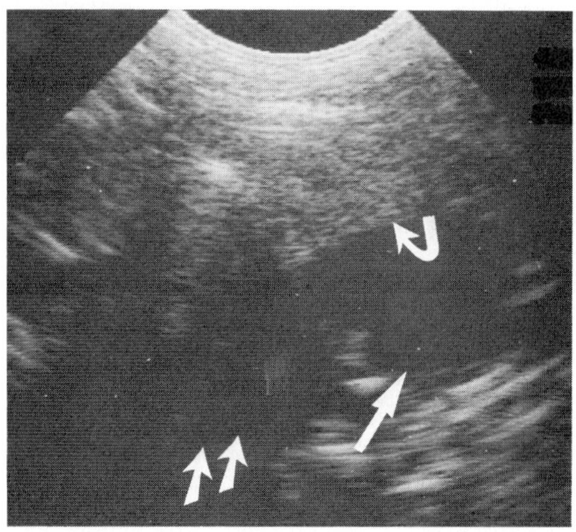

**FIGURE 25–4.** Sonolucent or cystlike adenoma of parathyroid (*straight arrow*) adjacent to trachea (*double arrows*) and normal thyroid (*curved arrow*).

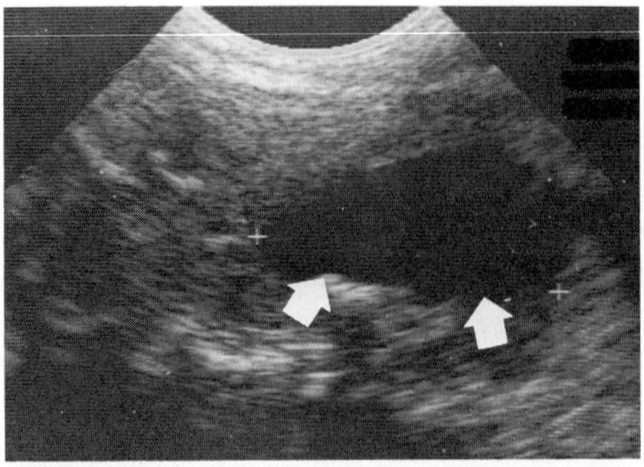

**FIGURE 25–5.** Lobulated sonolucent parathyroid adenoma (*arrows*).

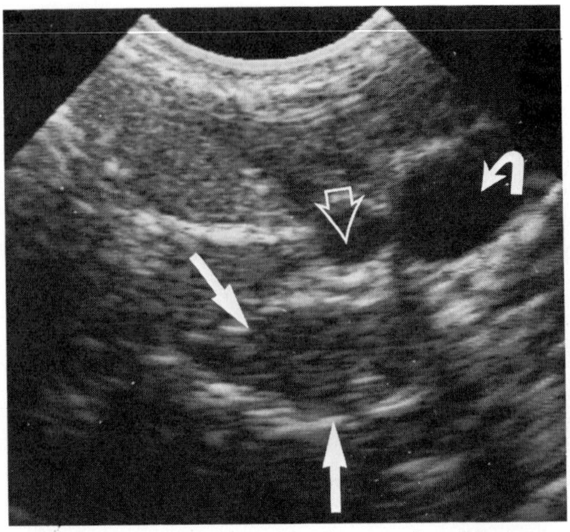

**FIGURE 25–7.** Parathyroid adenoma (*straight arrows*) adjacent to carotid artery (*open arrow*) and jugular vein (*curved arrow*).

lobulated, hypoechoic, and relatively large mass compared with an adenoma. However, the echogenicity and size of a carcinoma are as variable as they are for an adenoma, the only distinguishing feature being tissue invasion with carcinoma.[5]

Several factors limit the diagnostic accuracy of ultrasonography. Minimally enlarged glands are difficult to discern from adjacent thyroid (Figs. 25–6 and 25–7) and soft tissues of the neck. Simultaneous thyroid and parathyroid disease has been reported as high as 40 per cent, which decreases overall accuracy.[17] Ectopic locations may be missed when examination of the neck is not thorough, keeping in mind the embryologic migratory pathways of the parathyroid glands. Adequate evaluation cannot be made in areas of acoustic shadowing (behind the air-filled trachea, in the retroesophageal area, or in the mediastinum).[21, 25] Multiplicity of parathyroid tumors is another source of error, particularly when the examination is not complete.[17] The full participation of an interested radiologist is necessary for interpretation of data and to supervise the creation of meaningful images.

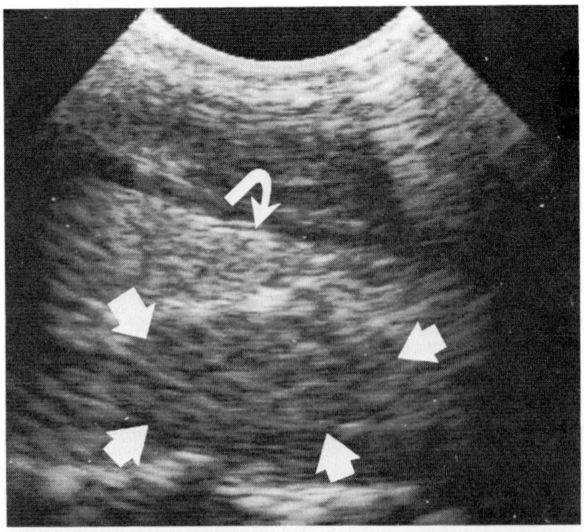

**FIGURE 25–6.** Ultrasonographic study showing parathyroid adenoma (*straight arrows*) with only slightly different echogenicity compared with the normal thyroid (*curved arrow*).

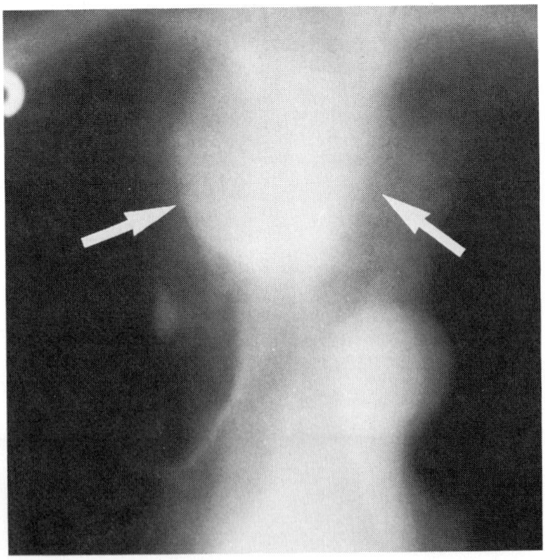

**FIGURE 25–8.** Conventional tomogram in anteroposterior projection of mediastinum demonstrating a large retrosternal parathyroid adenoma (*arrows*).

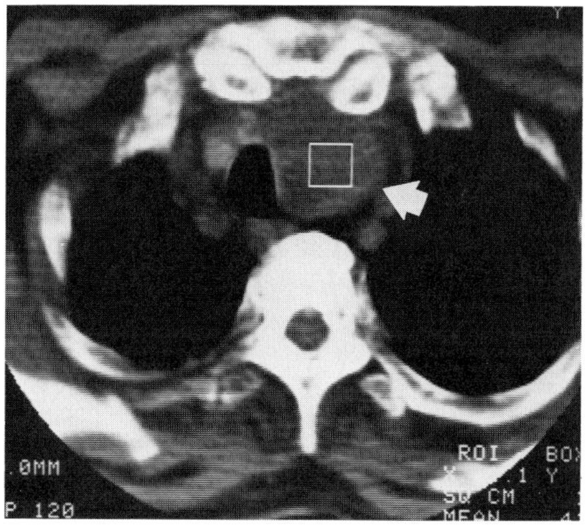


**FIGURE 25–9.** Computed tomogram demonstrating large substernal adenoma (*arrow*) with the cursor (*box*) measuring a computed tomography density of 41 Hounsfield units.

## COMPUTED TOMOGRAPHY

When ultrasonography or scintigraphy fails to localize a mass in the usual parathyroid locations, computed tomography of the neck and mediastinum should be the next diagnostic effort. The accuracy of computed tomography is not limited by the location of a tumor. Parathyroid disease in retrotracheal and retroesophageal as well as ectopic locations throughout the neck and mediastinum (Fig. 25–8) can easily be defined by means of computed tomography. Stark and colleagues[21, 22] found that state-of-the-art computed tomography could equal the accuracy of high-resolution sonography for localization of parathyroid disease. Tumor size is more of a limitation for detection by computed tomography (Fig. 25–9) than it is for ultrasonography. Cervical lymph nodes, tortuous vessels, a collapsed esophagus, and concomitant thyroid disease may be mistaken for parathyroid disease. The overall sensitivity of computed tomographic localization of parathyroid tumors is from 50 to 77 per cent.[1, 21] Computed tomography is limited considerably in its ability to distinguish the parathyroid glands from the thyroid gland and clavicles because of shoulder-streak artifact[2] caused by the bulk of tissue in the plane of the body at the level of the shoulders. Although contrast agents may be useful in identifying regional vessels, identification of tumors is limited because only 25 per cent of parathyroid adenomas are enhanced after administration of iodinated contrast material.[23]

Computed tomography is especially effective in evaluating patients with persistent or recurrent hyperparathyroidism. In one series,[20] computed tomography localized 63 per cent of cervical parathyroid disease in patients who have had prior surgery compared with 47 per cent detected by ultrasonography. In patients who have had prior surgery, the sensitivity of ultrasonography was 50 to 63 per cent after a review of three separate studies.[15] A combination of computed tomography, ultrasonography, and scintigraphy detected an adenoma between 75 and 78 per cent of the time in several studies.[2, 8, 15] In one study,[2] 75 per cent of the elusive tumors were identified with a combination of noninvasive studies, and 75 per cent of the tumors not localized by noninvasive methods were found by selective venous catheterization for parathyroid hormone.

The success rate for parathyroid reexploration is approximately 62 per cent[9] because patients who have undergone previous neck surgery have distorted anatomic landmarks, scarring, and adhesions that complicate surgical procedures. Percutaneous fine needle aspiration biopsy with either ultrasonographic or computed tomographic guidance may help to determine whether tissue identified with an imaging technique is consistent with parathyroid tissue.[4, 9] One group[11] even used this technique for percutaneous destruction of parathyroid tissue with alcohol injection. Fine needle aspiration biopsy techniques may permit a safer, more successful surgical procedure in the previously explored patient.

## MAGNETIC RESONANCE IMAGING

Although the role of magnetic resonance imaging of the parathyroid glands has yet to be defined, early studies indicate that this rapidly emerging technology has a great deal of promise in parathyroid imaging (Fig. 25–10). Improved resolution obtained with the use of surface coils for signal reception has

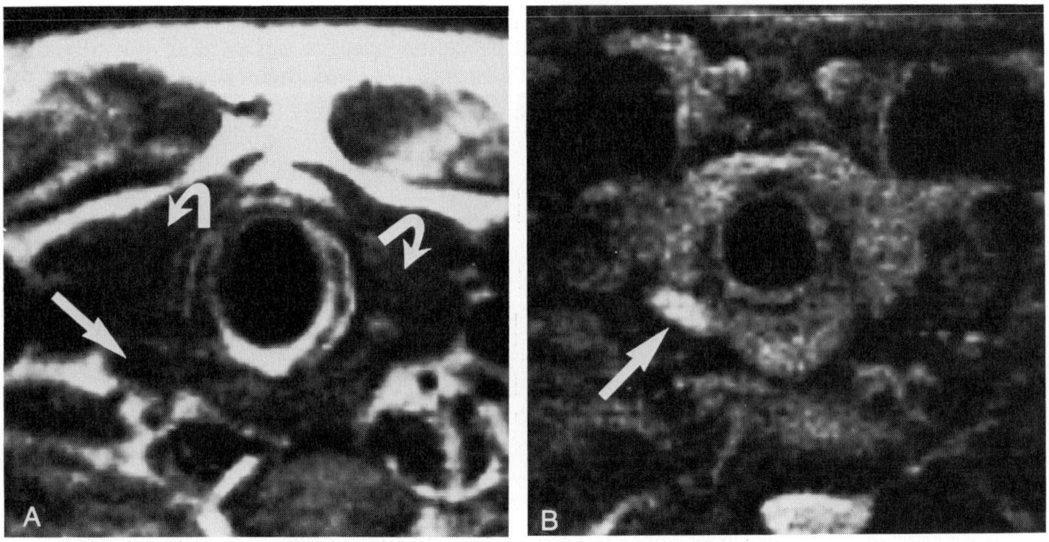


**FIGURE 25–10.** *A,* Magnetic resonance scan using T1 sequence in transaxial plane. Curved arrows indicate both lobes of thyroid gland. The straight arrow shows a parathyroid adenoma, which has a low signal on T1. *B,* Magnetic resonance image using T2–weighted sequence of same patient. The parathyroid adenoma (*arrow*) now has a high signal, confirming its presence.

produced high contrast in defining a parathyroid tumor, regional blood vessels, and adjacent soft tissues, making magnetic resonance imaging an attractive alternative to computed tomography. Most centers with magnetic resonance imaging capabilities are still in the early stages of their learning curve as evident by a 64 per cent detection rate prospectively and 83 per cent by retrospective postoperative film review by one group.[16]

Identification of lesions as small as 0.5 cm

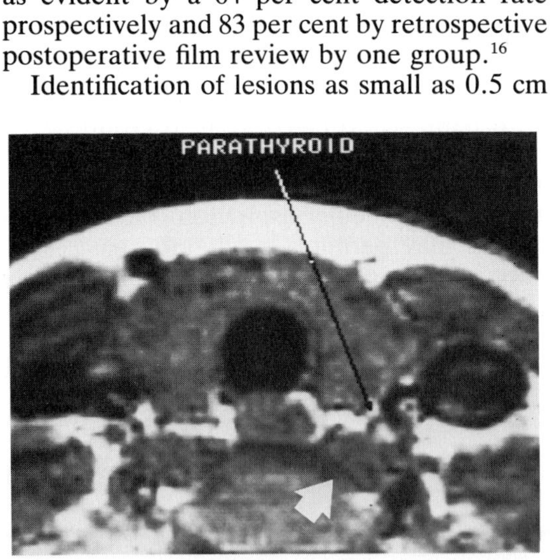


**FIGURE 25–11.** Magnetic resonance image of neck demonstrating the normal thyroid and probable normal parathyroid gland (*straight arrow*) in front of the longus colli muscle (*arrowhead*).

has been reported[23] using a high-field strength and surface coil. The high-signal intensity of these tumors on T2–weighted sequences permits excellent contrast resolution from surrounding tissues. Studies[6, 7, 12] of other neck tumors have shown that magnetic resonance imaging was superior to computed tomography in showing the relationship between recurrent tumors and muscle and in demonstrating vascular anatomy when no intravenous contrast material was used. Factors limiting magnetic resonance imaging include isointensity of signal with the thyroid gland, thyroid adenomas confused with parathyroid adenomas, and artifacts of respiration.[13, 23] Many of these factors will be less of a problem with improvements in technology. For some patients who have difficulty with a closed environment, claustrophobia is a problem in the magnetic resonance imaging chamber. Magnetic resonance imaging (Fig. 25–11) may eventually be the procedure of choice; however, larger series of studies are necessary to define its role in parathyroid disease.

## REFERENCES

1. Butch, R. J., Simeone, J. F., and Mueller, P. R.: Thyroid and parathyroid ultrasonography. Radiol. Clin. North Am., *23*:57–71, 1985.

2. Clark, O. H., Okerlund, M. D., Moss, A. A., et al.: Localization studies in patients with persistent or recurrent hyperparathyroidism. Surgery, *98:*1083–1094, 1985.
3. Crocker, E. F., Bautovich, G. J., and Jellins, J.: Gray-scale echographic visualization of a parathyroid adenoma. Radiology, *126:*233–234, 1978.
4. DeRaimo, A. J., Kane, R. A., Katz, J. F., and Rolla, A. P.: Parathyroid cyst: Diagnosis by sonography and needle aspiration. A.J.R., *142:*1227–1228, 1984.
5. Edmonson, G. R., Charboneau, J. W., James, E. M., et al.: Parathyroid carcinoma: High-frequency sonographic features. Radiology, *161:*65–67, 1986.
6. Glazer, H. S., Niemeyer, J. H., Balfe, D. M., et al.: Neck neoplasms: MR imaging. Part I. Initial evaluation. Radiology, *160:*343–348, 1986.
7. Glazer, H. S., Niemeyer, J. H., Balfe, D. M., et al.: Neck neoplasms: MR imaging. Part II. Post-treatment evaluation. Radiology, *160:*349–354, 1986.
8. Gooding, G. A., Okerlund, M. D., Stark, D. D., and Clark, O. H.: Parathyroid imaging: Comparison of double-tracer (Tl-201, Tc-99m) scintigraphy and high-resolution US. Radiology, *161:*57–64, 1986.
9. Gooding, G. A., Clark, O. H., Stark, D. D., et al.: Parathyroid aspiration biopsy under ultrasound guidance in the postoperative hyperparathyroid patient. Radiology, *155:*193–196, 1985.
10. Graif, M., Itzchak, Y., Strauss, S., et al.: Parathyroid sonography: Diagnostic accuracy related to shape, location and texture of the gland. Br. J. Radiol., *60:*439–443, 1987.
11. Karstrup, S., Holm, H. H., Torp-Pedersen, S., and Hegedüs, L.: Ultrasonically guided percutaneous inactivation of parathyroid tumours. Br. J. Radiol., *60:*667–670, 1987.
12. Kier, R., Herfkens, R. J., Blinder, R. A., et al.: MRI with surface coils for parathyroid tumors: Preliminary investigation. A.J.R., *147:*497–500, 1986.
13. Kneeland, J. B., Krubsack, A. J., Lawson, T. L., et al.: Enlarged parathyroid glands: High-resolution local coil MR imaging. Radiology, *162:*143–146, 1987.
14. Krudy, A. G., Doppman, J. L., Shawker, T. H., et al.: Hyperfunctioning cystic parathyroid glands: CT and sonographic findings. A.J.R., *142:*175–178, 1984.
15. Miller, D. L., Doppman, J. L., Shawker, T. H., et al.: Localization of parathyroid adenomas in patients who have undergone surgery. Part I. Noninvasive imaging methods. Radiology, *162:*133–137, 1987.
16. Peck, W. W., Higgins, C. B., Fisher, M. R., et al.: Hyperparathyroidism: Comparison of MR imaging with radionuclide scanning. Radiology, *163:*415–420, 1987.
17. Reading, C. C., Charboneau, J. W., James, E. M., et al.: High-resolution parathyroid sonography. A.J.R., *139:*539–546, 1982.
18. Sample, W. F., Mitchell, S. P., and Bledsoe, R. C.: Parathyroid ultrasonography. Radiology, *127:*485–490, 1978.
19. Simeone, J. F., Mueller, P. R., Ferrucci, J. T., Jr., et al.: High-resolution real-time sonography of the parathyroid. Radiology, *141:*745–751, 1981.
20. Stark, D. D., Gooding, G. A., and Clark, O. H.: Noninvasive parathyroid imaging. Semin. Ultra. C.T. M.R., *6:*310–320, 1985.
21. Stark, D. D., Gooding, G. A., Moss, A. A., et al.: Parathyroid imaging: Comparison of high-resolution CT and high-resolution sonography. A.J.R., *141:*633–638, 1983.
22. Stark, D. D., Moss, A. A., Gooding, G. A., and Clark, O. H.: Parathyroid scanning by computed tomography. Radiology, *148:*297–299, 1983.
23. Spritzer, C. E., Gefter, W. B., Hamilton, R., et al.: Abnormal parathyroid glands: High-resolution MR imaging. Radiology, *162:*487–491, 1987.
24. Takebayashi, S., Matsui, K., Onohara, Y., and Hidai, H.: Sonography for early diagnosis of enlarged parathyroid glands in patients with secondary hyperparathyroidism. A.J.R., *148:*911–914, 1987.
25. Winzelberg, G. G.: Parathyroid imaging. Ann. Intern. Med., *107:*64–70, 1987.

# 26

# INVASIVE RADIOLOGIC EVALUATION OF HYPERPARATHYROIDISM

*Kenneth R. Stokes, M.D.*

In patients with hyperparathyroidism without previous operation, the greater than 90 per cent success rate of surgical exploration and, if needed, the high sensitivity of noninvasive evaluation with ultrasonography, nuclear medicine, and computed tomography obviate the need for invasive vascular localization.[22, 38] In patients with persistent or recurrent hyperparathyroidism after operation, however, reoperation is difficult because loss of normal tissue planes and possible ectopic parathyroid location lower the surgical success rate and increase the complication rate.[2, 3, 38] To improve the success of reoperation, extensive noninvasive evaluation and, in some instances, invasive evaluation are required before reexploration.

Prior operation greatly reduces the reliability of noninvasive testing. In patients with previous surgery, computed tomography has only a 44 to 47 per cent sensitivity, with a false-positive rate of 2 to 12 per cent.[7, 26, 30] The sensitivity of ultrasonography ranges from 36 to 63 per cent, with a false-positive rate of 11 to 14 per cent.[6, 7, 30, 36] Relatively limited experience with magnetic resonance imaging reveals a 65 to 75 per cent sensitivity, with an 18 per cent false-positive rate.[1, 26] Thallium chloride 201 and technetium 99m pertechnetate scintigraphy have a sensitivity of 27 to 49 per cent and a false-positive rate of 6 to 27 per cent.[7, 30, 44]

A false-positive noninvasive result may be caused by a thyroid nodule or tumor, enlarged lymph node, sympathetic ganglion, muscle, tortuous vessel, or collapsed esophagus.[4, 45] In 75 to 78 per cent of these patients, abnormal parathyroid tissue will be localized with at least one noninvasive study. Because of the relatively high false-positive rate, however, the location of a parathyroid adenoma in a patient who has undergone operation should be confirmed by two noninvasive studies or by one noninvasive study coupled with aspiration biopsy and cytology or biopsy and parathyroid hormone assay or by invasive vascular examination.[6, 17, 30, 37] In only 30 per cent of patients who have undergone operation is the location of the abnormal parathyroid gland confirmed by two noninvasive examinations.[30, 39] When the suspected ectopic parathyroid tissue is cervical in location, it may be accessible to aspiration biopsy for parathyroid hormone assay or cytology, eliminating the need for angiography and venous sampling.[5, 16, 43] The specificity of biopsy is nearly 100 per cent, with the sensitivity approaching that of the localizing modality used.[20]

Up to 20 per cent of glands missed at surgery are situated in the mediastinum. Some of these glands can be evaluated noninvasively with computed tomography, but invasive vascular localization is often required. Nuclear medicine has limited usefulness in identifying mediastinal glands. Invasive radiologic studies for evaluating patients with primary hyperparathyroidism include conventional angiography, digital subtraction angiography, and parathyroid venous sampling. Overall, these invasive localization procedures have a 95 per cent sensitivity.[28]

## PARATHYROID ANGIOGRAPHY

Angiography of the parathyroid gland can be performed by intravenous digital subtraction angiography, either selective or nonselective intra-arterial digital subtraction angiography or selective conventional angiography. Because of poor resolution, increased contrast injection, and motion artifacts, intravenous digital subtraction angiography is inferior to arterial studies and is not recommended. Nonselective intra-arterial digital subtraction angiography is performed by injection of the aortic arch and by injection of both common carotid arteries and both subclavian arteries, with filming of the cervical region and mediastinum. This examination is technically easier to perform than conventional angiography because it does not require superselective arterial catheterization and consequently is associated with shorter catheterization time and fewer complications. In addition, after surgical ligation of the thyroid arteries, the parathyroid gland may be supplied only by collateral vessels or by the thyroidea ima artery. Vascular routes may then be opacified only by nonselective digital subtraction angiography and not by conventional studies. On the other hand, the sensitivity of nonselective intra-arterial digital subtraction angiography in patients with previous surgery is 40 to 49 per cent compared with the 60 to 77 per cent sensitivity of conventional selective angiography.[18, 29, 34] Consequently, nonselective digital subtraction angiography should be performed before conventional angiography. When results are equivocal, selective angiography or selective intra-arterial digital subtraction angiography can be performed at the same time.[30] Digital subtraction angiography also facilitates venous sampling of parathyroid hormone by accurately mapping the venous drainage of the neck, which may be distorted from previous surgery.

Selective angiography can be performed by either conventional techniques or by selective digital subtraction. Both require injection of both internal mammary arteries, either both thyrocervical trunks or both inferior thyroid arteries and, if necessary, both superior thyroid arteries.[13, 15] Sensitivities of the two techniques are similar, although selective intra-arterial digital subtraction angiography may be more sensitive for mediastinal glands.[27] Although unusual, serious neurovascular complications and even death can occur with selective catheterization. Inadvertent injection of the spinal branch of the costocervical trunk or the occasional spinal branch arising from the thyrocervical trunk may damage the spinal cord.[22, 31, 40] The superior thyroid artery arises from the external carotid artery, and extensive manipulation can cause internal carotid embolization and stroke.

Angiographic findings of parathyroid adenoma are a round tumor stain or blush, enlarged supplying artery, and displacement of adjacent vasculature[11, 33] (Fig. 26–1). False-positive results (less than 5 per cent) are caused by dense staining of muscle, normal thyroid, a thyroid adenoma, or lymph node. With angiography, an intrathyroid parathyroid adenoma may be obscured by the normal thyroid blush and cannot be differentiated from a thyroid adenoma. Consequently, when noninvasive examinations reveal a nodule, aspiration biopsy and parathyroid hormone assay should precede angiography and venous sampling.

## PARATHYROID HORMONE VENOUS SAMPLING

Parathyroid venous sampling is the most sensitive (69 to 80 per cent) of the invasive

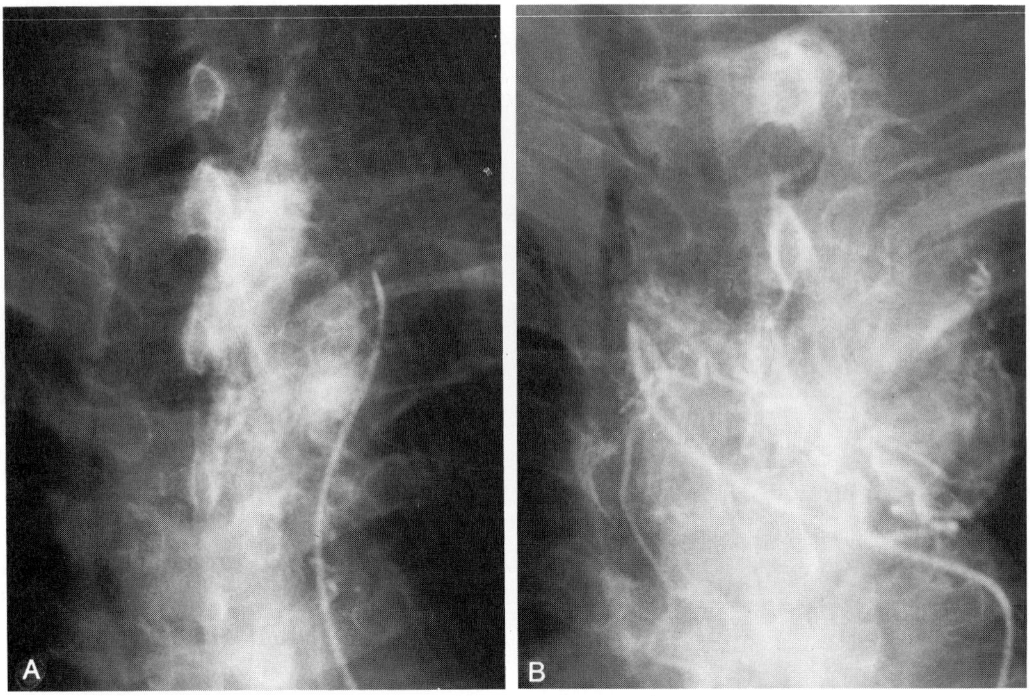


**FIGURE 26–1.** Recurrent hypercalcemia in a 50-year-old man after removal of a right parathyroid adenoma. *A,* Capillary phase after injection of the left inferior thyroid artery reveals a large adenoma beneath the left clavicular head. *B,* Injection of aberrant artery arising from the right innominate artery reveals the inferior portion of the adenoma.

techniques.[9, 12, 29, 32, 46] A parathyroid hormone level, as measured by radioimmunoassay or bioassay, that is twice the peripheral venous level is considered significant. Adenomas are associated with unilateral elevation of the parathyroid hormone level, while hyperplasia results in bilateral elevation of the parathyroid hormone level.[47] Venous samples should be obtained from all patent thyroid veins and the vertebral, thymic, and internal mammary veins.[8] Because the inferior, medial, and superior thyroid veins form a plexus and drain irregularly, an elevated level of parathyroid hormone from a single vein lateralizes the abnormal parathyroid gland but does not identify its exact location. Differentiation between mediastinal and cervical location may not be possible because mediastinal glands may drain into the inferior thyroid vein, brachiocephalic vein, or mediastinal veins, such as the thymic or azygos vein.[10, 14, 24] In addition, anastomosis between the thymic vein and the inferior thyroid vein may exist.[15, 21]

During cervical exploration, the middle thyroid veins and often the inferior thyroid veins are ligated, resulting in collateral venous drainage. These collaterals and any accessory veins should also be sampled, if possible. When a thyroid vein has been catheterized, careful venography will facilitate subsequent catheterizations and may identify the abnormal parathyroid gland.[41] Nonselective venous sampling of the jugular and brachiocephalic veins should be avoided because the sensitivity is only 56 per cent.[35, 42]

Venous sampling is technically difficult, time consuming, and costly, and anomalous drainage may confound the results. For these reasons, the procedure should be performed by experienced personnel only. An alternative to venous sampling may be parathyroid aspiration for parathyroid hormone levels directed by angiography.[25]

## TRANSCATHETER PARATHYROID ABLATION

In patients with hyperparathyroidism and mediastinal adenoma transcatheter ablation is an alternative to median sternotomy and resection. At this time, radiographic contrast appears to be the best ablative agent.[9, 19, 28] After the catheter is wedged into the feeding artery, enough contrast material is injected to maintain an intense stain for 20 to 30 minutes. Using this technique, Miller et al.[28] reported a 71 per cent clinical success rate at 9 years. Two of their 24 patients became chronically hypocalcemic, a complication associated with previous removal of three parathyroid glands. Acute complications associated with embolization of thyroid arteries include acute transient thyroiditis in one patient, bradycardia in one patient, and bradycardia with respiratory arrest in one patient (the patient was successfully resuscitated). This last complication was probably related to irritation of the vagus nerve by the contrast medium.[23] For this reason, embolization is principally recommended for treatment of patients with mediastinal adenomas. Experience is, however, limited.

## REFERENCES

1. Auffermann, W., Gooding, G. A. W., Okerlund, M. D., et al.: Diagnosis of recurrent hyperparathyroidism: Comparison of MR imaging and other imaging techniques. A.J.R., *150:*1027–1033, 1988.
2. Brennan, M. F., Doppman, J. L., Krudy, A. G., et al.: Assessment of techniques for preoperative parathyroid gland localization in patients undergoing reoperation for hyperparathyroidism. Surgery, *91:*6–11, 1982.
3. Brennan, M. F., Doppman, J. L., Marx, S. J., et al.: Reoperative parathyroid surgery for persistent hyperparathyroidism. Surgery, *83:*669–676, 1978.
4. Clark, O. H.: Parathyroid localization. Med. Times, *110:*95–105, 1982.
5. Clark, O. H., Gooding, G. A. W., and Ljung, B. M.: Locating a parathyroid adenoma by ultrasonography and aspiration biopsy cytology. West. J. Med., *135:*154–158, 1981.
6. Clark, O. H., Stark, D. D., Gooding, G. A. W., et al.: Localization procedures in patients requiring reoperation for hyperparathyroidism. World J. Surg., *8:*509–521, 1984.
7. Clark, O. H., Okerlund, M. D., Moss, A. A., et al.: Localization studies in patients with persistent or recurrent hyperparathyroidism. Surgery, *98:*1083–1094, 1985.
8. Doppman, J. L.: Parathyroid localization: Arteriography and venous sampling. Radiol. Clin. North Am., *14:*163–188, 1976.
9. Doppman, J. L.: The treatment of hyperparathyroidism by transcatheter techniques. Cardiovasc. Intervent. Radiol., *3:*268–276, 1980.
10. Doppman, J. L., and Hammond, W. G.: The anatomic basis of parathyroid venous sampling. Radiology, *95:*603–610, 1970.
11. Doppman, J. L., Hammond, W. G., Melson, G. L., et al.: Staining of parathyroid adenomas by selective arteriography. Radiology, *92:*527–530, 1969.
12. Doppman, J. L., Brown, E. M., Brennan, M. F., et al.: Angiographic ablation of parathyroid adenomas. Radiology, *130:*577–582, 1979.
13. Doppman, J. L., Marx, S. J., Brennan, M. F., et al.: The blood supply of mediastinal parathyroid adenomas. Ann. Surg., *185:*488–490, 1977.
14. Doppman, J. L., Mallette, L. E., Marx, S. J., et al.: The localization of abnormal mediastinal parathyroid glands. Radiology, *115:*31–36, 1975.
15. Doppman, J. L., Wells, S. A., Shimkin, P. M., et al.: Parathyroid localization by angiographic techniques in patients with previous neck surgery. Br. J. Radiol., *46:*403–418, 1973.
16. Doppman, J. L., Krudy, A. G., Marx, S. J., et al.: Aspiration of enlarged parathyroid glands for parathyroid hormone assay. Radiology, *148:*31–35, 1983.
17. Duh, Q.-Y., Sancho, J. J., and Clark, O. H.: Parathyroid localization: Clinical review. Acta Chir. Scand., *153:*241–254, 1987.
18. Eisenberg, H., Pallotta, J., and Sherwood, L. M.: Selective arteriography, venography and venous hormone assay in diagnosis and localization of parathyroid lesions. Am. J. Med., *56:*810–820, 1974.
19. Geelhoed, G. W., Krudy, A. G., and Doppman, J. L.: Long-term follow-up of patients with hyperparathyroidism treated by transcatheter staining with contrast agent. Surgery, *94:*849–862, 1983.
20. Gooding, G. A. W., Clark, O. H., Stark, D. D., et al.: Parathyroid aspiration biopsy under ultrasound guidance in the postoperative hyperparathyroid patient. Radiology, *155:*193–196, 1985.
21. Kato, T., Hattori, T., Miura, K., and Sato, M.: Application of thyroid lymphography to preoperative localization of hyperfunctioning parathyroid adenomas. Ann. Surg., *179:*378–381, 1974.
22. Krementz, E. T., Yeager, R., Hawley, W., and Weichert, R.: The first 100 cases of parathyroid tumor from Charity Hospital of Louisiana. Ann. Surg., *173:*872–883, 1971.
23. Krudy, A. G., Doppman, J. L., Marx, S. J., et al.: Failure of ablation of a mediastinal parathyroid adenoma by repeated contrast staining. Radiology, *140:*63–65, 1981.
24. Krudy, A. G., Doppman, J. L., Brennan, M. F., et al.: The detection of mediastinal parathyroid glands by computed tomography, selective arteriography, and venous sampling: An analysis of 17 cases. Radiology, *140:*739–744, 1981.
25. Krudy, A. G., Doppman, J. L., Marx, S. J., et al.: Parathyroid aspiration directed by angiography: An alternative to venous sampling. Radiology, *152:*207–208, 1984.
26. Levin, K. E., Gooding, G. A. W., Okerlund, M., et al.: Localizing studies in patients with persistent or recurrent hyperparathyroidism. Surgery, *102:*917–925, 1987.
27. Miller, D. L., Chang, R., Doppman, J. L., and Norton, J. A.: Localization of parathyroid adenomas: Superselective arterial DSA versus superselective conventional angiography. Radiology, *170:*1003–1006, 1989.

28. Miller, D. L., Doppman, J. L., Chang, R., et al.: Angiographic ablation of parathyroid adenomas: Lessons from a 10-year experience. Radiology, *165:*601–607, 1987.
29. Miller, D. L., Doppman, J. L., Krudy, A. G., et al.: Localization of parathyroid adenomas in patients who have undergone surgery. Part II. Invasive procedures. Radiology, *162:*138–141, 1987.
30. Miller, D. L., Doppman, J. L., Shawker, T. H., et al.: Localization of parathyroid adenomas in patients who have undergone surgery. Part I. Noninvasive imaging methods. Radiology, *162:*133–137, 1987.
31. Mishkin, M. M., Baum, S., and Di Chiro, G.: Emergency treatment of angiography-induced paraplegia and tetraplegia (Letter). N. Engl. J. Med., *288:*1184–1185, 1973.
32. Müller, H.-W., Montz, R., Schneider, C., et al.: Lokalisationsdiagnostik vergrösster Nebenschilddrüsen: die 201T1-99mTc-Subtraktionsszintigraphie im Vergleich zur 5-MHz-Sonographie. R.O.F.O., *142:*543–547, 1985.
33. Newton, T. H., and Eisenberg, E.: Angiography of parathyroid adenomas. Radiology, *86:*843–850, 1966.
34. Obley, D. L., Winzelberg, G. G., Jarmolowski, C. R., et al.: Parathyroid adenomas studied by digital subtraction angiography. Radiology, *153:*449–451, 1984.
35. Powell, D., Shimkin, P. M., Doppman, J. L., et al.: Primary hyperparathyroidism: Preoperative tumor localization and differentiation between adenoma and hyperplasia. N. Engl. J. Med., *286:*1169–1175, 1972.
36. Reading, C. C., Charboneau, J. W., James, E. M., et al.: Postoperative parathyroid high-frequency sonography: Evaluation of persistent or recurrent hyperparathyroidism. A.J.R., *144:*399–402, 1985.
37. Rosoff, L., Sr.: Presidential address: Hyperparathyroidism, hypergraphia, and just plain hype. Surgery, *98:*989–994, 1985.
38. Satava, R. M., Jr., Beahrs, O. H., and Scholz, D. A.: Success rate of cervical exploration for hyperparathyroidism. Arch. Surg., *110:*625–628, 1975.
39. Saxe, A. W., and Brennan, M. F.: Strategy and technique of reoperative parathyroid surgery. Surgery, *89:*417–423, 1981.
40. Seldinger, S. I.: Localization of parathyroid adenomata by arteriography. Acta Radiol., *42:*353–366, 1954.
41. Shimkin, P. M., Doppman, J. L., Powell, D., et al.: Demonstration of parathyroid adenomas by retrograde thyroid venography. Radiology, *103:*63–67, 1972.
42. Shimkin, P. M., Powell, D., Doppman, J. L., et al.: Parathyroid venous sampling. Radiology, *104:*571–574, 1972.
43. Solbiati, L., Montali, G., Croce, F., et al.: Parathyroid tumors detected by fine-needle aspiration biopsy under ultrasonic guidance. Radiology, *148:*793–797, 1983.
44. Stark, D. D., Gooding, G. A. W., Moss, A. A., et al.: Parathyroid imaging: Comparison of high-resolution CT and high-resolution sonography. A.J.R., *141:*633–638, 1983.
45. van Heerden, J. A., James, E. M., Karsell, P. R., et al.: Small-part ultrasonography in primary hyperparathyroidism: Initial experience. Ann. Surg., *195:*774–780, 1982.
46. Wang, C. A.: Parathyroid re-exploration: A clinical and pathological study of 112 cases. Ann. Surg., *186:*140–145, 1977.
47. Wells, S. A., Jr., Ketchum, A. S., Marx, S. J., et al.: Preoperative localization of hyperfunctioning parathyroid tissue: Radioimmunoassay of parathyroid hormone in plasma from selectively catheterized thyroid veins. Ann. Surg., *177:*93–98, 1973.

# 27

# SURGERY OF PARATHYROID GLANDS

*Ricardo L. Rossi, M.D., and Blake Cady, M.D.*

The basic requirements for success in parathyroid surgery are an accurate diagnosis, absolute hemostasis because blood-stained tissue can make identification of parathyroid tissue difficult, complete exposure that requires extensive elevation of the skin flap up to the notch of the thyroid cartilage and down to the suprasternal notch and clavicle (the strap muscles are divided routinely), an unhurried time schedule, knowledge of the anatomy and embryology of the parathyroid glands and experience in visual identification of parathyroid tissue, and systematic exploration in an attempt to identify all glands. In addition to the actual technical maneuvers in parathyroid surgery, a successful operation also depends on knowledge acquired by the surgeon long before entering the operating room.

## INDICATIONS FOR OPERATION

Almost all patients with complications related to primary hyperparathyroidism should be advised to undergo operation. Although general constraints must be considered, morbidity and mortality rates after exploration of the neck approach zero. A more controversial issue is the management of patients with mild hypercalcemia who have no complications attributable to the disease. Some patients remain in this category for years and perhaps indefinitely; in other patients, complications can develop with such dramatic suddenness that kidney function is compromised. The risk in an individual patient cannot be determined accurately. Scholz and Purnell[26] reported on 147 asymptomatic patients with primary hyperparathyroidism and mild hypercalcemia (serum calcium, 10.2 to 11.0 mg/dl) followed up in a prospective study for 10 years. Most of their 26 patients who underwent operation did so during the first 5 years of the follow-up period. The indications for operation were increased calcium levels in 11 patients, lithiasis in eight patients, decreased renal function in six patients, bone disease shown by radiography in four patients, and psychiatric manifestations in four patients. Because 13 per cent of the patients were lost to follow-up study, concerns about the effectiveness of long-term follow-up as a means of management of the asymptomatic patient are raised. The authors[26] could not identify any finding that could predict the development of symptoms or complications and the need for operation. These observations and the high cost of long-term medical care are arguments proposed for operation as the initial treatment.

## PREOPERATIVE LOCALIZATION OF PARATHYROID GLANDS

In approximately 95 per cent of patients who undergo operation for primary hyperparathyroidism, the disease will be treated successfully[9, 23] without the need for preoperative localization. High-resolution ultrasonography[30] has detected up to 76 per cent of parathyroid lesions, but wider experience with this technique is necessary. Conventional computed tomography[6] has detected abnormal parathyroid glands in approximately 50 per cent of patients. The capability of detecting tumors has increased to more than 70 per cent when a specially designed patient-positioning device and the new imaging method of dynamic scanning and intravenous administration of a bolus of contrast material are used.[28] Double-tracer scanning using technetium $^{99m}$pertechnetate and thallium 201 as chloride has increased the ability to detect abnormal parathyroid glands compared with previous radioisotope techniques.[14] Although further research on noninvasive procedures is justified, unless these studies are used to decrease operative time and morbidity and improve the success rate, they will probably not be used or will not be cost effective in patients being operated on for the first time by an experienced surgeon. Selective venous sampling for parathyroid hormone and selective arteriography, which are invasive, time consuming, costly, and are associated with complications, are also not indicated when exploration of the neck is being performed for the first time.

The cure rate is lower[8, 32] and the morbidity rate is higher in patients who have had previous neck exploration for hyperparathyroidism than in patients operated on for the first time. The operative report and pathologic findings of the initial operation should be reviewed when hyperparathyroidism persists or recurs. The diagnosis of primary hyperparathyroidism should be confirmed and the possibility of nonparathyroid hypercalcemia considered. The degree of hypercalcemia and the presence or absence of symptoms or complications determine whether the patient will be observed, evaluated aggressively, or undergo reexploration. Evaluation and treatment are necessary for symptomatic or progressive disease. Studies are carried out to locate the parathyroid tumor before reexploration, especially when the initial surgical procedure was performed by a surgeon with expertise in parathyroid surgery and when four parathyroid glands were identified in the neck at the original operation. We begin our search with noninvasive studies, such as the technetium thallium subtraction scan,[14] cervical ultrasonography,[30] and, if needed, mediastinal computed tomography.[6, 28] Invasive studies, such as digital subtraction angiography,[13] venous catheterization with sampling for parathormone assays, and selective arteriography, are used selectively. When exploration of the neck was not performed by an experienced surgeon or all glands were not identified in the neck, reexploration without previous invasive studies is an acceptable option, although mediastinotomy may be required. In most patients, reoperation is accomplished successfully through the neck, and mediastinotomy is not required. The reported success rate for reexploration varies between 70 and 90 per cent.[8, 10, 12, 27]

## TECHNIQUE OF NECK EXPLORATION

No substitute exists for experience in identification and assessment of the macroscopic appearance of all parathyroid tissue because adenomatous, hyperplastic, and normal glands may coexist.[4] Identification of normal glands is of great value in the search for the missing adenoma because exploration can be performed in a logical sequence based on anatomic and embryologic knowledge. The operation has to be meticulous, hemostasis must be absolute, and exposure must be superior.

We have divided exploration of the neck for parathyroid glands into several steps.

*Step one* is exposure and dissection of the posterior thyroid capsule. The incision and the technique of exposure of the thyroid are similar to those illustrated for thyroidectomy. Skin flaps are elevated extensively both upward to the notch in the thyroid cartilage and downward to the suprasternal notch and clavicles. The strap muscles are divided routinely. Steady, strong medial traction on the thyroid lobe after division of the middle thyroid veins should be countered by retraction of the carotid artery laterally. In this way, the inferior thyroid artery will be placed on a slight stretch. The recurrent laryngeal nerve is exposed easily, and the entire posterior thyroid capsule is demonstrated for ease in identifying the parathyroid glands. A cross-sectional view of the neck (Fig. 27–1) makes apparent the degree of organ dislocation required for exposure of the general area of the parathyroid glands. The region where the recurrent laryngeal nerve and the inferior thyroid artery cross is inspected carefully. Three quarters of the lower glands will be found adjacent to the lower one third of the thyroid inferior, posterior, or lateral to the thyroid pole or anteriorly high up on the thyroid lobe closely attached to the thyroid capsule. In about one fourth of the patients, the inferior parathyroid glands are closely associated with the superior thymus. Approximately 80 per cent of the superior parathyroid glands are located within a circumscribed 2 cm area about 1 cm above the intersection of the recurrent laryngeal nerve and the inferior thyroid artery. The glands are frequently concealed in the connective tissue fibers posteriorly that bind the posterior edge of the thyroid lobe to the larynx. These tissue fibers should be divided. The posterior thyroid capsule superiorly should be incised when the upper gland is not seen external to the capsule. Division of the superior pole vessels permits complete inspection of this region when the upper glands are not properly visualized and better inspection of the upper posterior capsular area.

Most of the glands are found in a regular and symmetric fashion and location in relation to the thyroid. Therefore, careful exploration of the common locations with meticulous technique is advised before an unusual position is searched for. When an abnormal gland is not found, the opposite side is examined, and the disease will often be apparent. Identification of normal glands is important because exploration for a specific missing gland can be conducted in a logical sequence based on knowledge of the anatomy and embryology of the parathyroid glands. An awareness of the frequency of ectopic adenomas and their usual locations is helpful.

*Step two* is dissection of the superior mediastinum after clearing the inferior poles of the thyroid. This consists of clearing the entire lower pole of the thyroid glands, identifying thymic tissue, and dissecting all tissue within 2 or 3 cm of the thyroid gland inferiorly. Of inferior glands, 15 per cent or more will be found in this region, which is usually

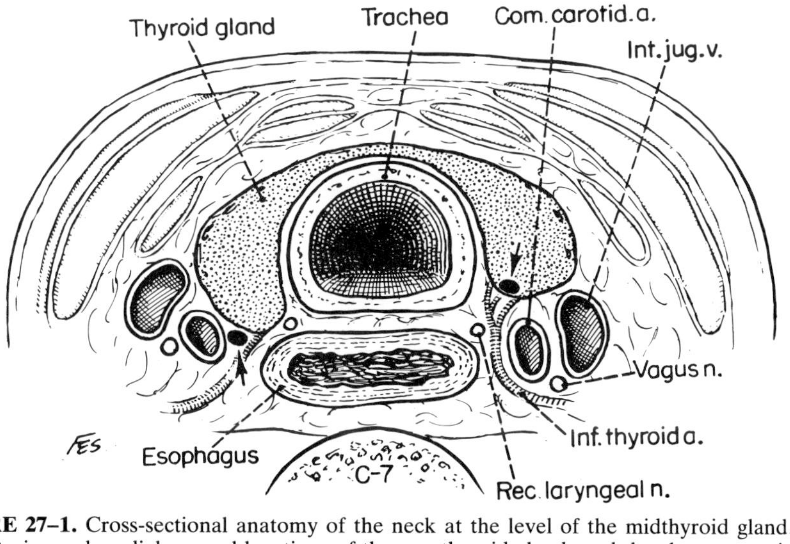


**FIGURE 27–1.** Cross-sectional anatomy of the neck at the level of the midthyroid gland. Note the posterior and medial general locations of the parathyroid glands and the close approximation of the esophagus.

the thoracic inlet and adjacent to the thymus. When a brief preliminary dissection designed to reveal any large or obvious glands is not helpful, this tissue should be removed en bloc. The lower parathyroid glands are almost always adjacent to the thymus when they are at a considerable distance from the thyroid gland.

*Step three* is dissection of the relative avascular paraesophageal, paralaryngeal, retroesophageal, and retropharyngeal regions when the abnormal gland has not been identified.

*Step four* is total thyroid lobectomy on the side without normal parathyroid anatomy. Although the incidence of a true intrathyroid or parathyroid gland is about 2 per cent, some parathyroid glands may be so closely attached to the thyroid gland or within the thyroid capsule that thyroid lobectomy may be required to identify and remove such a gland.

*Step five* is incision of the carotid sheath. Occasionally, glands may reside in or near the carotid sheath as high as the carotid bifurcation.

*Step six* is mediastinotomy and mediastinal dissection. We usually reserve this step for a second operation because most missing abnormal glands will still be present in the neck and because 3 to 4 hours of operating time may have elapsed and the anatomy and tissues may have been distorted. This makes identification of abnormal parathyroid tissue difficult. Mediastinal exploration will not be required in more than 2 per cent of patients and should not be performed at the initial procedure unless special circumstances exist, such as severe hypercalcemia or preoperative studies that have suggested the presence of a mediastinal tumor. Most ectopic glands located in the thymus can be removed through transcervical thymectomy. In addition, when the patient has a relatively low level of hypercalcemia and does not have major complications from the disease, complications from mediastinotomy may outweigh those of the disease in severity.

In most instances, the pathologic process is not obscure, the gland is in a normal location, and the search should be started on the initial side by exposure and dissection of the posterior thyroid capsule after the recurrent laryngeal nerve and inferior thyroid artery are displayed. When no abnormality is found, the search should be carried to the opposite side. The posterior thyroid capsule should be exposed and dissected, and the recurrent laryngeal nerve and inferior thyroid artery displayed before an entire stepwise search is begun because in most patients the abnormality will become apparent. This will avoid unnecessary extensive dissection and decrease operating time. On the other hand, when one adenomatous gland and one or two clearly normal glands are identified, we do not routinely look for the fourth gland because more than 95 per cent of patients will be cured when one adenomatous gland is removed and a clinically normal gland is confirmed histologically by biopsy.

## EXTENT OF PARATHYROID OPERATION

About 80 per cent of patients who are seen initially with primary hyperparathyroidism will have a single adenoma.[2, 29, 32] Hyperplasia occurs in 10 to 15 per cent of patients, and two adenomas are found in about 2 per cent of patients. We advocate a conservative approach that consists of excision of the adenoma and biopsy of one normal-appearing gland, preferably with identification of all four glands. We usually rely on the clinical findings when biopsy of a normal-appearing gland in a patient with an otherwise enlarged abnormal gland (adenoma) suggests the possibility of microscopic glandular hypercellularity. Most of the patients will be cured of the disease, and presently available data suggest that microscopic glandular hypercellularity may be of questionable clinical importance.[1, 21] We do not advocate routine use of subtotal parathyroidectomy when one gland is enlarged because this aggressive approach is likely to result in an increased incidence of iatrogenic disease.[17] Edis et al.[11] reported on a prospective study comparing this conservative approach with subtotal parathyroidectomy on the basis of presumed and proved microscopic hyperplasia. The study strongly supported the conservative management of these patients. Information suggests that patients with hyperparathyroidism may have defects in enzyme-regulating transcription and translation hormone synthesis in the parathyroid cells and that parathyroid adenomas may be of multicellular origin. This indicates a possible genetic predisposition for the development of primary hyperparathyroidism.[15, 16] Yet, the biologic and clinical importance of these findings remains unclear and does not support aggressive surgical therapy.

With conservative management, persistent or recurrent hyperparathyroidism can be expected in fewer than 5 per cent of patients with adenoma and usually represents failure to recognize the presence of multiple gland involvement or to identify the abnormal gland. Extensive dissection to identify all parathyroid glands and removal of more parathyroid tissue than needed are associated with an increased incidence of postoperative hypoparathyroidism.[17]

An uncommon problem is that of a patient with more than one but less than four glands involved. In such patients, we prefer conservative therapy with removal of enlarged glands and identification and biopsy of remaining glands. An exception to this is the patient with multiple endocrine neoplasia syndrome Type I in whom subtotal parathyroidectomy is preferred.

Management of patients with hyperplastic glands remains controversial. This heterogeneous group includes familial hyperparathyroidism, multiple endocrine neoplasia syndrome Type I (parathyroid disease, islet cell tumor of the pancreas, and pituitary adenoma), multiple endocrine neoplasia syndrome Type IIA (parathyroid disease, medullary carcinoma of the thyroid, and pheochromocytoma), and secondary hyperparathyroidism caused by renal failure. The difficulties in treating patients with hyperplasia arise because all glands must be identified, and an adequate amount of viable parathyroid tissue must be left behind to preserve parathyroid function. When insufficient tissue is removed, persistent hypercalcemia results, and when excessive tissue is excised or the remaining tissue is not viable, permanent hypoparathyroidism will develop. The occurrence of a supernumerary fifth gland, which may be present in 1 to 6 per cent of patients and in an even higher percentage of patients with multiple endocrine neoplasia syndrome Type I, adds to the surgical difficulty.

For patients with sporadic hyperparathyroidism who have diffuse glandular involvement, subtotal parathyroidectomy is successful in approximately 92 per cent of patients[5, 10, 21] and is our procedure of choice. Early success rates are similar for both subtotal parathyroidectomy and total parathyroidectomy with autotransplantation, but a period of hypoparathyroidism occurs with the latter technique and is permanent in a few patients.[33] To avoid hypoparathyroidism at the time of subtotal parathyroidectomy (3.5 glands), the viability of the remaining parathyroid tissue must be ensured. One half of each of two glands is excised, and the two largest glands are removed completely. The two halves are inspected, and the half that appears to be in better condition is left behind and the other half is removed. The remaining half is marked with a clip or a long black silk suture. Current techniques of cryopreservation permit preservation of functioning parathyroid tissue in patients in whom subtotal parathyroidectomy or total parathyroidectomy with autotransplantation is being performed, thus ensuring that tissue will be available for future autotransplantation should hypoparathyroidism result.[7, 25] Cryopreserved tissue is estimated to function when autotransplanted in about 67 per cent of patients, but fresh glands, when autotransplanted, are estimated to function in as many as 92 per cent of patients.[25] Hypoparathyroidism after subtotal parathyroidectomy has been estimated to occur in approximately 4 per cent of patients.

Management of patients with multiple endocrine neoplasia syndrome is even more controversial. Hyperparathyroidism appears to develop eventually in essentially all patients with multiple endocrine neoplasia syndrome Type I[18, 31] but in only about 30 per cent of patients with Type IIA. Patients with multiple endocrine neoplasia syndrome Type I have uniform involvement of all parathyroid glands, but patients with Type IIA frequently have adenomatous disease. Persistent hypercalcemia has been reported[5, 22] in 30 to 50 per cent of patients with multiple endocrine neoplasia syndrome treated with subtotal parathyroidectomy. Hypercalcemia has also recurred in 30 per cent of patients treated with total parathyroidectomy and parathyroid autotransplantation.[33] Postoperative hypocalcemia occurs frequently in patients with multiple endocrine neoplasia syndrome Type IIA treated with subtotal parathyroidectomy but infrequently in patients with multiple endocrine neoplasia syndrome Type I in whom recurrent hypercalcemia is far more likely. Thus, conservatism and preservation of parathyroid tissue has been emphasized in the treatment of patients with multiple endocrine neoplasia syndrome Type IIA.

Arguments in favor of subtotal parathyroidectomy instead of total parathyroidectomy and autotransplantation in patients with multiple endocrine neoplasia syndrome[31] have stated that 20 to 30 per cent of patients (especially with multiple endocrine neoplasia syndrome Type IIA) will have adenomatous disease only and therefore excision of a single gland may potentially be curable, although long-term follow-up studies are required; that cryopreservation and future autotransplantation, if required, permit treatment of patients with hypoparathyroidism if the latter results from subtotal parathyroidectomy; and that the incidence of recurrent hyperparathyroidism after subtotal parathyroidectomy appears to be similar to that after total parathyroidectomy and autotransplantation. In a patient with multiple endocrine neoplasia syndrome Type IIA who is being operated on for medullary carcinoma of the thyroid, the approach to the parathyroid glands should be conservative, especially when the patient has normal levels of calcium in the blood, because clinical hyperparathyroidism usually will not develop. Only enlarged glands should be removed or biopsied in such patients.

The most frequent indications for parathyroid operation in patients with renal failure and secondary hyperparathyroidism are aggressive bone disease and persistent hypercalcemia. When performed by an experienced surgeon, the type of operation chosen, subtotal parathyroidectomy, removing 3.5 glands, or total parathyroidectomy with autografting, does not appear to affect success rate.[3, 20] Both operations are frequently associated at least temporarily with hypoparathyroidism, requiring supplementation of calcium and vitamin D.[33] Although some physicians have reported an increasing interest in the use of total parathyroidectomy with autotransplantation in these patients, the controversies continue.[19, 24] Functioning parathyroid tissue can be cryopreserved so that it can be used when long-term hypoparathyroidism results from operation.

At operation, when a parathyroid carcinoma is suspected because of a firm gland, fibrotic capsule, or obvious invasion, the gland should be removed en bloc with involved soft tissues. This can necessitate partial thyroid lobectomy on that side. However, without capsular invasion and only cytologic characteristics suggesting carcinoma, such patients will rarely die of recurrent disease. Therefore, more extensive surgery than total removal of the gland is probably not indicated, especially if it can result in vocal cord paralysis. When nodes are involved, modified neck dissection is performed.

## RESULTS OF OPERATION

The overall success rate of operation in the management of patients with primary hyperparathyroidism currently is between 95 and 97 per cent.[9, 23] For patients who undergo removal of an adenomatous single gland and biopsy of a normal gland, the expected incidence of persistent or recurrent hyperparathyroidism is about 1 per cent; of permanent hypoparathyroidism, less than 0.5 per cent; of major complications, about 1 per cent; and of death, approaching zero. Among patients having subtotal parathyroidectomy for multiple gland involvement, persistent or recurrent disease occurs in about 8 per cent of patients without multiple endocrine neoplasia syndromes and in as many as 30 to 50 per cent of patients with multiple endocrine neoplasia syndrome Type I.[5, 22] The incidence of permanent hypoparathyroidism after this operation is about 3.4 per cent, with major operative complications occurring in 1 per cent of patients, and an operative mortality approaching zero.

Of the last 104 patients operated on at the Lahey Clinic, 84 per cent had a single adenoma, 4 per cent had two adenomas, 12 per cent had diffuse hyperplasia, and 1 per cent had carcinoma. Hypercalcemia was treated successfully in 95 per cent of patients despite conservative therapy with excision of only one or two glands in 90 per cent of patients.

## REFERENCES

1. Badder, E. M., Graham, W. P., III, and Harrison, T. S.: Functional insignificance of microscopic

parathyroid hyperplasia. Surg. Gynecol. Obstet., *145:*863–868, 1977.
2. Barnes, A. D.: The changing face of parathyroid surgery. Ann. R. Coll. Surg. (Engl.), *66:*77–80, 1984.
3. Blake, D. P., O'Brien, T. J., Smith, C. L., et al.: Surgical treatment of renal hyperparathyroidism. Surg. Gynecol. Obstet., *157:*325–331, 1983.
4. Block, M. A., Frame, B., Jackson, C. E., et al.: Primary diffuse microscopical hyperplasia of the parathyroid glands: Surgical importance. Arch. Surg., *111:*348–353, 1976.
5. Block, M. A., Frame, B., Kleerekoper, M., and Rao, D. S.: Surgical management of persistence or recurrence after subtotal parathyroidectomy for primary hyperparathyroidism. Am. J. Surg., *138:*561–566, 1979.
6. Blum, M., Reede, D. L., Seltzer, T. F., et al.: Computerized axial tomography in the diagnosis and management of thyroid and parathyroid disorders. Am. J. Med. Sci., *287:*34–39, 1984.
7. Brennan, M. F., Brown, E. M., Spiegel, A. M., et al.: Autotransplantation of cryopreserved parathyroid tissue in man. Ann. Surg., *189:*139–142, 1979.
8. Brennan, M. F., Marx, S. J., Doppman, J., et al.: Results of reoperation for persistent and recurrent hyperparathyroidism. Ann. Surg., *194:*671–676, 1981.
9. Bruining, H. A., van Houten, H., Juttmann, J. R., et al.: Results of operative treatment of 615 patients with primary hyperparathyroidism. World J. Surg., *5:*85–89, 1981.
10. Clark, O. H., Way, L. W., and Hunt, T. K.: Recurrent hyperparathyroidism. Ann. Surg., *184:*391–402, 1976.
11. Edis, A. J., Beahrs, O. H., van Heerden, J. K., and Akwari, O. E.: "Conservative" versus "liberal" approach to parathyroid neck exploration. Surgery, *82:*466–473, 1977.
12. Edis, A. J., Sheedy, P. F., II, Beahrs, O. H., and van Heerden, J. A.: Results of reoperation for hyperparathyroidism, with evaluation of preoperative localization studies. Surgery, *84:*384–391, 1978.
13. Esselstyn, C. B., Jr., and Buonocore, E.: The use of digital subtraction angiography and computed tomography scanning in localization of parathyroid adenomas in secondary parathyroid operations: Preliminary observations. Surgery, *94:*869–872, 1983.
14. Ferlin, G., Borsato, N., Camerani, M., et al.: New prospectives in localizing enlarged parathyroids by technetium-thallium subtraction scan. J. Nucl. Med., *24:*438–441, 1983.
15. Fialkow, P. J., Jackson, C. E., Block, M. A., and Greenawald, K. A.: Multicellular origin of parathyroid "adenoma." N. Engl. J. Med., *297:*696–698, 1977.
16. Geelhoed, G. W., Krudy, A. G., and Doppman, J. L.: Long-term follow-up of patients with hyperparathyroidism treated by transcatheter staining with contrast agent. Surgery, *94:*849–862, 1983.
17. Kaplan, E. L., Bartlett, S., Sugimoto, J., and Fredland, A.: Relation of postoperative hypocalcemia to operative techniques: Deleterious effect of excessive use of parathyroid biopsy. Surgery, *92:*827–834, 1982.
18. Majewski, J. T., and Wilson, S. D.: The MEA-I syndrome: An all or none phenomenon? Surgery, *86:*475–482, 1979.
19. Mallette, L. E., Eisenberg, K. L., Schwaitzberg, S. D., et al.: Total parathyroidectomy and autogenous parathyroid graft placement for treatment of hyperparathyroidism due to chronic renal failure. Am. J. Surg., *146:*727–733, 1983.
20. Malmaeus, J., Åkerström, G., Johansson, H., et al.: Parathyroid surgery in chronic renal insufficiency: Subtotal parathyroidectomy versus total parathyroidectomy with autotransplantation to the forearm. Acta Chir. Scand., *148:*229–238, 1982.
21. Martin, J. K., Jr., van Heerden, J. A., Edis, A. J., and Dahlin, D. C.: Persistent postoperative hyperparathyroidism. Surg. Gynecol. Obstet., *151:*764–768, 1980.
22. Prinz, R. A., Gamvros, O. I., Sellu, D., and Lynn, J. A.: Subtotal parathyroidectomy for primary chief cell hyperplasia of the multiple endocrine neoplasia type I syndromes. Ann. Surg., *193:*26–29, 1981.
23. Purnell, D. C., Scholz, D. A., and Beahrs, O. H.: Hyperparathyroidism due to single gland enlargement: Prospective postoperative study. Arch. Surg., *112:*369–372, 1977.
24. Rothmund, M., and Wagner, P. K.: Total parathyroidectomy and autotransplantation of parathyroid tissue for renal hyperparathyroidism: A one-to-six-year follow-up. Ann. Surg., *197:*7–16, 1983.
25. Saxe, A. W., and Brennan, M. F.: Reoperative parathyroid surgery for primary hyperparathyroidism caused by multiple-gland disease: Total parathyroidectomy and autotransplantation with cryopreserved tissue. Surgery, *91:*616–621, 1982.
26. Scholz, D. A., and Purnell, D. C.: Asymptomatic primary hyperparathyroidism: 10-Year prospective study. Mayo Clin. Proc., *56:*473–478, 1981.
27. Shane, E., Baquiran, D. C., and Bilezikian, J. P.: Effects of dichloromethylene diphosphate on serum and urinary calcium in primary hyperparathyroidism. Ann. Intern. Med., *95:*23–27, 1981.
28. Stark, D. D., Moss, A. A., Gooding, G. A. W., and Clark, O. H.: Parathyroid scanning by computed tomography. Radiology, *148:*297–299, 1983.
29. Trigonis, C., Hamberger, B., Farnebo, L.-O., et al.: Primary hyperparathyroidism: Changing trends over fifty years. Acta Chir. Scand., *149:*675–679, 1983.
30. van Heerden, J. A., James, E. M., Karsell, P. R., et al.: Small-parts ultrasonography in primary hyperparathyroidism: Initial experience. Ann. Surg., *195:*774–779, 1982.
31. van Heerden, J. A., Kent, R. B., III, Sizemore, G. W., et al.: Primary hyperparathyroidism in patients with multiple endocrine neoplasia syndromes: Surgical experience. Arch. Surg., *118:*533–535, 1983.
32. Wang, C.-A.: Parathyroid re-exploration: A clinical and pathological study of 112 cases. Ann. Surg., *186:*140–145, 1977.
33. Wells, S. A., Jr., Gunnells, J. C., Lesley, J. B., et al.: Transplantation of the parathyroid glands in man. Transplant. Proc., *9:*241–243, 1977.

# Commentary

*Edward Paloyan, M.D., A.M. Lawrence, M.D., Ph.D., and Steven DeJong, M.D.*

As endocrine surgeons have been meeting around the globe and exchanging views for a decade, the world seems to be shrinking, as are the differences in approach to the diagnosis and operative treatment of patients with hyperparathyroidism. Although we are in basic agreement with the principles described by Rossi and Cady in their excellent chapter, we would like to highlight differences in our thoughts regarding hyperparathyroidism and our operative treatment based on a consecutive series of 705 patients.

It is becoming increasingly clear that in many patients with hyperparathyroidism the parathyroid glands are multicellular in origin, although some adenomas have been shown to be monoclonal. In addition to this genetic predisposition, a number of "triggers," such as exposure to low-dose head and neck irradiation and the coexistence of Hashimoto's thyroiditis, are responsible. These basic tenets imply that in many (if not most) patients in the early developing stages of hyperparathyroidism all four glands are involved, although it is clear that as the disease develops and progresses and the hypercalcemia becomes "fixed" and the neoplastic tissue becomes autonomous, a single dominant adenoma is found in 75 per cent of patients (excluding patients with the multiple endocrine neoplasia syndrome and the familial forms). Even in those patients, we frequently find that the contralateral (embryologic equivalent) gland is enlarged; therefore, its resection should be considered.

## CLINICAL FORMS OF HYPERPARATHYROIDISM

Patients with hyperparathyroidism have renal calculus disease, either nephrocalcinosis or renal lithiasis; bone disease with definite bone involvement, osteopenia, subperiosteal resorption, and osteitis fibrosa; a combination of calculus and bone disease; or chemical hyperparathyroidism. Although these clinical forms tend to overlap, a review of large series reveals discrete clinical forms of hyperparathyroidism.

Patients with chemical hyperparathyroidism (presumably the early stage of this disease) are seen in increasing numbers because of the automation of serum calcium determinations. These patients are usually without symptoms, although they may have such associated problems as peptic ulcer disease, hypertension, and psychologic problems in addition to such mild nonspecific symptoms as fatigue and listlessness. At least 20 per cent of patients with chemical hyperparathyroidism with mild hypercalcemia experience complications of the disease during the 3 years after the diagnosis is made. Surgical treatment should be recommended for most of these patients.

When an elevated serum calcium level is accompanied by increased parathyroid hormone secretion or an inappropriate level of circulating parathyroid hormone, the weight of the parathyroid parenchyma usually is increased. The theoretical possibility is that functioning parathyroid hormone-secreting cells do not perform up to capacity and that when demand for greater hormone production is present, the cells secrete parathyroid hormone in excessive quantities. However, it should be emphasized that hyperfunction without hyperplasia or hypertrophy is rarely observed in the clinical setting. Consequently, the purpose of parathyroidectomy for patients with primary hyperparathyroidism is to locate and resect the excessive parathyroid parenchyma.

In general, primary hyperparathyroidism is caused by a parathyroid carcinoma in 1 to 2 per cent of patients, hyperplasia (multiglandular disease) in 20 to 25 per cent of patients, and a single adenoma in 75 to 80 per cent of patients.

## DIAGNOSIS OF HYPERPARATHYROIDISM

The myriad of clinical signs and symptoms that accompany primary hyperparathyroidism permit this disorder to be viewed legitimately in the category of the "great masquerader." However, many or few clinical signs and symptoms may be present when the patient is first seen. The frequency with which such symptoms as tiredness, headache, somnolence, and constipation constitute the only complaints of such patients demonstrates the difficulty of diagnosis. The physician who sees a patient with established hypercalcemia with few signs and symptoms should consider thoroughly all causes of hypercalcemia. The simplest measure is to obtain an ultrasound examination of the neck. When a mass compatible with a parathyroid adenoma is demonstrated, the diagnosis is essentially made, and parathyroidectomy may follow. In the absence of a demonstrable parathyroid tumor in the neck by ultrasonography or a subsequent dual isotope thallium/technetium scan, primary hyperparathyroidism may still exist in many patients. The involved gland(s) may be smaller, and the disease may be caused by multiglandular adenomatous hyperplasia. Patients with recurring calcium renal calculi present a particular diagnostic challenge. When they fail to demonstrate hypercalcemia on repeated testing, they should undergo thorough investigation to exclude hyperparathyroidism. The laboratory procedures should include a variety of blood tests, particularly tests of renal handling of phosphorus and calcium; appropriate roentgenographic studies, including bone density measurements; parathyroid hormone assay after calcium suppression; and tests to exclude other causes of hypercalcemia.

The indications for parathyroidectomy are clear in patients with significant hypercalcemia (>11.0 mg/dl serum) or in patients who demonstrate such complications of hyperparathyroidism as renal lithiasis and osteopenia.

The problem of diagnosis resides in the group of patients with mild hypercalcemia (calcium levels of 10.4 to 11.0 mg/dl, the normal range being 8.6 to 10.4 mg/dl) who have no demonstrable complications attributable to hyperparathyroidism. Even though parathyroidectomy is still advised for these patients in a number of centers, the best evidence currently available indicates that in only 20 per cent of such patients (with asymptomatic or chemical hyperparathyroidism) will some of the classic complications of the disease develop within a few years.

## STEPS OF THE OPERATION

### *Anesthesia*

Tracheal intubation is necessary, and the introduction of an esophageal stethoscope is contraindicated because such instrumentation interferes with neck dissection and increases the likelihood of trauma to laryngeal structures. Local anesthesia may be dangerous because paralysis of the vocal cords and airway obstruction may result from diffusion of the local anesthetic to the recurrent laryngeal nerves or the vagal trunks from which they originate.

### *Position*

The position of the patient is the same as for thyroidectomy. The traditional marked hyperextension of the neck, which produces severe muscular spasm after operation, is not needed. Furthermore, patients with hyperparathyroidism have a high incidence of cervical arthritis with limitation of cervical motion. Elevation of the trunk to 25 degrees permits a drier field than is the case when the patient is flat. However, the legs also must be elevated and wrapped in elastic bandages.

### *The Incision*

A supraclavicular incision is planned, the skin and platysma are incised, the sternocleidomastoid muscle is dissected and retracted, and the strap muscles are divided transversely to permit better exposure. We have not been developing skin flaps in recent years.

### *Mobilization of Thyroid*

The lobes of the thyroid are exposed and dissected anteriorly. The middle thyroid vein is usually divided bilaterally, and the lobes of the thyroid are mobilized posteriorly.

### *Inspection and Palpation*

Exposed areas, including the superior mediastinum, thyroid gland, and thymus, are inspected visually and palpated for enlarged or adenomatous parathyroid glands. Superior parathyroid glands should be sought in their normal location at the superior end of the recurrent laryngeal nerves, in the retroesophageal space (posterior mediastinum), in the superior thyroid pedicles, within the thyroid gland, and along the carotid sheaths. The inferior parathyroid glands should be sought in their normal location near the inferior pole of the thyroid, within the thymus, within the thyroid gland, and in the superior, anterior, or posterior mediastinum.

### *Resection of Parathyroid Tissue*

When all four glands have been exposed, the surgeon has to decide which glands will be excised and which will remain in situ. Careful biopsies should be performed in the glands that remain in situ. Dissection should be minimal and blood supply preserved. The site of each remaining gland is marked with a single titanium clip.

### *Autotransplantation and Cryopreservation*

When the glands in situ are judged too small, autotransplantation of 50 to 75 mg of excised parathyroid parenchyma in the sternocleidomastoid muscle is recommended. The autotransplantation site is marked with a titanium clip. Cryopreservation of 100 to 150 mg of excised parathyroid—for future autotransplantation if necessary—is advisable when facilities are available. Supernumerary parathyroid glands should be sought in the locations listed previously.

### *Hemostasis Before Closure*

The patient is placed in a slight Trendelenburg position to increase hydrostatic pressure. The field is irrigated and flooded with saline solution to identify submerged bleeders with greater certainty.

The incision is closed by suturing strap muscles, platysma, and skin. Drains are not necessary.

To obtain better exposure or to deliver large tumors, it may be necessary in some instances to divide the superior or inferior thyroid vessels. In other instances, when an intrathyroid tumor is suspected, thyroid lobectomy is performed.

When pathologic findings are insufficient to explain the degree of hypercalcemia, the long-held practice of dividing all pedicles coursing from the thyroid to the mediastinum should be abandoned. Division of a pedicle that feeds a mediastinal parathyroid adenoma may not devascularize such a tumor. Furthermore, subsequent venous sampling localization procedures are invalidated when these pedicles are divided.

### *Interpretation of Biopsies*

Normal parathyroid glands, which in the adult contain about 50 per cent fat, are easily confused with fat lobules, especially in obese patients. A simple method of differentiating fat from parathyroid tissue, before the specimen is submitted to surgical pathologic examination, is to immerse the biopsy specimen in a cup filled with normal saline solution. Fat floats whereas parathyroid tissue usually sinks. Wang advocates the use of mannitol to obtain an estimate of the percentage of fat in a given sample.

Frozen section interpretation may be fraught with pitfalls when the pathologist bases the diagnosis on the microscopic examination of the biopsy specimen alone without knowledge of the size or estimated weight of the entire gland. Fat stains, which detect intracellular fat (a sign of normalcy), are useful. The best results are obtained when the surgeon reviews the frozen sections or the pathologist comes into the operating room to view the macroscopic findings.

## POSTOPERATIVE MANAGEMENT

The stress of the operation should be minimized as much as possible. Opiates should be avoided. Aluminum hydroxide gel antacids are given before and after operation to buffer acid secretion when an ulcer diathesis is not recognized and to neutralize the stimulating effect of gastric acid on pancreatic secretion. Furthermore, these gels bind dietary phosphates and blunt the symptoms of postoperative hypocalcemia in severe instances of "bone hunger."

Metabolic and clinical changes may be seen after successful parathyroidectomy. If hypocalcemia is going to develop, it may not occur for 12 to 72 hours, presumably because of the prolonged action of the parathyroid hormone and the availability of some parathyroid hormone secretion from remaining cells. The function of remaining glands or autotransplanted tissue falters temporarily with the onset of edema and associated inflammatory reaction, which impairs blood supply. Functional recovery of these tissues may therefore require several weeks. Symptoms of hypocalcemia become more noticeable to the patient with increase in dietary phosphate load after a normal postoperative diet is resumed. During the first week, patients may experience bizarre psychologic distress. The judicious use of sedatives and antianxiety drugs is effective in the treatment of this temporary phenomenon.

### *Management of Hypocalcemia*

The rare episode of bona fide acute tetany seen in the immediate postoperative period and often precipitated by hyperventilation is best treated with a slow intravenous infusion of 10 per cent calcium gluconate.

In the rare instances of prolonged and symptomatic hypocalcemia or repeated episodes of mild tetany, hospitalization is prolonged by 24 hours to start the administration of dihydrotachysterol (or 1,25 dihydroxyvitamin $D_3$) and calciferol (activated ergosterol). The administration of the two sterols is started simultaneously in doses of 0.375 mg every 6 hours and 50,000 units daily, respectively. Calcium carbonate tablets are added to ensure availability of calcium. Dihydrotachysterol gives relief of symptoms within a few hours. The serum calcium level usually returns to the normal range by 24 to 48 hours. The full effect of calciferol, which mainly enhances calcium absorption from the digestive tract, is not manifested for 7 to 10 days, at which time the administration of dihydrotachysterol and calcium supplements is gradually discontinued. Thereafter, the dose of calciferol can be reduced gradually over a period of several weeks. Because patients differ somewhat in their response to these sterols, serum calcium levels should be determined at appropriate intervals to detect hypercalcemia. Patients should be alerted to the symptoms of hypercalcemia, such as fatigue, thirst, and polyuria, and should contact the attending surgeon when such symptoms arise between clinic visits. The incidence of permanent hypoparathyroidism after the first parathyroidectomy is less than 1 per cent. Autotransplantation of cryopreserved tissue may reduce that number.

## REEXPLORATION AFTER PARATHYROIDECTOMY

A second exploration is indicated when the patient remains hypercalcemic after the first parathyroidectomy or when hypercalcemia recurs after a variable period of eucalcemia.

Assuming accuracy of the diagnosis of primary hyperparathyroidism, persistent or recurring hypercalcemia means that either insufficient hyperplastic tissue was removed or an undiscovered supernumerary gland is present in instances in which four glands had been identified histologically at the first operation.

After the diagnosis of hyperparathyroidism has been confirmed again, localization studies are indicated in almost all patients before a second operation, especially in instances in which an experienced endocrine surgeon had performed the first operation.

### *Localization Studies Before Reexploration*

Noninvasive localization studies are performed first. These include ultrasound examination of the neck, thallium/technetium scanning of the neck and chest, and magnetic resonance imaging of the neck and chest.[1] Although the arteriographic demonstration of a parathyroid tumor presents the most definite evidence of such a lesion, this technique is seldom used because of reported catastrophes, such as transient or permanent blindness and transverse myelitis. Venous catheterization for the retrograde demonstration of parathyroid tumors with contrast media and venous sampling for parathyroid hormone is practiced in a few centers. The identification of the site of a parathyroid hormone gradient provides a reasonably reliable guide for the localization of the tumor in question. However, after thorough neck exploration, with ligation of the thyroid veins and their tributaries, data regarding venous sampling gradient may be misleading because of the newly formed collateral circulation—misleading not only as to level but also as to the side.

### *Surgical Technique*

Reexploration is a relatively simple task when the tumor has been localized. In the absence of precise imaging, both lobes of the thyroid are mobilized and palpated. When parathyroid hormone data indicate that the tumor may be on a particular side, the corresponding lobe of the thyroid is excised because the tumor may be entirely embedded within the substance of the thyroid. When this fails, the neck is carefully reexplored with special attention to possible ectopic sites within the neck.

When careful and thorough exploration of the neck fails to disclose the aberrant gland, the surgeon proceeds with median sternotomy. This maneuver permits simultaneous visualization of the superior mediastinum from both the cervical and thoracic incisions.

The mediastinal lobes of the thymus are dissected, excised, and examined for intrathymic parathyroid tissue. The retroesophageal space is dissected and visualized as far down in the chest as possible. The pericardium is incised, and the aortopulmonary window is examined. When the missing gland is still not identified, the pleura must be entered bilaterally to permit visualization of the deeper retroesophageal space and the posterior surface of the trachea behind the carina. This procedure can be accomplished more easily when the azygos vein is divided and dissection of the posterior mediastinum can proceed from the right side.

When the missing gland is found and it is the only known parathyroid tissue remaining in the patient, a portion of this tissue should be sliced and transplanted into skeletal muscle or subcutaneous tissue as a single piece, in a single pocket, provided that the tumor appears perfectly benign on macroscopic and microscopic examination. A portion of the tumor is cryopreserved as well.

## CONCLUSION

Again, we would like to emphasize that our approach is similar to that of Rossi and Cady. The numbers speak for themselves because in most centers with interested and experienced endocrinologists and endocrine surgeons, 95 to 97 per cent of patients undergoing a first exploration are cured on a long-term basis.

Finally, in this era of cost consciousness, we believe that when a parathyroid tumor is demonstrated by ultrasonography, which is initially performed for diagnostic purposes (not for localization) in a patient with confirmed hypercalcemia, the diagnosis is established to such a degree that parathyroidectomy can be performed. Other studies may be considered confirmatory, baseline information, or even superfluous, depending on the setting.

### REFERENCE

1. Attie, J. N., Khan, A., Rumancik, W. M., et al.: Preoperative localization of parathyroid adenomas. Am. J. Surg., *156:*323–326, 1988.

# 28

# RECURRENT OR PERSISTENT HYPERPARATHYROIDISM: SURGICAL APPROACH

*Randall D. Gaz, M.D.*

The surgical management of patients with persistent or recurrent hyperparathyroidism can be one of the most challenging endeavors facing the endocrine surgeon. The initial operation for most patients with primary hyperparathyroidism is usually straightforward exploration of the neck for a solitary parathyroid adenoma in a common cervical location. On the other hand, the elusive, missing or supernumerary hyperfunctioning gland or the recurrence of hypercalcemia after prior exploration and subtotal parathyroidectomy presents a clinical riddle[42] that is often difficult to solve. The situation may require a complex reoperation in a scarred field and sternotomy with an increased risk of morbidity and a greater likelihood of failure. The embryologic vagaries and anatomic variations of parathyroid glands have been deceiving the surgeon since the days of the famous sea captain, Charles Martel, who underwent six unrewarding operations before a mediastinal tumor was successfully retrieved from the thymus gland through a median sternotomy by Cope and Churchill at the Massachusetts General Hospital in 1932.[9] Paloyan[28] has paraphrased Organ as saying "The second most difficult decision in surgery is to advise operation—the most difficult decision, though, is the one to reoperate!"

Persistent hyperparathyroidism is manifested by hypercalcemia (caused by hypersecretion of parathyroid hormone) returning within 6 months of initial parathyroid surgery. Recurrent hyperparathyroidism is manifested by return of supranormal levels of calcium after 6 months of normocalcemia. The outcome for patients with hyperparathyroidism should be successful in more than 95 per cent of initial operations. When performed by surgeons with experience, reoperations are successful in from 80 to 90 per cent of patients.[17] With as many as 16,000 parathyroid operations being performed per year in the United States, from 800 to 1,000 operations may be unsuccessful at the primary procedure, and thus reoperation becomes necessary.

Several large series[2–4, 6, 7, 13, 16, 17, 23, 31, 36] of patients undergoing reoperative surgical treatment of hyperparathyroidism have produced several common observations and recommendations. In the patient undergoing reoperation, questions or issues that must be addressed include the following: Has the diagnosis of hyperparathyroidism been confirmed? Is the disease severe enough to warrant reoperation at this time? What can we learn from the previous exploration(s) and pathologic findings? Where is (are) the remaining hyperfunctioning parathyroid gland(s) likely to be found? Which localization procedures will provide beneficial information? What surgical exposure approach should be employed? What is the role of subtotal excision, parathyroid cryopreservation, and immediate or delayed autotransplantation? How does one minimize the risks of permanent hypoparathyroidism and laryngeal nerve injury? What is the likelihood of a successful reoperation?

## CAUSES OF RECURRENT OR PERSISTENT HYPERCALCEMIA

Patients who have undergone prior parathyroid operations may have the return of elevated levels of calcium for many reasons[6, 8, 21, 33] (Table 28–1). As many as 2 to 10 per cent, depending on the series reported, of the surgical failures can be attributed to an error in diagnosis. Instead of or in addition to hyperparathyroidism, the patient may have some other cause of hypercalcemia, such as carcinoma, sarcoidosis, multiple myeloma, milk-alkali syndrome, or familial hypocalciuric hypercalcemia. Errors in surgical technique involving incomplete or inadequate excision of hyperfunctioning glands or rupture of the capsule with implantation or spillage of diseased tissue into the wound may result in residual disease.[29] Improper surgical management may be the result of failure to recognize multiple gland disease, incomplete excision of invasive carcinoma of a parathyroid gland, or failure to locate all of the parathyroid glands. Unusual parathyroid glands, including supernumerary glands and anomalous locations, are a common cause of difficulty.[15] Growth of residual parathyroid tissue from parathyroid hyperplasia after subtotal excision or autograft hyperfunction as well as parathyroid carcinoma implants or metastatic disease may produce recurrent disease.

**TABLE 28–1. Etiology of Persistent or Recurrent Hyperparathyroidism**

| |
|---|
| Error in diagnosis |
| Carcinoma with lytic osseous metastatic disease (breast, lung, prostate, or other carcinomas) |
| Humoral hypercalcemia of malignancy (pseudohyperparathyroidism) |
| Hematologic carcinomas involving bone (multiple myeloma, lymphoma, leukemia) |
| Granulomatous diseases (sarcoidosis, tuberculosis, berylliosis) |
| Paget's disease of bone |
| Immobilization |
| Acute renal failure |
| Aluminum intoxication during chronic dialysis |
| Hyperthyroidism |
| Adrenal insufficiency (addisonian crisis) |
| Familial hypocalciuric hypercalcemia |
| Idiopathic hypercalcemia of infancy |
| Thiazide diuretics |
| Milk-alkali syndrome |
| Vitamin D or A intoxication |
| Lithium therapy |
| Error in surgical technique or management |
| Incomplete or inadequate excision |
| Implantation or spillage of diseased tissue |
| Unrecognized multiple gland disease |
| Incomplete excision of invasive carcinoma |
| Failure to locate all parathyroid glands |
| Unusual elusive parathyroid glands |
| Supernumerary glands |
| Anomalous locations |
| Growth of residual parathyroid tissue |
| Parathyroid hyperplasia after subtotal excision |
| Parathyroid carcinoma implants or metastatic disease |
| Autograft hyperfunction |

## RECURRENCE RATES AND ADEQUATE POSTOPERATIVE FOLLOW-UP

Patients who have undergone parathyroidectomy for hyperparathyroidism should be observed for evidence of recurrent disease. Recurrent disease has been documented as long as 34 years after operative treatment. The true incidence of recurrent hyperparathyroidism may be higher than is thought because few patients have extended monitoring of the serum calcium.[7] Overall recurrence rates after parathyroidectomy for hyperparathyroidism are about 2 to 4 per cent in series[18] with careful long-term follow-up studies. The

**TABLE 28–2. Incidence of Recurrent Hyperparathyroidism**

| DIAGNOSIS | INCIDENCE, PER CENT |
|---|---|
| All instances of hyperparathyroidism | 4–16 |
| Adenoma | <1 |
| Primary hyperplasia | 3.5–13 |
| Familial hyperparathyroidism | 33 |
| Multiple endocrine neoplasia | 33–54 |
| Secondary hyperplasia | 6–17 |
| Carcinoma | 50 |

recurrence rates of various subsets of parathyroid disease are given in Table 28–2. At greatest risk for recurrent disease are patients with parathyroid carcinoma, multiple gland disease,[43] familial hyperparathyroidism, and multiple endocrine neoplasia syndrome. Parathyroid carcinoma, when not totally excised at the time of the initial operation, will inevitably recur. Parathyroid carcinoma will recur after 6 months to 3 years in as many as half of patients who are treated surgically.[38] Recurrence rates for patients with familial hyperparathyroidism or multiple endocrine neoplasia syndrome are as high as 33 per cent.[7] Patients with multiple gland disease have a 10 to 15 per cent risk of recurrent disease.[43] The recurrence rate for single gland disease should be less than 1 per cent. Patients with a history of parathyroid carcinoma, hyperplasia, familial hyperparathyroidism, or multiple endocrine neoplasia syndrome type I should have careful periodic monitoring of the serum calcium for at least 10 years. The importance of elevated postoperative parathyroid hormone levels with associated normocalcemia is not known at this time. However, these patients should be followed up closely as well because they may be at risk for the development of hypercalcemia and its complications.

## REEVALUATION FOR PERSISTENT OR RECURRENT DISEASE

After parathyroid surgery, recurrent symptoms or biochemical determinations may suggest the return of disease. Many times the surgeon will anticipate failure after an unsuccessful operation at which time only normal glands are encountered or not all parathyroid glands are identified. A period of observation with serial measurements of calcium, phosphorus, albumin, and parathyroid hormone may be beneficial to document the persistence of disease. Occasionally, pathologists will discover a hyperfunctioning gland in the specimen of tissue removed (thymus, thyroid) that may have been overlooked by the surgeon. Rarely, the patient's disease will abate despite the apparent lack of removal of any parathyroid tumor, perhaps because the blood supply to an undiscovered adenoma has been interrupted and the gland infarcted during the operative exploration.

Clear documentation of hyperparathyroidism with confirmation of the diagnosis is important. Many patients thought to have hypercalcemia caused by residual hyperparathyroidism actually have another disease that has erroneously been overlooked. Some patients may have more than one cause for hypercalcemia, such as hyperparathyroidism coexisting with carcinoma of the breast, multiple myeloma, lymphoma, sarcoidosis, or other disease. A carefully taken history and physical examination will often serve as a guide in the selection of diagnostic tests to confirm or exclude other causes of hypercalcemia. These may include roentgenography of the chest, computed tomography, excretory urography, serum and urine immunoelectrophoresis, bone scan, angiotensin-converting enzyme, prostatic acid phosphatase, peripheral blood smear, bone marrow biopsy, blood urea nitrogen, creatinine, magnesium, 24-hour urine for creatinine and calcium, fasting 8 AM cortisol, thyroid function tests, vitamin D, and urinary cyclic adenosine monophosphate (cAMP). The use of these tests should be tailored selectively to the individual patient. When the patient has been taking thiazide diuretics, vitamin A or D, lithium, or large amounts of antacids and milk, the patient should be reevaluated after an appropriate interval of time after these agents have been discontinued. In the case of a family history of endocrinopathy, nephrolithiasis, hypercalcemia, hyperparathyroidism, or multiple endocrine neoplasia syndrome. The diagnosis of parathyroid hyperplasia must be considered, and multiple gland disease should consequently be anticipated. Family screening may reveal other relatives with elevated serum levels of calcium and low urinary levels of calcium indicative of familial hypocalciuric hypercalcemia. The intact 1-84 parathyroid hormone assay appears to be an excellent means of excluding other causes of hypercalcemia. Rarely, the Dent test using exogenous administration of corticosteroids for several days with serial measurements of calcium will help detect patients with hypercalcemia resulting from causes other than hyperparathyroidism.

After the diagnosis has been verified, a clinical decision must be made about the relative severity of the disease and the indications for reoperation. The patient's individual situation is evaluated to ensure that reoperative intervention is warranted. In the asymptomatic patient with a serum level of calcium that has not been above 11 mg/dl, medical management and careful observation may be prudent. A diet low in calcium, adequate hydration, and phosphate therapy (when indicated) may be the most appropriate treatment for patients with mild disease or prohibitive operative risk. Alternatively, when the disease appears to be worsening, is accompanied by severe complications (nephrolithiasis or significant renal or bone disease), or severe hypercalcemia (>12 mg/dl), surgical intervention is indicated. The potential risks of untreated disease (hypercalcemic crisis, pathologic fractures, renal failure, ulcers, pancreatitis, deterioration of mental status, and other problems) must be weighed against the risks of reoperation (anesthetic complications, injury to the recurrent laryngeal nerves, permanent hypoparathyroidism).

When the severity of disease warrants intervention, a careful collection and review of information are paramount before reoperation.[28] A detailed analysis of prior operation(s) should indicate the extent of previous exploration, which areas were examined and which not examined, which glands were identified and their precise anatomic locations, which glands have undergone biopsy for histologic confirmation, and which viable glands or remnants of glands remain. A frank discussion with the surgeon who treated the patient previously may provide additional valuable information not available in the operative notes and hospital records. How experienced is the previous operator and how thorough was the exploration? Were the common locations of parathyroid glands examined? Were the ectopic locations of parathyroid glands exposed and explored? How many glands were actually identified? Were they marked with sutures or clips? Were they confirmed by biopsy? How many parathyroid glands were removed and how many remain? The pathologic specimens and slides should be reviewed to corroborate the surgical description. Of the surgical specimens removed, how many are truly parathyroid tissue? Do the surgical pathologic specimens appear to represent normal, atrophic, or diseased (hyperfunctioning) glands? Does the patient appear to have a missed adenoma (only normal-appearing parathyroid gland tissue seen on biopsy)? Does the patient have residual hyperplastic disease (manifested by previous hyperplastic biopsy specimens)?

The anatomic location of the previously identified glands and their relationship to the thyroid, thymus, and course of the recurrent laryngeal nerves is used to make a deduction of the side and position (superior or inferior) of the missing gland(s). For example, a patient in whom only three normal-appearing glands were identified may present with persistent hyperparathyroidism. The initial exploration hypothetically may have revealed a parathyroid gland posterior to the left upper lobe of the thyroid near the cricothyroid junction and superolateral to the recurrent laryngeal nerve. Two additional glands were identified in the right and left thyrothymic ligaments just inferior to the lower poles of the thyroid gland. These findings are consistent with identification of the left superior (posterior to upper pole, at the level of the cricothyroid junction, and superolateral to the course of the recurrent laryngeal nerve) and right and left inferior parathyroid glands (near the lower poles in association with thymic tissue). By the process of elimination, the missing gland is the right superior gland. The common locations of the superior gland are posterior to the superior pole (often beneath the capsule of the thyroid) and at the level of the cricothyroid junction. The previously identified contralateral gland may help infer the mirror image location of the missing gland. Alternatively, the pathologically enlarged gland may have migrated caudally into the superoposterior mediastinum or lie in the deep inferior cervical tracheoesophageal groove. Less likely are ectopic locations of parathyroid glands, such as undescended (high cervical), intrathyroidal, retrotracheal, retroesophageal, carotid sheath, or deep mediastinal positions.[15]

Review of the pathologic findings is crucial. The slides should be reexamined by a skilled endocrine pathologist to verify the findings. Often discrepancies will be identified indicating that some tissue removed that was originally thought to be parathyroid actually was not. Serial sectioning of paraffin-embedded thymic or thyroid specimens may reveal previously missed parathyroid glands. The diagnosis should be confirmed. Do the excised or biopsied parathyroid glands represent atrophic, normal, adenomatous, hyperplastic, or carcinomatous tissue? Do the previous pathologic findings correspond to the operative description?

After analysis of the results of the previous operation and deduction of the position (superior or inferior) and expected anatomic location of the missing or residual gland(s), the appropriate localization tests can be arranged, completing preoperative assessment of the patient.

## LOCALIZATION STUDIES

The most valuable method of locating elusive hyperfunctioning parathyroid glands is a skillful reexploration by an experienced endocrine surgeon. Radiologic examinations alone are not a substitute for sound surgical judgment and technical expertise. Many helpful preoperative and intraoperative localization procedures are available for the evaluation of patients with persistent or recurrent hyperparathyroidism.[22, 24] The currently employed techniques include noninvasive (ultrasonography, thallium scan, magnetic resonance imaging, and computed tomography), invasive (fine needle aspiration, selective venous catheterization, and angiography), and intraoperative (methylene blue,[12] ultrasonography,[34] urinary cAMP,[25] and parathyroid hormone assay[26]) procedures. Several excellent reviews[14, 22, 24] have described the use of the various methods. The individual tests are further described elsewhere in this text. For patients requiring parathyroid reoperations, preoperative localization is highly valuable. It provides an anatomic target for the reoperation, indirectly reconfirms the diagnosis, and reassures the patient and surgeon of a greater likelihood of finding the missing gland. Patients who have had prior unsuccessful operations have a greater incidence of multiple gland disease, supernumerary glands, and ectopic glands. In a scarred operative field, it is harder for the surgeon to find an elusive parathyroid tumor. Localization tests help shorten the search and limit dissection in unrewarding regions and thereby minimize the risk of recurrent laryngeal injury and other complications. The operative time is shortened, and the safety of the patient is maximized. Parathyroid localization procedures are best performed and interpreted by experienced technicians and radiologists in centers with expertise in treating patients with parathyroid disease.

In patients who have undergone a limited previous initial exploration, the missing gland will probably be found in the neck. Ultrasonography (10 MHz small parts) will detect as many as two thirds of the missed parathyroid glands in locations near the thyroid gland. It also detects associated thyroid nodules, which on rare occasions represent intrathyroidal parathyroid glands. It cannot visualize areas behind the trachea or clavicles. The technetium-thallium scan is helpful for detecting parathyroid glands farther away from the thyroid gland. Oblique views or expanded views, including the angle of the jaw and mediastinum, often reveal the locations of ectopic parathyroid tumors. The success rate for this scanning method in patients who then undergo reoperation is about 67 per cent. These two examinations (ultrasonography and thallium scan) complement each other and are helpful in the evaluation of the cervical region. When they are unrewarding, examination of the mediastinum by means of magnetic resonance imaging or computed tomography may be worthwhile. In the event that thorough diagnostic studies of the neck have not located a hyperfunctioning parathyroid gland, the mediastinum should be considered. Before mediastinotomy and mediastinal exploration are performed, it is helpful to document the presence of a mediastinal lesion that arouses suspicion. The noninvasive procedures of magnetic resonance imaging or computed tomography can be beneficial. When results of magnetic resonance imaging or computed tomography are unsuccessful, angiography with digital subtraction may be helpful in identifying a mediastinal parathyroid gland.[41] However, because of the risk of neurologic complications, its use should be restricted to complicated reoperative situations and its performance limited to highly skilled and experienced vascular radiologists in centers having a special expertise and proficiency with the procedure. Similarly, selective venous catheterization and sampling for measurements of parathyroid hormone may reveal a localized step–up in the concentration of parathyroid hormone, indicating the site of the hyperfunctioning gland in complex reoperative situations.[42]

Fine needle aspiration (guided by ultrasonography or computed tomography) to obtain tissue for cytologic examination or fluid for measurement of parathyroid hormone has been described. Because of the risk of rupturing the parathyroid tissue outside the gland, this maneuver may have some theoretical risks. Few clinical situations exist in which this procedure may add any useful information to radiologic localization alone. In other situations, this technique has been combined with alcohol injection ablation of hyperfunctioning parathyroid tumors in patients who are not operative candidates. Angiographic ablation of parathyroid tumors has also been tried. The risks and benefits of these nonoperative methods of treatment are not well established; therefore, their use should be restricted to investigational centers with patients in whom the operative risk is prohibitive and whose condition cannot be controlled adequately medically.

Several innovative intraoperative techniques have been described. They include intravenous methylene blue staining,[12] intraoperative ultrasonography using a sterile transducer,[34] intraoperative venous sampling for measurements of parathyroid hormone,[27] and urinary cAMP.[25] Because of scarring, loss of normal tissue planes, and distortion of the normal anatomy, the staining of parathyroid tissue may be masked or obscured. Therefore, the use of methylene blue dye may be less rewarding in the reoperative setting than with the initial operation. Its use may be most helpful in the setting of the first operation when difficulty in identifying a missing gland is encountered. Intraoperative ultrasonography may help identify the intrathyroid or retrothyroid parathyroid gland encased in thyroid parenchyma or scar tissue.[33] Examination of the region of the carotid sheath may also detect an ectopic gland. The success of this technique depends on the skill and experience of the ultrasound operator. Ultrasonography is predominantly helpful in the preoperative setting. With the availability of new rapid methods for measurement of intact 1-84 parathyroid hormone,[26] intraoperative venous sampling for parathyroid hormone during operation may enable the surgeon to confirm adequate removal of hyperfunctioning parathyroid tissue (>60 per cent drop from baseline) or actually to attribute a concentration step-up in parathyroid hormone to the hyperfunctioning gland. Measurement of intraoperative urinary cAMP (50 per cent drop from the median baseline) has been described[10] as an aid in predicting success.

At the time of this publication, no radiolabeled monoclonal antibody to parathyroid cell surface antigens is available that can be used for a parathyroid specific scan. Ideally, this would be a useful addition to the diagnostic armamentarium for reoperative situations.

## PREOPERATIVE PREPARATION

Before reoperation, it is important to verify the function of the vocal cords. Indirect laryngoscopy should be performed to document any preoperative deficits. In previous operations the recurrent laryngeal nerve may have been injured on one side without apparent hoarseness. When unilateral vocal cord palsy is identified, extreme care must be taken during the reoperation to avoid injury to the contralateral nerve. This might result in bilateral cord paralysis and airway obstruction necessitating temporary or permanent tracheostomy.

A discussion with the patient should include the potential risks and hazards of reoperation: recurrent laryngeal nerve injury, hypoparathyroidism, and failure to locate the diseased gland. The patient should be aware of the possible need for temporary or long-term therapy with calcium and vitamin D after operation. When median sternotomy is to be carried out during the same anesthesia period after an unrewarding neck exploration, the patient must be informed of this prospect. The consideration of immediate or delayed parathyroid autotransplantation should be entertained when appropriate.

The anesthetic management and patient positioning for reoperation are similar to those for initial operation. When mediastinotomy is a consideration, preparing and draping should be tailored to provide access to both the neck (from the mandibular angles bilaterally) and the entire anterior chest. Placement of the intravenous line in the right arm ensures that access will be available should the innominate vein be injured during operation. The availability of thoracic instruments, including Lebsche sternal knife or pneumatic saw and a pediatric Finochietto or other appropriate rib-spreading retractor to expose the mediastinum, should be confirmed before operation. When a long operation is anticipated, catheterization of the bladder may be indicated.

## OPERATIVE STRATEGY

When the diagnosis has been verified incontrovertibly, the severity of the disease determined to warrant intervention, the previous operation and pathologic findings carefully analyzed, and the appropriate localization procedures performed, the reoperative plan can be formulated. A series of strategic considerations and maneuvers often beneficial in the course of parathyroid reoperations is listed in Table 28–3. The operative anatomy and technique are described elsewhere.[39]

When the initial operation was limited or was performed by an inexperienced parathyroid surgeon, the odds are high that the missing gland is in the neck. As many as 70 to 80 per cent of elusive residual glands are retrievable through a cervical incision and neck reexploration.[17, 36] When the missing gland has not been localized by preoperative radiologic studies and the possibility of a cervical tumor still exists, neck reoperation is indicated. A low transverse collar incision is made using the previous operative incision if it was appropriately placed. Rather than entering the route of the previously scarred

**TABLE 28–3. Operative Strategy**

| |
|---|
| Exposure through lateral cervical approach avoiding scarred previously dissected areas |
| Examination of preoperative localization target site when studies have been rewarding |
| Examination of anticipated missing gland normal locations suggested by prior findings |
| Mobilization and reflection of thyroid gland to expose retrothyroid region |
| Consideration of cervical thymectomy |
| Exploration of unusual locations |
| Consideration of thyroid lobectomy or thyrotomy |
| Simultaneous versus delayed or staged mediastinal exploration through upper one third median sternotomy |
| Mediastinal thymectomy with serial tissue sectioning |
| Examination of aortic arch, hilar, carinal regions |
| Exploration of aortopulmonary window and pericardium |
| Cryopreservation of parathyroid tissue when appropriate |
| Consideration of immediate versus delayed transplantation |
| Reexamination of previously identified normal parathyroid glands when indicated |
| Any residual glands or remnants marked with metal clips or nonabsorbable sutures |

median raphe between the strap muscles, it is often much easier to select a "back door" approach that is lateral to the strap muscles and medial to the sternocleidomastoid muscle and carotid sheath (Fig. 28–1). A previously undissected virgin plane can often be entered that facilitates exposure of the tracheoesophageal groove and retrothyroid region where undiscovered glands often reside. Examination of the target area identified by preoperative studies is performed. When the localization studies are unrewarding, the area thought to contain the missing gland, as suggested by the previous operative findings, is examined.

The elusive inferior gland is commonly found in a normal location[35] on the posterior or lateral surface of the lower pole of the thyroid gland, in the thyrothymic ligament, or in the cervical or superior mediastinal thymus. Other unusual locations include within the carotid sheath, intrathyroidal, and undescended (high cervical parapharyngeal position above the level of the superior pole). A search along the embryologic descent migration path of the parathyroid glands is made from the angle of the mandible to the carotid bifurcation to the parapharyngeal region, down along the tracheoesophageal groove and carotid sheath, with the area examined inside and posterior to the carotid

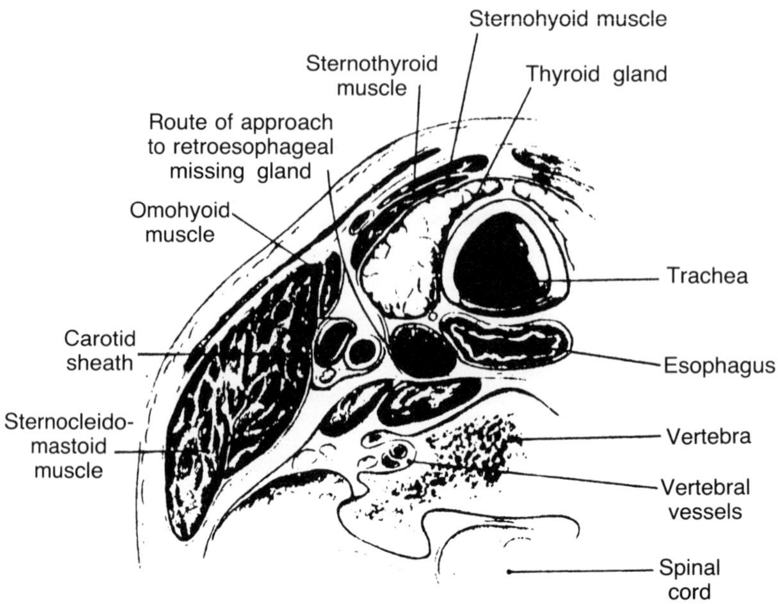


**FIGURE 28–1.** Alternative back door operative approach for parathyroid reoperations. (From Wang, C. A., and Guyton, S. P.: Reoperations for parathyroid disease. *In* Malt, R. A. (ed.): Complex Operations at Massachusetts General Hospital. Philadelphia, W. B. Saunders Co., 1983, p. 113.)

sheath, and if necessary, into the superior mediastinum. Division of the superior pole vessels and lateral thyroid vein may facilitate exposure of the posterior surface of the thyroid and the cleft between the thyroid and trachea where obscure parathyroid glands often are found. Resection of the cervical thymus and as much of the mediastinal thymus as can safely be mobilized through the neck incision often will yield a missing inferior intrathymic gland. When no other promising tissue is identified, scrutiny of the thyroid gland itself by thyrotomy or lobectomy may expose an intrathyroid parathyroid tumor. Palpation and examination of the retropharyngeal, retroesophageal, and retrotracheal regions may disclose a midline ectopic gland.

When methodical complete exploration fails to reveal the missing gland, consideration is given to contralateral exploration of the neck. When systematic thorough bilateral cervical search is unrewarding, it is usually appropriate to terminate the operation. Mediastinal localization procedures can then be executed and a staged mediastinal exploration performed. When the patient has hypercalcemic crisis, simultaneous mediastinotomy should be performed after completion of the cervical exploration. The majority of mediastinal parathyroid glands are intrathymic at or near the level of the innominate vein.[17, 41] Other rare locations include the aortic arch near the origin of the great vessels, the pulmonary hila, the tracheal carina, the aortopulmonary window, and within the pericardium.

Missing superior glands most often are found in the superoposterior mediastinum near the thoracic inlet along the tracheoesophageal groove. In the Massachusetts General Hospital series, in about one third of the reoperations enlarged parathyroid glands were identified in this location. Other common sites of missed glands include the normal locations behind the upper pole of the thyroid and along the tracheoesophageal groove posterior to the thyroid gland. Less common hiding places include the retrotracheal or retroesophageal midline, in the carotid sheath, under the thyroid capsule, and intrathyroidal.

Superior glands are usually located superolateral to the recurrent laryngeal nerve, and the inferior glands commonly are located inferomedial to the nerve. However, the enlarged diseased superior (arising from pharyngeal pouch III) gland may migrate down and actually be found lower or more caudal than the inferior (arising from pharyngeal pouch IV) parathyroid gland. When reexploration fails to locate the missing gland in an upper location, the lower locations are examined and vice versa.

Reoperations for patients with familial hyperparathyroidism, patients with multiple endocrine neoplasia syndrome type I, or patients with primary hyperplasia[7, 40] necessitate identification of all previously unidentified parathyroid glands, careful examination of the thymus gland, and consideration of possible supernumerary parathyroid glands.[20, 30] Identification and removal of a single hyperfunctioning gland may be insufficient or inadequate treatment for a disease that is known to involve all of the parathyroid glands in patients with these forms of parathyroid disease. Information from the previous operation is used to decide which missing glands must be sought, whether previously identified and biopsied glands should be reexamined, and whether a supernumerary parathyroid gland is expected.

When thymic examination was not previously performed, the thymus gland should be mobilized meticulously, scrutinized, and excised to eliminate the possibility of an additional evasive hidden gland. Care should be taken to leave 30 to 50 mg of viable tissue on the native vascular pedicle of one of the glands. Its position should be carefully marked with a metal clip or nonresorbable suture. Alternatively, when total (all glands) parathyroidectomy is planned or inadvertently performed at the time of reoperation, cryopreservation of tissue with simultaneous or delayed autotransplantation can be performed.

At times it is advantageous to delay transplantation to await the clinical postoperative response. Occasionally, a remaining unidentified supernumerary parathyroid gland may continue adequate calcium homeostasis without transplantation. When the patient has persistent hypercalcemia, transplantation is clearly not indicated. When mild hypocalcemia with hyperphosphatemia resulting from hypoparathyroidism develops after operation, observation with calcium replacement with or without vitamin D therapy may be appropriate. With time, the level of calcium may normalize without the need for transplantation. When profound persistent hypoparathyroidism is apparent, delayed transplantation of cryopreserved tissue can be performed.

How should recurrent or persistent secondary or tertiary hyperparathyroidism be managed?[1, 11, 32] Usually, the patient will have undergone previous subtotal parathyroidectomy with total removal of three glands and partial excision of the fourth gland. The location of the residual gland is known. When the disease is mild to moderate, reexploration with subtotal excision of the remnant or total excision with simultaneous transplantation of a portion of the tissue in the forearm may be appropriate. With severe disease, total excision and cryopreservation of a portion of the remaining gland may be indicated. The resultant hypocalcemia may be easier to manage than the complications of persistent hyperparathyroidism. When necessary, delayed transplantation can be performed.

Reoperations for parathyroid carcinoma involve removal of residual disease at the site of the original tumor (resulting from tumor spillage or incomplete excision at the time of the initial operation) or distant metastatic disease.[38] Radical en bloc resection of the malignant tumor and any adjacent invaded or adherent structures is indicated.

After parathyroid operations, the prior dissection, biopsies, and parathyroid gland excisions may remove, devitalize, or destroy all other parathyroid glands other than the residual hyperfunctioning gland. Therefore, excision of the remaining tumor may leave the patient with no remaining parathyroid tissue. In this situation, the sole remaining hyperfunctioning gland can be excised subtotally, with 30 to 50 mg of viable tissue left on the intact vascular pedicle. When the gland must be removed totally or is inadvertently devitalized during operation, a portion of the excised tissue should be cryopreserved. Delayed autotransplantation can be performed when severe hypoparathyroidism develops after operation and persists after 6 months. Alternatively, some surgeons have carried out simultaneous autotransplantation of a portion of the tissue to a muscle pocket in the forearm. However, when the patient has persistent hypercalcemia immediately after operation, the autograft may exacerbate the problems. Because of the possible erroneous transplantation of parathyroid carcinoma with resultant disastrous results, it may be prudent to cryopreserve a portion of the tissue and delay transplantation until careful final pathologic examination has been per-

**TABLE 28–4. Results of Reoperations for Hyperparathyroidism**

| AUTHOR, YEAR | NO. OF PATIENTS | SUCCESS RATE, PER CENT |
|---|---|---|
| Beazley et al., 1975[2] | 35 | 74 |
| Wang, 1977[36] | 112 | 91 |
| Bruining et al., 1981[6] | 53 | 81 |
| Granberg et al., 1982[16] | 53 | 83 |
| Brennan and Norton, 1985[4] | 175 | 90 |
| Grant et al., 1986[17] | 157 | 89 |
| Levin and Clark, 1989[21] | 81 | 95 |

formed and documentation of the patient's calcium response to the reoperation has taken place.

## OUTCOME

Referral centers[4, 5, 17, 19, 36] with extensive experience have described their results with parathyroid reoperative surgery. In hospitals with experienced radiologic personnel and highly skilled parathyroid surgeons, the success rate for reoperations is from 80 to 90 per cent (Table 28–4). As anticipated, the pathologic findings in reoperations vary when compared with results from initial operation (Table 28–5). Hyperplasia is found in about 10 to 15 per cent of primary operations for hyperparathyroidism. In reoperations, it represents about 25 to 30 per cent of patients. About 70 per cent of the reoperations (versus 85 per cent for initial operation) are for elusive adenomas. Fortunately, carcinoma is rarely encountered. Persistent disease and recurrent disease in patients who have undergone autografts are challenging because it is often not obvious whether the source of the disease resides in the forearm transplant or in a residual cervical gland. The anatomic locations of elusive hyperfunctioning glands found at reoperation have been well documented (Tables 28–6 and 28–7) and described (Fig. 28–2).[37]

From 10 to 20 per cent of parathyroid reoperations result in failure to cure the hypercalcemia. The incidence of unsuccessful operations is even higher for mediastinal explorations (30 to 40 per cent). The causes of failure with reoperations include errors in diagnosis, extremely unusual ectopic locations, unidentified supernumerary glands, an expected unsuccessful attempt to find a mediastinal tumor during neck reexploration, and parathyroid carcinoma. Reappearance of hypercalcemia after operation for parathyroid carcinoma denotes a poor prognosis (44 per cent 5-year survival and 22 per cent 10-year survival for patients with recurrent disease). Reoperation for control of recurrent malignant disease appears to prolong survival. (One patient reportedly survived 22 years after recurrent disease.) However, all patients ultimately die of the disease. The best treatment is aggressive meticulous total excision of the carcinoma at the time of the initial operation.[38]

Reported rates of complications encountered in parathyroid reoperations are listed in Table 28–8. Because of the scarring and proximity of the parathyroid glands to the recurrent laryngeal nerves, the incidence of vocal cord palsy resulting from injury to the recurrent laryngeal nerves is increased (about twice that of the initial operation). Detailed

**TABLE 28–5. Pathologic Findings in Parathyroid Reoperations**

| SERIES | ADENOMA | HYPERPLASIA | CARCINOMA | TOTAL |
|---|---|---|---|---|
| Massachusetts General Hospital | 66 | 29 | 7 | 102 |
| University of California at San Francisco | | | | |
| Persistent | 43 | 11 | 1 | 55 |
| Recurrent | 8 | 19 | 1 | 28 |
| Mayo Clinic | 119 | 19 | — | 138 |
| National Institutes of Health | 58 | 34 | 4 | 96 |
| Total | 294 | 112 | 13 | 419 |
| Per cent | 70 | 27 | 3 | 100 |

**TABLE 28–6. Anatomic Location of Residual Hyperfunctioning Glands at Reoperation (Massachusetts General Hospital Series)**

| LOCATION | NO. | PER CENT |
|---|---|---|
| Cervical | | |
| Posterior upper pole | 19 | 14 |
| Thymus | 17 | 13 |
| Lower pole | 17 | 13 |
| Posterosuperior mediastinum | 50 | 37 |
| Other unusual locations | 3 | 2 |
| Subtotal | 106 | 79 |
| Mediastinal | | |
| Intrathymic | 24 | 17 |
| Extrathymic | 5 | 4 |
| Subtotal | 29 | 21 |
| Total | 135 | 100 |

knowledge of the course of the external branch of the superior laryngeal nerve and the recurrent laryngeal nerve and the adjacent structures is crucial in avoiding injury to these structures. When possible, the nerves should be identified and spared as dissection proceeds into the region posteromedial to the superior pole vessels or the tracheoesophageal groove caudal to the inferior cornu of the thyroid cartilage.

As many as 10 to 20 per cent of patients undergoing reoperations will have continued hypercalcemia resulting from failure to locate and remove the hyperfunctioning gland. The risk of hypoparathyroidism with reoperations is appreciable. Transient postoperative hypocalcemia develops in as many as half of the patients undergoing parathyroid reoperations. Fortunately, most of these patients do not require long-term therapy with calcium or vitamin D. However, from 3 to 13 per cent of patients treated by experienced parathyroid surgeons may have permanent postoperative hypoparathyroidism. This risk is particularly great in patients undergoing mediastinal exploration where permanent hypoparathyroidism develops in from 9 to 21 per cent of patients. Therefore, techniques of subtotal resection, cryopreservation, and autotransplantation must often be employed.

**TABLE 28–7. Anatomic Location of Residual Hyperfunctioning Glands at Reoperation (Mayo Clinic Series)**

| LOCATION | NO. | PER CENT |
|---|---|---|
| Inferior | | |
| Normal | 34 | 22.5 |
| Cervical thymus | 3 | 2.0 |
| Mediastinal thymus | 18 | 11.9 |
| Within carotid sheath | 2 | 1.3 |
| Intrathyroid | 3 | 2.0 |
| Undescended | 1 | 0.7 |
| Subtotal | 61 | 40.4 |
| Superior | | |
| Normal | 15 | 9.9 |
| Tracheoesophageal groove | 15 | 9.9 |
| Posterosuperior mediastinum | 11 | 7.3 |
| Retrotracheal/retroesophageal | 10 | 6.6 |
| Medial to upper pole | 2 | 1.3 |
| In carotid sheath | 1 | 0.7 |
| Under thyroid capsule | 4 | 2.7 |
| Intrathyroid | 5 | 3.3 |
| Subtotal | 63 | 41.7 |
| Mediastinal | | |
| Mediastinal thymus | 19 | 12.6 |
| Aortic arch | 7 | 4.6 |
| Tracheal carina | 1 | 0.7 |
| Subtotal | 27 | 17.9 |
| Total | 151 | 100 |

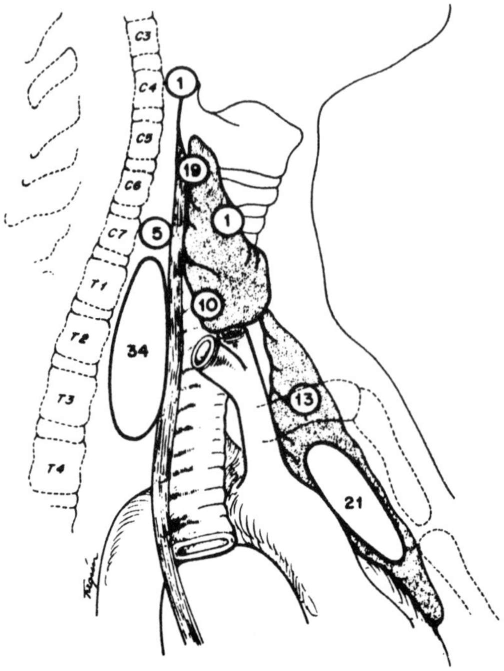


34 SUPERIOR POSTERIOR MEDIASTINUM
21 ANTERIOR MEDIASTINUM
19 BEHIND UPPER POLE OF THYROID
13 BEHIND CLAVICLE WITHIN THYMIC TONGUE
10 BEHIND LOWER POLE OF THYROID
5 BEHIND ESOPHAGUS
1 BEHIND ANGLE OF THE JAW
1 INTRATHYROIDAL

**FIGURE 28–2.** Anatomic locations of residual hyperfunctioning parathyroid glands. (From Wang, C. A.: Surgical management of primary hyperparathyroidism. Curr. Probl. Surg., *22*:37, 1985.)

Death associated with parathyroid reoperations is exceedingly rare (<1 per cent) and most often occurs from other unrelated concurrent systemic problems (carcinoma, infection, pulmonary, or cardiovascular causes). Because of the increased magnitude of operative difficulty and associated risks, these patients should be treated by endocrine surgical teams with established success and experience.

**TABLE 28–8. Complications of Reoperations for Hyperparathyroidism**

| COMPLICATION | INCIDENCE, PER CENT |
|---|---|
| Failure to cure hypercalcemia | 7–19 |
| Recurrent laryngeal nerve injury | 4–8 |
| Permanent hypoparathyroidism | 13–25 |
| Autograft failure | 6–50 |
| Autograft recurrence | 7 |
| Mortality | <1 |

What does the surgeon do in the event of an exhaustive reoperation with negative results? During operation, several maneuvers should be considered. The previously identified normal glands must be scrutinized carefully. Are they really normal or do they represent unrecognized residual disease or are they part of a larger underlying tumor? All identified parathyroid glands undergo biopsy and are marked to document what has been accomplished with the current operation. Have all unusual locations been exposed and examined? When thyroid lobectomy or thymectomy has not already been carried out, these procedures should be considered. Selective venous blood samples are obtained for measurement of parathyroid hormone from the appropriate exposed veins (upper and lower internal jugular; superior, middle, or inferior thyroid; innominate; internal mammary; superior vena cava). It might be worthwhile to ask an experienced nonfatigued colleague to review the situation and to assist in the exploration. When the point of diminishing returns arrives, the operation should be terminated. As the operative time lengthens the surgeon tires, and further dissection jeopardizes the recurrent laryngeal nerves and other structures. At this point terminating the operation is safer to the patient than continuing it: Primum non nocere. After operation, the diagnosis should be reconfirmed. Medical management of the ongoing hypercalcemia, when severe, may require use of hydration, furosemide, calcitonin, phosphate, diphosphonate, or mithramycin therapy. A period of observation should be considered with later reevaluation with repeated or more sophisticated localization procedures. Consultation with or referral to a center with reoperative expertise may be rewarding.

## SUMMARY

Reoperations for patients with recurrent or persistent hyperparathyroidism can be exceedingly challenging. They are accompanied by increased risk of failure, injury to the recurrent laryngeal nerves, and hypoparathyroidism. The majority (80 per cent) of missing hyperfunctioning parathyroid glands are in the neck region or accessible through a cervical incision. Only rarely does the elusive tumor reside in the deep mediastinum requiring sternotomy. Preoperative parathyroid localization examinations can be helpful in guiding the surgeon and may shorten operative time and minimize risks to the patient. Ultrasonography and thallium scanning appear to be the most useful procedures for elusive cervical parathyroid tumors. Magnetic resonance imaging or computed tomography may visualize a hyperfunctioning mediastinal gland. Invasive procedures, such as angiography, selective venous catheterization, and fine needle aspiration, should be reserved for selected complex reoperative situations. Because of the inherent difficulties and hazards of parathyroid reoperations, these patients are best treated in referral centers with special expertise.

As with many other medical problems, the best treatment is prevention. The need for reoperation could be circumvented in most patients if the initial exploration were carried out properly. The cardinal principles of parathyroid surgery include a thorough knowledge of parathyroid embryology and anatomy, a meticulous systematic exploration, identification of all parathyroid glands, recognition of the pathologic diagnosis, and adequate excision of the appropriate glands. In the hands of skilled endocrine surgical teams, application of the methods described can result in successful treatment of patients with persistent or recurrent hyperparathyroidism in more than 80 per cent of reoperations.

## REFERENCES


1. Alexander, P. T., Schuman, E. S., Vetto, R. M., et al.: Repeat parathyroid operation associated with renal disease. Am. J. Surg., *155*:686–689, 1988.
2. Beazley, R. M., Costa, J., and Ketcham, A. S.: Reoperative parathyroid surgery. Am. J. Surg., *130*:427–429, 1975.
3. Block, M. A., Frame, B., Kleerekoper, M., and Rao, D. S.: Surgical management of persistence or recurrence after subtotal parathyroidectomy for primary hyperparathyroidism. Am. J. Surg., *138*:561–566, 1979.
4. Brennan, M. F., and Norton, J. A.: Reoperation for persistent and recurrent hyperparathyroidism. Ann. Surg., *201*:40–44, 1985.
5. Brennan, M. F., Marx, S. J., Doppman, J., et al.: Results of reoperation for persistent and recurrent hyperparathyroidism. Ann. Surg., *194*:671–676, 1981.
6. Bruining, H. A., Birkenhäger, J. C., Ong, G. L., and Lamberts, S. W.: Causes of failure in operations for hyperparathyroidism. Surgery, *101*:562–565, 1987.
7. Clark, O. H., Way, L. W., and Hunt, T. K.: Recurrent hyperparathyroidism. Ann. Surg., *184*:391–402, 1976.
8. Cohn, K. H., and Silen, W.: Lessons of parathyroid reoperations. Am. J. Surg., *144*:511–517, 1982.
9. Cope, O.: The study of hyperparathyroidism at the Massachusetts General Hospital. N. Engl. J. Med., *274*:1174–1182, 1966.
10. Darling, G. E., Marx, S. J., Spiegel, A. M., et al.: Prospective analysis of intraoperative and postoperative urinary cyclic adenosine 3′,5′-monophosphate levels to predict outcome of patients undergoing reoperations for primary hyperparathyroidism. Surgery, *104*:1128–1136, 1988.
11. Delmonico, F. L., Wang, C. A., Rubin, N. T., et al.: Parathyroid surgery in patients with renal failure. Ann. Surg., *200*:644–647, 1984.
12. Devine, R. M., van Heerden, J. A., Grant, C. S., and Muir, J. J.: The role of methylene blue infusion in the management of persistent or recurrent hyperparathyroidism. Surgery, *94*:916–918, 1983.
13. Edis, A. J., Beahrs, O. H., and Sheedy, P. F., 2d: Reoperation for hyperparathyroidism. World J. Surg., *1*:731–738, 1977.
14. Edis, A. J., Sheedy, P. F., Beahrs, O. H., and van Heerden, J. A.: Results of reoperation for hyperparathyroidism, with evaluation of preoperative localization studies. Surgery, *84*:384–393, 1978.
15. Gaz, R. D., H'Doubler, P. B., and Wang, C. A.: The management of 50 unusual hyperfunctioning parathyroid glands. Surgery, *102*:949–957, 1987.
16. Granberg, P. O., Johansson, G., Lindval, N., et al.: Reoperation for primary hyperparathyroidism. Am. J. Surg., *143*:296–300, 1982.
17. Grant, C. S., van Heerden, J. A., Charboneau, J. W., et al.: Clinical management of persistent and/or recurrent primary hyperparathyroidism. World J. Surg., *10*:555–565, 1986.
18. Irvin, G. L., Newell, D. J., and Morgan, S. D.: Parathyroid metabolism after operative treatment of hypercalcemic (primary) hyperparathyroidism. Surgery, *102*:898–902, 1987.
19. Lafferty, F. W., and Hubay, C. A.: Primary hyperparathyroidism: A review of the long-term surgical and nonsurgical morbidities as a basis for a rational approach to treatment. Arch. Intern. Med., *149*:789–796, 1989.
20. Levin, K. E., and Clark, O. H.: Reoperative thyroid and parathyroid surgery. *In* Tompkins, R. K. (ed.): Reoperative Surgery. Philadelphia, J. B. Lippincott Co., 1988, pp. 509–524.
21. Levin, K. E., and Clark, O. H.: The reasons for failure in parathyroid operations. Arch. Surg., *124*:911–915, 1989.
22. Levin, K. E., Gooding, G. A. W., Okerlund, M., et al.: Localizing studies in patients with persistent or recurrent hyperparathyroidism. Surgery, *102*:917–925, 1987.
23. McGarity, W. C., and Goldman, A. L.: Reoperation for primary hyperparathyroidism. Ann. Surg., *194*:134–139, 1981.

24. Miller, D. L., Doppman, J. L., Shawker, T. H., et al.: Localization of parathyroid adenomas in patients who have undergone surgery. Part I. Noninvasive imaging methods. Radiology, *162* (1 Pt. 1):133–137, 1987.
25. Norton, J. A., Brennan, M. F., Saxe, A. W., et al.: Intraoperative urinary cyclic adenosine monophosphate as a guide to successful reoperative parathyroidectomy. Ann. Surg., *200*:389–395, 1984.
26. Nussbaum, S. R., Thompson, A. R., Hutcheson, K. A., et al.: Intraoperative measurement of parathyroid hormone in the surgical management of hyperparathyroidism. Surgery, *104*:1121–1127, 1988.
27. Nussbaum, S. R., Zahradnik, R. J., Lavigne, J. R., et al.: Highly sensitive two-site immunoradiometric assay of parathyrin, and its clinical utility in evaluating patients with hypercalcemia. Clin. Chem., *33*:1364–1367, 1987.
28. Paloyan, E.: Persistent/recurrent primary hyperparathyroidism. *In* van Heerden, J. A. (ed.): Common Problems in Endocrine Surgery. Chicago, Year Book Medical Publishers, 1989, pp. 183–190.
29. Rattner, D. W., Marrone, G. C., Kasdon, E., and Silen, W.: Recurrent hyperparathyroidism due to implantation of parathyroid tissue. Am. J. Surg., *149*:745–748, 1985.
30. Rizzoli, R., Green, J., 3d, and Marx, S. J.: Primary hyperparathyroidism in familial multiple endocrine neoplasia type I: Long-term follow-up of serum calcium levels after parathyroidectomy. Am. J. Med., *78*:467–474, 1985.
31. Roslyn, J. J., Mulder, D. G., and Gordon, H. E.: Persistent and recurrent hyperparathyroidism. Am. J. Surg., *142*:21–25, 1981.
32. Rothmund, M., and Wagner, P. K.: Reoperations for persistent and recurrent secondary hyperparathyroidism. Ann. Surg., *207*:310–314, 1988.
33. Russell, C. F., Edis, A. J., and Purnell, D. C.: The reasons for persistent hypercalcaemia after cervical exploration for presumed primary hyperparathyroidism. Br. J. Surg., *70*:198–201, 1983.
34. Sigel, B., Kraft, A. R., Nyhus, L. M.: Identification of a parathyroid adenoma by operative ultrasonography. Arch. Surg., *116*:234–235, 1981.
35. Wang, C. A.: The anatomic basis of parathyroid surgery. Ann. Surg., *183*:271–275, 1976.
36. Wang, C. A.: Parathyroid re-exploration: A clinical and pathological study of 112 cases. Ann. Surg., *186*:140–145, 1977.
37. Wang, C. A.: Surgical management of primary hyperparathyroidism. Curr. Probl. Surg., *22*:1–50, 1985.
38. Wang, C. A., and Gaz, R. D.: Natural history of parathyroid carcinoma: Diagnosis, treatment, and results. Am. J. Surg., *149*:522–527, 1985.
39. Wang, C. A., and Guyton, S. P.: Reoperations for parathyroid disease. *In* Malt, R. A. (ed.): Complex Operations at Massachusetts General Hospital. Philadelphia, W. B. Saunders Co., 1983, pp. 108–123.
40. Wang, C. A., Castleman, B., and Cope, O.: Surgical management of hyperparathyroidism due to primary hyperplasia. Ann. Surg., *195*:384–392, 1982.
41. Wang, C. A., Gaz, R. D., and Moncure, A. C.: Mediastinal parathyroid exploration: A clinical and pathologic study of 47 cases. World J. Surg., *10*:687–695, 1986.
42. Wang, C. A., Reitz, R. E., Pollard, J. J., et al.: Localization of hyperfunctioning parathyroids: The surgeon's riddle. Am. J. Surg., *119*:462–464, 1970.
43. Wells, S. A., Jr., Leight, G. S., Hensley, M., and Dilley, W. G.: Hyperparathyroidism associated with the enlargement of two or three parathyroid glands. Ann. Surg., *202*:533–538, 1985.

# 29

# CARCINOMA OF PARATHYROID GLANDS

*Ricardo L. Rossi, M.D.*

Parathyroid carcinoma has been found in 0.5 to 1 per cent of patients operated on for primary hyperparathyroidism.[3, 5, 7] The pathologic criteria for the diagnosis of parathyroid carcinoma are controversial, and, as in other endocrine carcinomas, histopathology is less definitive than evidence of involvement of tissues outside the parathyroid gland. Findings characteristic of malignant disease include invasion of the capsule and surrounding structures, metastasis to lymph nodes or other organs (for example, the lungs), blood vessel invasion, and cellular mitosis. However, when these characteristics are not present, the definitive diagnosis may not be made until local or nodal recurrent disease and hypercalcemia recur.

A definitive preoperative diagnosis of carcinoma is usually not possible in a patient with hyperparathyroidism. However, carcinoma is suspected in patients with severe hypercalcemia, in patients with a palpable mass in the neck, and in patients with unexplained paralysis of the vocal cord. Hypercalcemia of more than 14 mg/dl has been reported[2–4, 6, 8] in 39 to 75 per cent of patients who have proved parathyroid carcinoma. Complications of hyperparathyroidism are common in this group of patients. Bone disease has been a finding in 46 to 73 per cent of patients, renal disease in between 31 and 64 per cent of patients, and the coexistence of generalized fibro-osteitis and urolithiasis in 25 per cent of patients.[2, 3, 6, 8] A tumor in the neck has been palpable in 32 to 69 per cent of patients. Radiography of the hands will demonstrate subperiosteal resorption in half of the patients. An elevated level of serum immunoreactive parathormone excludes nonparathyroid carcinoma associated with hypercalcemia.

Ultrasonography, on occasion, discloses a hyperechogenic lesion, whereas most benign parathyroid tumors present a hypoechogenic lesion with sharp margins. When the diagnosis of parathyroid carcinoma is strongly suspected before operation, radiography of the chest, computed tomography of the neck and mediastinum, and a thallium-201 chloride scintiscan study of the neck, mediastinum, and lungs may identify metastatic disease. During the preoperative evaluation of the patient, medical therapy consists primarily of hydration with normal saline solution and administration of furosemide (Lasix) for a greatly elevated serum level of calcium. However, semiurgent surgery is the best approach in such patients.

At the time of operation when soft tissue invasion is not obvious, the parathyroid gland may appear to be surrounded by fibrosis and to be more adherent to the surrounding structures than is characteristic of a benign adenoma. The gland can be firm and pale white. Invasion of the thyroid gland, muscles, recurrent laryngeal nerve, esophagus, or other soft tissues of the neck may be present. When malignant disease is suspected at the time of operation, en bloc resection is attempted, which may require thyroid lobectomy, excision of the strap muscles, and sacrifice of the recurrent laryngeal nerve when it is involved by the tumor and when unilateral vocal cord paralysis is apparent preoperatively. Lymph node metastases are found in 11 to 32 per cent of patients, and when metastatic disease is present, a modified neck dissection should be performed. When a lesion removed at operation is pathologically thought to be carcinoma because of increased mitosis, no further operation is required in the absence of capsular or extracapsular invasion.

The natural course of parathyroid carcinoma tends to be that of a slow-growing tumor with episodes of acute and chronic hyperparathyroidism and with clinical deterioration usually caused by the severe hyperparathyroidism rather than by the local extent of the malignant tumor or distant metastatic disease. Recurrent cervical disease and pulmonary metastasis can occur. Local recurrent tumors have been seen in 31 to 65 per cent of patients and distant metastasis in 14 to 21 per cent of patients. Postoperatively, adjuvant chemotherapy or radiotherapy has not proved to be effective in the control of local disease or distant metastasis. Aggressive surgical therapy is indicated, when possible, because management of the recurrent disease can achieve control of the hypercalcemia. Operation often provides palliation and occasionally a cure.

Van Heerden and associates[7] reported a 5-year survival rate of 36 per cent, and Holmes et al.[3] reported 5-year and 10-year survival rates of 50 and 13 per cent, respectively. Prognosis is related to the biologic characteristics of the tumor in each patient. Patients with increased mitosis but no definite soft tissue invasion are likely to have a more favorable prognosis than patients with invasive disease.

Medical therapy for patients with nonoperable recurrent disease consists of the oral administration of a neutral phosphate solution, mithramycin, and diphosphonates.

After successful resection of parathyroid carcinoma with normalization of the serum level of calcium, serial calcium levels are obtained. If recurrent hypercalcemia becomes manifested, the recurrent tumor can be studied by means of a thallium-201 chloride scan, computed tomography, and standard radiographic techniques.[2]

The Lahey Clinic experience[1] from 1942 to 1981 includes eight patients whose average age was 55 years (19 to 60 years). The median serum calcium level was 14 mg/dl. All patients had symptoms of weakness and fatigue, and one patient had neuropsychiatric manifestations. Five patients had bone disease, two patients had a palpable mass in the neck, five patients had urolithiasis, and two patients had ulcer disease. Of the eight patients, one died of recurrent disease in the neck and lung 9 years after the original operation. A second patient presented with extensive recurrent disease in the neck, severe hypercalcemia, and bone disease with pathologic fractures. Treatment consisted of wide local excision of the tumor, total thyroidectomy, and segmental resection of the trachea and esophagus. The patient required prolonged treatment with supplements of calcium and vitamin D because of hypoparathyroidism. Five years after operation, the patient was well and had no signs of recurrent disease. He was lost to follow-up study. Two other patients treated before 1965 have been lost to follow-up study. The other five patients were known to be alive without signs of recurrent disease when the review was undertaken in 1981, with a follow-up time of less than 5 years.

It is important that the surgeon be aware of parathyroid carcinoma because identification at the time of initial operation permits en bloc resection that offers the patient the best possibility for cure.

## REFERENCES

1. Cohn, K., Silverman, M., Corrado, J., and Sedgwick, C.: Parathyroid carcinoma: The Lahey Clinic experience. Surgery, *98:*1095–1100, 1985.
2. Fujimoto, Y., Obara, T., Ito, Y., et al.: Localization and surgical resection of metastatic parathyroid carcinoma. World J. Surg., *10:*539–547, 1986.
3. Holmes, E. C., Morton, D. L., and Ketcham, A. S.: Parathyroid carcinoma: A collective review. Ann. Surg., *169:*631–640, 1969.
4. Levin, K. E., Galante, M., and Clark, O. H.: Parathyroid carcinoma versus parathyroid adenoma in

patients with profound hypercalcemia. Surgery, *101*:649–660, 1987.
5. Schantz, A., and Castleman, B.: Parathyroid carcinoma: A study of 70 cases. Cancer, *31*:600–605, 1973.
6. Shane, E., and Bilezikian, J. P.: Parathyroid carcinoma: A review of 62 patients. Endocr. Rev., *3*:218–226, 1982.
7. van Heerden, J. A., Weiland, L. H., ReMine, W. H., et al.: Cancer of the parathyroid glands. Arch. Surg., *114*:475–480, 1979.
8. Wang, C.-A., and Gaz, R. D.: Natural history of parathyroid carcinoma: Diagnosis, treatment, and results. Am. J. Surg., *149*:522–527, 1985.

# Commentary

*Barbara Kinder, M.D.*

This chapter on parathyroid carcinoma emphasizes the importance of recognizing this clinical entity at the time of first exploration when wide local excision, combined when indicated with dissection of the neck, offers the best chance of cure. Such characteristics as invasion of surrounding structures and a pale fibrotic appearance and firm texture are critical features that the operating surgeon can immediately appreciate. One exception to the rule that fibrotic-appearing parathyroid glands should be considered suspicious is in the patient receiving dialysis who is being operated on for secondary hyperparathyroidism. Glands in this setting often have areas of scarring, the result perhaps of intraglandular hemorrhage conceivably related to periods of heparinization or to uremic coagulopathy.

We have treated 11 patients with parathyroid carcinoma at Yale between 1960 and 1989, ten of whom were seen since 1977. Our data are similar to those of others in terms of age (25 to 88 years; median age, 59 years), serum calcium level (11 to 25 mg/dl; median, 13 mg/dl), and the presence in most patients of symptoms caused by urolithiasis, bone disease, or both. Our approach to treatment is much as outlined, with emphasis placed on adequate local excision at the first operation. We have had no experience with adjuvant chemotherapy but have used local radiotherapy in three patients: in two patients after resection of locally recurrent tumor and in one patient, in a true adjuvant sense, after initial en bloc resection of the thyroid lobe and adherent parathyroid carcinoma and central neck dissection (one positive node). This latter patient is interesting in that, although normocalcemia was achieved after operation, the parathyroid hormone values remained elevated until after the patient received 5,000 cGy to the neck and then declined gradually over a period of one and a half years until now, three years later, the parathyroid hormone and calcium levels are normal. One might speculate that this prolonged fall in the parathyroid hormone level could represent ongoing radiation damage to residual parathyroid tumor. Except for some hoarseness, which subsided a few months after cessation of treatment, the patient experienced no side effects from the radiation. The minimal morbidity and possible efficacy of this treatment have led us to conclude that radiation therapy should be considered in patients after primary resection of parathyroid carcinoma.

We agree that, as with other endocrine tumors, an aggressive approach to metastatic disease should be adopted. We have performed two median sternotomies for pulmonary metastatic disease and four reoperations for locally recurrent disease. The only complications were a hematoma of the neck and hypocalcemia. In all patients, surgical excision of tumor resulted in a beneficial lowering, at least temporarily, of the serum calcium level.

In patients with nonresectable disease, we have relied initially on vigorous hydration and salt loading. Calcitonin with and without glucocorticoids is often temporarily useful, and mithramycin can be given, although renal compromise is a limiting factor. In our experience and that of others, the oral diphosphonates have not been effective in reducing serum calcium levels.[1] We have used intravenously administered ethane hydroxydiphosphonate (EHDP [Didronel]) with good response. One patient responded transiently to intravenously administered gallium nitrate, which inhibits calcium release from bone.[2] This patient is alive with disease 18 years after initial treatment for parathyroid carcinoma and has also undergone resection of pulmonary metastatic disease, repeat neck exploration with central node dissection followed by radiation therapy, and irradiation of metastatic disease to bone.

Patients with parathyroid carcinoma continue to represent a challenge to surgeons and endocrinologists both in terms of early diagnosis, which permits appropriate local treatment initially, and in the devising of new treatments for the ravages of chronic hypercalcemia in this often indolent disease.

## REFERENCES

1. Shane, E., Jacobs, T. P., Siris, E. S., et al.: Therapy of hypercalcemia due to parathyroid carcinoma with intravenous dichloromethylene diphosphonate. Am. J. Med., *72:*939–944, 1982.
2. Warrell, R. P., Skelos, A., Alcock, N. W., and Bockman, R. S.: Gallium nitrate for acute treatment of cancer-related hypercalcemia: Clinicopharmacological and dose response analysis. Cancer Res., *46:*4208–4212, 1986.

# 30

# THYROID AND PARATHYROID DISEASE DURING PREGNANCY

*Mary Beth Hodge, M.D.*

## THYROID DISEASE

To detect and treat maternal thyroid disease during pregnancy, the physician must be aware of the normal changes in maternal thyroid function that take place during pregnancy. The hormonal changes and metabolic demands of pregnancy have an important effect on the thyroid gland, and alterations in maternal thyroid function may, in turn, influence gestation. Although the healthy pregnant woman is considered to be euthyroid, changes occur in the basal metabolic rate, radioactive iodine uptake, and size of the thyroid gland. Many of the changes seen in maternal thyroid function tests during pregnancy are secondary to an increase in thyroxine-binding globulin, which is attributable to an increase in estrogens.

### *Normal Thyroid Gland During Pregnancy*

The thyroid gland may be slightly enlarged in a pregnant woman as a result of hyperplasia of the glandular tissue and increased vascularity of the gland. The increased radioactive iodine uptake of the thyroid gland during pregnancy is believed to result from a relative iodine deficiency. An increase in the glomerular filtration rate results in increased excretion of iodide and a subsequent decrease in the maternal iodine pool.[9] The goiter of pregnancy appears to reflect and compensate for the lower level of circulating iodine available for synthesis of thyroxine[1] and the possible thyroid-stimulating effect of chorionic gonadotropin, which is at its highest level during the first trimester.

The basal metabolic rate is increased about 20 per cent during pregnancy as a result of the increase in total mass of body tissue (that is, the fetus, placenta, and uterus) and the increased work of the maternal heart.[11]

Serum levels of total thyroxine ($T_4$) and total triiodothyronine ($T_3$) increase during the first trimester and remain elevated until about the sixth week after delivery. The elevation in both total $T_4$ and total $T_3$ is caused by an increase in thyroxine-binding globulin that results from the increased secretion of estrogens.[25] The level of the serum total $T_3$ increases to a lesser extent than does the level of the serum total $T_4$, with the result that the T4 to $T_3$ ratio is greater than in the nonpregnant state.[49] The proportion of both the free $T_4$ and free $T_3$ is decreased relative to the total $T_4$ and total $T_3$, and thus the actual levels of free $T_4$ and free $T_3$ remain within normal limits.[9] As a result of the decrease in the proportion of free $T_4$, the volume of distribution and fractional rate of turnover of total $T_4$ are decreased, but the total daily disposal of the hormone remains essentially unchanged because of the increase in total $T_4$.[24, 49]

Because thyroxine-binding globulin is increased, the $T_3$ resin uptake is decreased into the hypothyroid range. The combination of an elevated serum level of total $T_4$ and a decreased serum level of $T_3$ resin uptake is characteristic of the increase in thyroxine-binding globulin that occurs in normal pregnancy. When the total $T_4$ is not elevated in a pregnant woman, the possibility of maternal hypothyroidism, thyroxine-binding globulin deficiency, or failure of thyroxine-binding globulin to rise should be considered. The increase in thyroxine-binding globulin is dependent on elevated levels of estrogens that occur because of an intact fetal-placental unit, and therefore failure of serum levels of $T_4$ to rise may also indicate fetal death.[79a]

The serum level of thyrotropin-stimulating hormone is slightly increased during early pregnancy and returns to normal by term.[65] The response of thyroid-stimulating hormone to thyrotropin-releasing hormone is accentuated relative to the nonpregnant state as a result of hyperestrogenemia.[9] The physiologic importance of this increased sensitivity to thyrotropin-releasing hormone remains undetermined, however. The increased response of thyroid-stimulating hormone to thyrotropin-releasing hormone in pregnancy may compensate for the increased binding of $T_4$ to thyroxine-binding globulin as a result of the increase in thyroxine-binding globulin.[9] As a compensatory phenomenon, a given amount of thyrotropin-releasing hormone results in a greater secretion of thyroid-stimulating hormone and, secondarily, the release of a larger amount of thyroid hormone from the thyroid gland.[9] These phenomena result in the maintenance of normal thyroid function during pregnancy. Despite alterations in the hypothalamic-pituitary thyroid axis, the normal pregnant woman remains euthyroid.

## *Thyroid Function in the Fetus*

The fetal hypothalamic-pituitary-thyroid system develops and functions independently of the maternal system.[30] The fetal thyroid is able to accumulate iodine by the 10th to 12th week of gestation[29] and can produce a small amount of thyroid hormone by the end of the first trimester.[85] Shortly after midgestation, the levels of fetal thyroid-stimulating hormone, fetal thyroid radioactive iodine uptake, and fetal serum free $T_4$ increase abruptly; this suggests that the fetal hypothalamic-pituitary thyroid-stimulating hormone control system begins to mature at about the 20th week of gestation.[30]

Results of studies[30] in humans and animals have shown that the placental transfer of $T_4$ and $T_3$ is severely limited in both the maternal-fetal and fetal-maternal directions. Little or no thyroid hormone traverses the placenta at physiologic serum levels. Although some maternal-fetal transfer of thyroid hormone may occur at extremely high serum levels, transfer is limited even in these circumstances.[12, 30, 56]

Placental transfer of thyroid-stimulating hormone was determined to be unimportant in all species studied.[28] Proposed mechanisms preventing the transfer of thyroid hormones across the placenta include the increased binding of the hormones in maternal serum and the poor solubility of hormones in the lipid-rich placental tissue.[16] The placenta was hypothesized to be an active site of deiodination of the inner ring (5′-deiodinase) of both $T_4$ and $T_3$ with the production of inactive iodothyronines, preventing the active hormones from reaching the fetal compartment.[81] Iodides easily cross the placenta from the mother to the fetus, and exposure of the fetus to iodine can result in fetal hypothyroidism and goiter.

## *Thyrotoxicosis*

Thyrotoxicosis occurs in about 0.2 per cent of pregnant women.[76] Without specific antithyroid treatment, the number of infants with a low birth weight and the neonatal mortality rate are increased.[76]

Graves' disease is the most common cause of thyrotoxicosis in women of childbearing age. Other less common causes include toxic adenoma, toxic multinodular goiter, subacute thyroiditis, Hashimoto's thyroiditis, trophoblastic tumors, and hydatidiform moles.

Thyrotoxicosis attributable to a hydatidiform mole is treated by surgical evacuation of the mole from the uterus. These patients should be treated with antithyroid medication, iodides, and beta blockers before operation to avoid serious complications during the surgical procedure.

Patients with toxic adenoma and toxic multinodular goiter can be managed with propylthiouracil during pregnancy. After delivery, consideration should be given to radioactive iodine as definitive treatment for these two types of hyperthyroidism. When large doses of propylthiouracil are required to maintain a euthyroid state during pregnancy, thyroidectomy should be performed during the second trimester.

Subacute thyroiditis results in a transient form of hyperthyroidism, usually lasting no more than 4 to 6 weeks. Transient hypothyroidism may develop later. Antithyroid drugs are inappropriate because thyroid inflammation blocks the uptake of iodine and the coupling reaction. Antithyroid drugs do not change the course or severity of this form of hyperthyroidism. Aspirin is contraindicated during pregnancy. Beta blockers should be used only when hyperthyroidism is severe or when arrhythmia is present. Most women tolerate subacute thyroiditis well.

Hashimoto's thyroiditis may also have a transient phase of hyperthyroidism. Treatment is not necessary when elevation of free $T_4$ is mild and when both mother and fetus are tolerating the hyperthyroidism. However, when the hyperthyroidism is severe, small doses of propylthiouracil can be given and may be necessary only for a month or two.

Patients with trophoblastic tumors, such as choriocarcinoma, need specific antitumor treatment. Antithyroid drugs should be used until the tumor is controlled. Thyroidectomy is not indicated for this type of thyrotoxicosis.

Women who have had Graves' disease before pregnancy may have a remission of thyrotoxicosis during pregnancy and an exacerbation during the postpartum period.[2] The immunologic changes that normally occur during pregnancy may be responsible for the fluctuations in the intensity of Graves' disease.

In a normal pregnancy, the fetus escapes immunologic rejection by the mother, although the fetus has antigens that are foreign to the mother (that is, paternal antigens). The reason the maternal immune system does not reject these foreign antigens may be that maternal immunoresponsiveness is decreased during gestation.[7, 20, 88] Decreased maternal immunoresponsiveness appears to be caused by increased activity of fetal suppressor T cells. This increased activity, which permits suppressor factors to cross the placenta, disappears after parturition.[7]

## *Diagnosis*

The clinical diagnosis of mild or moderate hyperthyroidism during pregnancy can be difficult to establish in some patients. Often, the diagnosis is missed because many of the symptoms and signs, such as heat intolerance, anxiety, tachycardia, and warm moist skin, observed in hyperthyroid patients are also frequently seen in healthy pregnant women. Weight loss and excessive tachycardia (that is, a resting heart rate of more than 100 beats a minute) are not seen in normal pregnancy, and therefore a diagnosis of thyrotoxicosis should be considered when either of these signs is present. Hyperemesis gravidarum, which can be a presenting feature of hyperthyroidism, resolves when thyrotoxicosis is treated.[26]

Because of estrogen-induced increases in thyroxine-binding globulin, the serum level of total $T_4$ is elevated in normal pregnancy. Likewise, $T_3$ resin uptake is normally decreased into the hypothyroid range. However, when the serum level of total $T_4$ is elevated (especially when the total $T_4$ is more than 15 μg/dl) and the level of $T_3$ resin uptake is in the euthyroid range provided that no deficiency exists in thyroxine-binding globulin, thyrotoxicosis should be suspected.

The serum free $T_4$ is the definitive test for making the diagnosis of hyperthyroidism during pregnancy. The serum level of free $T_4$ is elevated in hyperthyroid pregnant women, but the level is normal in euthyroid pregnant women.

The free $T_4$ should not be confused with the free thyroxine index. The free $T_4$ is a measure of the biologically active hormone, and it is not bound to thyroxine-binding globulin. The free thyroxine index is a calculated product of the total $T_4$ and $T_3$ resin uptake and is sometimes subject to error in interpretation. The free thyroxine index is usually elevated in hyperthyroid pregnant women and is usually normal in euthyroid pregnant women.

The 24-hour radioactive iodine uptake test is contraindicated during pregnancy but is often helpful in determining the type of thyrotoxicosis in nonpregnant patients.

## *Treatment*

The pregnant hyperthyroid woman should be treated because without therapy the risk of spontaneous abortion, premature labor, and fetal death is increased. The incidence of congenital malformations may be higher in the offspring of mothers who are hyperthyroid during the sensitive period of organogenesis.[71]

Antithyroid drugs (that is, propylthiouracil, methimazole, and carbimazole) and surgery are the two available treatment options. Radioactive iodine is contraindicated during pregnancy; it is concentrated in the fetal thyroid gland after the 10th or 12th week of pregnancy, and it destroys the gland. However, when radioactive iodine has inadvertently been administered early in pregnancy, it is not an indication for interruption of the pregnancy because Stoffer and Hamburger[89] showed that the rate of spontaneous abortion or incidence of congenital abnormalities was no higher in such patients.

The thionamides are effective in the treatment of thyrotoxicosis during pregnancy. The starting dose of propylthiouracil should be no more than 300 mg/day in divided doses. The starting dose of methimazole is about one tenth that of propylthiouracil. When control of thyrotoxicosis has been achieved, the dose of propylthiouracil should be decreased rapidly. Maintenance therapy should be as low a dose of propylthiouracil as possible, preferably less than 100 mg/day, to keep the free $T_4$ in the upper range of normal and to avoid fetal goiter and fetal hypothyroidism. The free $T_4$ level should be monitored monthly throughout the pregnancy.

Antithyroid drugs can easily cross the placenta and can inhibit production of thyroid hormone in the fetus, resulting in a secondary rise in fetal thyroid-stimulating hormone and subsequent development of fetal goiter. Only by using the least amount of antithyroid drug can the risk of fetal hypothyroidism and goiter be minimized.

Investigators[33, 46] proposed combination therapy with thionamides and thyroid hormones to treat the hyperthyroid mother and to prevent the development of fetal hypothyroidism. This approach was based on the assumption that some of the thyroid hormone given to the mother crossed the placenta to the fetus and prevented not only maternal hypothyroidism, which is deleterious to the pregnancy, but also hypothyroidism in the fetus. However, the placenta is now known to be relatively impermeable to thyroid hormone.[31, 81]

In addition, physiologic replacement doses of thyroid hormone in the mother may raise the level of maternal free $T_4$ and secondarily necessitate an increase in the dose of propylthiouracil to control hyperthyroidism. This defeats the purpose of giving thyroid hormone to the mother. Therefore, propylthiouracil should be used in the lowest possible dose to maintain a euthyroid state in the pregnant hyperthyroid woman rather than using combination therapy with propylthiouracil and thyroid hormone.

When hypothyroidism develops in a pregnant woman who is taking antithyroid medication, the drug should be discontinued temporarily, and thyroid hormone should be given. The serum thyroid-stimulating hormone is the most sensitive test to monitor for the development of maternal hypothyroidism. Results of studies[66] showed that the offspring of mothers with low serum levels of thyroid hormone during pregnancy had lower intelligence quotients at the age of 7 years. Results of thyroid screening programs in newborns suggest that early diagnosis and treatment of neonatal hypothyroidism prevent the sequelae of hypothyroidism in utero.[7] Thyroid function tests should be obtained on the cord blood of all neonates born to mothers who have had thyroid dysfunction during pregnancy.

The thionamides cross the placenta and may impair fetal thyroid function, resulting in fetal goiter and hypothyroidism.[6, 14] The placenta in rats and humans has been shown to be more permeable to methimazole than to propylthiouracil.[67] Results of this study suggest that propylthiouracil may be preferable to methimazole in the treatment of thyrotoxicosis during pregnancy because of a reduced incidence of fetal hypothyroidism. Propylthiouracil may also be preferable to methimazole for another reason: 11 cases of aplasia cutis of the scalp have been reported in infants born to mothers treated with methimazole.[4, 69, 75, 95]

Whether the thionamides cause other congenital defects is unclear. Of 243 infants whose mothers were treated with methimazole during pregnancy, two had congenital defects (that is, omphalocele and malformation of the ear lobe); no skin defects were found.[71]

Whether children exposed to antithyroid drugs in utero attain optimal intellectual development has been questioned.[10] However, results of intelligence tests administered to 28 children whose mothers took propylthiouracil during pregnancy and to 32 siblings who were not exposed to antithyroid drugs in utero revealed no significant differences between the two groups.[8]

### Use of Antithyroid Drugs During Lactation

A lactating hyperthyroid mother who is taking thionamides can transfer them to the baby in breast milk. Methimazole passes much more freely into breast milk than does propylthiouracil.[53, 60, 61] Lamberg and associates[60] studied the effect of thionamides on neonates who were being breast-fed by mothers taking antithyroid drugs. They concluded that breast-feeding was safe provided the daily dose of carbimazole did not exceed 15 mg (or 150 mg of propylthiouracil) and serum levels of $T_4$ and thyroid-stimulating hormone in the infant were monitored closely. Propylthiouracil is preferable to methimazole because it passes into breast milk only one tenth as well as methimazole. It is preferable that a lactating mother not take any medication. When a hyperthyroid mother requires moderate to large doses of thionamides, bottle-feeding is advisable to avoid the risk of neonatal hypothyroidism and its possible adverse effects on the intellectual development of the child.

### Beta Blockers

In nonpregnant hyperthyroid patients, beta blockers are often used in conjunction with the thionamides to control the symptoms of thyrotoxicosis. However, the use of beta blockers in pregnancy has been associated with a small placenta, intrauterine growth retardation, premature labor, impaired responses to anoxic stress, postnatal bradycardia, and postnatal hypoglycemia.[37, 42, 80] Rubin[82] suggested that adequate data are available to indicate that pregnant women can be treated safely with beta blocking agents. In general, beta blockers are not given to a pregnant hyperthyroid patient unless she is undergoing thyroidectomy or when thyroid storm is a concern.

### Iodides

Iodides are contraindicated during pregnancy unless the pregnant woman is being prepared for thyroidectomy or thyroid storm is present. Iodides easily cross the placenta and can cause fetal hypothyroidism and a large obstructing goiter.[91, 99] Fetal hypothyroidism occurs because large amounts of iodide acutely inhibit the incorporation of iodide into thyroglobulin (Wolff-Chaikoff effect) and also block the secretion of thyroid hormone.[31, 91]

### Surgery

Operation during pregnancy should be avoided because it carries the risk of spontaneous abortion and fetal anoxia in addition to the usual risks associated with thyroidectomy (that is, hypoparathyroidism and recurrent laryngeal nerve paralysis). When necessary, operation should be performed during the second trimester after organogenesis has occurred. The mother must be prepared for operation with antithyroid drugs and a short course of iodides (supersaturated solution of potassium iodide, 5 drops a day for 10 days) to avoid thyroid storm during the procedure.

Thyroidectomy during pregnancy should usually be reserved only for patients in whom hypersensitivity to the antithyroid drugs develops, patients who are noncompliant with the medication, patients who require large doses of antithyroid drugs to maintain a euthyroid state, and in the rare instance of an individual who is unresponsive to antithyroid medication.[50] Surgery does not alleviate the risks of neonatal or fetal thyrotoxicosis because transplacental passage of thyroid-stimulating immunoglobulins can still occur.

## *Neonatal Thyrotoxicosis*

Neonatal thyrotoxicosis is a self-limited illness that results from the transplacental passage of high titers of thyroid-stimulating immunoglobulins from the mother to the fetus.[68, 100] It occurs in about 1 to 2 per cent of infants born to mothers with Graves' disease, and the infant mortality rate is about 10 to 20 per cent.[68a] Neonatal thyrotoxicosis can also occur in the infants of mothers who have had successfully treated Graves' disease in the past and who remained euthyroid during pregnancy. The mother may still have appreciable amounts of thyroid-stimulating immunoglobulins that cross the placenta and stimulate the fetal thyroid.

Pregnancy is one of the few conditions in which measurement of thyroid-stimulating immunoglobulins in the mother is clinically helpful. High maternal titers indicate that the neonate is at an increased risk for the development of neonatal thyrotoxicosis.[7, 23] Thyroid function tests should be performed on the infant immediately after birth. The transient nature of neonatal thyrotoxicosis, which has a duration of about 3 to 4 weeks, is the result of the decrease in circulating maternal thyroid-stimulating immunoglobulin in the neonate. When the mother has taken antithyroid drugs during pregnancy, the onset of neonatal thyrotoxicosis may be delayed until 7 to 10 days after birth. As the effect of these drugs wears off, the elevated thyroid-stimulating immunoglobulins stimulate the infant's thyroid to produce too much thyroid hormone.[7]

Fetal thyrotoxicosis should be suspected when the fetal heart rate is more than 160 beats a minute and the serum levels of maternal thyroid-stimulating immunoglobulins are high.[7] Because of the increased risk of complications (that is, low birth weight for gestational age and premature labor), the administration of antithyroid drugs to the mother with the aim of treating the fetus should be considered.[7, 13, 70, 96] Treatment of neonatal thyrotoxicosis is required for at least 3 to 4 weeks after birth.

## *Thyroid Storm*

Thyroid storm is a life-threatening exacerbation of thyrotoxicosis. It is rare but usually occurs during stressful events or in the untreated hyperthyroid patient. Precipitating factors include labor, cesarean section, and infection in pregnancy.[41] Thyroid storm must be treated immediately with antithyroid drugs, iodides, beta blockers, intravenous fluids, and steroids (to block the conversion of $T_4$ to $T_3$ and help decrease the hyperthermia).

## *Postpartum Thyrotoxicosis*

The development of postpartum thyrotoxicosis in a woman with a past history of Graves' disease that has been in remission for several months or years is usually the result of an exacerbation of the Graves' disease. On the other hand, when postpartum thyrotoxicosis arises in the absence of a previous history of thyroid dysfunction, postpartum painless thyroiditis must be considered. This transient type of thyrotoxicosis behaves similarly to subacute thyroiditis, but pain over the thyroid is absent (that is, it is a silent thyroiditis). Although the exact etiologic factor is unclear, postpartum thyroiditis appears to be caused by a subclinical variant of autoimmune thyroiditis that becomes activated after delivery by peripartum changes in the maternal immune system.[43, 98] Results of various surveys[3, 19, 94] revealed an incidence of 1 to 5.5 per cent. One wonders how many women with postpartum depression actually have postpartum painless thyroiditis.

Postpartum painless thyroiditis usually develops about 1 to 3 months after delivery and is characterized by the abrupt onset of thyrotoxicosis that may last 2 to 4 months followed by transient hypothyroidism that can last 2 to 4 months. In most instances, the patient becomes euthyroid without any specific treatment.[98] Postpartum painless thyroiditis tends to recur in subsequent pregnancies. Often, no specific therapy is required, but when symptoms arise, treatment with beta blockers or thyroid hormone may be needed in the hyperthyroid or hypothyroid phases, respectively. The use of antithyroid drugs should be avoided because of the transient nature of the thyrotoxicosis and the possibility of rapidly inducing hypothyroidism.[98]

Physical examination reveals a small nontender goiter in about 50 per cent of patients, and results of laboratory tests performed during the hyperthyroid phase show elevated serum levels of thyroid hormone and low thyroid uptake of radioactive iodine.[7, 36] The serum level of thyroid hormone is decreased, and serum thyroid-stimulating hormone is increased in the hypothyroid phase. As the gland begins to recover, thyroid uptake of radioactive iodine is elevated. Despite its similarities to subacute thyroiditis, the thyroid is not painful, fever is not present, and the sedimentation rate, leukocyte count, and antiviral titers are not elevated.[98] Often, a high titer of antimicrosomal antibodies may persist on long-term follow-up evaluation.[43] Needle biopsy of the thyroid during the hyperthyroid phase shows evidence of lymphocytic thyroiditis.[98]

When postpartum thyrotoxicosis develops, the most important step is to determine the type of thyrotoxicosis. A 24-hour radioactive iodine uptake test performed while the patient is hyperthyroid is the one test that distinguishes whether the thyrotoxicosis is the result of Graves' disease (elevated values on radioactive iodine uptake test) or postpartum painless thyroiditis (decreased or undetectable values on radioactive iodine uptake test). When Graves' disease is established, initial treatment should be with antithyroid drugs. On the other hand, when thyrotoxicosis results from painless thyroiditis, a conservative approach, such as observation alone or beta blockers, is the preferred form of treatment.

## *Hypothyroidism During Pregnancy*

The majority of women who are hypothyroid have great difficulty becoming pregnant because of a high rate of anovulation.[39] An increased frequency of spontaneous abortions, perinatal deaths, congenital anomalies, and depressed intellectual development has been reported in the offspring of hypothyroid women.[40, 52, 66] However, as noted by Montoro and colleagues,[74] the actual thyroid status of many of the mothers in the previously mentioned reports[40, 52, 66] was not entirely clear because results of free $T_4$ and thyroid-stimulating hormone assays were unavailable. Instead, the diagnosis of hypothyroidism was based on failure of protein-bound iodine or the butanol-extractable iodine to increase as expected during pregnancy.[74]

The well-documented cases of nine hypothyroid women who had a total of 11 pregnancies were described by Montoro and colleagues.[74] Seven of the nine patients first presented after the 24th week of gestation. The only patient with preeclampsia had one stillborn infant. Another infant had Down's syndrome, but the mother was 41 years old. The remaining nine infants were normal at birth. Although follow-up study of seven of these infants for up to 3 years showed normal thyroid function and central nervous system and somatic development, several more years of follow-up are needed to determine whether intellectual function remains normal.

The results of this report[74] are more consistent with the fact that development of the fetal hypothalamic-pituitary-thyroid axis is independent of the thyroid status of the mother because thyroid hormone does not cross the placenta. Any thyroid hormone necessary for fetal growth must come from the mother until about 12 weeks' gestation, but whether maternal thyroid hormone is necessary for fetal development is unclear.[74] Montoro and colleagues[74] concluded that when maternal hypothyroidism affects the fetus at all, it must do so indirectly in ways that have yet to be shown.

To diagnose hypothyroidism during pregnancy, results should be obtained for serum free $T_4$ and thyroid-stimulating hormone. Because pregnancy causes an increase in serum thyroxine-binding globulin, the serum total $T_4$ may be normal but probably will not be elevated. The serum free $T_4$ index is decreased in maternal hypothyroidism.

When a diagnosis of hypothyroidism is confirmed, the mother should be treated with thyroid hormone. Thyroid hormone does not harm the fetus because it does not cross the placenta.

Some pregnant patients have subclinical hypothyroidism, characterized by low to normal free $T_4$ and mildly elevated thyroid-stimulating hormone. It is probably best to consider treating these women with thyroid hormone because of the possibility that hypothyroidism can develop insidiously, which may have an adverse effect on the fetus.

## *Summary*

Thyroid dysfunction during pregnancy is common, and knowledge of which tests to order is essential for successful detection of hyperthyroidism and hypothyroidism. The elevated thyroxine-binding globulin that occurs during pregnancy can yield misleading results in thyroid function tests. The free $T_4$ provides an accurate assessment of maternal thyroid function. When hyperthyroidism is confirmed, the mother should be treated with one of the thionamides, preferably propylthiouracil, because it does not cross the placenta as well as methimazole. The lowest possible dose of propylthiouracil should be used to achieve a euthyroid state in the mother while avoiding the risk of fetal hypothyroidism. The neonate should be monitored closely for a few weeks after birth for the development of thyrotoxicosis. The ability to recognize and differentiate the types of postpartum thyrotoxicosis is essential to determine which patients require treatment.

## HYPERPARATHYROIDISM

The incidence of primary hyperparathyroidism in women of childbearing age is about eight cases per 100,000 population per year.[45] Primary hyperparathyroidism is diagnosed infrequently during pregnancy. About 73 cases of hyperparathyroidism associated with pregnancy have been reported to date, and its actual incidence during pregnancy is probably greater than that reported in the literature.[15, 17, 21, 22, 34, 38, 47, 57, 59, 62, 63, 77, 84, 92, 97] The discrepancy between the number of expected and the number of reported cases of hyperparathyroidism during pregnancy probably exists because many patients with hyperparathyroidism are asymptomatic, and the tendency is to report on only those patients in whom complications have developed.[17] Hyperparathyroidism remains undetected unless a complication develops, neonatal hypocalcemia occurs, or an elevated level of serum calcium is detected as part of a routine chemistry profile.

Primary hyperparathyroidism during pregnancy can be associated with serious maternal and neonatal complications and fetal loss.[17, 21, 63, 72, 84] A review of the literature[17, 21, 63, 72, 84] revealed a 45 to 80 per cent incidence of complications in pregnancies associated with maternal hyperparathyroidism. For this reason, many investigators[17, 21, 59] recommend parathyroidectomy after the first trimester of pregnancy in women with primary hyperparathyroidism.

### *Calcium Metabolism During Normal Pregnancy*

About 25 to 30 gm of calcium is transferred across the placenta from the mother to the fetus,[18, 32] thus providing the necessary amount of calcium needed for fetal skeletal formation. The majority of calcium is transferred to the fetus during the third trimester. The human placenta normally maintains the fetal levels of serum total and ionized calcium slightly greater than the corresponding levels in the mother.[21, 32, 93]

In addition to late loss of maternal calcium to the fetus, urinary excretion of calcium is sometimes increased in early pregnancy, probably because of the increase in the maternal glomerular filtration rate.[21, 55, 58] Calcium losses of this magnitude would lead to a negative maternal calcium balance were it not for the increased intestinal calcium absorption, which begins to occur as early as the second trimester.[21, 44]

As pregnancy progresses, the maternal serum level of total calcium decreases. This decrease is believed to result from physiologic hypoalbuminemia, increased extracellular fluid volume, and the transport of calcium to the fetus.[64] Maternal ionized calcium also decreases to the lower range of normal by about the 21st week of gestation and remains in this range until term.[17, 78, 90] As the level of maternal serum calcium decreases, the maternal immunoreactive parathyroid hormone level begins to increase at about the 20th week to the 25th week of gestation, and it remains elevated until term,[18, 78] resulting in an increase in intestinal calcium absorption and a decrease in urinary calcium loss. The elevation in maternal parathyroid hormone, which does not result in maternal hypercalcemia, has been referred to as "the physiologic hyperparathyroidism of pregnancy."[17, 18, 27]

The level of maternal serum calcitonin is increased during pregnancy.[27, 83] This increase may provide protection to the maternal skeleton during the latter half of pregnancy when the level of parathyroid hormone is elevated.[17, 27] Two groups of investigators[35, 54] showed that circulating calcitonin levels in the fetus exceeded those of the mother, a possible result of relative fetal hypercalcemia.[54] Hypercalcitoninemia in the fetus is believed to play an important role in fetal bone mineralization. Although calcium crosses the placenta, several investigators[35, 54, 79] showed that neither parathyroid hormone nor calcitonin crosses the placenta.

## Diagnosis

Primary hyperparathyroidism should be suspected in any pregnant woman with a history of renal calculi, osteopenia, recurrent peptic ulcer disease, pancreatitis, or routine levels of serum calcium greater than 10.5 mg/dl.[21] An unusual family history of these illnesses should also arouse suspicion because primary hyperparathyroidism is occasionally familial when associated with the multiple endocrine neoplasia syndromes.[21] A personal or family history of other components of the multiple endocrine neoplasia syndrome should also make the physician suspect the possible existence of primary hyperparathyroidism. A woman who has had an infant with neonatal hypocalcemia or seizures or who has a history of previous miscarriage should also be evaluated for hyperparathyroidism.[21]

The most reliable diagnostic method is the documentation of persistent hypercalcemia in the absence of any other apparent cause (that is, thyrotoxicosis, malignancy, or overdose of vitamin D or vitamin A, sarcoidosis, thiazide diuretics, or immobilization).[21] Detection of parathyroid hormone in the patient's blood despite continued hypercalcemia can provide important confirmatory evidence.[21] Hypercalcemia normally suppresses parathyroid hormone in the blood of chronically hypercalcemic patients, and therefore its presence is evidence of abnormal parathyroid function.[21] The use of parathyroid hormone levels alone may result in occasional diagnostic errors because of the adaptive hyperparathyroidism that occurs in normal pregnancy.[21]

## Maternal Hyperparathyroidism and Neonatal Hypocalcemia

Maternal primary hyperparathyroidism can be tolerated well by both mother and fetus and results in a normal delivery and neonatal period. However, maternal primary hyperparathyroidism can also be associated with spontaneous abortion, neonatal hypocalcemia and tetany, stillbirth, and maternal hypercalcemic crisis.[15, 17, 21, 62, 84] In 1962, Ludwig[63] reviewed the literature and found a complication rate of 50 per cent in 40 pregnancies in 21 mothers with primary hyperparathyroidism. Spontaneous abortion, stillbirth, and neonatal death accounted for 31 per cent, and neonatal tetany accounted for 19 per cent. A review of the literature[21] from 1962 to 1975 revealed an 80 per cent rate of fetal and neonatal complications during 15 pregnancies in 13 patients with primary hyperparathyroidism who were not treated surgically. Of the eight patients reported between 1947 and 1974 who underwent exploration of the neck during pregnancy, the complications were minimal and consisted of one episode of neonatal hypocalcemia and one spontaneous abortion that occurred in a woman 18 hours after emergency parathyroid surgery.[21]

Maternal hyperparathyroidism causes hypercalcemia, which facilitates increased placental transport of calcium and consequently abnormally high levels of serum calcium in the fetus.[17] This can suppress function of the fetal parathyroid gland.[32] At delivery, the baby is suddenly deprived of the maternal source of calcium and is unable to mobilize calcium from bone because of a low level of parathyroid hormone and an elevated level of calcitonin. This series of events can lead to acute neonatal hypocalcemia,[17, 32] and when it is untreated, tetany can result, usually at 5 to 14 days of age.[73] Low fetal levels of circulating parathyroid hormone and 1,25-dihydroxyvitamin D have been identified in the cord blood of these infants.[32, 54]

The actual incidence of neonatal tetany resulting from a hyperparathyroid pregnancy is difficult to determine. Some mothers are not identified as having primary hyperparathyroidism until tetany develops after birth in their infants.[21] This can yield a falsely elevated incidence of neonatal tetany. Neonatal hypocalcemia is believed to occur when severe hypercalcemia is present in the mother.[62] However, neonatal complications have been reported even in mothers with asymptomatic hyperparathyroidism.[84]

Hypocalcemia in an infant can usually be managed successfully by supplementary calcium and vitamin D in addition to dietary phosphate restriction. Transient hypoparathyroidism resolves within 3 to 5 months.[17, 84]

Maternal hyperparathyroidism can cause fetal and neonatal complications and hypercalcemic crisis in the mother. The mother is especially at risk in the immediate postpartum period when the maternal efflux of calcium to the fetus is suddenly discontinued. In some instances of primary hyperparathyroidism and pregnancy, the maternal complications were lowest in the third trimester.[21, 51, 64] Maternal levels of serum calcium have been shown to decrease in the third trimester in some instances of maternal hyperparathyroidism.[48, 64] Possibly, hypercalcemia is milder in advanced pregnancy because this is the period of most rapid fetal skeletal growth. Therefore, pregnancy could improve maternal hypercalcemia during the third trimester when the maternal calcium flux toward the fetus is large.[64]

## *Management of Hyperparathyroidism During Pregnancy*

Management of maternal primary hyperparathyroidism diagnosed during pregnancy should be individualized and is based on the patient's symptoms, severity of the disease, and gestational age of the fetus. Pregnancy should not be terminated because maternal hyperparathyroidism is discovered early in gestation.[17]

Mild primary hyperparathyroidism in which the level of serum calcium remains stable or can be controlled with orally administered phosphate therapy may be well tolerated by both mother and fetus throughout pregnancy.[62, 73] One report,[59] however, described nine pregnant women with asymptomatic hyperparathyroidism. Of these women, six who did not undergo neck exploration during pregnancy had a much higher incidence of complicated births (mostly neonatal tetany) than did the three women who underwent parathyroidectomy.

An extensive review of the literature[59] revealed a total of 73 reported cases of primary hyperparathyroidism in 102 pregnancies from 1930 to 1983. Of the 102 pregnancies, normocalcemia was achieved in 23 patients through parathyroidectomy during pregnancy, and the mothers remained hypercalcemic throughout a total of 79 pregnancies. The risk of complicated births (neonatal tetany, stillbirth, abortion) in the hypercalcemic group was 53 per cent versus 24 per cent in the patients who underwent surgery. Perinatal death occurred in 15 per cent of the offspring in the group of women who did not undergo operation and in 9 per cent of the offspring of the group who underwent operation.

To rule out the possibility that the difference in rates of complications between the two groups did not result from a general improvement in obstetric care, these investigators[59] compared the fetal complications in the two groups during the last 15 years of the study period (1968 to 1983). Thirty-two patients with primary hyperparathyroidism during pregnancy were reported on from 1968 to 1983; 17 patients underwent operation, and 15 were treated conservatively. Neonatal hypocalcemia and tetany occurred in the offspring of 29 per cent of the 17 patients who were operated on and in 73 per cent of the offspring of mothers who did not undergo operation.[59]

Thus, the significant risk of serious maternal, fetal, and neonatal complications has led most investigators[17, 21, 54, 59] to recommend parathyroidectomy after the first trimester of pregnancy. It is preferable to try to delay maternal parathyroid surgery until the second trimester because by the 16th week of gestation all fetal organs are fully developed and the risks of anesthesia and surgery are decreased.[59, 87] The danger of spontaneous abortion after general anesthesia appears to be minimal,[59, 86] although the danger of precipitating premature labor is increased during the third trimester. The most threatening risks of surgery for the mother are postoperative hemorrhage that results in airway obstruction and the potential development of hypoparathyroidism in the mother.[21] The general venous dilatation during pregnancy makes meticulous hemostasis imperative.[21] Postoperatively, maternal calcium must be monitored closely. Permanent maternal hypoparathyroidism must be treated because it can result in fetal hyperparathyroidism and cystic changes in bone.[5, 21]

When a pregnant woman has symptomatic hypercalcemia and surgery is medically contraindicated or the patient refuses surgery, orally administered phosphate therapy has proved to be a safe and effective therapeutic alternative to decrease serum calcium provided that renal failure is not present.[73] The recommended dose of phosphate is 1.5 to 2.5 gm of inorganic phosphorus a day administered in divided doses.[73]

## *Summary*

The management of patients with primary hyperparathyroidism during pregnancy must be individualized. In the majority of pregnant women, primary hyperparathyroidism remains undetected, and these women have uncomplicated pregnancies. When the hypercalcemia is mild and asymptomatic, the mother can be observed closely and treated with orally administered phosphates when necessary. The neonate must be monitored closely because of the risk of the development of hypocalcemia and tetany. Only women with greatly elevated serum levels of calcium whose disease does not respond to oral administration of phosphates should be operated on during pregnancy, preferably in the second trimester.

The surgical treatment of primary hyperparathyroidism should be recommended to any young woman who is contemplating pregnancy in the future.

## REFERENCES


1. Aboul-Khair, S. A., Crooks, J., Turnbull, A. C., and Hylten, F. E.: The physiological changes in thyroid function during pregnancy. Clin. Sci., *27:*195–207, 1964.
2. Amino, N., Tanizawa, O., Mori, H., et al.: Aggravation of thyrotoxicosis in early pregnancy and after delivery in Graves' disease. J. Clin. Endocrinol. Metab., *55:*108–112, 1982.
3. Amino, N., Mori, H., Iwatani, Y., et al.: High prevalence of transient post-partum thyrotoxicosis and hypothyroidism. N. Engl. J. Med., *306:*849–852, 1982.
4. Bachrach, L. K., and Burrow, G. N.: Aplasia cutis congenita and methimazole (Letter). Can. Med. Assoc. J., *130:*1264, 1984.
5. Bronsky, D., Kiamko, R. T., Moncada, R., and Rosenthal, I. M.: Intra-uterine hyperparathyroidism secondary to maternal hypoparathyroidism. Pediatrics, *42:*606–613, 1968.
6. Burrow, G. N.: Neonatal goiter after maternal propylthiouracil therapy. J. Clin. Endocrinol. Metab., *25:*403–408, 1965.
7. Burrow, G. N.: The management of thyrotoxicosis in pregnancy. N. Engl. J. Med., *313:*562–565, 1985.
8. Burrow, G. N., Klatskin, E. H., and Genel, M.: Intellectual development in children whose mothers received propylthiouracil during pregnancy. Yale J. Biol. Med., *51:*151–156, 1978.
9. Burrow, G. N., Palackwich, R., and Donabedian, R.: The hypothalamic-pituitary thyroid axis in normal pregnancy. *In* Fisher, D. A., and Burrow, G.N. (eds.): Perinatal Thyroid Physiology and Disease. New York, Raven Press, 1975, pp. 1–10.
10. Burrow, G. N., Bartsocas, C., Klatskin, E. H., and Grunt, J. A.: Children exposed in utero to propylthiouracil: Subsequent intellectual and physical development. Am. J. Dis. Child., *116:*161–165, 1968.
11. Burwell, C. S.: Circulatory adjustments to pregnancy. Bull. Johns Hopkins Hosp., *95:*115–129, 1954.
12. Carr, E. A., Jr., Bierwaltes, W. H., Raman, G., et al.: The effect of maternal thyroid function on fetal thyroid function and development. J. Clin. Endocrinol. Metab., *19:*1–18, 1959.
13. Check, J. H., Rezvani, I., Goodner, D., and Hooper, B.: Prenatal treatment of thyrotoxicosis to prevent intrauterine growth retardation. Obstet. Gynecol., *60:*122–124, 1982.
14. Cheron, R. G., Kaplan, M. M., Larsen, P. R., et al.: Neonatal thyroid function after propylthiouracil therapy for maternal Graves' disease. N. Engl. J. Med., *304:*525–528, 1981.
15. Clark, D., Seeds, J. W., and Cefalo, R. C.: Hyperparathyroid crisis and pregnancy. Am. J. Obstet. Gynecol., *140:*840–842, 1981.
16. Comite, F., Burrow, G. N., and Jorgensen, E. C.: Thyroid hormone analogs and fetal goiter. Endocrinology, *102:*1670–1674, 1978.
17. Croom, R. D., III, and Thomas, C. G.: Primary hyperparathyroidism during pregnancy. Surgery, *96:*1109–1118, 1984.
18. Cushard, W. G., Jr., Creditor, M. A., Canterbury, J. M., and Reiss, E.: Physiologic hyperparathyroidism in pregnancy. J. Clin. Endocrinol. Metab., *34:*767–771, 1972.
19. Dahlberg, P. A., and Jansson, R.: Different aetiologies in post-partum thyroiditis? Acta Endocrinol. (Copenh.), *104:*195–200, 1983.
20. Davies, T. F., and Weiss, I.: Autoimmune thyroid disease and pregnancy. Am. J. Reprod. Immunol. Microbiol., *1:*187–192, 1981.
21. Delmonico, F. L., Neer, R. M., Cosimi, A. B., et al.: Hyperparathyroidism during pregnancy. Am. J. Surg., *131:*328–337, 1976.
22. Deutsch, A. A., Zager, M., Berheim, J., et al.: The diagnosis and management of hyperparathyroidism during pregnancy. Postgrad. Med. J., *56:*333–335, 1980.
23. Dirmikis, S. M., and Munro, D. S.: Placental transmission of thyroid-stimulating immunoglobulins. Br. Med. J., *2:*665–666, 1975.
24. Dowling, J. T., Appleton, W. G., and Nicoloff, J. T.: Thyroxine turnover during human pregnancy. J. Clin. Endocrinol. Metab., *27:*1749–1750, 1967.
25. Dowling, J. T., Freinkel, N., and Ingbar, S. H.: Thyroxine-binding by sera of pregnant women, newborn infants, and women with spontaneous abortion. J. Clin. Invest., *35:*1263–1276, 1956.
26. Dozeman, R., Kaiser, F. E., Cass, O., and Pries, J.: Hyperthyroidism appearing as hyperemesis gravidarum. Arch. Intern. Med., *143:*2202–2203, 1983.

27. Drake, T. S., Kaplan, R. A., and Lewis, T. A.: The physiologic hyperparathyroidism of pregnancy: Is it primary or secondary? Obstet. Gynecol., *53:*746–749, 1979.
28. Dussault, J. H., Hobel, C. J., and Fisher, D. A.: Maternal and fetal thyroxine secretion during pregnancy in the sheep. Endocrinology, *88:*47–51, 1971.
29. Evans, T. C., Kretzschmer, R. M., Hodges, R. E., and Song, C. W.: Radioiodine uptake studies of the human fetal thyroid. J. Nucl. Med., *8:*157–165, 1967.
30. Fisher, D. A.: Thyroid function in the fetus. *In* Fisher, D. A., and Burrow, G. N. (eds.): Perinatal Thyroid Physiology and Disease. New York, Raven Press, 1975, pp. 21–29.
31. Fisher, D. A., and Klein, A. H.: Thyroid development and disorders of thyroid function in the newborn. N. Engl. J. Med., *304:*702–712, 1981.
32. Fleischman, A. R.: Fetal parathyroid gland and calcium homeostasis. Clin. Obstet. Gynecol., *23:*791–802, 1980.
33. Fraser, R., and Wilkinson, M.: Simplified method of drug treatment for thyrotoxicosis using uniform dosage of methylthiouracil and added thyroxine. Br. Med. J., *1:*481–484, 1953.
34. Friedrichsen, C.: Hypocalcämie bei einem Brustkind und Hypercalcämie bei der Mutter. Monatsschr. Kinderheilkd., *75:*146–149, 1938.
35. Garel, J. M., Care, A. D., and Barlet, J. P.: A radioimmunoassay for bovine calcitonin: An evaluation of calcitonin secretion during gestation, lactation, and fetal life. J. Endocrinol., *62:*497–509, 1974.
36. Ginsberg, J., and Walfish, P. G.: Post-partum transient thyrotoxicosis with painless thyroiditis. Lancet, *1:*1125–1128, 1977.
37. Gladstone, G. R., Hordaf, A., and Gersony, W. M.: Propranolol administration during pregnancy: Effects on the fetus. J. Pediatr., *86:*962–964, 1975.
38. Goldsmith, R. E., Zalme, E., and Weinstein, A. S.: Clinical experience with primary hyperparathyroidism: Evaluation of treatment. Acta Endocrinol. (Copenh.), *52:*221–238, 1966.
39. Goldsmith, R. E., Sturgis, S. H., Lerman, J., and Stanbury, J. B.: Menstrual pattern in thyroid disease. J. Clin. Endocrinol., *12:*846–855, 1952.
40. Greenman, G. W., Gabrielson, M. O., Howard-Flanders, J., and Wessel, M. A.: Thyroid dysfunction in pregnancy: Fetal loss and follow-up of surviving infants. N. Engl. J. Med., *267:*426–431, 1962.
41. Guenter, K. E., and Friedland, G. A.: Thyroid storm and placenta previa in a primigravida. Obstet. Gynecol., *26:*403–407, 1965.
42. Habib, A., and McCarthy, J. S.: Effects on the neonate of propranolol administered during pregnancy. J. Pediatr., *91:*808–811, 1977.
43. Hamburger, J. I., and Miller, J. M. (eds.): Controversies in Clinical Thyroidology. New York, Springer-Verlag, 1981, pp. 31–36.
44. Heaney, R. P., and Skillman, T. G.: Calcium metabolism in normal human pregnancy. J. Clin. Endocrinol. Metab., *33:*661–670, 1971.
45. Heath, H., 3d, Hodgson, S. F., and Kennedy, M. A.: Primary hyperparathyroidism: Incidence, morbidity, and potential economic impact in a community. N. Engl. J. Med., *302:*189–193, 1980.
46. Herbst, A. L., and Selenkow, H. A.: Combined antithyroid-thyroid therapy of hyperthyroidism in pregnancy. Obstet. Gynecol., *21:*543–550, 1963.
47. Hess, H. M., Dickson, J., and Fox, H. E.: Hyperfunctioning parathyroid carcinoma presenting as acute pancreatitis in pregnancy. J. Reprod. Med., *25:*83–87, 1980.
48. Hutchin, P., and Kessner, D. M.: Neonatal tetany: Diagnostic lead to hyperparathyroidism in the mother. Ann. Intern. Med., *61:*1109–1115, 1964.
49. Ingbar, S.: The thyroid gland. *In* Wilson, J. D., and Foster, D. W. (eds.): Williams Textbook of Endocrinology. 7th Edition. Philadelphia, W.B. Saunders Co., 1985, pp. 682–815.
50. Innerfield, F., and Hollander, C. S.: Thyroidal complications of pregnancy. Med. Clin. North Am., *61:*67–87, 1977.
51. Johnstone, R. E., 2d, Kreindler, T., and Johnstone, R.E.: Hyperparathyroidism during pregnancy. Obstet. Gynecol., *40:*580–585, 1972.
52. Jones, W. S., and Man, E. B.: Thyroid function in human pregnancy. VI. Premature deliveries and reproductive failures of pregnant women with low serum butanol-extractable iodines: Maternal serum TBG and TBPA capacities. Am. J. Obstet. Gynecol., *104:*909–914, 1969.
53. Kampmann, J. P., Johansen, K., Hansen, J. M., and Helweg, J.: Propylthiouracil in human milk: Revision of a dogma. Lancet, *1:*736–737, 1980.
54. Kaplan, E. L., Burrington, J. D., Klementschitsch, P., et al.: Primary hyperparathyroidism, pregnancy, and neonatal hypocalcemia. Surgery, *96:*717–722, 1984.
55. Kerr, C., Loken, H. F., Glendening, M. B., et al.: Calcium and phosphorus dynamics in pregnancy. Am. J. Obstet. Gynecol., *83:*2–8, 1962.
56. Keynes, G.: Obstetrics and gynaecology in relation to thyrotoxicosis and myasthenia gravis. J. Obstet. Gynecol., *59:*173–182, 1952.
57. Kirby, C. A., and Read, M. D.: Primary hyperparathyroidism in pregnancy. Aust N.Z. J. Obstet. Gynecol., *22:*121–122, 1982.
58. Knapp, E. L.: Studies on Urinary Excretion of Calcium. Doctoral thesis. Department of Chemistry, State University of Iowa, Iowa City, 1943.
59. Kristoffersson, A., Dahlgren, S., Lithner, F., and Jarhault, J.: Primary hyperparathyroidism in pregnancy. Surgery, *97:*326–330, 1985.
60. Lamberg, B. A., Ikonen, E., Österlund, K., et al.: Antithyroid treatment of maternal hyperthyroidism during lactation. Clin. Endocrinol., *21:*81–87, 1984.
61. Low, L. C., Lang, J., and Alexander, W. D.: Excretion of carbimazole and propylthiouracil in breast milk (Letter). Lancet, *2:*1011, 1979.
62. Lowe, D. K., Orwoll, E. S., McClung, M. R., et al.: Hyperparathyroidism and pregnancy. Am. J. Surg., *145:*611–614, 1983.
63. Ludwig, G.: Hyperparathyroidism in relation to pregnancy. N. Engl. J. Med., *267:*637–642, 1962.
64. Lueg, M. C., and Dawkins, W. E.: Primary hyperparathyroidism and pregnancy. South. Med. J., *76:*1389–1392, 1983.
65. Malkasian, G. D., and Mayberry, W. E.: Serum total and free thyroxine and thyrotropin in normal and pregnant women, neonates, and women receiving progestogens. Am. J. Obstet. Gynecol., *108:*1234–1238, 1970.

66. Man, E. B.: Maternal hypothyroxinemia: Development of 4- and 7-year-old offspring. *In* Fisher, D. A., and Burrow, G. N. (eds.): Perinatal Thyroid Physiology and Disease. New York, Raven Press, 1975, pp. 117–132.
67. Marchant, B., Brownlie, B. E. W., McKay, H. D., et al.: The placental transfer of propylthiouracil, methimazole and carbimazole. J. Clin. Endocrinol. Metab., *45:*1187–1193, 1977.
68. McKenzie, J. M.: Neonatal Graves' disease. J. Clin. Endocrinol. Metab., *24:*660–669, 1964.
68a. Mestman, J.: The thyroid in pregnancy. Emerg. Med., *14*:177–186, 1982.
69. Milham, S., and Elledge, W.: Maternal methimazole and congenital defects in children. Teratology, *5:*125, 1972.
70. Momotani, N., Noh, J., Oyanagi, H., et al.: Antithyroid drug therapy for Graves' disease during pregnancy: Optimal regimen for fetal thyroid status. N. Engl. J. Med., *315:*24–28, 1986.
71. Momotani, N., Ito, K., Hamada, N., et al.: Maternal hyperthyroidism and congenital malformation in the offspring. Clin. Endocrinol. (Oxf.), *20:*695–700, 1984.
72. Monteleone, J. A., Lee, J. B., Tashjian, A. H., Jr., and Cantor, H.: Transient neonatal hypocalcemia, hypomagnesemia, and high serum parathyroid hormone with maternal hyperparathyroidism. Ann. Intern. Med., *82:*670–672, 1975.
73. Montoro, M. N., Collea, J. V., and Mestman, J. H.: Management of hyperparathyroidism in pregnancy with oral phosphate therapy. Obstet. Gynecol., *55:*431–434, 1980.
74. Montoro, M., Collea, J. V., Frasier, S. D., and Mestman, J. H.: Successful outcome of pregnancy in women with hypothyroidism. Ann. Intern. Med., *94:*31–34, 1981.
75. Mujtaba, Q., and Burrow, G. N.: Treatment of hyperthyroidism in pregnancy with propylthiouracil and methimazole. Obstet. Gynecol., *46:*282–286, 1975.
76. Niswander, K. R., and Gordon, M.: The Women and Their Pregnancies. Philadelphia, W. B. Saunders Co., 1972.
77. Petit, D. W., and Clark, R. L., Jr.: Hyperparathyroidism and pregnancy. Am. J. Surg., *74:*860–866, 1947.
78. Pitkin, R. M., and Gebhardt, M. P.: Serum calcium concentrations in human pregnancy. Am. J. Obstet. Gynecol., *127:*775–778, 1977.
79. Pitkin, R. M., Reynolds, W. A., Williams, G. A., and Hargis, B. K.: Calcium metabolism in normal pregnancy: A longitudinal study. Am. J. Obstet. Gynecol., *133:*781–790, 1979.
79a. Pritchard, J., and MacDonald, P.: Williams Obstetrics. 15th Edition. New York, Appleton-Century-Crofts, Inc., 1976, p. 197.
80. Pruyn, S. C., Phelan, J. P., and Buchanan, G. C.: Long-term propranolol therapy in pregnancy: Maternal and fetal outcome. Am. J. Obstet. Gynecol., *135:*485–489, 1979.
81. Roti, E., Fang, S. L., Green, K., et al.: Human placenta is an active site of thyroxine and 3,3′,5-triiodothyronine tyrosol ring deiodination. J. Clin. Endocrinol. Metab., *53:*498–501, 1981.
82. Rubin, P. C.: Beta-blockers in pregnancy. N. Engl. J. Med., *305:*1323–1326, 1981.
83. Samaan, N. A., Anderson, G. D., and Adam-Mayne, M. E.: Immunoreactive calcitonin in the mother, neonate, child and adult. Am. J. Obstet. Gynecol., *121:*622–625, 1975.
84. Shangold, M. M., Dor, N., Welt, S. I., et al.: Hyperparathyroidism and pregnancy: A review. Obstet. Gynecol. Surv., *37:*217–228, 1982.
85. Shepard, T. H.: Onset of function in the human fetal thyroid: Biochemical and radioautographic studies from organ culture. J. Clin. Endocrinol. Metab., *27:*945–958, 1967.
86. Shnider, S. M., and Webster, G. M.: Maternal and fetal hazards of surgery during pregnancy. Am. J. Obstet. Gynecol., *92:*891–900, 1965.
87. Smith, B. E.: Teratology in anesthesia. Clin. Obstet. Gynecol., *17:*145–163, 1974.
88. Sridama, V., Pacini, F., Yang, S. L., et al.: Decreased levels of helper T cells: A possible cause of immunodeficiency in pregnancy. N. Engl. J. Med., *307:*352–356, 1982.
89. Stoffer, S. S., and Hamburger, J. I.: Inadvertent $^{131}I$ therapy for hyperthyroidism in the first trimester of pregnancy. J. Nucl. Med., *17:*146–149, 1976.
90. Tan, C. M., Raman, A., and Sinnathyray, T. A.: Serum ionic calcium levels during pregnancy. J. Obstet. Gynaecol., *79:*694–697, 1972.
91. Theodoropoulos, T., Braverman, L. E., and Vagenakis, A. G.: Iodide-induced hypothyroidism: A potential hazard during perinatal life. Science, *205:*502–503, 1979.
92. Thomason, J. L., Sampson, M. B., Farb, H. F., and Spellacy, W. N.: Pregnancy complicated by concurrent primary hyperparathyroidism and pancreatitis. Obstet. Gynecol., *57*(Suppl. 6): 34S–36S, 1981.
93. Tsang, R. C., Chen, I. W., Friedman, M. A., and Chen, I.: Neonatal parathyroid function: Role of gestational age and postnatal age. J. Pediatr., *83:*728–738, 1973.
94. Turney, S., Nikolai, T., and Roberts, R.: The prevalence and clinical course of postpartum lymphocytic thyroiditis. Abstract 557, 63rd Annual Meeting, American Endocrine Society, San Francisco, 1982.
95. van Dijke, C. P., Heydendael, R. J., and De Kleine, M. J.: Methimazole, carbimazole, and congenital skin defects. Ann. Intern. Med., *106:*60–61, 1987.
96. Volpé, R., Ehrlich, R., Steiner, G., and Row, V. V.: Graves' disease in pregnancy years after hypothyroidism with recurrent passive-transfer neonatal Graves' disease in offspring: Therapeutic considerations. Am. J. Med., *77:*572–578, 1984.
97. Wagner, G., Transbol, I., and Melchior, J. C.: Hyperparathyroidism and pregnancy. Acta Endocrinol. (Copenh.), *47:*549–564, 1964.
98. Walfish, P. G., and Chan, J. Y. C.: Post-partum hyperthyroidism. Clin. Endocrinol. Metab., *14:*417–447, 1985.
99. Wolf, J.: Iodide goiter and pharmacologic effects of excess iodine. Am. J. Med., *47:*101, 1969.
100. Zakarija, M., and McKenzie, J. M.: Pregnancy-associated changes in the thyroid-stimulating antibody of Graves' disease and the relationship to neonatal hyperthyroidism. J. Clin. Endocrinol. Metab., *57:*1036–1040, 1983.

# 31

# SURGICAL COMPLICATIONS AND THEIR MANAGEMENT

*Laura E. Sanders, M.D., Ricardo L. Rossi, M.D., and Blake Cady, M.D.*

Postoperative complications may be as unimportant as edema of the flap or as dangerous and life-threatening as hemorrhage or respiratory obstruction. Today, fortunately, because of better preoperative preparation, postoperative complications are few. Most are preventable. The proper management of the patient with a thyroid disorder and the surgical technique of thyroidectomy as described previously keep complications at a minimum. With proper preoperative management, the patient will be euthyroid at the time of operation. When the patient is hyperthyroid, thyroid storm may occur; when the patient is hypothyroid, laryngeal edema may result, producing respiratory obstruction. Careless technique may result in hemorrhage, recurrent laryngeal or superior laryngeal nerve paralysis, or both, causing respiratory embarrassment. Lack of experience or of attention to technical details may result in removal of too little or too much thyroid tissue or possibly all parathyroid glands, resulting in hypothyroidism, recurrent hyperthyroidism, or parathyroid deficiency. Postoperative complications are related to the wound, hemorrhage, respiratory difficulties, nerve paralysis, recurrent hyperthyroidism or hypothyroidism, or parathyroid deficiency.

## POSTOPERATIVE MORTALITY

Death has become an extremely rare complication of thyroid or parathyroid surgery. Before Lister introduced antisepsis and Kocher refined the technique of thyroidectomy in the late 19th century, thyroidectomy was infrequently performed, and a 40 per cent mortality rate was reported. Today, postoperative deaths are far below 1 per cent. At the Lahey Clinic,[8] in a series of 309 patients undergoing thyroidectomy for differentiated carcinoma, only one death, which occurred in the 1960s, was from a cardiovascular cause 1 week after operation.

## WOUND COMPLICATIONS

Wound complications include edema of the flap, accumulation of serum, hematoma, or infection. Edema of the flap is secondary to trauma and division of the prethyroid muscles. It occurs most often after thyroidectomy for chronic thyroiditis. Accumulation of serum or blood usually occurs on the fourth or fifth day after operation and is evident by fluctuant swelling; it may be relieved by aspiration or opening the wound edges and evacuating a clot when the hematoma is not liquid. Frank infection is unusual[6] except when associated with tracheostomy. When surrounding cellulitis occurs, heat, drainage, and antibiotics are indicated.

## HEMORRHAGE

The most serious complication of thyroid surgery is postoperative hemorrhage. The danger from this is tracheal compression. All patients having thyroid or parathyroid operations should be observed closely in the recovery room for 3 or 4 hours because the majority of significant hemorrhages with tracheal compression occur within this period. When unusual bleeding has occurred or when dissection was extensive, an overnight stay in the recovery room may be considered. Any symptoms of stridor or hypoxia, distention, or bulging of skin flaps should indicate prompt return to the operating room where evacuation of the hematoma can be performed. In truly emergency situations, skin clips are removed in the recovery room with prompt evacuation of clot, and, if necessary, emergency tracheostomy or endotracheal intubation is performed before transfer to the operating room. In the unusual situation of accumulation of hematoma with no respiratory compromise of any kind, evacuation can be performed without accompanying tracheostomy at reexploration.

Hemorrhage may be immediate or delayed. Immediate hemorrhage is the more serious and must be recognized early. It frequently occurs during the postanesthetic period when the endotracheal tube is removed. Its origin may be arterial or venous, such as from a tear in a large vein. The patient may cough or vomit, producing increased venous pressure, which permits insecure sutures to dislodge or insignificant vessels to bleed profusely. The surgeon or the assistant must remain with the patient until the endotracheal tube is removed and the patient is breathing quietly. Smooth extubation without coughing should be the goal of good anesthesia.

Profuse hemorrhage may also occur during the several hours after surgery. It becomes apparent from swelling of the neck and from stridor. Blood accumulates beneath the prethyroid muscles, producing pressure on the trachea with subsequent respiratory obstruction. The wound can be opened immediately to release the blood and to permit adequate respiratory exchange. An endotracheal tube may be inserted immediately and the patient returned to the operating room when respiratory embarrassment is present. With the patient under anesthesia, the wound is carefully explored and irrigated, and hemostasis is ensured. When considerable edema is present or vocal cord paralysis has occurred, tracheostomy should also be performed.

Delayed bleeding may occur 2 or 3 days after operation and is usually the result of oozing from small veins. The neck will appear swollen, and the patient may complain of tightness in the neck. Usually, respiratory difficulty is not evident. Serum and liquid whole blood may be aspirated, but clots should be evacuated through an opening in the incision.

The potential disasters that may arise from such post-thyroidectomy hemorrhage can almost be eliminated by meticulous attention to hemostasis at operation, careful monitoring in the recovery room, appreciation of the subtle signs of respiratory distress and hypoxia (restlessness and mild degree of stridor), willingness to admit that complications occur, and return of the patient to the operating room promptly when necessary. Two further technical features useful in evaluating and managing patients after thyroid and parathyroid operations are the omission of drains and dressings. The presence of drains tends to decrease the concern of the recovery room and surgical teams about hemorrhage and hematoma; their absence heightens concern about the patient's status and thus leads to earlier willingness to reexplore the operative area as well as to stimulate a more thorough attention to hemostasis by the surgeon. Frequently, a clot forms and prevents egress of blood from the drains. Most patients returned to the operating room for hemorrhage have had drains in place. When concerns arise about the completeness of operative hemostasis, we use medium Hemovac suction catheters or the smallest Jackson-Pratt drain brought out through the ends of the collar incision and placed beneath the muscles and into the deep compartment of the neck. Our usual policy, however, is to avoid use of any drains and to observe the patient closely in the recovery room.

The second technical modification is to avoid all dressings so that the incision and the contour of the neck may be inspected and evaluated quickly, closely, and repeatedly. We have not used dressings for many years, and during this time no wound infections have been encountered. Indeed, it has been demonstrated conclusively that wound infections originate not from the incision after sutures or clips have been placed but from the nasopharynx or the skin of the operating team or circulating bacteria of the patient while the wound is open. The absence of dressings has major advantages and no theoretic or practical disadvantages despite the enormous weight of custom and bias among surgeons, nurses, and patients. Of course, the absence of dressings is only practical in the absence of drains—another reason for the elimination of drains.

## RESPIRATORY OBSTRUCTION

Respiratory obstruction may result from hemorrhage, as described earlier, and from edema to the larynx and vocal cord paralysis. Edema of the larynx, vocal cords, and uvula, producing an inadequate airway, is most frequently seen in patients with severe or untreated hypothyroidism, particularly secondary to chronic thyroiditis, or in patients who have been overprepared with antithyroid drugs. A clue to laryngeal edema may be seen by the anesthesiologist at the time of intubation. It must be emphasized that the margin of safety permitting an adequate airway is not great. The patient may have an adequate exchange with a relatively small aperture between the edematous vocal cords. A slight increase of edema may produce sudden obstruction. A tracheostomy must be performed or preferably an endotracheal tube placed at the slightest indication of respiratory embarrassment. On occasion, a patient will be anxious and nervous and will complain of difficulty in breathing with no evidence of stridor. Steam inhalation and sedation may be all that is necessary. A patient with cardiac disease may not tolerate respiratory embarrassment.

## THORACIC DUCT FISTULA

A thoracic duct fistula occurred in one of the 309 patients in the Lahey Clinic series.[8] When the thoracic duct is damaged during operation, it should be identified and ligated. A chylous leak, which is noticed after operation and does not seal within 48 to 72 hours, may respond to a trial of discontinuing drainage and a pressure dressing. Occasionally, the patient must be returned to the operating room so that the leaking duct can be identified and ligated.[1]

## NERVE INJURY

Injury to the superior laryngeal nerve is not as devastating to the voice as an injury to the recurrent laryngeal nerve. However, it interferes with the standing tension of the vocal cord, which can cause a fatigued voice. While the difference may be subtle, the alteration in timbre can create difficulty for the patient who sings or speaks in public professionally. The vocal cords appear normal at rest but on phonation become asymmetric as the paralyzed side remains shorter and less tense. Bilateral superior laryngeal nerve paralysis is infrequent and produces a weak, breathy, low-pitched voice. When the sensory branch of the superior laryngeal nerve is injured, aspiration may occur secondary to anesthesia of the larynx. The superior laryngeal nerve is likely to be injured during mobilization of the upper thyroid as it accompanies the superior thyroid artery. The nerve, sometimes running within the constrictor muscle at that level,[7] cannot always be identified. However, ligation of the superior thyroid vessels individually under direct vision and as close to their entrance into the thyroid gland by passing instruments from medial to lateral while protecting the recurrent laryngeal nerve as well minimizes risk of injury. Patients with isolated superior laryngeal nerve palsy can usually compensate well enough not to need treatment. The incidence of superior and recurrent laryngeal nerve damage was the same (0.3 per cent) in the last Lahey Clinic series.[8]

Damage to the recurrent laryngeal nerve is a more serious complication because it causes vocal cord paralysis. The ipsilateral vocal cord is fixed in a paramedian position. The patient cannot close the glottis completely to speak or cough. The voice is weak and breathy.

The vocal cords should be evaluated before operation in patients being reoperated on and in patients with voice changes or other signs of vocal cord disease. This will document whether the vocal cord palsy that occurs after operation is old or new. Routine preoperative vocal cord evaluation is not required when the voice is normal and a strong cough can be generated.

The recurrent laryngeal nerve should routinely be identified during thyroidectomy or parathyroidectomy. Ligation of the inferior thyroid artery or its branches where the nerve may be intertwined should be avoided altogether. When the recurrent laryngeal nerve is routinely seen and dissected out from the level of the lower pole of the thyroid up to its entrance into the larynx, nerve injury should be rare. No structures in the area lateral to the thyroid should be ligated until the surgeon is completely confident of the visualization of the nerve. Traction on the nerve combined with endotracheal tube trauma can produce transient postoperative hoarseness, although this condition should resolve in a few days to a week.

Bilateral recurrent laryngeal nerve paralysis is dangerous because it may lead to respiratory obstruction. Both vocal cords are paralyzed in slight abduction so the patient may, paradoxically, have a relatively normal voice but be unable to cough. The airway is severely compromised, however, and the patient will have some stridor and is in danger of respiratory obstruction. Damage to both the superior and the recurrent laryngeal nerve causes a distorted larynx with the cricoid cartilage rotated under the thyroid with a shortened paralyzed vocal cord on that side.[2] This complication of thyroid or parathyroid surgery is unusual and occurs more often with other types of head and neck surgery.

Treatment of the injured recurrent laryngeal nerve has evolved in the last few years. The most pressing problem is maintenance and protection of the airway. Bilateral vocal cord paralysis will require tracheostomy to establish a stable airway. A tracheostomy may also be required for unilateral paralysis, especially when laryngeal edema from hypothyroidism or endotracheal tube trauma is present. When a tracheostomy tube has been placed for unilateral paralysis, it may be plugged when postoperative edema has subsided in a few days. In most patients with unilateral cord paralysis, the tracheostomy tube can be removed within 1 or 2 weeks when respiratory stridor is not present.

When the recurrent laryngeal nerve is transected during operation, immediate direct repair of the nerve can be performed, but results have not been good. Only occasional slight mass movement of the vocal cord has been achieved and no return of sophisticated function. A number of new techniques, however, have been used in recent years. Holl-Allen[5] explored paralyzed nerves in 26 patients and noted some return of nerve function when sutures on an intact nerve could be removed or when surrounding fibrosis was present and neurolysis could be performed. The nerve should be explored as soon as possible after palsy is noted. Holl-Allen[5] had much less success if this procedure were performed more than 6 months after the initial operation.

When nerve paralysis is not the result of a correctable lesion, such as a suture, the presumed neurapraxia may resolve over a few months. For permanent unilateral vocal cord paralysis, Teflon injection of the paralyzed vocal cord can be performed to stiffen it and to hold it closer to the midline. This permits the undamaged cord to adduct against the stiff injected cord, partially restoring the voice. Temporary injections can be given in a similar manner with glycerine.[1]

Several attempts have been made at reinnervating the larynx, the best known of which is Tucker's nerve-muscle flap from the sternohyoid implanted into the larynx. None of these procedures have achieved the general acceptance or success of Teflon injection.[2]

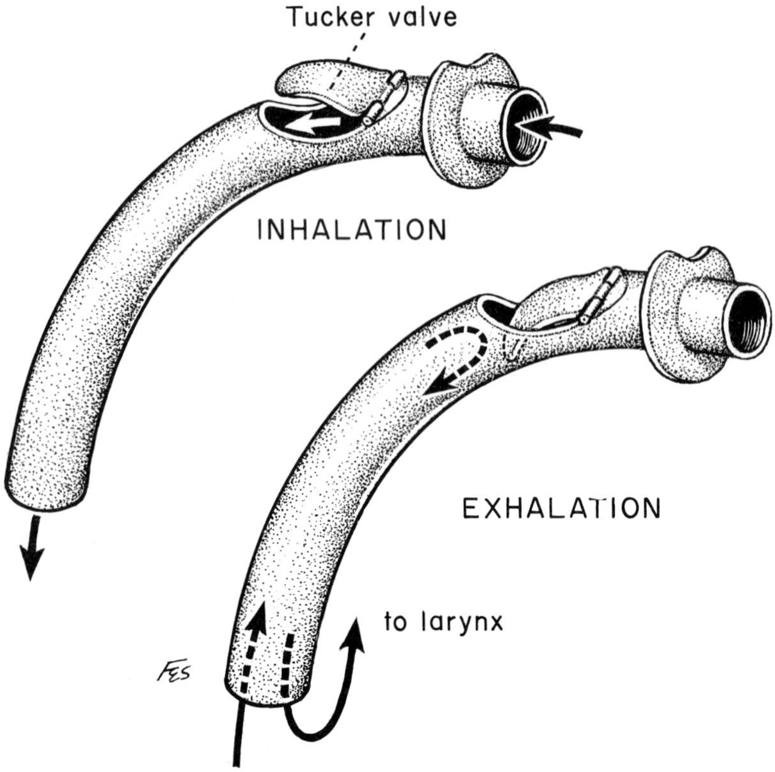


**FIGURE 31–1.** Tracheostomy tube modified to permit one-way airflow.

Several otolaryngologic procedures have been developed to correct bilateral vocal cord paralysis. Often, however, patients will require a permanent valved tracheostomy that permits them to breathe easily and speak clearly (Tucker valve*; Figs. 31–1 and 31–2). Fortunately, this complication is extremely unusual. In the last Lahey Clinic series[8] of more than 300 thyroid operations, only one instance of transient and one of permanent recurrent laryngeal nerve paralysis occurred, and no instance of bilateral laryngeal nerve paralysis was encountered.

## HYPOPARATHYROIDISM

Hypoparathyroidism is related to removal and devascularization of the parathyroid glands. The incidence of this complication rises when previous operations have been performed and with more extensive surgery, such as total thyroidectomy. Subtotal thyroidectomy rather than total thyroidectomy has been associated with a much lower incidence of hypoparathyroidism.[8]

During thyroidectomy, the parathyroid glands can be removed inadvertently with the thyroid or they may be devascularized during removal of the thyroid. Careful preservation of the inferior thyroid artery and its branches will preserve the blood supply of the parathyroid glands. Meticulous dissection of the parathyroid glands is critical when total thyroidectomy is performed. Sometimes after removal of the thyroid, the surgeon may note that the parathyroid gland has been removed inadvertently or is contained within the specimen. The tissue should be confirmed histologically as being parathyroid, cut into minute fragments, and inserted into an adjacent muscle pocket that can be closed with a suture to avoid displacement.[3, 4]

After parathyroid surgery, hypoparathyroidism can result from a metabolic or an anatomic cause. Prolonged hypercalcemia from a parathyroid adenoma can cause

*Tucker valve is obtained from the Pilling Company, 420 Delaware Drive, Ft. Washington, PA 19034.

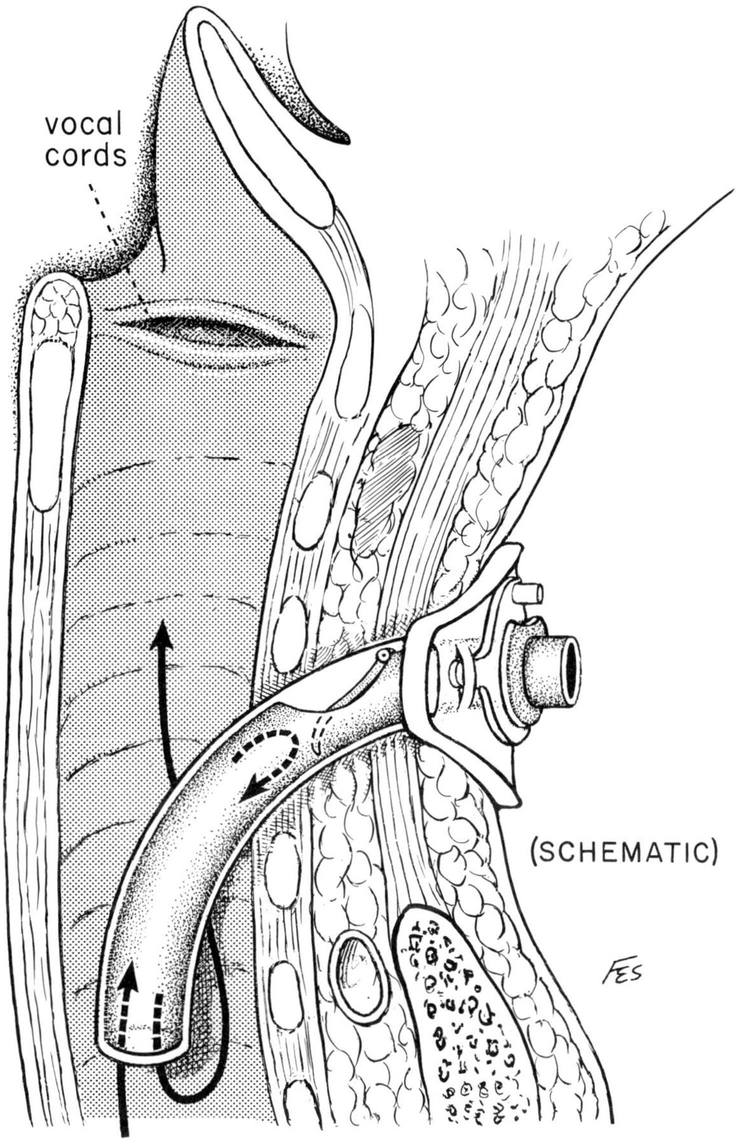


**FIGURE 31–2.** Placement of the one-way valve in the trachea.

suppression of the remaining glands, resulting in transient hypoparathyroidism until the suppressed glands resume function. "Hungry bone syndrome," a separate entity, results from the rapid deposition of calcium in bones in which calcium has been leached while the patient had hyperparathyroidism. In transient hypoparathyroidism, the level of calcium will be low and the level of phosphorus will be high, whereas with "bone hunger," the level of phosphorus will be low as well.[9]

Hypoparathyroidism can also result from overzealous biopsy of normal glands during exploration for hyperparathyroidism as the surgeon attempts to rule out hyperplasia. In the treatment of primary parathyroid hyperplasia or for secondary or tertiary hyperparathyroidism resulting from renal failure, the usual practice is to remove 3½ glands. The safest technique is to remove two glands and then two half glands. After observation for 10 minutes or so the final half gland can be excised. This obviates the discouraging finding of devascularization of the only remaining one half gland. The residual portion of gland is preferably left in situ but may be autotransplanted into muscle. The technique of autotransplantation in the forearm has been described by Wells and associates[10] in detail. The parathyroid specimen to be transplanted is kept on ice while the arm site is prepared. An incision is made over the antecubital fossa, and several muscle pockets are created in each of which is planted a thin slice (1 mm maximum) of parathyroid gland. Each site is closed with a suture of black silk and marked with a small metallic clip for easy relocation should recurrent hyperparathyroidism develop. Some parathyroid tissue should also be cryopreserved where it can be kept for up to 18 months in the event the first graft fails.[10]

The patient's calcium, phosphorus, and albumin levels should be checked at least daily after bilateral thyroidectomy or parathyroidectomy. The nadir of hypocalcemia usually occurs 48 to 72 hours after operation but occasionally may be later. The patient may have subjective symptoms of circumoral or toe and finger paresthesias. Chvostek's sign should be elicited, keeping in mind that the result is positive in 10 per cent of normal persons. Chvostek's sign is most readily demonstrated by tapping the patient in the preauricular area and observing the lip twitching. Trousseau's sign, elicited by inflating the blood pressure cuff between the venous and arterial pressure and checking for carpopedal spasm, is less sensitive and more disagreeable to the patient. Carpopedal spasm, laryngeal spasm, and seizures can complicate severe hypocalcemia.

For tetany or other severe symptoms, the patient is given calcium gluconate, 1 ampule, over 5 to 10 minutes. For moderate symptoms or for a calcium less than 7 mg/dl, an intravenous drip may be mixed of calcium gluconate, 4 ampules, and dextrose in water, 250 ml, given over 4 to 8 hours. This infusion is repeated if necessary, titrating to signs and symptoms and the level of serum calcium, which is rechecked at frequent intervals. The patient is given an oral calcium, which may also be used for treatment of mild symptoms. Oral calcium carbonate, which is 40 per cent elemental calcium, is used in a dose that provides 2 gm of elemental calcium daily. When the patient is still hypocalcemic after several days of taking calcium supplements, the administration of rocaltrol (the active form of vitamin D) may be started at 0.25 mg twice daily. The dose can be increased if needed on an outpatient basis, but the vitamin D should not be given if prompt return of parathyroid function is anticipated.

## LATE COMPLICATIONS

Later complications are usually minor but include wound hematoma or seroma, which can be handled by simple aspiration; wound infection, which is rare and treated by drainage; and hypothyroidism or recurrent hyperthyroidism in Graves' disease. Over the years, we have tended to preserve between 6 and 8 gm of thyroid tissue in operations for Graves' disease. The incidence of hypothyroidism in such patients is low, as is the incidence of recurrent hyperthyroidism. Recently, we have left between 8 and 10 gm of thyroid tissue in an attempt to reduce the rate of hypothyroidism without generating recurrent hyperthyroidism. Hypothyroidism requires only oral medication for treatment, but recurrent hyperthyroidism usually requires further operation because the reasons for avoiding use of radioactive iodine still exist. Thus, any bias in surgical resection in Graves' disease should be toward preventing recurrence.

Hypothyroidism may occur after significant resection of the thyroid gland and perhaps should not be considered a complication. When subtotal thyroidectomy is performed for multiple colloid adenomatous goiter owing to its size, symptoms, or unattractive appearance or for thyroiditis, these patients almost certainly will require thyroid hormone therapy because their residual thyroid gland may well be incompetent. Alertness for hypothyroidism should be maintained throughout the life of the patient because it may develop many years later.

## REFERENCES

1. Caldarelli, D. D., and Hollinger, L. D.: Complications and sequelae of thyroid surgery. Otolaryngol. Clin. North Am., *13*:85–97, 1980.
2. Croft, C. B., McKelvie, P., Fairley, J. W., et al.: Treatment of paralysis of the vocal cords: A review. J. R. Soc. Med., *79*:473–475, 1986.
3. Falk, S. A., Birken, E. A., and Baran, D. T.: Temporary postthyroidectomy hypocalcemia.

Arch. Otolaryngol. Head Neck Surg., *114*:168–174, 1988.
4. Freeman, J. L., Dindzans, L. J., and Noyek, A. M.: Management of the parathyroids in surgery for advanced malignancy of the larynx and hypopharynx. J. Otolaryngol., *14*:387–390, 1985.
5. Holl-Allen, R. T.: A new approach to the surgical management of paralysis of the laryngeal nerve after thyroidectomy. Surg. Gynecol. Obstet., *163*:543–546, 1986.
6. Johnson, J. T., and Wagner, R. L.: Infection following uncontaminated head and neck surgery. Arch. Otolaryngol. Head Neck Surg., *113*:368–369, 1987.
7. Lennquist, S., Cahlin, C., and Smeds, S.: The superior laryngeal nerve in thyroid surgery. Surgery, *102*:999–1008, 1987.
8. Rossi, R. L., Cady, B., Silverman, M. L., et al.: Current results of conservative surgery for differentiated thyroid carcinoma. World J. Surg., *10*:612–622, 1986.
9. Tiegs, R. D.: Postoperative hypocalcemia—treatment. *In* van Heerden, J. A. (ed.): Common Problems in Endocrine Surgery. Chicago, Year Book Medical Publishers, Inc., 1989, pp. 201–204.
10. Wells, S. A., Jr., Ross, A. J., 3d, Dale, J. K., and Gray, R. S.: Transplantation of the parathyroid glands: Current status. Surg. Clin. North Am., *59*:167–177, 1979.

# Commentary

*Joseph N. Attie, M.D.*

## HEMORRHAGE

Although serous collections and hematomas are sometimes seen after thyroidectomy, hemorrhage necessitating intervention is a rare complication today. Collections of serum or blood that develop over a period of days usually do not cause respiratory embarrassment. Although such seromas and hematomas would eventually be absorbed, they may become infected and are best controlled by repeated aspiration using a No. 20 or No. 18 gauge needle.

Uncontrolled bleeding within the wound causes rapid swelling, usually immediately after operation or within a few hours, and may result in respiratory distress. In such instances, the patient should undergo reintubation and be taken to the operating room where the wound is reopened and examined for a source of bleeding, which is usually arterial in nature. The bleeding vessel or vessels must be clamped and ligated, smaller bleeders controlled with the electrocautery, and the wound closed. Unless an accompanying narrowing of the glottis is the result of edema or accidental injury to the recurrent laryngeal nerve, tracheostomy is rarely needed.

Certain conditions increase the risk of postoperative hemorrhage. The thyroid gland in Graves' disease and in some patients with Hashimoto's thyroiditis is often friable and brittle, and the tissue is hard to compress with clamps or to tie. The cut surfaces of such glands are vascular, and the bleeding is not controlled by the electrocautery. Figure-of-eight or mattress sutures of 2-0 chromic catgut will effectively control the bleeding surface. Suturing of the oozing thyroid stump to the perichondrium of the trachea gives excellent hemostasis. Carcinoma invading the trachea, cricoid, thyroid cartilage, or the membranes between them requires partial resection of these structures, which may be vascular.

Surgery for patients with substernal goiter carries a greater risk of hemorrhage. Large glands in the mediastinum may cause the superior vena cava syndrome with engorgement of the cervical veins and severe congestion of all the tissues. Until the gland is delivered from the chest and the venous compression relieved, bleeding is increased throughout the dissection. The inferior and lateral thyroid veins may be torn during delivery of the gland from the mediastinum, and laceration of the innominate veins may occur. At times, a friable substernal thyroid gland may rupture during delivery, resulting in brisk bleeding. Postoperative bleeding from such torn mediastinal vessels may result in a substernal hematoma, which can be difficult to detect.

Technical points to avoid hemorrhage include meticulous attention to hemostasis during the procedure, avoidance of mass ligatures that include thyroid tissue with major vessels, ligation in continuity before cutting a vessel rather than the clamp-cut-tie technique, and the use of drains when oozing cannot be controlled adequately. Occasionally, the bleeding results from abnormal clotting factor deficiencies in the patient.

## INJURY TO RECURRENT LARYNGEAL NERVES

The two recurrent laryngeal nerves have different courses and anatomic relationships and have different risks of injury. The right recurrent laryngeal nerve arises from the vagus low in the neck, passes around the innominate artery, and ascends in the tracheoesophageal groove. It, therefore, has a more lateral course than the left nerve and is more susceptible to injury. The left recurrent laryngeal nerve arises from the vagus in the chest, passing behind the aorta at the point of attachment of the ligamentum arteriosum. Idiopathic paralysis of the left recurrent laryngeal nerve is sometimes seen because of inflammation or scarring of mediastinal nodes.

When one cord is paralyzed, the patient may or may not exhibit hoarseness. This emphasizes the importance of routine preoperative examination of the vocal cords before thyroidectomy. When idiopathic paralysis of the left vocal cord is apparent in adduction and only a right hemithyroidectomy is performed with injury to the right recurrent laryngeal nerve, bilateral paralysis with respiratory obstruction may ensue.

Bilateral paralysis of the vocal cords caused by bilateral nerve injury during thyroidectomy usually (but not invariably) results in respiratory obstruction manifested by stridor, usually requiring tracheostomy. Respiratory distress may not be manifested immediately; sometimes it may occur after several days. Immediate examination of the vocal cords on extubation by the anesthesiologist may not be a reliable evaluation of the mobility or ultimate position of the vocal cords. In rare instances, the patient may function adequately without respiratory difficulty for months or years despite bilateral nerve injury. An acute respiratory infection or superimposed laryngeal edema will precipitate acute respiratory obstruction.

The relationship of the recurrent laryngeal nerves and inferior thyroid arteries is variable, up to 60 different variations having been described. Arterial branching is variable, and the nerve on one or both sides may pass anterior, posterior, or between the branches of the artery. The nerve lies between arterial branches in 50 per cent, behind the artery in 25 per cent, and in front of the artery in 25 per cent of patients. In instances in which the nerve is anterior to the artery, delivery of the lobe into the wound during thyroidectomy may stretch the nerve.

Temporary or permanent damage to the nerve may result from stretching, pinching, clamping, or actual division. Stripping the nerve from surrounding structures may destroy its blood supply and cause loss of function. Occasionally, none of these conditions exist, and neurapraxia is temporary or permanent. A rare cause of trauma has been described in which the nerve is compressed between the arytenoid and cricoid by the pressure of the endotracheal tube used to administer anesthesia. Finally, respiratory obstruction may be the result of edema of the cords or compression of the trachea by collapse of the tracheal rings (tracheomalacia) or by extrinsic pressure on the trachea by hematoma.

On the right side, the nerve may be anomalous and "nonrecurrent" because of absence of an innominate artery on that side. I have encountered this anomaly in 12 patients. Failure to recognize this anomaly may result in nerve injury.

When the nerve is stretched over a large goiter, delivery of the gland may result in injury to the nerve, and separation of the nerve from such a gland may be extremely difficult. Rarely, pressure on the nerve—especially in the presence of a large substernal goiter—even though it is benign, may result in paralysis. Delivery of a large substernal thyroid from the mediastinum is especially hazardous to the nerve.

The recurrent laryngeal nerve may pass through a carcinoma of the thyroid and yet not show clinical dysfunction. Such nerves often have to be sacrificed. Patients should be alerted to the possibility that an apparently functioning nerve may be involved by carcinoma.

The recurrent laryngeal nerves may enter the larynx as single trunks or divide into two (usually) or more (up to 12) branches before passing through the cricothyroid membrane. Visualizing a small nerve should make the surgeon suspect that it may only be one of several branches. The branches do not necessarily have different functions (abduction, adduction). Most often the branches contain mixed fibers. Consequently, the type of paralysis (abductor, adductor) cannot be predicted on the basis of the branch injured.

The recurrent laryngeal nerve occasionally passes through the capsule of the thyroid gland, and in rare instances the nerve passes through the ligament of Berry. In my experience with more than 5,000 thyroidectomies, I have not encountered a single instance in which the nerve goes through either of these two structures but always lateral to the ligament. By dissecting the nerve away by blunt dissection, it is always possible to divide the ligament of Berry with no risk to the nerve.

## INJURY TO SUPERIOR LARYNGEAL NERVE

The external branch of the superior laryngeal nerve supplies the cricothyroid muscle. Injury to the nerve changes the timbre of the voice, weakens it, and at times lowers the pitch—a change that is devastating to singers (the soprano Amelia Galli-Curci was forced to give up a career in opera). The nerve passes from the vagus in close proximity to the superior thyroid vessels to enter the muscle laterally. In 17 per cent of patients, the nerve runs between branches of the superior arteries. The vessels must be ligated individually rather than as mass ligatures, preferably low on the superior pole of the thyroid, to avoid injury to the nerve. Injury to the internal laryngeal nerve, which is sensory, causes difficulty in swallowing, especially liquids.

## HYPOPARATHYROIDISM

When two or more of the parathyroid glands are removed during thyroidectomy or their blood supply is interfered with, hypoparathyroidism may result. Most persons have four parathyroid glands; 3 to 4 per cent of patients have five glands. In nearly all patients, both the superior and inferior parathyroid glands obtain their blood supply from the inferior thyroid arteries. Occasionally, the superior parathyroid gland will get its blood supply from the superior thyroid artery. In instances in which the inferior parathyroid gland lies within the thymus, it may obtain an independent blood supply from the internal mammary artery. In most subjects, however, the previous common practice of ligating the inferior thyroid arteries laterally to control bleeding will destroy the blood supply to both parathyroid glands on that side. The reason for the low incidence of hypothyroidism in the early years is that the parathyroid glands were left attached to large thyroid remnants and received their collateral blood supply by means of the minute vessels running between the thyroid and parathyroid glands.

The most difficult task in preserving parathyroid glands is the identification of the parathyroid glands and distinguishing them from fat, lymph nodes, and thyroid nodules. They are usually identified by their golden brown color and size. Their position is variable. Locating them is difficult when they are embedded in much fat or within the thyroid lobe.

The parathyroid glands have a separate capsule and can nearly always be separated from the thyroid by the use of a fine clamp after the surgeon divides the thin layer of pretracheal fascia that envelops both glands and ligates or cauterizes the fine intervening vessels. The use of magnifying loupes, good lighting, and a meticulous dry field will facilitate this dissection. Blunt dissection is used throughout.

I usually identify and dissect the parathyroid glands, place them laterally with their intact blood supply, and sometimes suture them to adjoining structures (to prevent accidentally wiping them away) before exposure and dissection of the recurrent laryngeal nerves.

The reported incidence of permanent hypoparathyroidism remains high after total thyroidectomy, varying from 2 to 33 per cent in different clinics. This complication has been the most important deterrent to the use of total thyroidectomy in the treatment of patients with thyroid carcinoma. In my experience with more than 600 total thyroidectomies, the incidence of permanent hypoparathyroidism is less than 2 per cent; in the last 350 patients, only one instance of hypoparathyroidism occurred.

## SUGGESTED READING

Attie, J. N.: Pitfalls in thyroid surgery. Probl. Gen. Surg., *3:*15–25, 1986.

Attie, J. N.: Modified neck dissection in treatment of thyroid cancer: A safe procedure. Eur. J. Cancer Clin. Oncol., *24:*315–324, 1988.

Attie, J. N., and Khafif, R. A.: Preservation of parathyroid glands during total thyroidectomy. Am. J. Surg., *130:*399–404, 1975.

# INDEX

Note: Page numbers in *italics* refer to illustrations; page numbers followed by t refer to tables.